Pathophysiology and treatment of Paget's disease of bone

Metabolic Bone Disease

Series Editor: Ignac Fogelman, BSc, MD, FRCP

Pathophysiology and treatment of Paget's disease of bone

John A Kanis

Department of Human Metabolism
and Clinical Biochemistry, University
of Sheffield Medical School
Sheffield, UK

MARTIN DUNITZ

First published in the United Kingdom in 1991
by Martin Dunitz Ltd, 7–9 Pratt Street, London NW1 0AE

British Library Cataloguing in Publication Data
Kanis, John A.
Pathophysiology and treatment of Paget's disease of bone.
1. Man. Bones. Paget's disease
I. Title
616.712

ISBN 0-948269-73-1

Phototypeset by Scribe Design, Gillingham, Kent
Printed and bound in Singapore by Kyodo Printing Co (S'pore) Pte Ltd

CONTENTS

ACKNOWLEDGEMENTS

I am indebted to my clinical colleagues who have over the years sustained my interest in Paget's disease of bone at home and abroad. These include Olav Bijvoet, Pierre Meunier, Charles Nagant de Deuxchaisnes, Graham Russell, Fred Singer, Roger Smith, John Strong and Colin Woods.

I am most grateful to Wendy Pontefract for typing the manuscript, to Monique Benéton for extensive proof reading and to George Molnar for his help in providing a library service. Much of the previously unpublished research presented in this book was done by those who worked with me during the time of writing. These include Monique Benéton, Dereck Bickerstaff, Neveen Hamdy, Eugene McCloskey, Declan O'Doherty and Maniccam Thavarajah, and I thank them for their efforts and their patience.

I am grateful to the following colleagues for permission to use their original illustrations.

J Aaron, Department of Anatomy, University of Leeds, UK (Figures 2.6, 2.9, 2.10)

A Barrington, Department of Radiology, Royal Hallamshire Hospital, Sheffield, UK (Figures 3.21, 6.1, 6.2, 6.4, 6.7, 6.9, 6.16)

H Bone and Diana Cody, Henry Ford Hospital, Detroit, USA (Figure 8.18)

G Dickson, Department of Pathology, The Queen's University, Belfast, N Ireland (Figure 9.5)

D Douglas, Department of Orthopaedics, Royal Hallamshire Hospital, Sheffield, UK (Figures 3.4, 3.23, 3.31, 3.33, 3.34, 3.37, 3.42, 5.25, 5.34, 6.28, 8.21, 8.26)

C Gennari and G Agnusdei, Department of Medical Semiotics, University of Siena, Italy (Figure 3.66)

S Harris, Department of Pathology, Stafford General Infirmary, Stafford, UK (Plate 20)

B Maldague and J Malghem, Department of Radiology, Catholic University of Louvain, Belgium (Figures 2.23, 3.16, 3.36, 3.48, 3.59, 3.73, 3.74, 5.14, 6.6, 6.18, 6.22, 6.25, 6.29, 7.39, 7.40, 8.31)

C Nagant de Deuxchaisnes, Department of Rheumatology, Catholic University of Louvain, Belgium (Figures 8.12, 8.13, 8.14, 8.23)

I G Rennie, Department of Ophthalmology, Royal Hallamshire Hospital, Sheffield, UK (Plate 23)

J Rogers, Department of Paleopathology, University of Bristol, UK (Figure 1.7)

C J Smith and C Franklin, Dental Hospital, University of Sheffield, UK (Figures 3.43, 5.20, 5.21 and Plate 12)

M P Whyte and W A Murphy, Washington University School of Medicine, St Louis, Missouri, USA (Figures 3.6, 8.9, 8.10, 8.11)

C J Woods, Department of Pathology, Nuffield Orthopaedic Centre, Oxford, UK (Plates 17, 18, 19, 21, 22)

The following figures are reproduced with permission of the editors of:

American Journal of Medicine (Figures 3.6, 5.23, 8.9, 8.10, 8.11)
Arthritis and Rheumatism (Figures 4.20, 4.22, 7.18, 7.61)
Australian and New Zealand Journal of Medicine (Figures 5.22, 7.62, 8.39)
Bone (Figures 3.75, 4.5, 7.31, 7.33, 8.33, 8.38, 9.3)
British Journal of Preventative and Social Medicine (Figure 1.2)
British Medical Journal (Figures 1.5, 7.12, 7.36)
Clinical Orthopedics and Related Research (Figures 3.12, 7.17, 7.27, 8.16, 8.19)
Clinical Science (Figures 4.8, 7.32, 7.38, 7.45)
Hospital Practice (Figure 2.4)
International Orthopedics (Figure 5.12)
Journal of Bone and Joint Surgery (B) (Figures 5.24, 8.34, 8.35)
Journal of Bone and Mineral Research (Figure 7.46)
Journal of Clinical Investigation (Figure 4.19)
Lancet (Figures 7.64, 8.36, 9.6)
Medicine (Baltimore) (Figure 7.63)
New England Journal of Medicine (Figures 2.1, 4.1)
Revue du Practicien (Paris) (Figures 2.23, 3.16, 3.36, 3.48, 3.59, 3.73, 3.74, 5.14, 5.27, 5.28, 6.6, 6.18, 6.25, 6.29, 7.39, 7.40, 8.31)
Triangle (Figure 7.21)

The following figures were reproduced with the permission of:

Armour Pharmaceutical Company, Eastbourne, UK (Figures 3.29, 3.69, 8.28, 8.29)
W Heinemann Medical Books, London, UK (Figure 7.3)
Hans Huber, Berne (Figures 7.8, 7.22)
Masson Italia Editori, Milan, Italy (Figures 7.6, 7.20)
National Gallery, London, UK (Figure 1.6)
W B Saunders, Philadelphia, USA (Figures 8.12, 8.13, 8.14, 8.23)

FOREWORD

In 1876 Sir James Paget presented his classic paper 'On a form of chronic inflammation of bones (Osteitis Deformans)' before the Royal Medical and Chirurgical Society of London. In this paper, published in *Medico-Chirurgical Transactions* in 1877, Paget described the 22-year evolution of a skeletal disease in a patient from the North of England whose initial complaint was aching pains in his thighs and legs and whose first noticeable physical abnormality was a misshapen left shin. Over the ensuing years Paget noted enlargement and bowing of the patient's left femur and an increase in the circumference of the skull which necessitated a nearly annual increase in the size of his Yeomanry Corps helmet and his hat. His spine became curved and nearly rigid. Over time his height decreased from 6 feet 1 inch to 5 feet 9 inches, and Paget observed that when standing his posture was simian-like. During the last six years of his life the patient developed a severe effusion of his left knee joint, partial loss of hearing, partial loss of vision due to retinal haemorrhages, signs of mitral valve insufficiency, and lower extremity cramps. In early 1876 the patient experienced pain in his left forearm and elbow, followed shortly by the explosive development of a mass emanating from the proximal third of the left forearm. Within three months of the onset of his forearm pain he became emaciated, developed a pleural effusion and died. The postmortem examination done by Paget revealed extraordinary thickening of the skull with numerous vascular channels and areas which were porous in nature. The long bones involved were also markedly thickened and in some areas quite dense. A large malignant tumour arising from the left radius was found with metastatic nodules in the pleurae, mediastinum and skull. Mr HT Butlin was asked to provide a report of the microscopic examination of the diseased bones. His report and marvellous drawings were included in the manuscript and revealed the chaotic nature of the osseous microstructure, the high vascular character of the bone and a high degree of cellularity in the specimens examined. Mr Butlin recognized that numerous osteoblasts were present and also described round or oval cells which were similar in appearance to leucocytes. In Figure 10 he illustrated an oval multinucleated cell which was adjacent to a scalloped border of bone. He was apparently unaware that in 1873 Kolliker had proposed that such cells were responsible for resorption of bone and suggested that they be termed 'osteoclasts'. Butlin and Paget felt that the microscopic changes that were present were best accounted for by a chronic inflammatory process, hence the term 'osteitis deformans' was proposed as a short descriptive name. The only comment concerning treatment of this disorder was that iodine of potassium and liquor potassii were prescribed for this patient but were found ineffective.

In the more than 100 years since Paget brilliantly delineated many of the clinical and pathological aspects of Paget's disease, an enormous amount of new information has been generated at the clinical as well as the laboratory level. In this book Dr Kanis has done an outstanding job in gathering the relevant data and presenting it in a logical and lucid manner. He has provided the means for understanding, to a great extent, how the disease evolves into its highly variable clinical form. The use of roentgenographic and nuclear medicine techniques, as well as biochemical assessment of the patients, is comprehensively reviewed. Particularly useful to the clinician is the excellent summary of the variety of drugs now being used to treat patients with Paget's disease.

It is no surprise that Dr Kanis has been able to produce such an excellent review of the pathophysiology and treatment of the disease. He has been an outstanding student of the disease since early in his career and has made many significant contributions to the understanding of the nature of the problem and to the control of its manifestations. One could only surmise how pleased and grateful Sir James Paget would be if he were able to read Dr Kanis's exposition of the events that have ensued since Paget made public the unfortunate story of his patient from the North of England.

Frederick R Singer, MD
Cedars-Sinai Medical Center
Los Angeles
California

PREFACE

In the UK and many Western countries, Paget's disease of bone is the second most common disorder of bone, outstripped only by osteoporosis. Although it had been described earlier (Wilks, 1869, 1909), the first adequate clinical description of Paget's disease dates from 1877 when the disorder was described by Sir James Paget. He coined the term 'osteitis deformans', previously and probably coincidentally also used by Czerny (1873) to describe a different disorder.

Despite the excellent clinical descriptions of Sir James Paget and the wealth of information derived thereafter, we still know little about its natural history and know nothing of its cause. At best, we know that it is not an inflammation of bone, and neither does it necessarily induce deformity, and it seems appropriate, therefore, that the term 'Paget's disease of bone' be retained in use.

Where significant progress has been made is in our understanding of the nature of the disorder, particularly the way in which skeletal remodelling is disturbed. In addition, there is a much greater understanding of the way in which pagetic bone is modified by therapeutic intervention. These developments have arisen largely in the past 20 years; the extensive monograph by Barry (1969) states that 'no effective means have been found to make any significant change in the course of the disease', a sentiment concluded by Hutchinson (1889) 80 years previously. Indeed, less than five pages of Barry's text are devoted to treatment.

The purpose of this monograph is to redress that imbalance in the light of increased knowledge of the pathophysiology of the disorder and its response to therapeutic intervention.

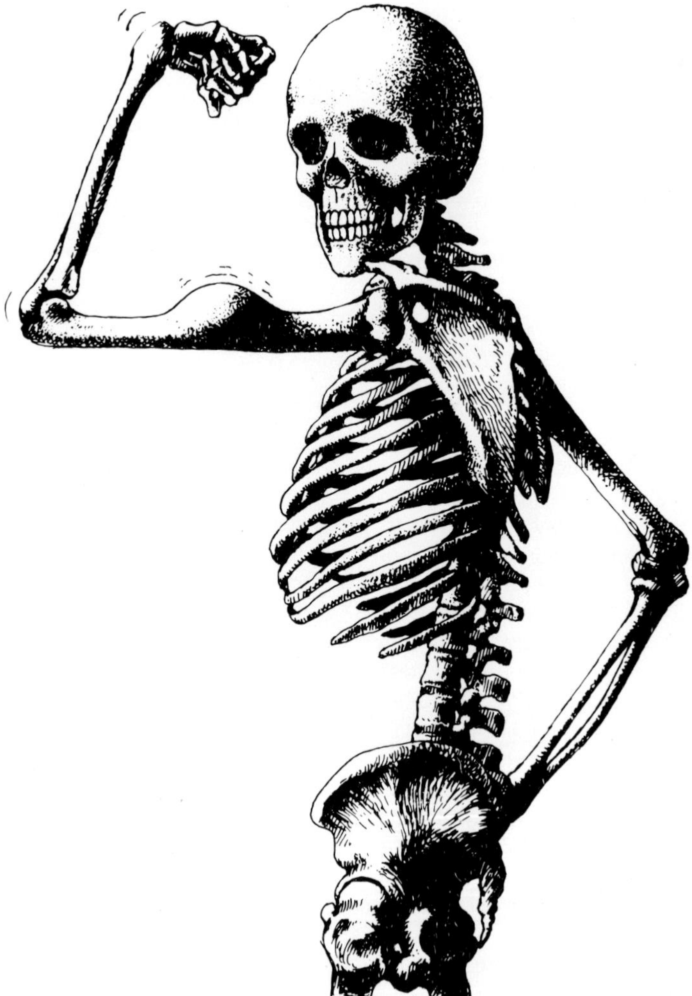

CHAPTER 1

Epidemiology

Paget's disease of bone is a focal disorder which may affect few or many skeletal sites. In addition, it is commonly asymptomatic. These factors present some difficulties for the acquisition of accurate data concerning its prevalence and incidence. Moreover, the prevalence appears to vary markedly around the world, making the comparison of various estimates difficult when different methods of data acquisition are used.

Studies of the prevalence of Paget's disease have been carried out largely in Europe and the USA from large-scale radiographic and autopsy surveys. These surveys have different inherent biases which variously over- or underestimate the prevalence. Important sources of bias are discussed where appropriate, but nevertheless, there is a measure of agreement between these surveys which indicate fascinating differences around the world and, if not providing insight into its aetiology, provide a framework on which aetiologic theories may be tested.

Prevalence

The disorder is well described but rarely presents before the age of 40 (Galbraith et al, 1977; Whyte et al, 1985; Harinck et al, 1986; Osterberg et al, 1988). In most hospital surveys patients under the age of 45 account for less than 1 per cent of the patient population (for example, 16 of 2630 patients in the series of Barry, 1969; Table 1.1) but in some series it is as high as 9 per cent (Dickson et al, 1945), probably related to referral biases. Thereafter it is found with increasing frequency with advancing age. For this reason prevalences have been commonly expressed as a proportion of the population aged 40 or more.

Several early estimates of prevalence were derived from hospital statistics and underestimate the prevalence, but two early studies on thousands of samples suggested a prevalence of about 3–4 per cent of the population at the age of 40 or greater. One was based on a very large autopsy series in Germany (Schmorl, 1932) and the other on a limited (spine and pelvis) radiographic survey in the UK (Pygott, 1957). Collins (1956), in a smaller autopsy series, estimated that the diagnosis was known pre-mortem in less than one-third of patients and less than 5 per cent had been admitted to hospital for the disorder. The similarities in apparent prevalence are probably fortuitous, but they all show an age-dependent increase in apparent prevalence. Both types of survey are subject to selection bias, but, nevertheless, indicate that the prevalence with age roughly doubles each decade after the age of 50, and by the age of 95 affects upwards of 10 per cent of the population (Figure 1.1). This exponential increase raises an interesting notion that Paget's disease of bone is an ubiquitous disorder in the UK that might affect the whole population were it to live long enough.

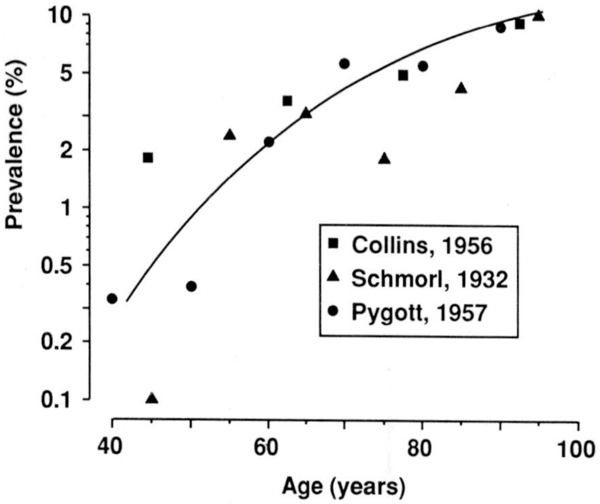

Figure 1.1

Prevalence of Paget's disease as judged from radiographic (Pygott, 1957) or autopsy surveys (Schmorl, 1932; Collins, 1956). Note the exponential rise in prevalence with age.

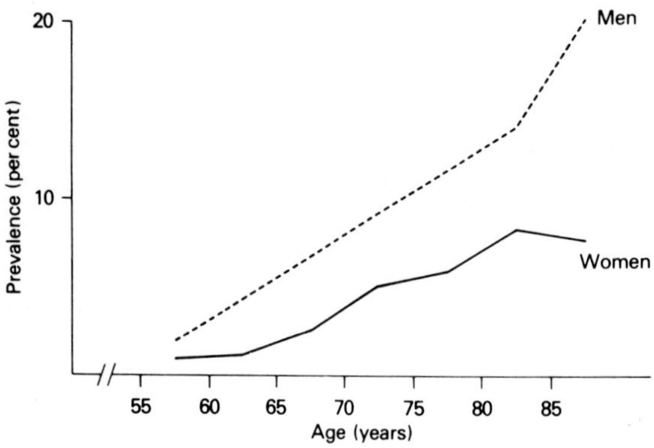

Figure 1.2

Prevalence of Paget's disease by age and sex (from Barker and Gardner, 1974).

The most comprehensive surveys have been based on limited skeletal surveys of hospital radiographs (Barker, 1981). This type of survey is also based on a number of assumptions (discussed later), and may underestimate the true prevalence by 25 per cent (Merrick and Merrick, 1985). The surveys in the UK indicate a prevalence of 5 per cent in the population over the age of 55, and suggest that there are about 750 000 patients with radiographic evidence for Paget's disease in England and Wales.

There have been no studies reported which examine the incidence of the disorder, but its prevalence might suggest a rising incidence with age with an average of 0.3 per cent pa in the population aged 55 or more. There are a number of reservations concerning such estimates. These relate not only to uncertainties concerning true prevalence, but more to gaps in our knowledge of its natural history. There is, for example, little evidence for the occurrence of new lesions (in contrast to their extension) in symptomatic Paget's disease. The evidence for this is reviewed later, but if true, this might indicate a high modal incidence in early middle age which declined rapidly thereafter, but with a variable latency between the onset of the disorder and its radiographic or clinical expression.

Sex

Most surveys indicate that the disease is more prevalent among men than among women, but in both sexes the prevalence increases with age (Schmorl, 1932; Pygott, 1957). Estimates of the male-to-female sex ratio generally range from 1.4 to 1.9 in favour of men (Schmorl, 1932; Collins, 1956; Pygott, 1957; Barker et al, 1980; Figure 1.2). A preponderance of males is commonly, but not invariably, seen in total hospital populations (Dickson et al, 1945; Barry, 1969; Harinck et al, 1986; Polednak, 1987). In our own referral population, women outnumber men (Table 1.1), and in other hospital studies it is of interest that the male/female ratio is commonly less than non-hospital surveys. This is due, in part, to the increased longevity of women, but the age- and sex-adjusted prevalence of patients residing within the Sheffield postal area (Table 1.2) suggests that this is not so. If the population-based estimates of prevalence are to be believed, it might suggest the more vigorous referral of symptomatic women.

Table 1.1 Age and sex distribution of patients presenting with Paget's disease at the Sheffield Metabolic Bone Unit over an 8-year period (1980–9). Note the slight predominance of women (M/W = 0.91).

Age range (years)	*Men*	*Women*	*Men and women*	*% of all patients*
40–49	2	0	2	0.5
50–59	24	8	32	8.1
60–69	34	37	71	17.9
70–79	68	80	148	37.3
80+	61	83	144	36.3
45+	187	208	395	99.5

Familial incidence

Three types of investigation have been undertaken to explore genetic factors in Paget's disease. One approach has been based on pedigree studies and a second on the frequency with which family members are affected in populations with Paget's disease. Finally, several studies have investigated HLA antigen associations which are reviewed in Chapter 9.

There have been several reports of Paget's disease affecting several members of the same family (Barry, 1969). It has been described in children, siblings and in parents; and in such families appears to have an autosomal dominant pattern of inheritance (McKusick, 1972). Only five pairs of identical twins have been reported in the medical literature (Melick and Martin, 1975), and from the known incidence of Paget's disease, far more cases of the disease should perhaps have been observed. Jones and Reed (1967) describe a family with six cases in three generations, and others describe families with between seven and nine affected relatives in the one generation (Evens and Bartter, 1968; Singer, 1977b).

We ourselves have seen a family with 40 affected members in five generations (Osterberg et al, 1988; Figure 1.3). The disorder in this family has been termed 'familial expansile osteolysis' but it has many of the features of Paget's disease. It is focal and shares many of the radiographic and histological features. In addition, multinucleated giant cells are present which bear viral-like inclusion particles identical to those observed in classical Paget's disease (Dickson et al, 1991). The family is distinctive mainly in the age of presentation, which ranges from 18 to 45 years, and in the distribution of the disorder. For this reason it has been given the term 'expansile osteolysis', but can more justifiably be considered as a variant of Paget's disease.

It is our experience that those patients with a positive family history (excluding the family described above) have the more widespread Paget's disease, but present at the same age as those with no family history (Table 1.3). Similar conclusions have been inferred by others (Irvine, 1953; Evens and Bartter, 1968). The more marked disease is due principally to an increase in the

Table 1.2 Sex and age at diagnosis of patients with Paget's disease residing within Sheffield postal districts. Note the increase in prevalence with age in both sexes ($p < 0.001$; logistic regression). There was no significant difference in prevalence rates between men and women when taking age into account (log-linear regression).

Age range (years)	*Number of patients*		*Prevalence (/100 000)*			
	Men	*Women*	*Men*	*Women*	*Men and women*	*M/W*
40–49	4	1	13	3	9	4.3
50–59	8	9	26	28	27	0.9
60–69	15	27	53	81	68	0.7
70–79	28	41	168	159	162	1.1
80+	6	15	157	152	153	1.0
All ages	61	93	24	34	29	0.7
40+	61	93	56	72	64	0.8

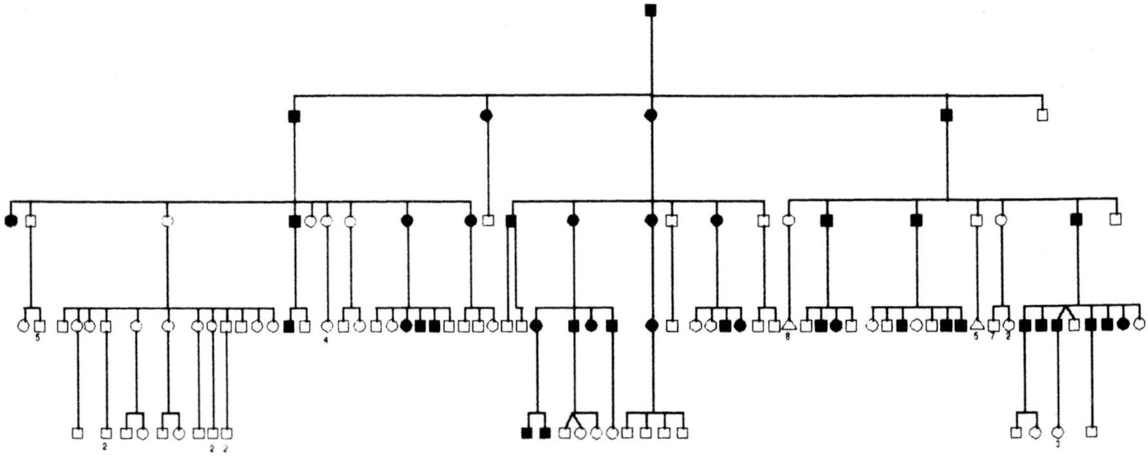

Figure 1.3

Pedigree chart of a family with 'expansile osteolysis' showing affected (solid symbols) and unaffected (open symbols) members (□ male, ○ female, △ sex unknown). Numbers below symbols refer to the number of unaffected siblings. Note the autosomal dominant pattern of inheritance (after Osterberg et al, 1988).

Table 1.3 Characteristics of 197 patients with and without a family history of Paget's disease (sib, parent or child); mean ± SEM.

	Family history n = 27)	*No family history (n = 170)*	*p<*
Male/female	10/17	69/101	NS
Age at first symptom (years)	61.5 ± 1.0	61.5 ± 1.0	NS
Age at presentation (years)	70.3 ± 0.7	70.1 ± 1.8	NS
Serum alkaline phosphatase (IU/l)	490 (404–594)	282 (265–300)	0.0002
Urine hydroxyproline (mmol/mol creatinine)	112 (93–135)	63 (60–66)	0.0002
Number of lesions/patient	11.0 ± 2.0	5.8 ± 0.4	0.001
Skeletal involvement (%)	23.2 ± 3.6	12.9 ± 0.7	0.0001
Scintigraphic index	75 ± 14	42 ± 3	0.001

NS: not significant

number of pagetic foci rather than to more extensive disease at each focus.

A positive family history is reported in several series of pagetic patients. Estimates vary from 1 to 25 per cent (Dickson et al, 1945; Rozenkrantz et al, 1952; Rauis, 1974; Canfield et al, 1977; Galbraith et al, 1977; Sofaer et al, 1983; Harinck et al, 1986). In our own patients a positive family history was obtained in 13.7 per cent of patients, a figure substantially higher than the prevalence of Paget's disease in the community (Table 1.2). Sofaer et al (1983) undertook an interesting survey based on a postal questionnaire. They found that parents and siblings of affected patients had a 10-fold greater chance of having Paget's disease compared with parents and siblings of the normal spouse (Table 1.4). Although the awareness of family members may be greater amongst index cases than spouses, these data, nevertheless, suggest that a genetic susceptibility

Table 1.4 Prevalence of awareness of Paget's disease (at 55 years and above) (from Sofaer et al, 1983).

	With Paget's disease	*Without Paget's disease*	*%*
Parents and siblings of index cases	57	1450	3.93
Parents and siblings of normal spouses	3	823	0.36
Relative risk			10.91

exists, conforming to a dominant autosomal pattern of inheritance.

A relatively small proportion of cases can be explained on the basis of a strict autosomal dominant inheritance. However, the majority of patients with Paget's disease are asymptomatic and there are no family studies based on radiography or biochemical investigation which can give reliable estimates on the importance of genetic factors. It is, therefore, likely that genetic factors could be more important than generally assumed. The question arises whether such findings are related to true inheritance, to a common environment or to a multiple aetiology. This is a question that is discussed further in Chapter 9.

Geographic variation

Documented cases of Paget's disease have come from many races and different parts of the world. Most clinical observations suggest, however, that the disease is far more common in Europe, North America and Australasia (Barry, 1969; Reasbeck et al, 1983). This has been studied in some detail by a series of radiographic surveys measuring the prevalence of Paget's disease in stored films at hospital departments of radiography. Radiographic surveys include the pelvis, lumbosacral spine and femoral heads. Estimates of prevalence are based on evidence (Barker et al, 1977; Detheridge et al, 1983) that one or more of these sites are affected in 95 per cent of people with Paget's disease. Before considering the geographic variation, it is worth questioning the assumptions on which the results are based.

The first assumption is that Paget's disease, when present, will be identifiable in 95 per cent of cases from X-ray scans of the pelvis. In our own hospital population, this is certainly an overestimate and only 85 per cent of our patients have pagetic lesions at these sites (Figure 1.4). This would have the effect of underestimating the prevalence of the disorder from pelvic films alone. It is of particular interest that the prevalence of 'pelvic' disease in the pagetic population increases with age. Thus, a pelvic film will capture nearly all patients aged 80 or more, but miss a quarter of pagetic patients less than the age of 70 (Figure 1.4). Thus a limited skeletal survey would underestimate the prevalence in the young. The possible reasons for the change in pelvic prevalence are discussed later.

A second assumption of these kinds of radiographic surveys is that mild asymptomatic disease has a similar distribution to that of symptomatic disease. This is probably not true. It seems likely that the prevalence of monostotic disease is higher in the general community than in the hospital population (Merrick and Merrick, 1985; Harinck et al, 1986).

A final assumption is that the distribution of pagetic lesions within patients does not differ between communities. This has never been tested, but there is some evidence, reviewed at the end of this chapter, that the pattern of distribution of lesions is changing with time. The power of population surveys of radiographs rests on the basis that most (but probably not all) radiographs will have been taken because of disorders unrelated to Paget's disease. Although the frequency of the disorder will be subject to bias, its bias may be similar at the different geographic locations examined and estimates of prevalence are probably relatively accurate (±25 per cent) compared with the differences observed.

The results of such a survey in 31 British towns is shown in Figure 1.5. Six towns in close proximity are found within a relatively small area of Lancashire. In these towns the prevalence exceeds 6.3 per cent (Table 1.5). Elsewhere the prevalences are substantially lower (Barker et al, 1980) with an average of 5 per cent in the urban

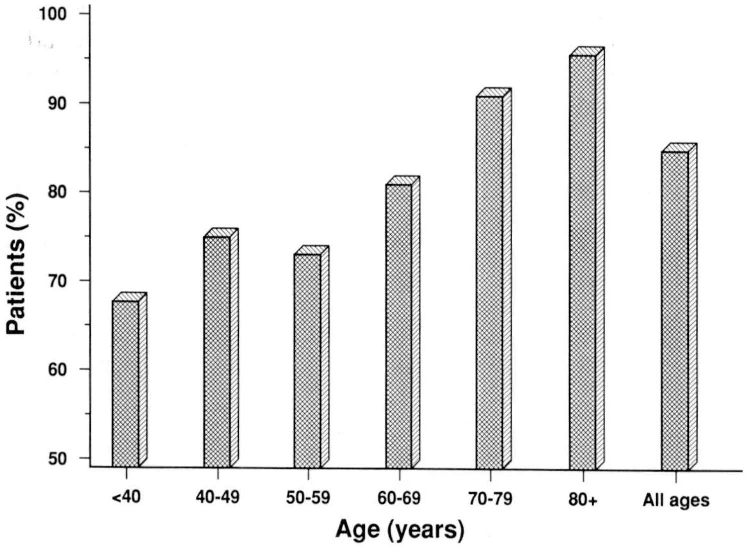

Figure 1.4

Prevalence of Paget's disease on pelvic radiographs in 197 patients grouped according to their age at diagnosis. Note the marked increase in prevalence with age. There were no differences between men and women at any age. The pelvic film included the pelvis, sacrum, proximal femora and the lower lumbar vertebrae (L3–L5).

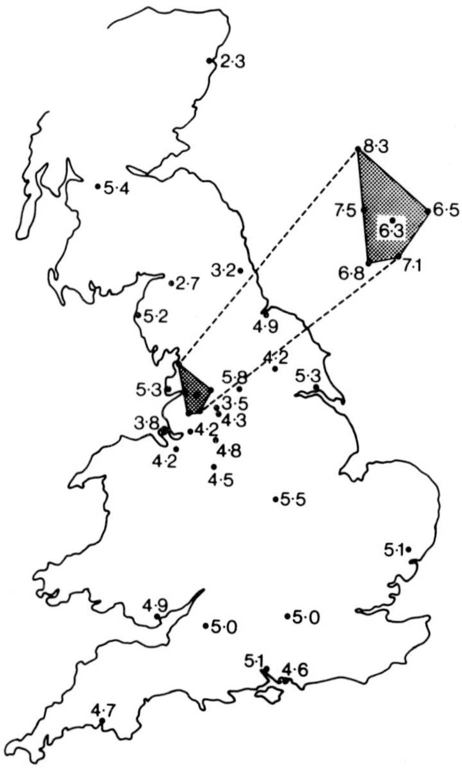

Figure 1.5

Age- and sex-standardized prevalences (percentages) of Paget's disease among hospital patients aged 55 years or more in 31 British towns (Barker et al, 1980).

population over the age of 55. There appears to be no relationship between prevalence and latitude or industrialization.

Using similar techniques in 15 towns in Europe, the age- and sex-standardized prevalence of Paget's disease appears to be much greater in the UK than in other European cities (Table 1.6). As in the UK, there are apparent variations in prevalence within European countries and, for example, the Sierra de la Cabrera in Spain has a significantly higher prevalence than its adjacent territories (Piga et al, 1988). It seems possible that other foci of high prevalence might exist elsewhere which could provide valuable clues concerning its aetiology.

Paget's disease of bone also appears to be common in countries such as Australia (Barry, 1969), New Zealand (Reasbeck et al, 1983), South Africa (Pompe et al, 1976; Guyer and Chamberlain, 1988) and the USA where significant British immigration occurred in the past. In Perth, the prevalence is 4 per cent amongst British-born immigrants over the age of 54, but is lower in the native-born Australian white population (Gardner et al, 1978; Table 1.7). When the same technique is utilized, the prevalence in Atlanta is 0.9 per cent, suggesting that there are geographical

Table 1.5 Age-standardized prevalence of Paget's disease in hospital patients aged 55 or more in Lancashire towns and in the 31 towns examined (refer to Figure 1.5) (from Barker et al, 1980).

Town	*Number of patients*	*Number affected*	*Prevalence*			*M/W*
			Men	*Women*	*Both sexes*	
Lancaster	626	58	6.5	10.0	8.3	0.63
Preston	1 000	82	8.6	6.3	7.5	1.36
Bolton	602	42	7.7	6.4	7.1	1.2
Wigan	600	42	8.1	5.4	6.8	1.3
Burnley	979	74	8.2	4.9	6.5	1.67
Blackburn	595	39	8.8	3.8	6.3	2.3
31 towns	29 054	1516	6.2	3.9	5.0	1.59

variations within the USA as well as in Europe (Table 1.8). It is of particular interest that Paget's disease is seen in a significant proportion of blacks in the USA (Tables 1.8 and 1.9; Guyer and Chamberlain, 1980; Polednak, 1987), South Africa (Pompe et al, 1976; Guyer and Chamberlain, 1988) and Jamaica (Lawrence, 1970), whereas the disorder appears to be less frequent in some black African races (Bohrer, 1970; van Meedervoort and Richter, 1976; Dahniya, 1987) and Asian Indians (Kumar, 1986). The disorder seems to be extremely rare in the Nordic countries, the Arab Middle East, China and Japan, and among Australian aboriginals (Falch, 1979; Barker, 1981; Bloom et al, 1985).

These remarkable variations in geographic distribution have to be accommodated when considering the aetiology of the disorder (Chapter 9). It has been suggested that the low prevalence in second-generation Australians and the higher prevalence in American blacks indicate a more marked importance of environmental than genetic factors (Barker, 1981, 1984). This conclusion may not be warranted since many immigrants to these countries are not of UK stock, so that an appropriate control population has not been studied.

Table 1.6 Age- and sex-standardized prevalence of Paget's disease among hospital patients aged 55 years and over in 15 European towns (Detheridge et al, 1982).

	Prevalence (%)
UK (31 towns)	4.6
France	
Bordeaux	2.7
Rennes	2.4
Nancy	2.0
Ireland	
Dublin	1.7
Galway	0.7
Spain	
Valencia	1.3
Portugal	
Porto	0.9
West German	
Essen	1.3
Italy	
Palermo	1.0
Greece	
Athens	0.5
Crete	0.5
Sweden	
Malmo	0.4

Table 1.7 Prevalence of Paget's disease in Perth, Australia and in 31 British towns in hospital patients aged 55 or more according to place of birth and residence (from Barker, 1984).

Place of birth	*Place of residence*	*No of radiographs*	*Age-standardized prevalence (%)*		
			Men	*Women*	*Both sexes*
Australia	Australia	1 203	3.5	2.8	3.2
UK	Australia	942	5.7	2.3	4.0
UK	UK	29 054	6.2	3.9	5.0

Table 1.8 Age-standardized prevalence of Paget's disease among hospital patients aged 55 years and over in the USA (from Guyer and Chamberlain, 1980).

Site	*Ethnic group*	*Prevalence (%)*			
		M	*F*	*M + F*	*M/F*
New York	Black	3.2	2.0	2.6	1.6
New York	White	5.2	2.5	3.9	2.1
Atlanta	Black	1.9	0.6	1.2	3.2
Atlanta	White	0.9	0.8	0.9	1.1

Table 1.9 Annual rates of hospital discharge (per 100 000) among New York State residents with Paget's disease (from Polednak, 1987).

Age	*White*		*Black*	
	Male	*Female*	*Male*	*Female*
20–59	0.3	0.4	0.4	0.6
60–9	4.3	4.2	3.8	4.3
70–9	10.3	9.2	9.1	10.2
>80	19.6	13.8	46.1	25.3

Secular trends

Very little information is available. The data on geographical distribution might suggest that the incidence would decrease in Australia or the USA, whether this be due to environmental factors or to racial admixture. The major difficulty in acquiring such information is that the disease is largely asymptomatic and requires invasive methods of population sampling such as radiographs or biochemical measurements. These have not been done.

The disorder undoubtedly existed for many years before the descriptions of Sir James Paget in 1877. The 'ugly duchess: a grotesque old woman' after Quinten Massys (1465–1530), copied from a drawing by Leonardo da Vinci, has some features of Paget's disease (DeQueker, 1989; Figure 1.6) and it has been suggested that Ludwig van Beethoven's deafness was due to Paget's disease (Naiken, 1971). Paget described 23 patients without the benefit of radiography, suggesting that it was not a rare disorder in London at that time (Paget, 1882, 1889).

There are a number of reports which claim to have demonstrated the disorder in isolated bones from antiquity found in the USA, Egypt and France (Hutchinson, 1889; Pales, 1929; Denninger, 1933; Fisher, 1935; Astre, 1957). In most instances the evidence is not convincing, and the finds have occurred in geographical areas or races where the disease is apparently rare. A notable exception to this is an intact skeleton excavated from Jarrow Monastery with the classic distribution and morphological and radiological features dated to about AD 950 in an Anglo-

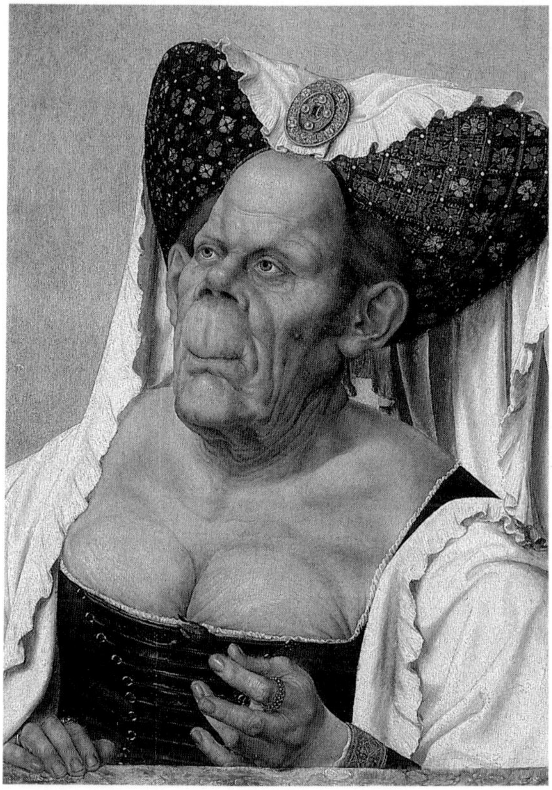

Figure 1.6

Painting after Quinten Massys (1465–1530), copied from a cartoon by Leonardo da Vinci. Note the marked maxillary hypertrophy, but also the enlarged clavicles, particularly the distal end of the right clavicle. (Reproduced by courtesy of the Trustees, The National Gallery, London.)

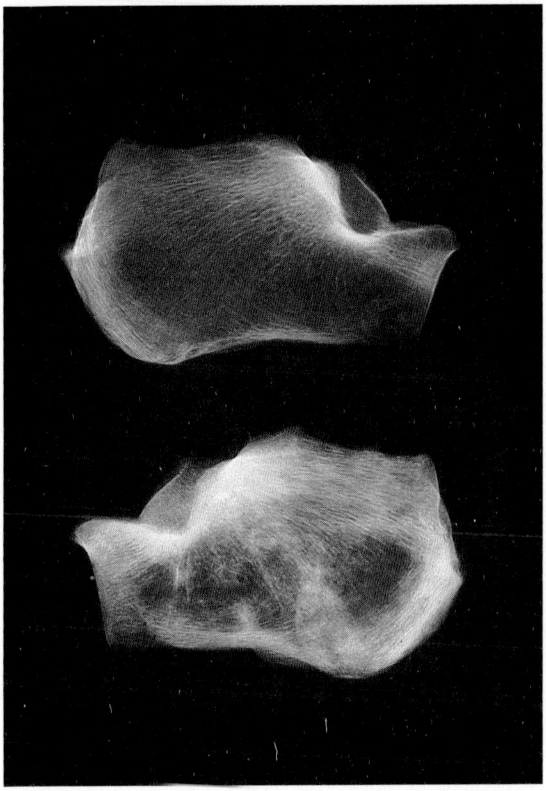

Figure 1.7

Radiograph of the os calces of a skeleton dating from the sixteenth century found at Wells (courtesy of Dr Juliet Rogers).

Saxon burial ground (Wells and Woodhouse, 1975). Other Saxon finds dated between AD 900 and 1066 include a pagetic skull and assorted bones at Winchester (Price, 1975).

We have recently had the opportunity of examining suspected cases of metabolic bone disease from a sixteenth-century burial ground in Wells. X-rays of both calcanea in one of the skeletons clearly show the thickened trabecular structure on the one side (Figure 1.7). This has been confirmed by quantitative histological observations showing woven bone, increased trabecular density and thickness, and increased resorption cavities highly characteristic of the disorder (Figure 1.8). These well-documented findings in the UK are consistent with the known geographical distribution, further suggesting an Anglo-Saxon origin for the disorder. It is, of course, not possible to know whether the prevalence amongst the Anglo-Saxon community was similar to that presently documented since the life expectancy was so different.

There is some indirect evidence that the incidence of Paget's disease is falling in the UK and

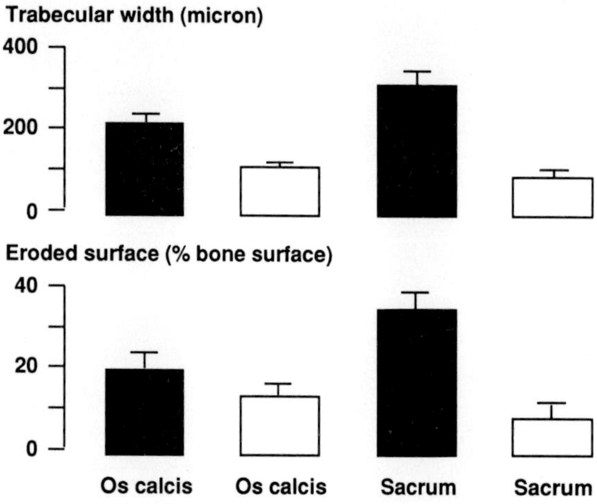

Figure 1.8

Quantitative histology of bone (mean values ± SEM) on medieval and post-medieval bones. Shaded areas denote values found in bones affected by Paget's disease on X–ray examination (see Figure 1.7). (Aaron J et al, unpublished work.)

Table 1.10 Death rates per million attributed to Paget's disease (from Barker, 1981).

	1951–5	*1956–60*	*1961–5*	*1966–70*
England and Wales	3.7	3.6	3.4	3.2
Scotland	2.9	2.4	2.2	1.4

the USA. The evidence is based on the decreasing number of deaths recorded on death certificates as attributable to Paget's disease (Barker and Gardner, 1974; Gardner and Barker, 1978; Table 1.10). In addition, if successive generations born from 1880 onwards are analysed, progressively lower death rates from Paget's disease are observed at any particular age. There are obvious difficulties in the interpretation of such data. Paget's disease is not normally a fatal disorder, and the declining frequency could be due to an increase in realization that patients do not commonly die from the disorder. On the other hand, a significant proportion of adult osteogenic sarcoma is associated with Paget's disease and it has been pointed out that the mortality of primary tumours of bone which occur over the age of 40 is also decreasing in parallel. This would be an expected consequence of a true decrease in incidence (Barker and Gardner, 1974).

There is circumstantial evidence to suggest that the pattern of Paget's disease might be changing. The prevalence of Paget's disease on pelvic radiographs appears to increase with age in the pagetic population (refer to Figure 1.4). The obvious explanation is the later occurrence of Paget's disease at the pelvis in the natural history of the disorder. There is evidence, however, that the number of pagetic foci does not increase markedly with age in the same population (Chapter 3). On the assumption that pagetic lesions rarely disappear, this suggests that the pattern of distribution is changing over the years with less

Table 1.11 Probability (percentage ± 95 per cent confidence interval) of disease involvement at the sites shown in 197 patients with Paget's disease divided by age.

Site	*Age < 70 (n = 102)*	*Age > 69 (n = 102)*	*Odds ratio*	*p <*
Tibia	31.6 ± 5.1	15.7 ± 3.6	2.01	0.008
Scapula	27.4 ± 4.6	11.8 ± 3.2	2.33	0.006
Foot (excluding os calcis)	22.1 ± 4.3	8.8 ± 2.8	2.51	0.01
Humerus	21.1 ± 4.3	12.7 ± 3.3	1.65	0.05
Sternum	17.9 ± 3.9	9.8 ± 2.9	1.83	0.05
Os calcis	11.6 ± 3.3	5.9 ± 2.3	1.97	
Radius	6.3 ± 2.5	2.0 ± 1.4	3.22	
Face	6.3 ± 2.5	2.0 ± 1.4	3.22	
Fibula	5.3 ± 2.3	1.0 ± 1.0	5.37	
Ulna	4.2 ± 2.1	1.0 ± 1.0	4.29	

pelvic foci, but more at other sites. Indeed, lesions at several sites appear to be more common in the young, particularly at the tibia and scapula, both relatively common sites of involvement (Table 1.11). When patients are divided by date of birth, a secular trend is apparent, showing secular differences in distribution (Table 1.12). Population studies would be needed to determine to what extent the apparent shift in the distribution (rather than number) of lesions was due to a heightened awareness and altered referral pattern in the younger population. If, however, these findings were due to a true change in the pattern of distribution of Paget's disease, they cloud still further our knowledge of the prevalence and geographic distribution of Paget's disease which is largely based on limited skeletal radiography.

Table 1.12 Frequency (per cent) of disease involvement at the sites shown in 197 patients with Paget's disease divided into quartiles according to their date of birth. The prevalence of disease at the lumbosacral spine decreases progressively with date of birth. The converse is true at the tibiae and scapulae.

Site	*<1909*	*1909–13*	*1914–20*	*>1920*
Lumbar spine	62.7	56.0	50.0	37.0
L1	23.5	28.0	23.8	9.3
L2	23.5	20.0	26.2	18.5
L3	29.4	30.0	23.8	16.7
L4	27.5	28.0	26.2	18.5
L5	33.3	28.0	14.3	13.0
Sacrum	41.2	26.0	28.6	16.7
Tibia	11.8	22.0	23.8	35.2
Scapula	15.7	18.0	21.4	22.

CHAPTER 2

Pathophysiology and histopathology

Paget's disease of bone is a focal disorder of bone remodelling, resulting in a number of important architectural abnormalities. Detailed accounts of bone remodelling are provided elsewhere (Frost, 1973; Albright and Skinner, 1979; Parfitt, 1983; Eriksen, 1986) but it is appropriate to review briefly the manner in which normal bone is remodelled and skeletal architecture is preserved (as distinct from skeletal growth) before identifying the way in which this is disrupted in Paget's disease. Bone subserves both metabolic (Parfitt, 1976) and structural functions, but it is the latter which are of primary concern in Paget's disease.

Structure of normal bone

Bone is comprised principally of a collagen matrix, but there are many other important proteins, including proteoglycans, glycoproteins and osteocalcin, which are incorporated within the collagen matrix. Under normal circumstances bone matrix is nearly fully mineralized. The collagen of adult bone is type I which is laid down by osteoblasts in a lamellar arrangement. Type I collagen is a heterotrimer comprising two alpha I (I) chains and one alpha 2 (I) chain encoded on chromosomes 17 and 7 respectively. During the process of collagen assembly and maturation procollagen undergoes a number of transformations including the cleavage of amino and carboxyterminal extension peptides, glycosylation and the formation of cross-links with other collagen molecules (Prockop et al, 1979a and b; Figure 2.1). Evidence of such activity can be measured in serum and may provide non-invasive indices of skeletal metabolism of value in the assessment of Paget's disease (Chapter 4). Collagen fibres comprise cross-linked molecules of collagen between which is found the mineral phase of bone. The mineral phase is mainly calcium, phosphate and carbonate (10:6:1) arranged as crystals predominantly in the form of hydroxyapatite.

In the adult there are broadly two types of bone, namely cortical (compact) and trabecular (spongy or cancellous) bone. Most bones have a cortical casing comprising an outer (periosteal) and inner (cortical endosteal) surface which encloses the trabecular bone and marrow space (Figure 2.2). In the adult with a total body calcium of approximately 1 kg, 80 per cent of skeletal mass is cortical. The remaining (trabecular) bone comprises plates and rods of tissue which interconnect with one another and with the inner aspect of the cortex (Figure 2.3). The turnover of bone is predominantly a surface-based phenomenon, and the several different types of bone surface available in the skeleton are summarized in Table 2.1 (see also Figure 2.2). The surface available for remodelling includes the trabecular and cortical

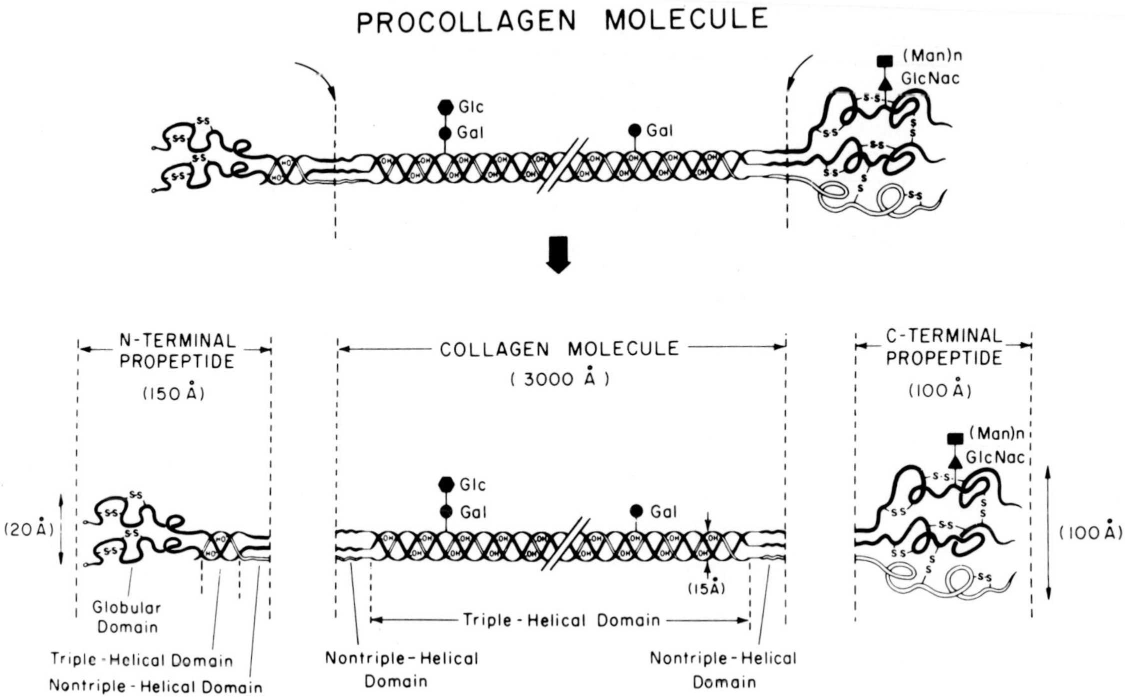

Figure 2.1

Structure of collagen and procollagen (Prockop et al, 1979a,b).

Table 2.1 Some characteristics of the normal skeleton (adapted from Johnson, 1966).

Surface	m^2
Cortical bone	3.5*
Trabecular bone	9*
Osteocyte	90
Lacunar and cannalicular	1200
Mass	g
Cortical bone	4000
Trabecular bone	1000
Total skeleton	5000
Surface*-to-mass ratio	cm^2/g
Cortical bone	8.75
Trabecular bone	90.0
Total skeleton	25.0

* Surface available for remodelling.

endosteal surface and the vascular channels within bone. This is considerably less than the surface available for mineral exchange which in addition includes the lacunae and canaliculi.

All these surfaces are covered by cells with distinct morphological and functional features (Plate 1). These include osteoblasts responsible for matrix synthesis and mineralization, osteoclasts which resorb mineralized bone and less active lining cells (thought to be resting osteoblasts). It is of interest that bone cells of the periosteal and endosteal surfaces respond differently to pathophysiologic insults, to hormones and to therapeutic intervention. There are also differences between endocortical and trabecular endosteal cells.

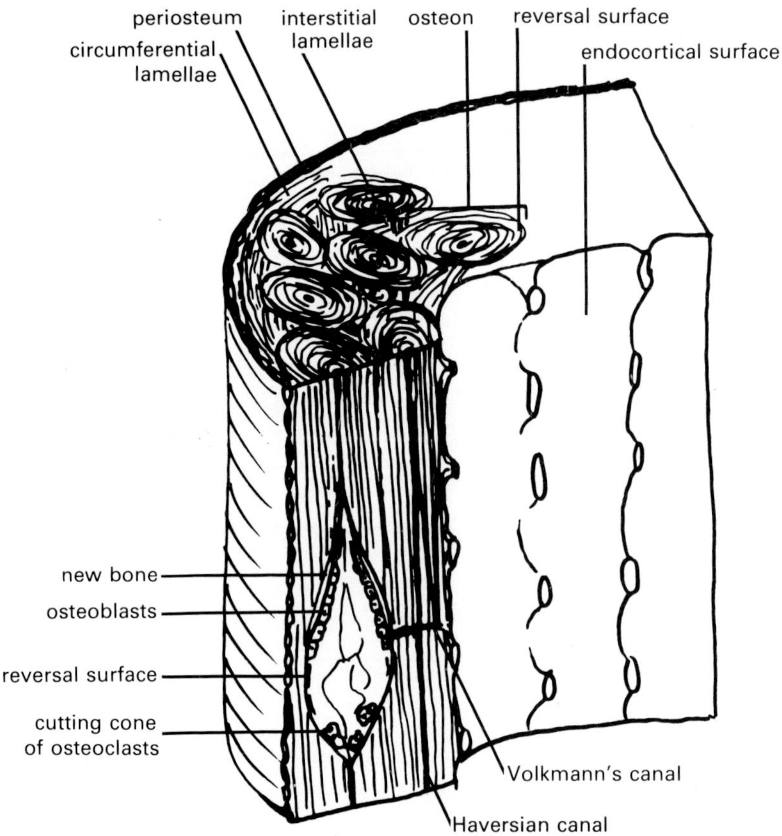

Figure 2.2

Schematic diagram of diaphyseal cortical bone showing the transverse and longitudinal arrangement of osteons.

The endosteal surface is covered by cells, the majority of which are flat and 'inert-looking', termed 'lining cells' or 'inactive osteoblasts' (surface osteocytes). It is thought that these cells are predominantly concerned with calcium transport in concert with the osteocytes and their extensive cell processes lying in the canalicular network. Even though cortical bone comprises three-quarters of the total skeletal tissue, the surfaces available in cortical bone are much lower than those of trabecular tissue. Indeed, the surface-to-mass ratio of trabecular bone is 8–10-fold greater than that of cortical bone (Table 2.1). Since bone remodelling is a surface-based event, remodelling activity is greater on trabecular than on cortical surfaces.

In the adult who is neither increasing nor decreasing in skeletal size, the skeleton is in zero balance. Despite this equilibrium, bone is continuously being turned over. In the adult these changes in focal skeletal balance comprise modelling and remodelling events. Modelling refers to changes in the architecture or size of bones that result from uninterrupted formation or resorption of bone, and is a conspicuous feature of growth. In the adult the gradual increase in the diameter

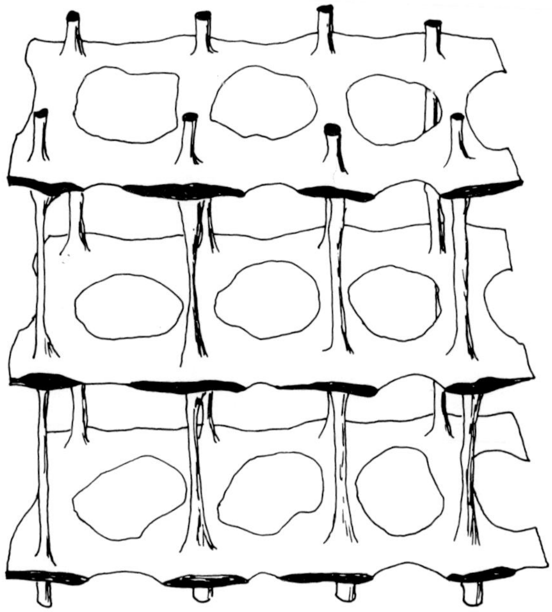

Figure 2.3

Schematic representation of cancellous bone showing a series of perforated trabecular plates connected by trabecular rods.

of some long bones (the metacarpal for example) is a form of modelling, but accounts for less than 5 per cent of all skeletal turnover. Remodelling comprises the process of bone resorption followed by bone formation and accounts for more than 95 per cent of skeletal turnover in the mature adult. This provides a mechanism for self-repair and adaptation to stress. Indeed, if turnover is halted experimentally or in disease this may give rise to pathological fracture without inducing changes in the amount of bone present (Frost, 1973; Flora et al, 1980).

Normal remodelling of trabecular bone

Bone remodelling is largely mediated by the activity of bone-forming (osteoblasts) and bone-resorbing cells (osteoclasts) and is a prominent feature of endosteal sites. At any one time osteoclasts and osteoblasts normally occupy the minority of the bone surface (10–15 per cent), most of which is covered by quiescent lining cells. Bone turnover is a series of discrete cellular events organized both in time and space on the surface. The steps involved have been well characterized both in health and in Paget's disease, the latter largely from the examination of bone biopsies from the ilium (Figure 2.4).

(1) Activation

The first visible step of normal bone remodelling is the attraction of osteoclasts to the quiescent surface. Osteoclast precursors are, however, present for several days beforehand close to the quiescent surface (Baron et al, 1983). It is not known how or if this process is regulated, but fat tissue is associated with low turnover rates and may decrease the availability of osteoclast precursors for activation. The origins of osteoclasts are still controversial but they can be formed from cells of the monocyte/macrophage lineage. The factors that determine the site for the focal attraction of a team of osteoclasts are not known, but it is possible that fatigue damage to bone could be a stimulus. Other structural, electrical and biochemical signals may also be important.

(2) Resorption

Osteoclasts, which may be mononucleated or, more often, multi-nucleated, are cells capable of undertaking bone resorption by the secretion of protons and lysosomal enzymes beneath their ruffled borders, which become closely applied to bone tissue (Figure 2.5). A team of osteoclasts can cut a depth of up to 20 μm/day. Osteoclasts preferentially resorb fully mineralized bone, but may sometimes be found on osteoid when this is abundant. Osteoclasts are motile both in vitro and in vivo with a small geographical domain, and working in concert they create a resorption or erosion cavity in bone. Their nuclear life span has been estimated at about 4–12 days and is similar to the duration of active bone resorption

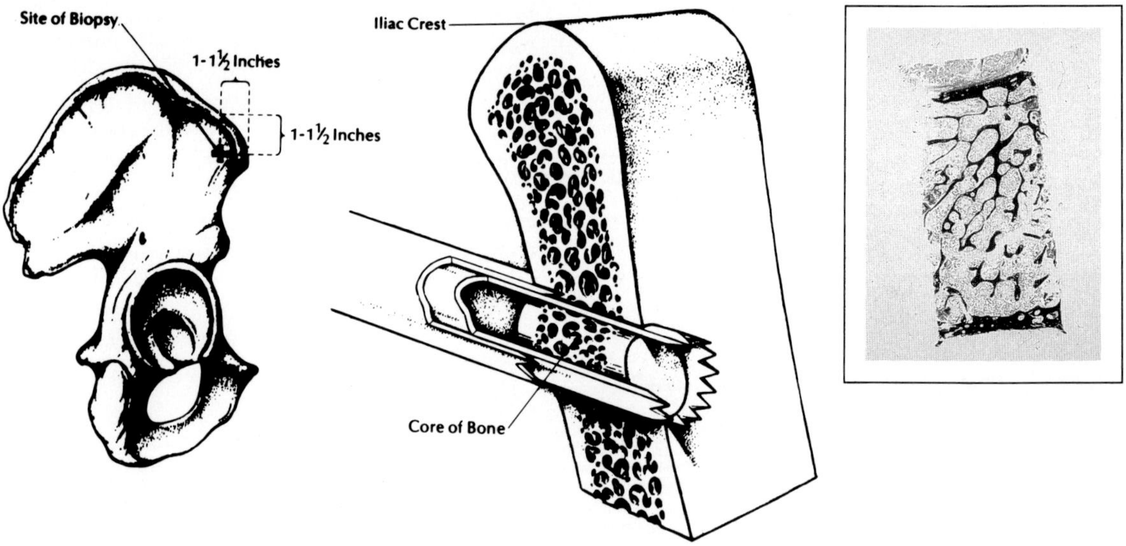

Figure 2.4

Site of bone biopsy and details of the trephine commonly utilized for the assessment of bone turnover and therapeutic intervention. The inset shows a stained section from a biopsy (× 2.5) in a normal subject to show the inner and outer cortex separated by an interconnecting lattice of cancellous bone. (From Mundy, 1978.)

(Jaworski and Hooper, 1980; Baron et al, 1983). During this time the osteoclast team excavates the erosion cavity to a depth of 40–60 μm (Eriksen, 1986; Plate 2). Since the life-span of the osteoclast nucleus is similar to the duration of resorption, it is possible that this determines the duration of resorption. If so, it suggests that nuclear recruitment to the osteoclast pool does not continue once osteoclasts begin to start resorption.

(3) Reversal

Later in the process of bone resorption, multinucleated cells disappear and are replaced by mononuclear cells which appear to be capable of some resorption and smooth off the resorption cavity (Baron et al, 1983; Eriksen, 1986). Over the next 7–10 days a layer of cement substance is deposited which is rich in proteoglycans, glycoproteins and acid phosphatase (Baron et al, 1983) but poor in collagen. This is termed the reversal phase, which describes the time interval between the cessation of osteoclast-mediated bone resorption and bone formation (Baron et al, 1981). The bed of the resorption cavity can be identified as a reversal or cement line by histological techniques even after subsequent bone formation has infilled the resorption cavity (Plate 2).

(4) Matrix synthesis

Once a resorption cavity is complete the process termed 'coupling' attracts osteoblasts to the resorbed surface which thereafter synthesize an

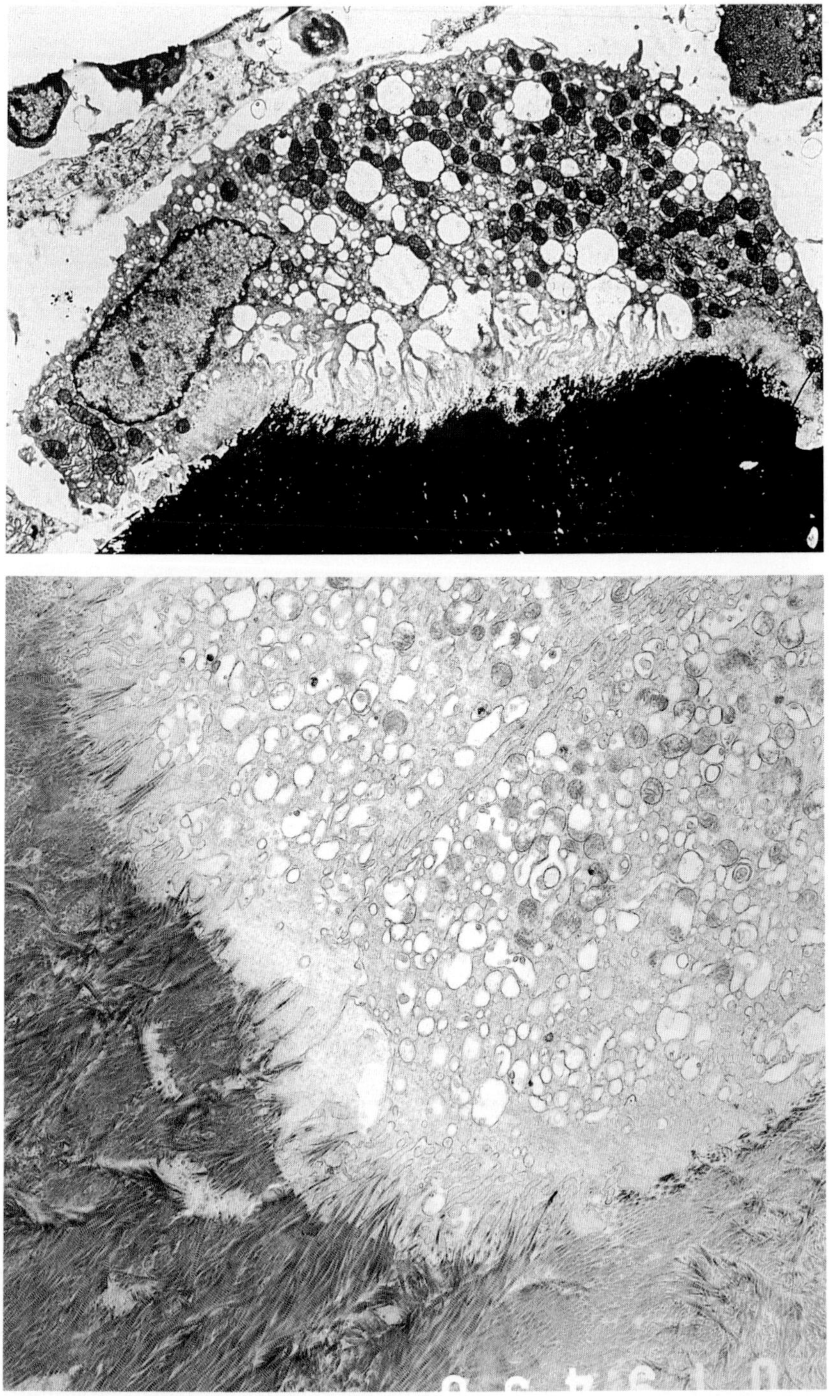

Figure 2.5

Electron micrographs showing a normal multi-nucleated osteoclast closely applied to the mineralized bone surface. The high power (B, × 46500) shows the ruffled border and clear zone at the mineral interface where resorption of fully mineralized bone is occurring.

osteoid matrix (Plate 2). The factors which determine the number of osteoblasts recruited to the reversal surface is not known, but may be critical in determining whether a resorption cavity is infilled adequately. The osteoblasts form a sheet of cells beneath which they synthesize layers of osteoid matrix which comprise unmineralized bone tissue. The newly formed osteoid has a well-ordered lamellated arrangement of collagen bundles because of periodic changes in the orientation of collagen bundles (Marotti and Muglia, 1988). These are well visualized under polarized light. In cancellous bone the lamellae are usually parallel to the trabeculae. In cortical bone the lamellae are more frequently arranged as concentric rings around vascular channels. There are, however, interconnections of collagen between lamellae which decrease the risk of slippage and increase, therefore, the mechanical competence of bone. It is clear that the construction of a lamellar sheet requires the concerted action of a team of osteoblasts but, as in the case of osteoclast teamwork, the processes which regulate this are not understood.

(5) Mineralization

A few days after the onset of matrix formation by osteoblasts, the newly formed osteoid undergoes mineralization (Eriksen, 1986). The time interval between the onset of matrix synthesis and the start of mineralization is about 10 days when the osteoid seam is 8–20 μm in width. The delay accounts for the appearance of osteoid in normal bone. During this period, maturation of collagen occurs and probably involves the incorporation of other bone proteins. The junction between mineralized bone and osteoid is sharply demarcated (the calcification front) indicating the rapidity of the initial rate of mineralization. It can be detected by stains such as toluidine blue or by ultraviolet fluorescence when bone is labelled with tetracycline (Plate 2). Tetracycline is localized and bound by calcium salts at critical concentrations both in vivo and in vitro, and the administration of a short course of tetracycline (generally 2–4 days) permits the visualization of the extent of the bone surface undergoing mineralization at any one time. If two courses of tetracycline are given, but separated by a known time interval, both the extent and the rate of mineralization can be measured. The combined measurements can give an estimate of the rate of mineralized bone formation.

Some osteoblasts, perhaps 30 per cent in trabecular and half as many in cortical bone, become buried within the osteoid matrix to become osteocytes within bone (Figure 2.6). The fate of the remaining cells is not known. Osteocytes have extensive canaliculi which form a network between other osteocytes and surface osteoblasts. They probably function in mineral transport and the surrounding bone is less mineralized. When cell death occurs the bone mineral density adjacent to the osteocyte increases giving rise to micropetrosis.

Mineralization of osteoid occurs rapidly to begin with and is three-quarters complete within a few days. In contrast, it takes many months to become fully mineralized. After 3 months osteoid is no longer visible as unmineralized bone on conventional staining, but further mineralization and maturation of the crystal phase may account for a further 10–20 per cent increase in bone mineral density over one or two years. The decreased bone mineral density of young bone can be detected by microradiography.

(6) Quiescence

When synthesis of matrix is complete, the morphology of the osteoblast changes. During mineralization they become elongated and when this is complete the resting osteoblasts become flattened (Miller and Jee, 1987).

The sequence of resorption, formation and mineralization occurs on the minority of the bone surface, and at any one time 90 per cent or so of available surfaces are inert. The moiety of bone at its completion, termed a bone structural unit (BSU), takes several months to be synthesized and mineralized. In contrast, the process of osteoclastic bone resorption is nearly complete in 3 or 5 days. This explains why formation surfaces on bone are more abundant than resorption surfaces. The fact that bone formation rates can be measured by tetracycline labelling, as well as the surface extent of formation, means that the time period of all events on bone surfaces can be

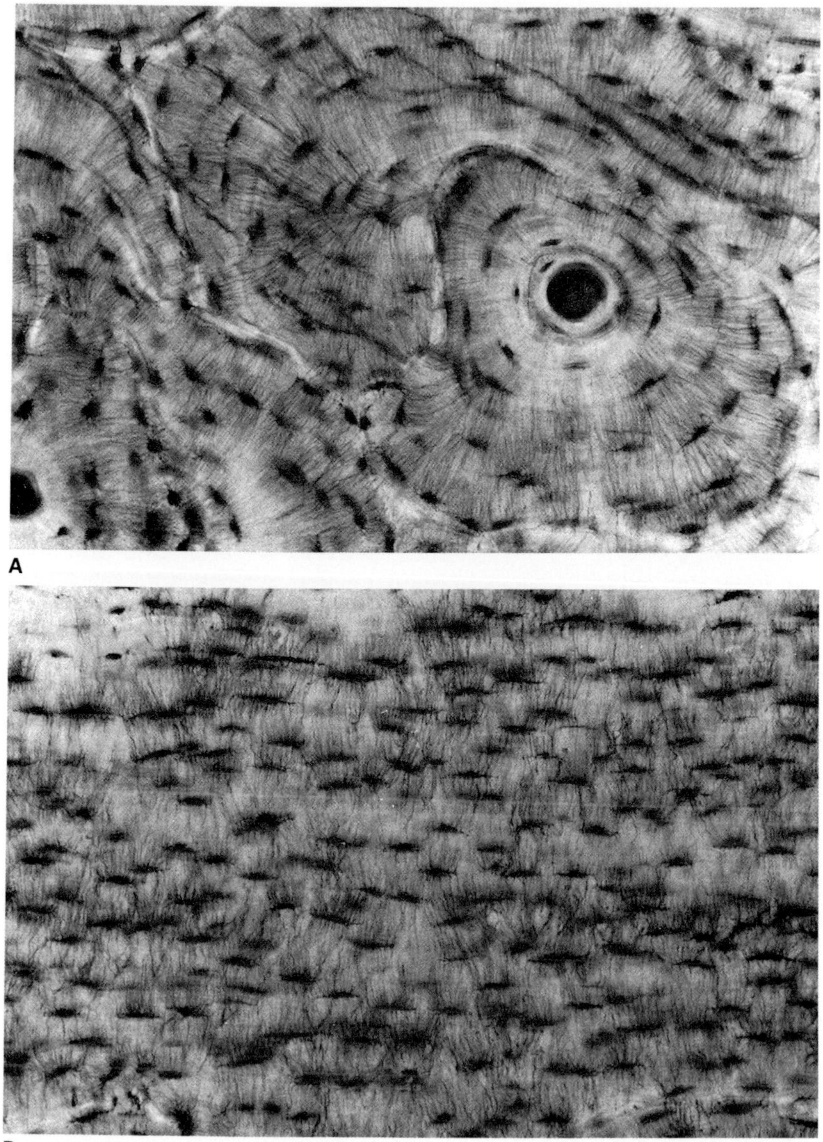

A

B

Figure 2.6

Cross- and longitudinal (B) section of cortical bone showing the osteocytes and their extensive cannicular arrangement. (A) shows that the orientation of osteocytes is concentrically arranged around the Haversian canal. In trabecular bone their orientation is parallel to the bone surface (basic fuschin; × 130).

measured. For example, if the time taken to form a new BSU is 4 months and these events occur on the minority of the bone surface (usually 10 per cent), then the average quiescent interval on any bit of bone surface is 40 months.

Cortical bone remodelling

The remodelling sequence is summarized in Figure 2.7 for trabecular tissue. A similar sequence of events occurs in cortical bone (Figure 2.8). Cortical bone has a system of interconnecting canals orientated in a plane longitudinal to the long axis of osteons and long bones (Haversian canals) as well as perpendicular channels (Volkmann's canals). The canals contain blood vessels, lymphatics, nerves and connective tissue so that all bone cells lie within 150 μm of the blood supply. At the initiation of bone remodelling osteoclasts gather together, often within a Haversian canal, and excavate a cylindrical tunnel through the cortical bone at a rate comparable to that in trabecular bone (20 μm/day; Figure 2.9). Behind the advancing resorption cone the tunnel is infilled several days later after the reversal phase by the products of osteoblast activity. Newly synthesized unmineralized bone matrix is arranged by these osteoblasts in concentric lamellae. The innermost lamella surrounds a new Harvesian system with its own blood supply, lymphatic, neural and connective tissue. Its subsequent mineralization creates a long cylindrical bone structural unit termed an osteon. Interstitial lamellae in cortical bone (Figures 2.2 and 2.10) represent the remnants of earlier osteons.

BRUs and BSUs

The remodelling sequence in both trabecular and cortical bone involves an organized and focal series of cellular events, which comprises a 'bone multicellular unit' (Frost, 1973) or 'bone remodelling unit' (BRU; Rasmussen and Bordier, 1974). The completion of activity of a bone remodelling unit results in the creation of a bone structural unit (Jaworski, 1976; BSU, also termed a 'bone

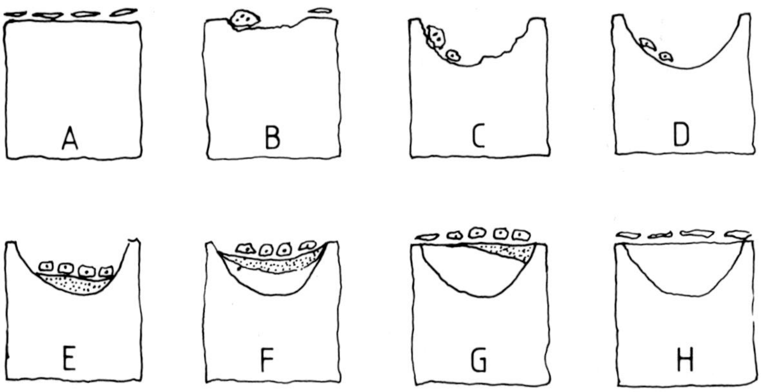

Figure 2.7

Schematic diagram to show the stages in the remodelling sequence of trabecular bone. (A) Quiescent bone surface. (B) The activation of bone resorption by the focal attraction of osteoclasts. (C) The creation by osteoclasts of a resorption cavity. (D) Smoothing of resorption cavities by mononuclear cells (reversal). (E) The differentiation of osteoblasts within resorption cavities (coupling). (F) The onset of matrix synthesis and mineralization. (G) The completion of matrix synthesis. (H) The completion of the remodelling sequence where the bone surface is covered by lining cells once more.

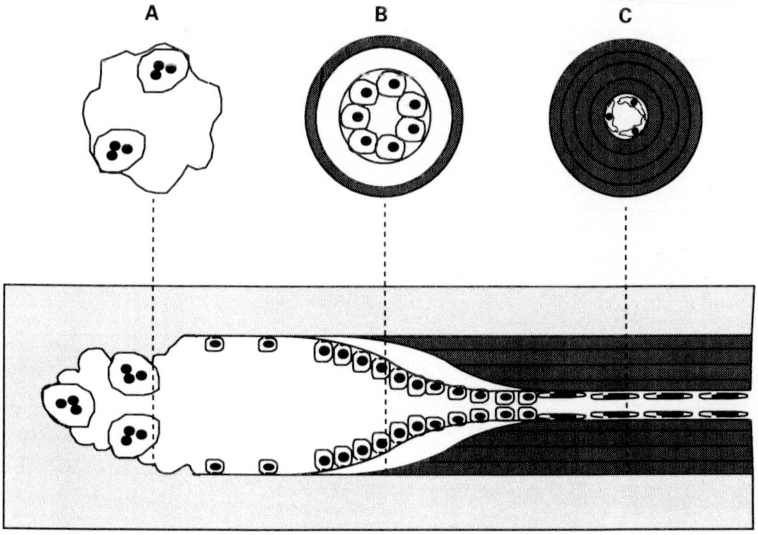

Figure 2.8

Schematic diagram of a bone remodelling unit in cortical bone. Osteoclasts tunnel in the long axis of the cortex to create a cutting cone (A). The resorption cavity is smoothed off during the reversal phase. Thereafter, osteoblasts synthesize an osteoid matrix in the form of concentric lamellae (B) which infill the resorption cavity (C) leaving a new Haversian canal. Note that unlike trabecular bone the resorption cavity cannot be markedly overfilled.

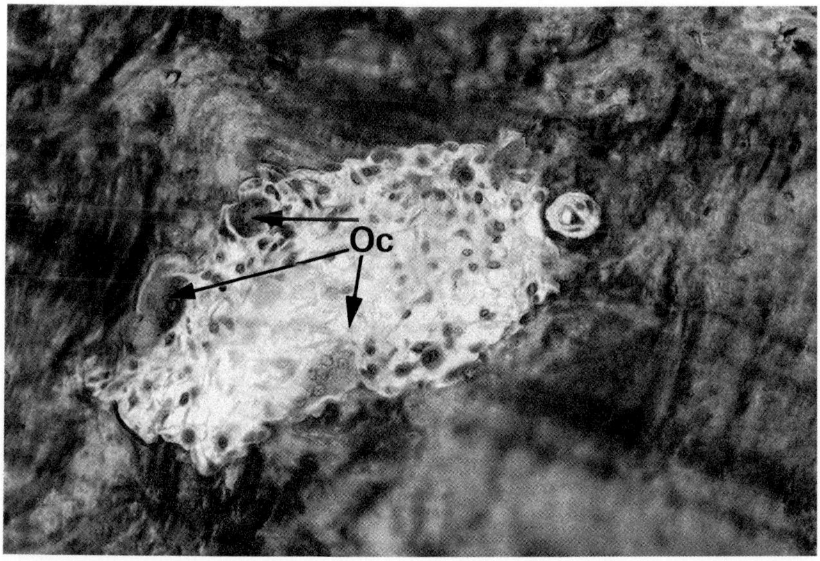

Figure 2.9

Cross-section through a cutting cone in cortical bone. Multi-nucleated osteoclasts (arrows) have tunnelled through fully mineralized bone (stained blue), (toluidine blue; × 170).

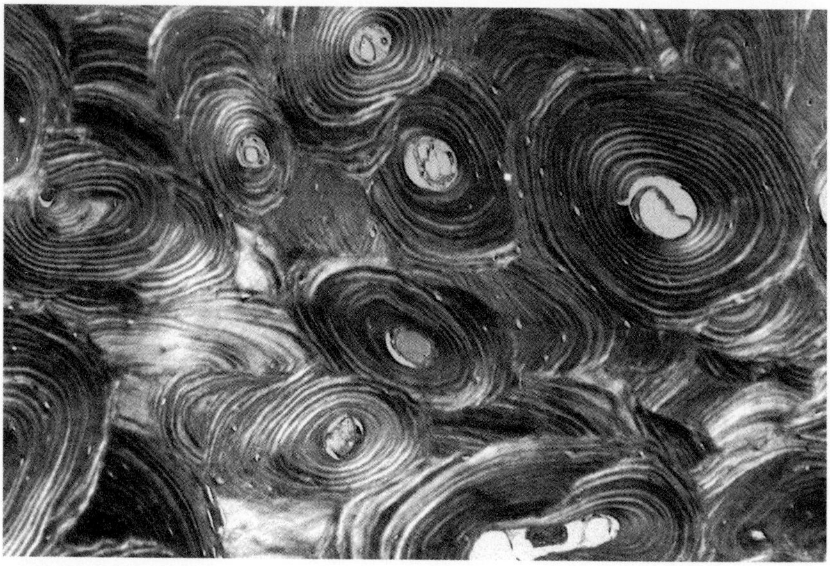

Figure 2.10

Cross-section through cortical bone showing Haversian systems. Note the concentric arrangement of lamellae surrounding Haversian canals. Interstitial lamellae represent the remnants of previous osteons (× 55; haematoxylin and eosin, partially polarized).

metabolic unit'). In the case of cortical bone the BSU is a secondary osteon or Haversian system. It is cylindrical in shape, 100–300 μm in diameter and several mm in length. In trabecular bone the BSU is flat, 40–60 μm thick with an area of 0.5–1 mm^2 (Table 2.2).

Thus, skeletal tissue comprises a series of BSUs which in adult man have been estimated at 35 million in number, of which 40 per cent are in trabecular bone (Parfitt, 1983). Where BSUs are in contact they are separated by the cement line or reversal surface which are not traversed by osteocytic canaliculi.

Bone turnover in Paget's disease

Paget's disease is characterized by an exuberant increase in metabolic activity of bone which can be readily demonstrated by bone microscopy. As indicated previously, bone remodelling normally occurs on 10 per cent or less of the bone surface. The proportion of bone surface involved in remodelling at any one time is a function of the number of remodelling units present, their size and also the duration of time between the onset of resorption and the completion of formation. Thus

$$\text{prevalence} = \text{incidence} \times \text{duration}$$

A considerable body of morphological evidence suggests that increased activity of bone in Paget's disease is predominantly due to an increase in the incidence of bone remodelling units (termed an increase in activation frequency). All aspects of the remodelling sequence are found with greater frequency so that up to 100 per cent of the bone surface can be occupied by active events (Jowsey, 1966; Meunier et al, 1980; Plate 3). Provided

Table 2.2 Some characteristics of normal bone structural units (BSUs) and bone remodelling units (BRUs) (from Parfitt, 1983).

	Cortex	*Trabecular bone*	*Cortical and trabecular bone*
BSUs			
Number (millions)	21	14	35
Volume (mm^3)	0.065	0.025	0.048
Total volume (cm^3)	1365	350	1715
Total calcium	800	200	1000
Calcium (μg/BSU)	38	14	
BRUs			
Number (thousands)	280	1400	1680
Number (% BSUs)	1.3	10	4.8
Number (/cm^3 bone tissue)	205	4000	1000
Total resorption space (cm^3)	5.6	7.1	12.6
Resorption space (g calcium)	3.4	4.2	7.6
Resorption space (% total volume)	0.4	2.0	0.72

that the time taken to complete each remodelling cycle is unaltered, the turnover rate of bone can be increased 10-fold or so. Parfitt (1983) has calculated that activation normally occurs once every 10 seconds in the normal adult, so that in Paget's disease this may rise to once per second.

There are few data concerning the remodelling period in Paget's disease (for technical reasons), but histological sections utilizing double tetracycline labelling (Meunier et al, 1980) suggest that the increased frequency with which cellular events are observed on bone are due principally to an increase in activation frequency. There is some evidence, discussed later, that the time relationships between resorption, reversal, formation and mineralization are disturbed in Paget's disease, in that resorption and reversal occupy a longer time than formation and mineralization compared with normal bone.

Osteoclasts and bone resorption

The number of osteoclasts in pagetic bone may be increased up to 100-fold (Table 2.3; Meunier et al, 1980). As well as an increased number of osteoclasts, the size and the number of nuclei of pagetic osteoclasts are increased (Rasmussen and Bordier, 1974; Meunier et al, 1980; Kanis et al, 1985a; Figure 2.11). This is a phenomenon seen in many disorders associated with increased bone remodelling (such as hyperparathyroidism), but in Paget's disease nuclearity is most marked with up to 100 nuclei per cell. As might be expected, osteoclasts are larger than normal and may reach 200 μm in diameter so that they are capable of engulfing thin trabeculae or small islands of bone (Plate 4).

Within the past few years many additional morphological abnormalities of pagetic osteoclasts have been noted. In many instances it is not clear to what extent these are specific for Paget's disease or related to the increase in their activity (Rebel et al, 1987). The most striking observation has been that the giant osteoclast characteristically found in this disorder contains virus-like nuclear and cytoplasmic inclusions (Rebel et al, 1974, 1975; Mills and Singer, 1976; Figure 2.12). These comprise micro-cylinders found as loose filaments or arranged tightly in a paracrystalline configuration and with the size and periodicity characteristic of paramyxoviral nucleocapsids (Malkani et al, 1976; Howatson and Fournasier, 1982). When cytoplasmic inclusions are abundant

Table 2.3 Bone cell surfaces and counts in Paget's disease of bone. Histomorphometric measurements were made (mean ± SEM) on trabecular bone from transiliac biopsies from 16 pagetic and 11 non-pagetic sites. (Benéton and Kanis, unpublished work.)

	Site of biopsy		*Ratio*	*p* <
	Involved	*Non-involved*		
Active osteoblast surface (% bone surface)	7.73 ± 1.05	0.96 ± 0.4	8.1	0.001
Osteoblast density (/mm bone surface)	5.23 ± 0.70	0.68 ± 0.22	7.7	0.001
Osteoclast surface (% bone surface)	5.40 ± 1.03	0.21 ± 0.12	26	0.001
Osteoclast density (/mm bone surface)	0.93 ± 0.15	0.04 ± 0.02	23	0.005
Active eroded surface* (% bone surface)	7.78 ± 1.28	0.35 ± 0.13	22	0.001
Total eroded surface (% bone surface)	28.67 ± 2.18	8.64 ± 1.50	3.3	0.001

* Includes mononuclear cells.

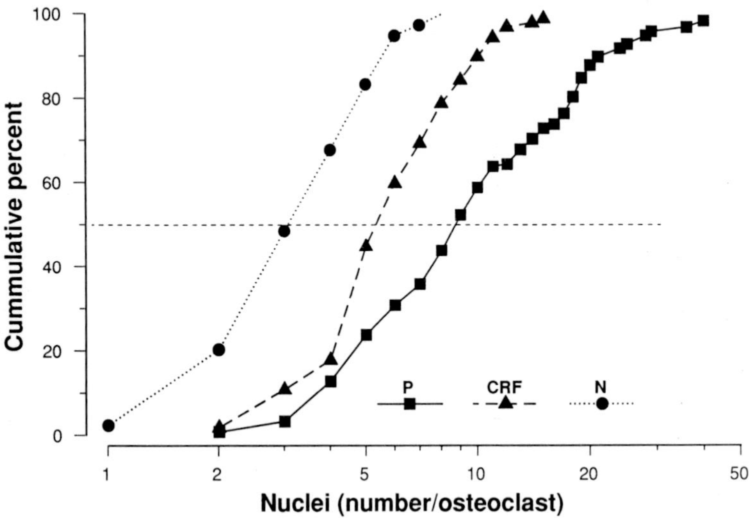

Figure 2.11

Frequency distribution showing the number of nuclei in pagetic osteoclasts (P) compared to normal subjects (N) and patients with secondary hyperparathyroidism due to chronic renal failure (CRF). The horizontal dotted line denotes the fiftieth percentile. Fifty per cent of pagetic nuclei have more than seven osteoclast nuclei and 10 per cent have more than 20.

the nuclei of osteoclasts show an unusual polychromasia visible on light microscopy (Plate 5). Subacute sclerosing panencephalitis is associated with similar inclusions in the nuclei and cytoplasm of brain cells of affected patients which have been identified as viral nucleocapsids (Oyanang et al, 1971; Raine et al, 1973; Iwasaki and Koprowski, 1974; Fraser and Martin, 1978). These findings have led to speculation that Paget's disease is due to a slow viral infection affecting osteoclasts.

Support for this notion has also come from indirect immunofluorescence using a variety of antisera. Positive reactions were shown for sera

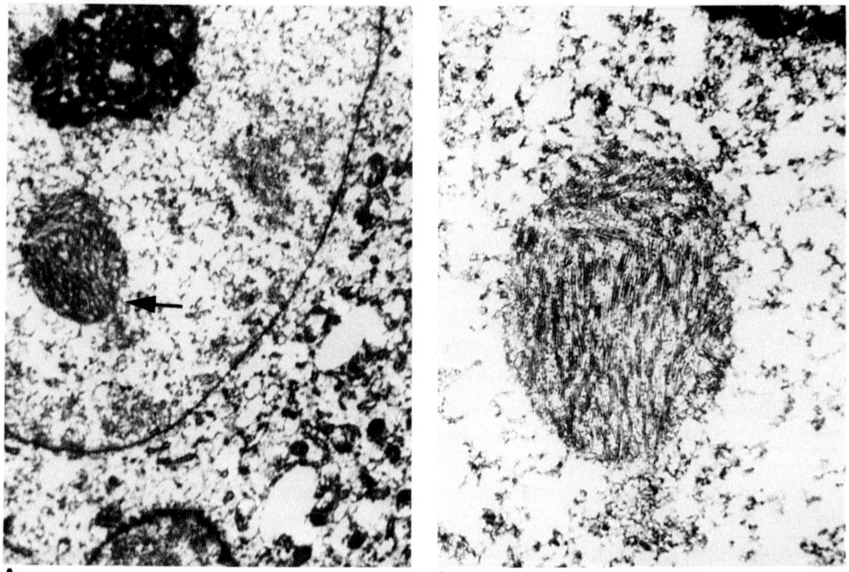

Figure 2.12

Electron micrograph showing an intranuclear inclusion in the osteoclast (arrow) of a patient with Paget's disease. Under high power (B) they share the morphological characteristics of the paramyxoviridae (× 30000).

containing antibody against paramyxoviridae, including antisera raised against measles (Rebel et al, 1980a), respiratory syncitial virus (Mills et al, 1980, 1981) or both (Mills et al, 1984). Measles virus mRNA has been shown in pagetic tissue by in situ hybridization (Baslé et al, 1986). In this study, viral RNA was demonstrated in other cells in addition to osteoclasts, even though inclusions have only been noted in osteoclasts. The canine distemper virus also belongs to the paramyxoviridae and specific probes have detected RNA of the nucleocapsid in some patients (Gordon et al, 1991).

A causal link between the viral inclusions and Paget's disease has not been established, and it has been difficult to passage these inclusions in bone-cell cultures or to infect experimental animals (Mills et al, 1980).

Viral-like inclusions have been found in all Paget's disease patients examined (Harvey et al, 1982; Singer and Mills, 1983) but not in all osteoclasts nor in all nuclei of affected osteoclasts (Harvey et al, 1982; Table 2.4). They have not been observed in osteoblasts, osteocytes or marrow cells (Mills et al, 1980: Rebel et al, 1980b) although viral RNA of measles has been detected in osteoblasts (Baslé et al, 1986). The paramyxoviridal inclusions are widely regarded as specific for Paget's disease, but this view is being increasingly challenged since they are observed in some

Table 2.4 Some characteristics of pagetic osteoclasts and their inclusions (from Kanis et al, 1985a).

Osteoclast density (number/mm^2 bone area)	10.0 ± 2.3
Number of nuclei/osteoclast	11.8 ± 1.3
Proportion of osteoclasts with inclusions (%)	86 ± 15*
Proportion of nuclei with inclusions (%)	31 ± 5*

* 95 per cent confidence intervals.

other bone disorders (Chapter 9). It is not known whether they occur in juvenile hyperphosphatasia, but this would be of interest to determine. The satisfactory explanation for its aetiology is discussed in Chapter 9.

The stimulus for an increase in osteoclast nuclearity and the increase in the activation frequency of bone remodelling units is unknown. Fusion of infected osteoclasts with non-infected mononuclear cells seems to be a likely mechanism for the replication of the virus. Inclusion bodies have not been observed in mononuclear cells, either in the marrow or in the peripheral circulation (Horton and Kanis, unpublished), but viral RNA has been observed in mononuclear cells of the marrow.

It is notable that Paget's disease is a very patchy disorder and once the diagnosis is established it is extremely rare to see new foci of pagetic involvement. This suggests that cells of the monocyte/macrophage series which fuse to form osteoclasts are either non-infected or only able to express viral protein at specific sites. A plausible explanation is that the osteoclast is 'immortal'. Osteoclasts are a syncitial structure and normally recruit and shed nuclear material. The normal nuclear turnover is approximately 8 per cent/day (Jaworski and Hooper, 1980). There could be local infection of an osteoclast that recruits normal osteoclast precursor cells from outside. If true, this suggests that the osteoclast, once formed, can be present for life with a fairly closely defined territory. This notion is supported by the finding that reactivation of Paget's disease following successful treatment invariably occurs at sites previously shown to be affected and that new pagetic lesions have never been convincingly demonstrated in patients after presentation (Chapter 3).

A notable feature of active Paget's disease is the finding of osteoclasts within the marrow cavity (Plate 6). The view has been forwarded that these represent osteoclasts which are no longer active and have moved from resorption cavities (Singer, 1977a). The finding of osteoclasts eroding osteoid rather than mineralized bone (Plate 6) suggests that their production can exceed the available mineralized surface, and perhaps more arguably that they can be formed within the marrow cavity rather than in resorption bays. This phenomenon is not specific for Paget's disease, but is also observed in other disorders where there is extensive surface coverage of trabecular bone with osteoid.

Whereas there is no doubt that overall rates of resorption are increased, it is by no means certain that the functional activity of osteoclasts is increased. Indirect evidence would suggest the contrary and is based on evidence that osteoblast performance is normal (discussed later), and observations that the osteoclast/osteoblast density is more than three times greater in Paget's disease than in healthy bone (Table 2.3). If these patients were in skeletal balance then the amount of bone formed would equal that resorbed but with three times the number of osteoclasts. This would imply a 65 per cent decrease in the functional capacity of osteoclasts. If bone formation was exceeding bone resorption (as is likely in these sclerotic patients), then this calculation of the functional impairment of osteoclasts would be an underestimate.

A characteristic difference between normal and pagetic resorption is the irregularity of the resorption cavities formed in the latter case. Their scalloped edges contribute to the 'mosaic appearance' of bone because of the irregularity of the cement lines representing the limits of previous osteoclastic bone resorption (Plate 7). The appearances are most striking when the newly formed bone is lamellar rather than woven. In the case of cortical bone resorption, an early feature of Paget's disease is the loss of the longitudinal orientation of osteons (Milgram, 1977) due to the non-polarized activity of osteoclasts.

Whereas the histological evidence clearly implicates abnormalities in osteoclast morphology and behaviour, and indeed might suggest a slow viral infection of osteoclasts, it is important to recognize that many of the clinical consequences of Paget's disease are related to the exuberant and anarchic bone formation occurring at endosteal and periosteal sites.

Osteoblasts and bone formation

As in normal bone remodelling, resorption by the giant osteoclasts of Paget's disease is followed by a wave of new bone formation. The ultrastructure of active osteoblasts does not show nuclear or cytoplasmic viral-like inclusions (Mills and Singer, 1976), but displays pleomorphism with variable invaginations of the nuclear border, and intranuclear abnormalities have been described (Rasmussen and Bordier, 1974; Singer, 1977a). As in the case of some of the alterations described in osteoclast morphology, these may represent non-specific changes since similar abnormalities are found in other disorders associated with rapid bone turnover such as secondary hyperparathyroidism.

The numbers of osteoblasts are greatly increased, but it is not known whether the performance of individual osteoblasts is greater than normal. Bone explants from pagetic bone synthesize more collagen in tissue culture (Cheung et al, 1980) which appears to be all of type I, but may be due to the increased numbers of osteoblasts (Lee, 1967). Quantitative bone histology suggests that the increase in osteoblast numbers matches the increase in bone formation rate (Tables 2.3 and 2.5). This suggests that the functional capacity of osteoblasts is quite normal. Also, there is a close correlation between alkaline phosphatase activity and the extent of the disease (Chapter 3; Meunier et al, 1987). This further suggests that variations in disease activity are more related to the number of osteoblasts than to variations in their synthetic performance.

The new bone formed by osteoblasts may be woven or lamellar in type. Woven bone is not normally present in the adult, except during fracture repair, but is found in other disorders associated with rapid rates of bone formation such as hyperparathyroidism, renal bone disease and fluorosis. It is characterized by a more random disposition of collagen fibres than in lamellar bone. It also has a lower and more variable mineral content. The osteocyte lacunae vary in size and shape and are more numerous. Osteocyte density (normally 20 000/mm^3) may be increased 4-fold and their canalicular arrangement is less organized. Thus, woven bone lacks much of the structural organization of lamellar bone and hence has greater flexibility and consequently less resistance to deformation. All degrees of disorganization can be found. When marked, all evidence of lamellar birefringence is lost on polarized light microscopy (Plate 8).

Woven bone formation is a characteristic but not invariant feature of Paget's disease and presumably reflects some defect in the co-ordination of collagen assembly by osteoblasts or perhaps the lack of cell polarity. Alternatively, it may result from defective collagen cross-linking during the early phase of maturation. There are many degrees of spatial disorientation, even on light microscopy. Woven bone occupies more space because the collagen fibres are less compactly arranged: thus even when the balance between bone resorption and formation is unaffected this would provide a mechanism for

Table 2.5 Indices of osteoid and bone formation in Paget's disease of bone. Histomorphometric measurements were made (mean ± SEM) on trabecular bone from transiliac biopsies from 16 pagetic and 11 non-pagetic sites. Note the increase in osteoid volume is associated with an increase in osteoid surface rather than its thickness. (Benéton and Kanis, unpublished work.)

	Site of biopsy		*Ratio*	$p <$
	Involved	*Non-involved*		
Osteoid volume (% bone volume)	2.95 ± 0.39	1.84 ± 0.51	1.6	0.001
Osteoid surface (% bone surface)	29.9 ± 2.9	11.7 ± 3.3	2.6	0.001
Osteoid thickness (μ)	13 ± 1	12 ± 2	1.1	NS
Mineral apposition rate (μ/day)	0.93 ± 0.10	0.48 ± 0.05	1.9	0.005
Bone formation rate (mm^2/mm^3/year)	0.137 ± 0.017	0.021 ± 0.005	6.5	0.001

NS: not signficant.

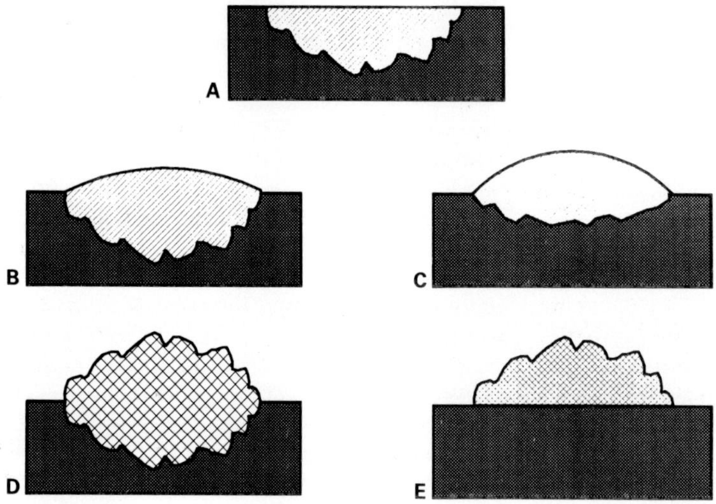

Figure 2.13

Mechanisms for the induction of trabecular osteosclerosis in Paget's disease. (A) depicts normal bone remodelling with the infilling of a resorption cavity with an equal volume of lamellar bone. (B) and (C) depict an imbalance between the amount formed and resorbed at each remodelling site in favour of net bone formation. In the latter example (C), a normal volume of new bone is deposited within a shallow resorption cavity. If the new bone formed is woven (D), trabecular osteosclerosis may arise without necessarily an increase in the amount of collagen (or calcium) due to the loosely packed collagen. Osteosclerosis may also arise from uncoupling (E) where new bone formed is laid down independently of previous resorption.

an increase in bone tissue volume and a distortion of trabecular architecture (Figure 2.13).

Woven bone formation need not be marked. More frequently a lamellar arrangement of matrix production is preserved but the lamellae themselves may be malorientated in that they no longer follow the orientation of trabecular surfaces. The formation of lamellar bone with variable orientation, together with irregular cement lines, accentuates the mosaic appearance so characteristic of pagetic bone (Plate 7).

Mineralization

The amount of osteoid present in pagetic bone is generally greater than that seen in healthy bone. This does not necessarily imply the presence of osteomalacia or a defect in the mineralization process. Accelerated bone turnover will increase the frequency of all events on bone surfaces, including the surface coverage with osteoid. Indeed, Paget's disease is characterized more by an increase in the surface coverage of bone by osteoid than by an increase in its width (Table 2.5). Where lamellar bone is being formed, the mean osteoid seam width is not increased in Paget's disease. Indeed, the finding of an increase in osteoid seam width and more than five osteoid lamellae should alert one to the possibility of co-existing osteomalacia, not an infrequent problem in the elderly. Pagetic bone appears to mineralize normally, though rates of mineralization are increased (Lee, 1967; Meunier et al, 1980; Table 2.5; Plate 9). The uptake of tetracycline is patchy and diffuse throughout the osteoid seam in the presence of woven bone formation. Again this should not be confused with the diffuse or defective uptake of tetracycline found in lamellar bone in the presence of co-existing osteomalacia.

Bone marrow

A conspicuous characteristic of Paget's disease of bone is the replacement of haemopoietic elements by fibrous tissue which may be very vascular (Plate 10; Table 2.6). Again, this does not appear to be a specific feature of Paget's disease, but is observed in many states where turnover is accelerated. Indeed, marrow fibrosis confined to resorption cavities may be found in immobilization, and in this sense seems to be related more to osteoclastic rather than osteoblastic activity. Nevertheless, fibrosis may be very marked but anaemia due to marrow replacement has not been described, even with extensive Paget's disease.

A further feature of pagetic marrow is a striking increase in marrow vascularity which may contribute to bone pain. It has been suggested on this basis that Paget's disease has a vascular aetiology (Cone, 1922) but, as for marrow fibrosis, the increased vascularity is usually thought to be a result rather than a cause of the disorder. This notion is supported by the observation that diphosphonates used in the treatment of the disorder are associated with a decrease in vascularity which occurs slowly and in parallel with the inhibition of bone formation. In addition, the diphosphonates (unlike calcitonin) have no known activity on vascular tissue.

No anatomic evidence exists for the presence of arterio-venous shunts (Rhodes et al, 1972).

The presence of fibroblasts and undifferentiated mesenchymal cells within the marrow may provide the framework for uncoupled bone formation and might arguably contribute to the dense osteosclerosis which is commonly observed. At this time the marrow becomes less vascular and is reoccupied by haemopoietic tissue or fat cells. When osteosclerosis is dense the surface to volume ratio of *trabecular* tissue approaches that of normal *cortical* bone (Plate 11; Table 2.6). For this reason, the surface available for bone remodelling progressively decreases.

Remodelling and focal skeletal balance

It is useful to draw a distinction between skeletal balance and the coupling of bone formation to

Table 2.6 Some structural characteristics (mean ± SEM) of iliac trabecular bone in female patients with Paget's disease and in normal women (unpublished work).

	Site of biopsy		*p <*
	Involved (n = 20)	*Non-involved (n = 20)*	
Degree of marrow fibrosis (0–3)	2.5 ± 0.7	0.55 ± 0.5	0.001
Maximum number of osteoid lamellae	3.75 ± 1.2	3.0 ± 1.0	NS
Bone volume (% of tissue volume)	41.9 ± 14.1	15.3 ± 3.9	0.001
Trabecular width (μ)	209 ± 37	131 ± 25	0.001
Trabecular density (number/field)	40 ± 12	24 ± 6	0.005
Surface/volume ratio (mm^2/mm^3 bone tissue)	13.2 ± 5.7	16.9 ± 3.2	NS

bone resorption. Uncoupling implies the dissociation of these two processes; either the creation of resorption cavities without subsequent attraction of osteoblasts, as is sometimes seen in neoplasia, or conversely, the deposition of new bone at sites other than sites of previous resorption (see Figure 2.13). The latter occurs conspicuously in various tumours such as metastatic bone disease due to prostatic carcinoma. The extent to which uncoupled resorption or formation occurs in the healthy adult is not known, but it is likely to be a very small component of turnover (Jaworski et al, 1972), perhaps principally in the repair of microfractures.

A characteristic feature of Paget's disease is focal areas of sclerosis and lysis. In the case of trabecular bone, biopsies from affected and unaffected sites indicate that areas of osteopaenia do occur, but that osteosclerosis is more commonly found, at least in the ilium (Figure 2.14). This can arise in a number of ways. Since the majority of skeletal turnover in the adult is accounted for by bone remodelling, large changes in bone-tissue volume are the result of imbalances at sites of remodelling between the amount of bone resorbed and that formed. Since cortical bone is a near solid structure, the amount of bone formed during each remodelling sequence cannot greatly exceed that resorbed (by less than 1 per cent). The same is not true at trabecular sites where resorption cavities can be infilled with an increased volume of trabecular tissue (for example with fluoride treatment by 25 per cent). In contrast, bone loss due to an imbalance between the amount resorbed and that formed at each remodelling unit may occur at both cortical and trabecular sites. It would be expected, however, that if the number of bone remodelling units did not change, then the rate of bone loss would be greater at trabecular than at cortical sites due to the larger numbers of remodelling units per unit volume of bone operational at any one time at trabecular sites (Table 2.2).

In the case of Paget's disease there is little evidence for uncoupled bone formation even in the presence of dense osteosclerosis. Unlike prostatic carcinoma, where condensation of marrow fibrosis may give rise to new trabecular elements, the trabecular density in Paget's disease is often normal even in the presence of dense osteosclerosis (Table 2.6). The osteosclerosis is therefore largely attributable to an increase

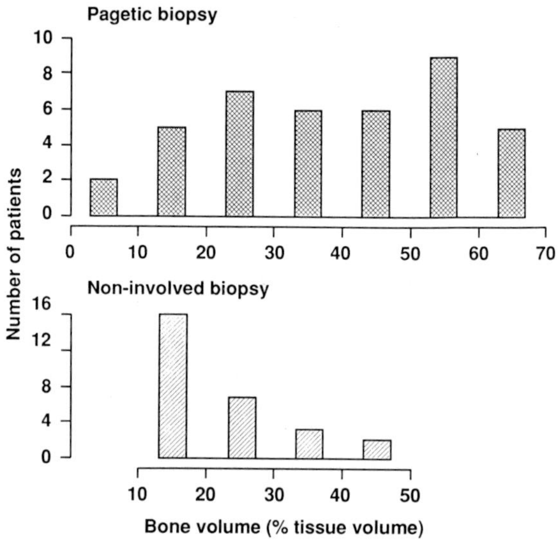

Figure 2.14

Distribution of trabecular bone volume (percentage of tissue volume) of the ilium in patients with Paget's disease. Note the large range in bone volume observed in biopsies taken from affected sites. The majority of biopsies showed osteosclerosis.

in the thickness of trabecular elements rather than their number. This indicates that if uncoupled bone formation did occur, this would have to arise on quiescent bone surfaces, which are conspicuously absent in active disease. In addition, the morphology of the reversal lines suggests that if this did occur it must be infrequent.

This conclusion accords with the close relationship between bone formation and resorption found in kinetic, histological and biochemical measurements in untreated disease, despite large changes in turnover which are more plausibly explained by a coupled rather than an uncoupled disorder. Finally, the response of pagetic bone to therapeutic intervention indicates the coupled nature of the disorder. These treatments which change bone resorption are followed by changes in bone formation–to be expected if coupling were preserved (Chapter 7).

These considerations suggest that steady-state changes in bone-tissue volume are due to focal imbalances at remodelling sites, related in turn to the functional capacity of osteoblast and osteoclast teams involved in the BRU. The measurement of wall thickness (the depth of BSUs on bone surfaces after the completion of bone formation) provides an index of the balance between formation and resorption at trabecular BRUs. Wall thickness is markedly increased in Paget's disease (Figure 2.15), indicating that the balance between the amount formed and that resorbed at each remodelling site is tipped in favour of net bone formation at this site. If at each remodelling sequence there is focal imbalance (that is a finite deficit or increment between the amount resorbed and that formed of say 10 000 μm^3, approximately 40 per cent of a trabecular BSU), then the rate of change of bone volume will depend on the activation frequency (Figure 2.16). If the rate of bone turnover is increased 5-fold then the rate of change of bone tissue volume will increase 5-fold, assuming that

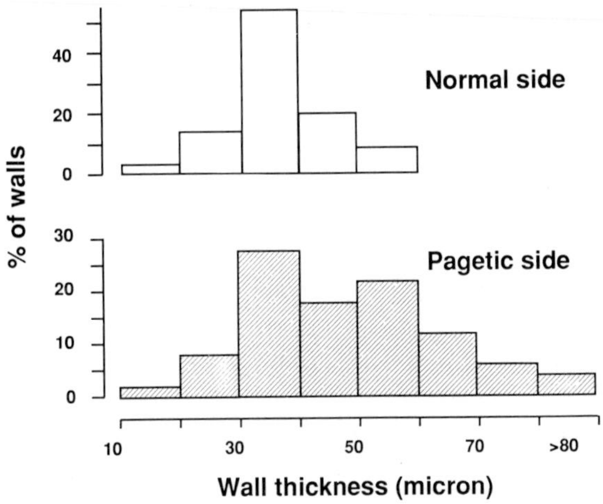

Figure 2.15

Frequency distribution of wall thickness at 50 trabecular sites in Paget's disease (hatched areas) compared to wall thickness measured at 35 sites unaffected by Paget's disease. Wall thickness was significantly higher at pagetic than at non-pagetic sites (50 $\mu m \pm$ SD 18 μm vs 36 $\mu m \pm$ 9 μm respectively; $p < 0.001$).

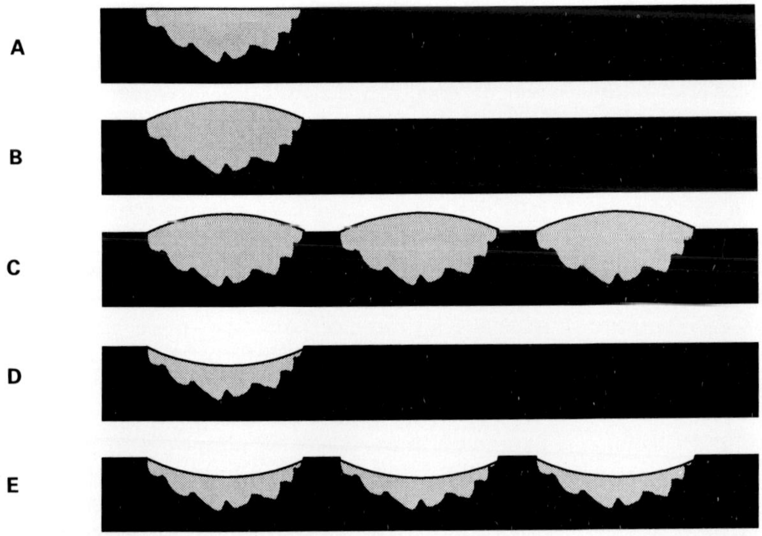

Figure 2.16

The effect of activation frequency and bone balance on bone volume. (A) depicts normal bone turnover. When the balance between bone formation and resorption is disturbed, each remodelling sequence results in a finite gain (B) or loss (D) of bone. The rate of gain or loss will be amplified in proportion to the frequency of activation of new remodelling units (C) and (E) respectively).

the duration of each BRU remains unchanged. In addition, the production of woven bone occupying more space (but less mineral and collagen density) may have important consequences on bone-tissue volume and density which may differ at different sites (see Figure 2.13).

At trabecular sites the deposition of a normal quantity of collagen matrix within a resorption cavity would occupy more space when woven. This would induce osteosclerosis (an increase in trabecular bone volume) without necessarily an increase in the total amount of collagen and mineral incorporated at each BSU. In the case of cortical bone, the geometric constraints of the osteoclastic cutting cone mean that resorption cavities cannot be overfilled. Thus, the deposition of woven bone would result in a loss of bone matrix and mineral density but without changes in the volume of skeletal tissue (see Figure 2.8).

An increase in turnover of bone has several additional consequences. Since the process of bone remodelling implies a net deficit of bone (until resorption cavities are completely infilled) the skeletal volume missing at any one time will increase proportionately according to the number of functional bone remodelling units (Figure 2.17). This skeletal deficit, termed the resorption space, is approximately 5.6 cm^3 at cortical sites and 7.1 cm^3 at trabecular sites. This is equivalent to 3.4 and 4.2 g calcium respectively, amounting at both sites to 7.6 g or 0.76 per cent of total body calcium (Tables 2.2 and 2.7). From these considerations Parfitt (1983) has calculated that a 5-fold increase in bone turnover would produce a negative calcium balance of 30 g or a decrease in total body bone volume of 3 per cent under steady-state conditions. The change in bone volume will, of course, depend on the prevailing rate of bone turnover, and will be correspondingly greater at trabecular than at cortical sites. Clearly if bone formation and bone resorption are not exactly balanced then an increase in bone remodelling will result in continued and accelerated skeletal losses or gains.

A further consequence of increased skeletal remodelling relates to the turnover time of the skeleton. The amount of calcium normally removed by bone resorption is 250 mg daily from a total body calcium of 1000 g. Thus, for the whole skeleton the average turnover time is 11 years or 9 per cent per annum. It is, however, much shorter at trabecular sites (4 years or 25 per cent per annum) than at cortical sites (30 years or 3 per cent per annum) due to the higher surface activity of the former. In addition, bone remodelling in trabecular bone is not random (it occurs on surfaces) so that the turnover time of trabecular tissue near the endosteal surface may vary between 3 and 15 months. As mentioned previously, mineralization is not complete, even after the completion of a new bone structural unit, and proceeds for many months thereafter. If bone turnover is accelerated, a proportionately greater amount of bone volume is occupied by young rather than by old BSUs. Consequently, the proportion of immature and incompletely mineralized bone will increase (Table 2.7).

A third consequence of increased remodelling is that the osteoid in the incompletely formed BRUs at any one time is not mineralized. Thus the 'calcium space' exceeds the resorption space by a proportion recently computed by Frost (1989).

For these three reasons the mineral content of bone may be profoundly influenced by changes in bone turnover. In the trabecular bone of the ilium, the resorption space is approximately 5 per cent of the bone volume. Consequently, a 5-fold increase in turnover would decrease the actual bone volume by 20 per cent and the mineral content by nearly double (see Figure 2.17), a process which is entirely reversible when bone turnover is decreased. The effects at cortical sites will be less, but if new bone is woven then the mineral density will be decreased still further. Such effects on bone density are within the detection limits of radiography, and explain in part the patchy osteolysis and intracortical bone resorption visible on X-ray examination.

It is important to recognize that the above considerations apply to the steady state (that is unchanging rates of bone resorption and formation). In the natural history of the extension of Paget's disease there is a sharp demarcation between normal and floridly abnormal bone. Extension is by waves of abnormal osteoclastic resorption followed only later by osteoblastic formation. Thus, the resorption space at an advancing front is considerably greater (3 to 5 times) than the average resorption space of pagetic bone tissue. This suggests that changes in bone turnover account in large measure for the 'osteolytic' resorption front so characteristic of early Paget's disease (Chapter 3).

Others have suggested that the resorption front

is due to unopposed resorption occurring for several years before formation occurs. The evidence for this view is based on the radiographic appearance of osteoporosis circumscripta at the skull (Chapter 3), where radiotranslucency may persist for many years without osteosclerosis appearing behind the front. Scintigraphic uptake is, however, almost invariably enhanced and, with the few histological data available (Milgram, 1977), this indicates the presence of osteoblasts. This suggests that all the steps of remodelling occur but that bone mineral density remains reduced due to increased turnover and the associated mineral deficit, a focal imbalance between formation and resorption in favour of the latter, or both.

Table 2.7 The reversible skeletal deficit of calcium due to bone remodelling. Note the greater deficits at trabecular bone associated with the greater bone turnover. (From Parfitt, 1980.)

	Cortical bone	*Trabecular bone*	*Cortical and trabecular bone*
Bone turnover (% pa)	3.0	28.0	8.0
Resorption space (g)	3.4	4.2	7.6
Osteoid tissue (g)	1.4	3.5	4.9
Low density bone (g)	1.1	2.5	3.6
TOTAL (g)	5.9	10.2	16.1
TOTAL (% skeletal calcium)	0.7	4.8	1.5

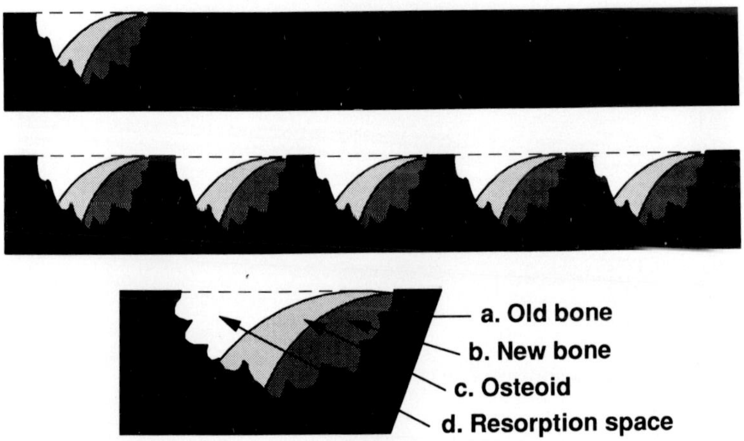

Figure 2.17

Effect of bone turnover on bone and calcium balance. The upper panel depicts normal bone remodelling activity occurring on 15 per cent of the trabecular surface. The resorption space (d) occupies 2 per cent of the bone volume and a somewhat smaller amount is occupied by osteoid, 1.5 per cent, accounting for 3.5 per cent of the bone volume. When turnover is increased five-fold (without affecting the balance between formation and resorption) the resorption space and osteoid space increase to 17.5 per cent of bone volume. In addition, new bone formed at each site is not completely mineralized, increasing the mineral deficit so that the apparent trabecular mineral density is decreased by 20 per cent.

Modelling of pagetic bone

In contrast to bone remodelling during the process of modelling, such as occurs during growth, resorption and formation occur at different skeletal surfaces and continue at the same surface without interruption. The width of long bones may increase by periosteal apposition and the medullary cavity by cortical endosteal resorption. Whereas in the adult, longitudinal growth has ceased, periosteal apposition continues throughout life so that the width of several tubular bones normally increases with age.

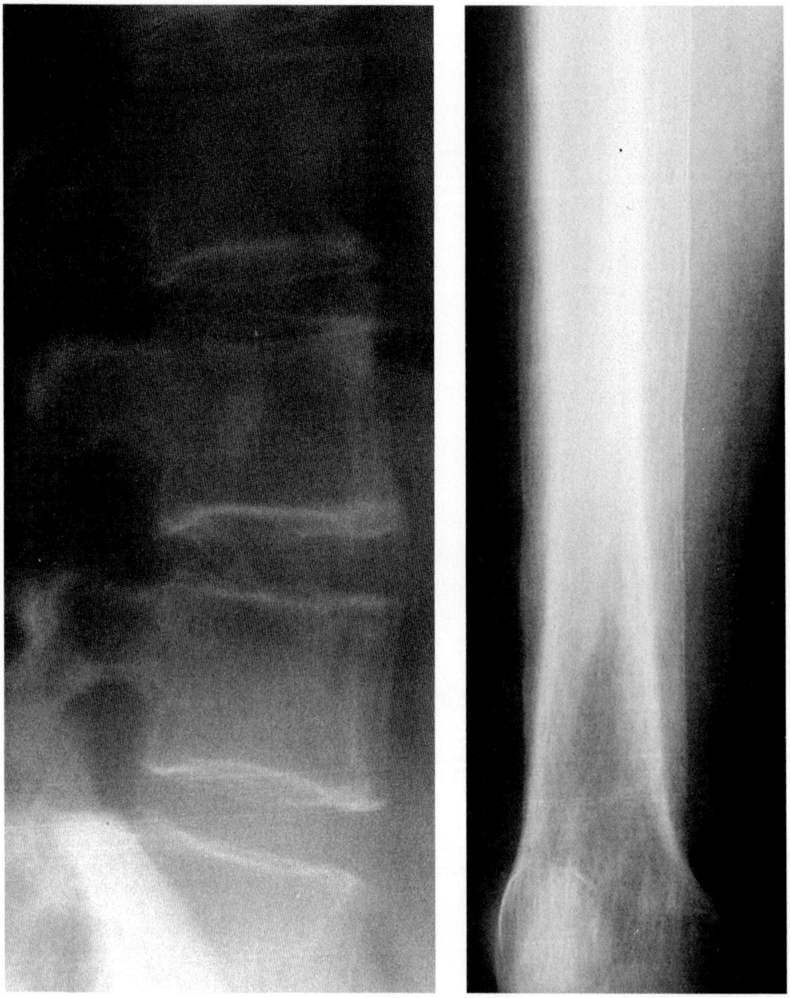

A B

Figure 2.18

'Bone within bone' appearance in two patients with Paget's disease. (A) The lateral radiograph of the lumbar spine (L1–3) shows cortical end-plates which appear to be normal and no obvious accentuation of trabecular markings. The diameters of the vertebral bodies have increased due to periosteal neostosis to give a double shadow or bone within bone appearance. (B) The radiograph of the femur shows marked neostosis and the external diameter of the shaft was 70 per cent greater than the unaffected site, representing a three-fold increase in cross-sectional area.

Paget's disease is commonly associated with bony enlargement and there are several possible mechanisms for this. The marked changes in size, shape and cortical thickness that occur suggest that modelling of bone is an important feature of the disorder. A dramatic but rare clinical example is the marked tooth migration which may occur in an affected jaw. This might imply, therefore, continued bone formation or resorption at specific periosteal or endocortical sites. The extent to which this represents uncoupling of formation and resorption is not known and it could represent extreme imbalances at resorption sites. There is some evidence for this view in that long-term treatment with inhibitors of bone resorption cause bone shape and size to decrease towards normal (Chapter 8). On the other hand, it is possible that Paget's disease amplifies the process whereby some tubular bones normally increase in diameter with age. This slow periosteal growth occurs by the apposition of lamellar bone, but in rapid growth is achieved by the formation of woven bone (Johnson, 1964). Sometimes spicules of bone are formed perpendicular to the surface and fuse to form lamellar bone. In Paget's disease, periosteal new bone formation may be very marked where the production of less dense woven bone at periosteal sites may give a 'bone within bone' appearance (Figure 2.18; see also Chapter 3).

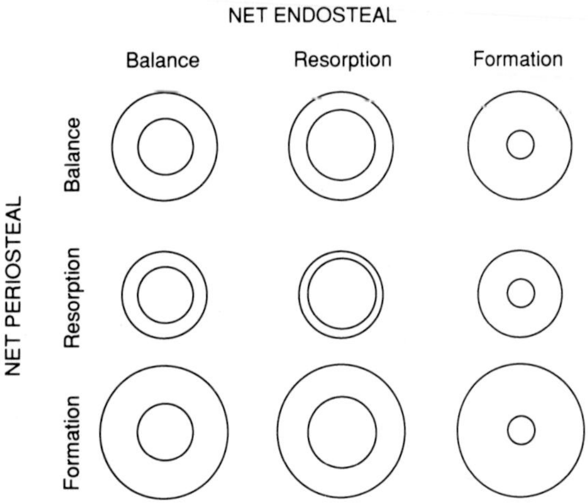

Figure 2.19

Schematic diagram to illustrate the patterns of change in cortical cross-section of a tubular bone due to changes in net endosteal and periosteal bone balance.

The majority of pagetic bones accessible to measurement show changes in cortical dimensions (73 per cent; Lander and Hadjipavlou, 1986a). Theoretically, endosteal net resorption rates can be increased, decreased or remain unchanged, as can the net rates of periosteal bone formation. This gives rise to nine possible permutations (Figure 2.19) of which several are commonly observed. The majority of bones show an increase in net periosteal formation, most frequently with an increase in cortical thickness. This is, however, usually associated with an increase in medullary width. Other common permutations are shown in Figures 2.20 and 2.21. A decrease in outer cortical diameter has been described in the forearm bones with or without a decrease in medullary width (Lander and Hadjipavlou, 1986a), but is exceedingly rare. More commonly (but still unusual), there may be a focal difference in net periosteal apposition which gives rise to a lumpy appearance (Figure 2.22). This is most commonly seen at the radius. The importance of the observation is that a decrease in outer cortical diameter is used as a criterion for radiographic improvement (Doyle et al, 1974a), but is clearly not entirely specific.

Remodelling throughout the cortex increases its porosity and blurs the distinction between cortical and trabecular bone. Osteosclerosis of trabecular elements will further contribute to this phenomenon. The relative contribution of endosteal and trabecular phenomena to bones with uniform density (for example Figures 2.23 and 2.24) is not therefore amenable to examination.

Stages of Paget's disease

Paget's disease has often been described in terms of phases or stages (Collins, 1966). The first phase is represented by abnormal destruction of bone. A second phase is represented by the formation of woven bone and a vascular marrow fibrosis.

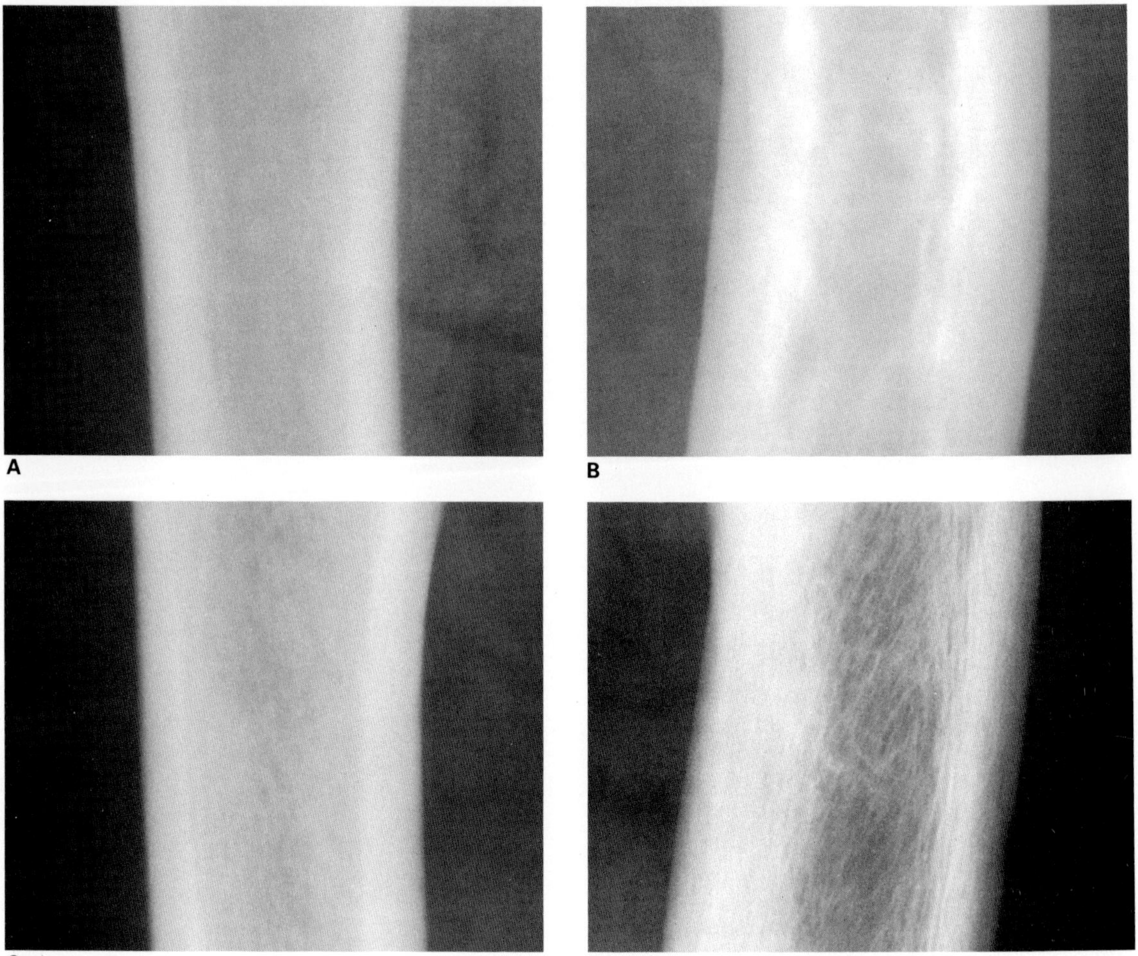

A B C D

Figure 2.20

Radiographs of the subtrochanteric region of the femur of two patients with Paget's disease. The affected side is compared with the uninvolved contralateral femur. Both show an increase in cortical width due to an increase in net periosteal apposition, the one associated with no change in medullary width (A) (B) and the other with a decrease in medullary width (C) (D).

The third phase describes established Paget's disease with waves of bone resorption and formation and a final phase of intense sclerosis where the marrow becomes less vascular and reoccupied by normal marrow elements. It seems likely that woven bone can be replaced by lamellar bone in the course of remodelling, so that late in the disorder osteosclerosis is commonly associated with a prominent mosaic appearance. An additional stage is neoplastic transformation (Chapter 5).

Similar classifications have been put forward by others in an attempt to find relationships between radiographic and histological findings (Khairi et al, 1974b; Milgram, 1977; Hamdy, 1981). With the exception of the resorption front and

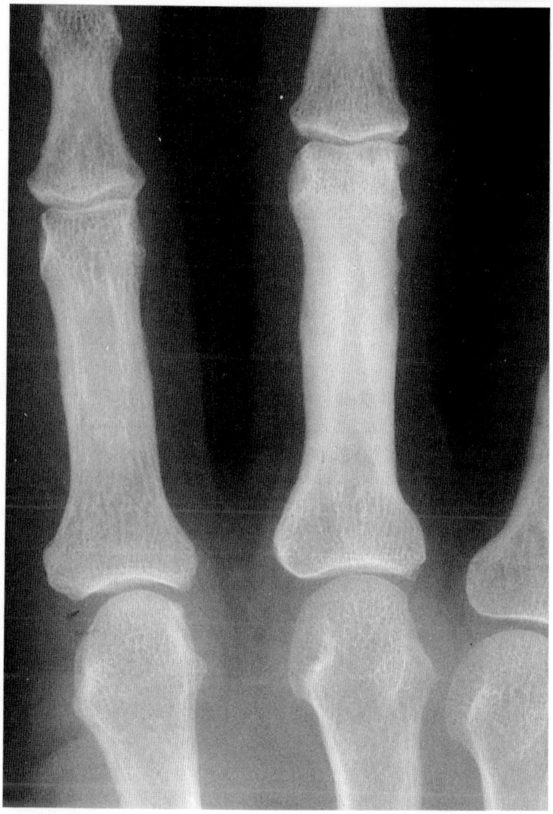

Figure 2.21

Radiograph showing Paget's disease of the proximal phalanx. The width of the phalanx is not markedly enlarged and the marked increase in cortical width is due to net endosteal apposition.

intense osteosclerosis all changes, however, coexist and are entirely explicable by the known disturbances in skeletal modelling and remodelling. Thus, the consideration of stages of Paget's disease is largely based on radiographic interpretation and may have less significance than is widely believed for the understanding of the natural history of Paget's disease.

Deformity and mechanical competence of bone

Changes in the shape of bone, its architecture, turnover and quality have obvious implications for its competence. Despite frequent increases in bone size, fracture and deformity are common. The mechanisms by which deformity arise are not known but could be related to increased plasticity of pagetic bone and the reaction to biochemical, torsional and compressive forces at various skeletal sites. It is likely that bowing deformity is due to focal changes in bone balance on periosteal and inner cortical surfaces. If so, it would seem that tension on the lateral convex surface stimulates net periosteal apposition with a variable degree of endosteal activity. Marked changes (increase or decrease) in cortical width are observed at this site. Conversely, compressive forces on the concave side appear to stimulate net periosteal resorption and endosteal apposition.

If this schema is correct, it would suggest that the responsiveness of bone remodelling and modelling to compression and tension is impaired. Nevertheless, deformity does not invariably occur and, when present, is not invariably progressive so that buttressing of cortical and trabecular bone may be appropriate and is accentuated at lines of stress (Chapter 3). The view that bones bend only because they are soft seems less plausible.

Irrespective of the mechanism, it is clear that weight-bearing forces are insufficient to account for all deformities since bones not exposed to weight bearing may be markedly deformed. The extent to which these deformities arise from normal biomechanical forces is unknown, but the characteristic nature of deformities at specific sites suggests that these forces are involved.

There seems to be a closer relationship between deformity and the length of long bones than between tubular diameter and length. Bones not subject to a bowing deformity do not generally increase in length. An example is the vertebral body in which very marked changes in width occur without an increase in length (that is height). Similarly, long bones may become markedly enlarged but in the absence of deformity retain their normal length (Figure 2.24; see also Figure 2.23). This would suggest that true longitudinal bone growth rarely if ever occurs and

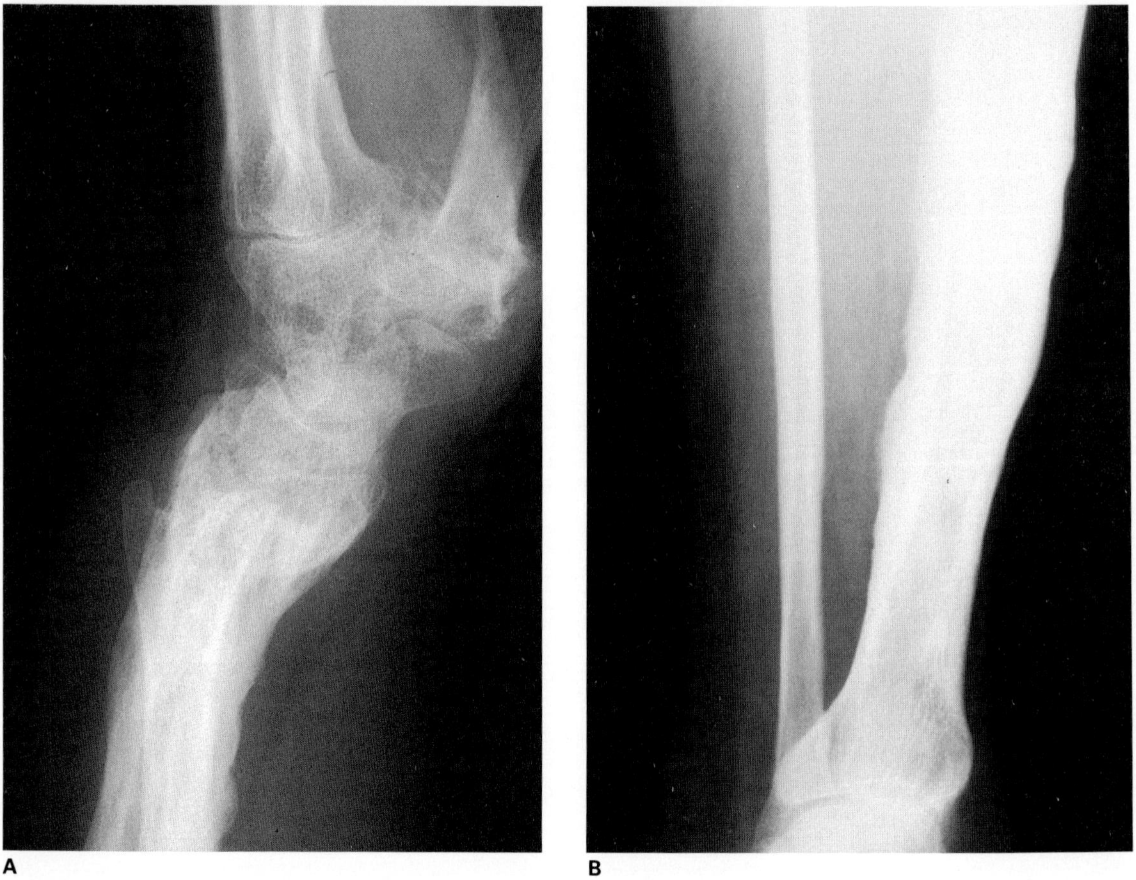

Figure 2.22

Radiograph of the wrist (A) and tibia (B). Note the lumpy appearance of the external cortex due to focal differences in the rates of net periosteal apposition.

that the increase in length is mediated by the abnormal radial diaphyseal modelling which increases the length of bone without increasing the interepiphyseal distance (Figure 2.25).

The unaffected skeleton

The junction between pagetic and normal bone is extremely well defined (Chapter 3). Preceding the resorbing bone there is an area of bone which demonstrates increased osteocytic death on microscopy (Johnson, 1964), suggestive of premature senescence in pre-pagetic bone. The extent to which this is a feature of Paget's disease or an accentuation of osteocytic changes during normal resorption is unknown.

Histological evidence for increased turnover has commonly been observed at biopsy sites distant from pagetic lesions (Meunier et al, 1980). Our own experience suggests that this is more

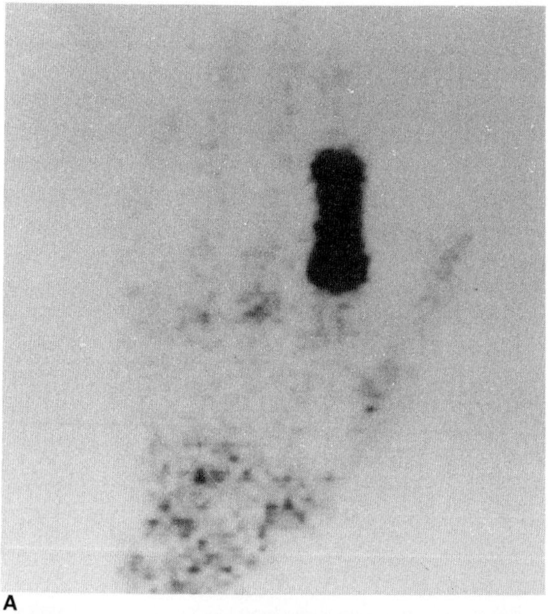

A

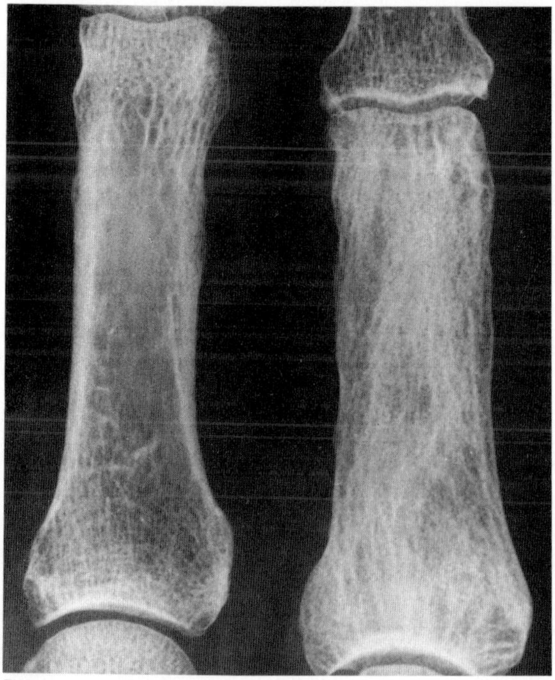

B

Figure 2.23

Scintigraph (A) and radiograph (B) of the proximal phalanges. Note the marked homogeneous scintigraphic fixation of the whole phalanx without affecting surrounding bones. The X-rays show skeletal enlargement, loss of differentiation between cortical and trabecular bone due to intracortical resorption, but normal length.

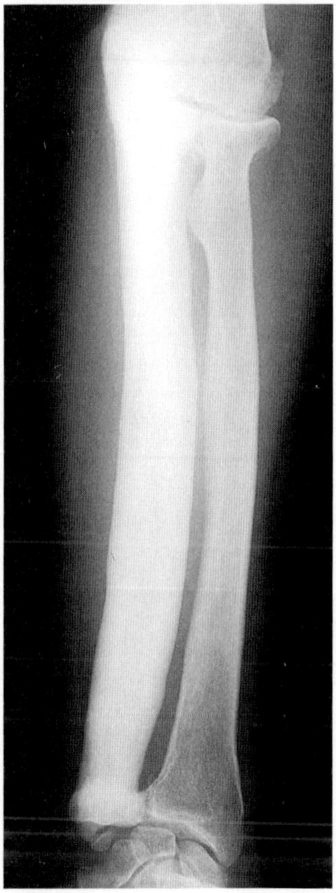

Figure 2.24

Radiograph showing dense osteosclerosis of the ulna. Note the marked increase in ulnar width but the normal ulnar length in the absence of a bowing deformity.

marked when bone disease is more extensive. A number of studies have now documented increased circulating concentrations of PTH in Paget's disease, and in our own studies this was confined to patients with extensive disease activity (Chapter 4). Studies by Meunier suggest that this is a consequence of focal imbalances between bone formation and bone resorption. An imbalance in favour of net bone formation would decrease the net efflux of calcium from bone, and thereby decrease serum calcium concentrations

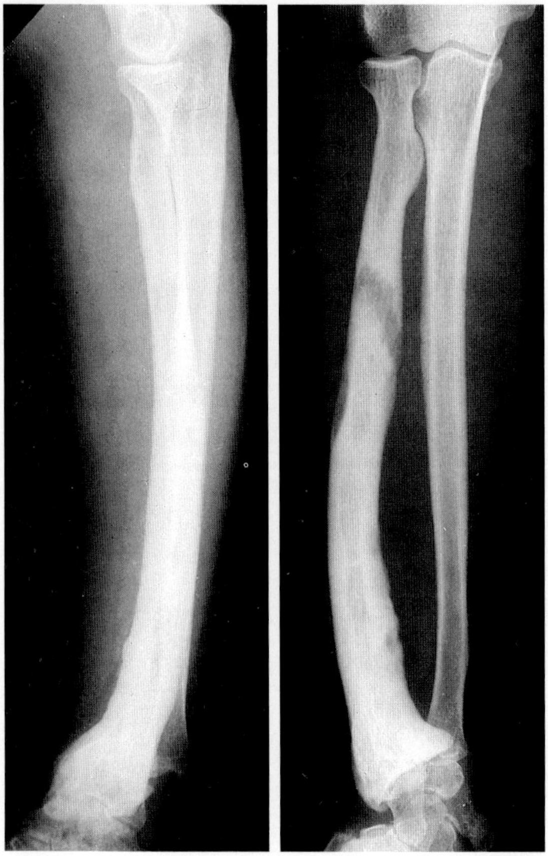

and increase the secretion of PTH. Since PTH activates bone remodelling, this would provide a plausible mechanism for the increased bone remodelling found at non-pagetic sites. It is not known whether this is associated with significant loss of normal bone, but if so, might increase the risk of fracture at non-pagetic sites.

Figure 2.25

Marked pagetic deformity of the radius. Compare with Figure 2.24. Note also the medullary stenosis and the 'osteolytic' resorption front.

CHAPTER 3

Radiological features

Introduction

Conventional radiography and scintigraphy are important tools in the diagnosis and evaluation of Paget's disease. These techniques can also be used to assess response to treatment, but radiographic changes in particular require careful and cautious interpretation (Chapter 8). They have also been helpful as epidemiological tools in assessing the distribution of the disease. As reviewed in Chapter 1, most of our knowledge of the geographic distribution of Paget's disease is dependent on the finding that the lumbar spine, pelvis and femoral heads are affected in the majority of patients. In this chapter the focal distribution of the disorder is reviewed together with the major radiological features.

Skeletal distribution of the disorder

The skeletal distribution of Paget's disease has been investigated principally by radiographic techniques, but early surveys were generally limited to parts of the skeleton (Gutman and Kasabach, 1936; Newman, 1946; Rosenkrantz et al, 1952; Barry, 1969; Guyer, 1981). Some of the early surveys were also based on post-mortem findings. Irrespective of the manner of investigation, the extent of disease involvement is markedly heterogeneous. It may involve only one bone at any site and it is described even in the sesamoids. More frequently, multiple sites are involved, typically in an asymmetric distribution. The most common sites for involvement are the pelvis, lumbar spine and femur (Dickson et al, 1945; Guyer, 1981) and one or more of these sites are involved in more than 75 per cent of cases irrespective of the sampling methods or the manner of diagnosis (Table 3.1).

The extent of skeletal involvement can be quantitated from radiographs or more readily from bone scans. The proportion of each bone affected is calculated and multiplied by the skeletal volume or weight at that site (Table 3.2). In addition, the number of sites can be documented. Not surprisingly, there is a wide variation in the number of lesions (1 to 45 in our series) and in the extent of skeletal involvement (1 to 80 per cent). The average patient has six lesions affecting 14 per cent of the skeleton (Figure 3.1). As might be expected, there is a close relationship between the anatomical spread of the disorder and the number of affected sites (Figure 3.2). For each additional site affected there is approximately a further one and a half per cent increase in the extent of the disease.

Not surprisingly, there are differences in the apparent distribution of the disorder dependent on the techniques used. For example, the pattern of distribution at post mortem (Table 3.3; Schmorl, 1932; Collins, 1956) does not conform

Table 3.1 Distribution of Paget's disease showing the proportion of patients (percentage of 170 patients) with pagetic lesions at the sites indicated. The patients were assessed concurrently by the two techniques. (From Salson, 1981.)

Site	*Scintigraphy*	*Radiography*	*Ratio*
Pelvis	72.3	68.2	1.06
Lumbar vertebrae	58.2	48.8	1.08
Femora	55.3	54.7	1.01
Thoracic vertebrae	44.7	37.1	1.20
Sacrum	43.5	40.6	1.07
Skull	41.7	44.1	0.94
Tibiae	34.7	30.6	1.13
Humeri	31.2	28.8	1.08
Scapulae	23.5	19.4	1.21
Cervical vertebrae	14.1	12.9	1.09
Ribs	11.7	0	
Sternum	11.1	0	
Clavicles	11.1	9.4	1.18
Facial bones	11.1	8.2	1.35
Os calces	10.0	6.4	1.56
Patellae	7.0	3.5	2.00
Hand bones	6.4	5.2	1.23
Foot bones (excluding talus and os calcis)	5.1	3.5	1.46
Tali	4.7	4.1	1.14
Radii	3.5	4.1	0.85
Fibulae	2.3	1.1	2.09
Total number of foci	863	727	

Table 3.2 Scoring methods for calculating the extent of disease involvement on radiographs and bone scans.

Site	*Coutris et al (1975)*		*Howarth (1953)*	
	Each	*Total*	*Each*	*Total*
Skull and face	12	12	11	11
Pelvis	5	10	5	10
Femur	5	10	8	16
Lumbar spine	1	5	–	–
Dorsal spine	1	12	–	–
Cervical spine	1	7	–	–
Whole spine	–	–	–	11
Sacrum	5	5	3	3
Tibia	4	8	5	10
Scapula	0.5	1	1.5	3
Humerus	3	6	3.5	7
Sternum	1	1	1	1
Ribs	0.25	6	–	9
Foot	1	2	4	8
Clavicle	0.5	1	0.5	1
Radius	2	4	1	2
Ulna	2	4	1	2
Hand	1	2	1.5	3
Patella	–	–	0.5	1
Fibula	2	4	1	2

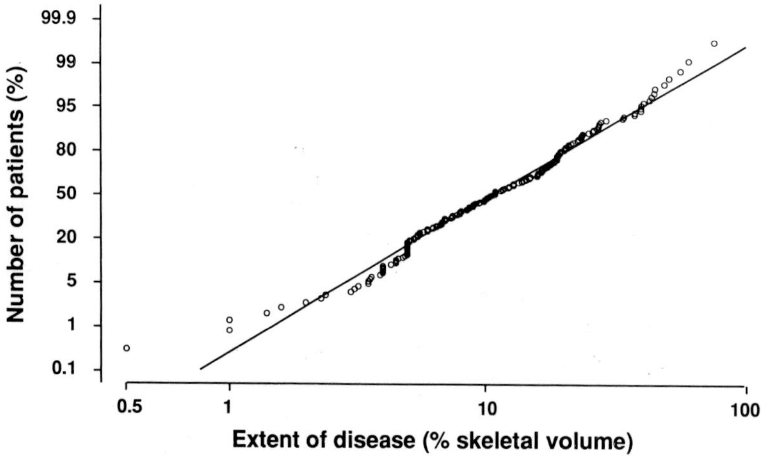

Figure 3.1

Distribution of the extent of disease in 197 untreated patients shown on a probability scale. The extent of disease, assessed as the per cent skeletal involvement, conforms to a single log-normal distribution. The median extent of disease was 14 per cent of the skeleton and 95 per cent of patients had less than 40 per cent affected.

Table 3.3 Distribution of Paget's disease based on a large necropsy series (Schmorl, 1932).

Site	*% patients*
Sacrum	56
Spine	50
Femur	46
Skull	28
Sternum	23
Pelvis	22
Clavicle	13
Ribs	7
Scapula	0

closely with that obtained either by scintigraphy or radiography, although there is a general measure of agreement. These differences may reflect population biases as well as differences in the sensitivity of each technique to detect pagetic lesions at different sites.

Radiography and scintigraphy are by no means mutually exclusive. Radiography is the principal technique utilized to give information concerning the distribution and extent of disease involvement. In addition, it gives information on the focal abnormalities of skeletal architecture not provided by scintigraphic or biochemical investigation. On the other hand, scanning agents such as ^{99m}Tc-labelled polyphosphonates or diphosphonates (Fogelman and Carr, 1980; Fogelman et al, 1981a) may reveal areas apparently normal on conventional radiographs. They also have the advantage of imaging the whole skeleton, which is not often completely achieved during radiographic skeletal surveys.

In large surveys of patients there is a close relationship between the scintigraphic and radiographic distribution (Salson, 1981; Meunier et al, 1987; Table 3.1). As a general rule, scintigraphy is more sensitive than radiography, and in one large survey 8 per cent of lesions considered to be pagetic were not picked up by radiography (Salson, 1981). In various series, radiography has underestimated the number of pagetic sites by 5–30 per cent (Khairi et al, 1974b; Wellman et al, 1977; Fogelman and Carr, 1980; Vellenga et al, 1984b; Meunier et al, 1987). On the other hand, it should not be assumed that scintigraphy is always more sensitive than radiography and well documented sites are described showing classical radiographic features in which no hyperfixation of scanning agents is found (Figure 3.3; see also Figure 3.67). In the survey shown in Table 3.1 this occurred in 2–3 per cent of pagetic lesions.

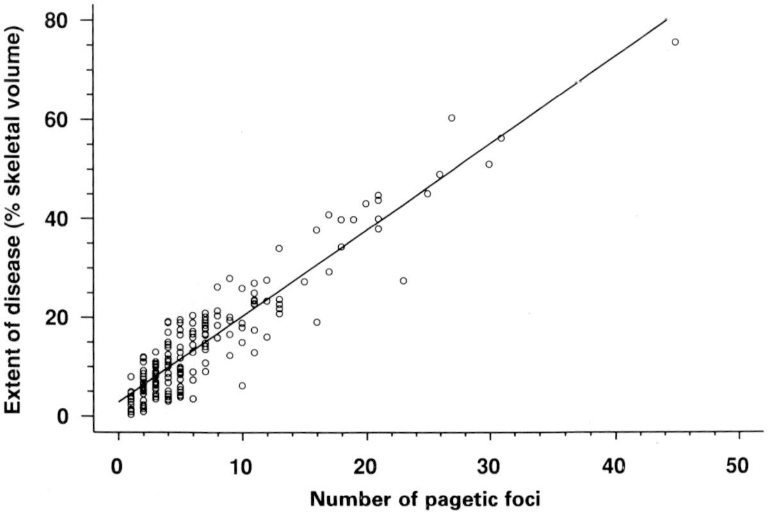

Figure 3.2

Relationship between the extent of disease and the numbers of skeletal lesions assessed by scintigraphy in 197 patients ($r = +0.83$ on log-transformed data).

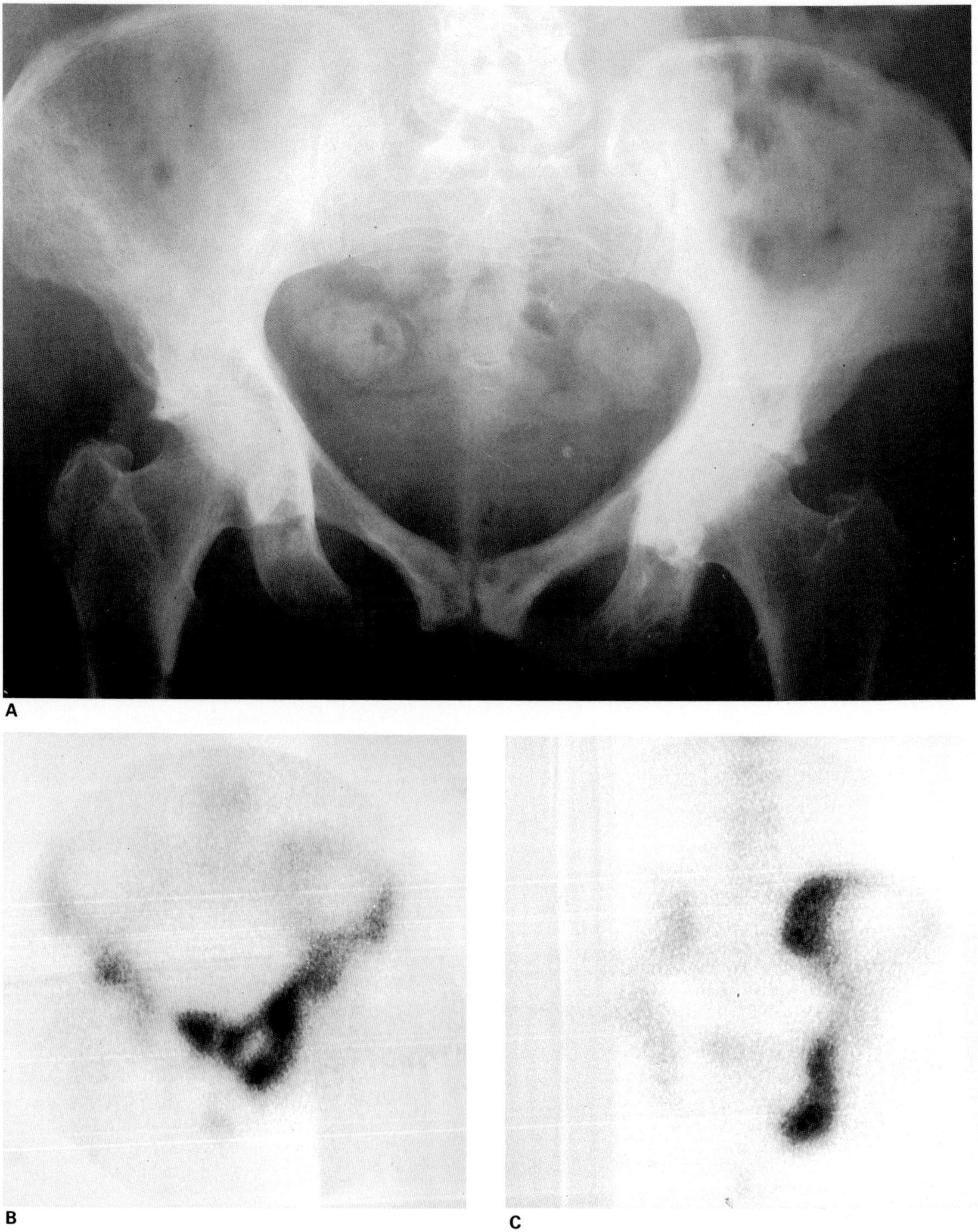

Figure 3.3

Pelvic radiograph (A) and anterior (B) and posterior (C) bone scan in an untreated patient with Paget's disease. Note the bilateral pelvic disease on radiography but lack of scintigraphic uptake on the left.

Some authors have found no differences in radiographic appearance between scan-positive and scan-negative lesions (Vellenga et al, 1984b). Others have found scan-negative lesions either in association with osteoporosis circumscripta or more usually with marked osteosclerosis (Fogelman et al,. 1981; Guyer, 1981; Lander and Hadjipavlou, 1986a). Biopsies from such sites have shown sclerotic bone with little evidence for bone-cell activity and the absence of scintigraphic uptake is not therefore surprising (Lander and Hadjipavlou, 1986a). This phenomenon accounts only in part for the discrepancies between scintigraphic and radiographic distribution. The major reason for the discrepancy is that scanning is particularly sensitive in the detection of Paget's disease in the ribs and sternum, sites which are difficult to detect by conventional radiographic techniques (Figure 3.4). A similar, though less marked sensitivity of scintigraphy over radiography is shown for the patella, os calcis and scapula and for the facial bones (Figure 3.1). These discrepancies between the techniques are reduced when radiographic technique and views are optimized, and findings interpreted in the presence of the bone scan.

There are also some differences in the apparent distribution if one uses the same techniques in different populations. For example, in scintigraphic surveys of hospital populations (generally for neoplastic disease and therefore detecting asymptomatic Paget's disease) the frequency of involvement of sites other than the pelvis is lower than that found in symptomatic patients (Khairi et al, 1974b; Fogelman and Carr, 1980; Meunier et al, 1987). It is not known whether the distribution of disease differs in different countries, but this may well be so. If true, this might variously over- or underestimate the relative prevalence of Paget's disease in geographical surveys (Chapter 1) since these have relied on limited skeletal surveys.

The distribution of the disease may differ in patients with a strong family history of the disorder. In our family of 40 patients (expansile osteolysis), the disorder spares the axial skeleton almost completely (Table 3.4), in marked contrast to the distribution otherwise expected. Patients

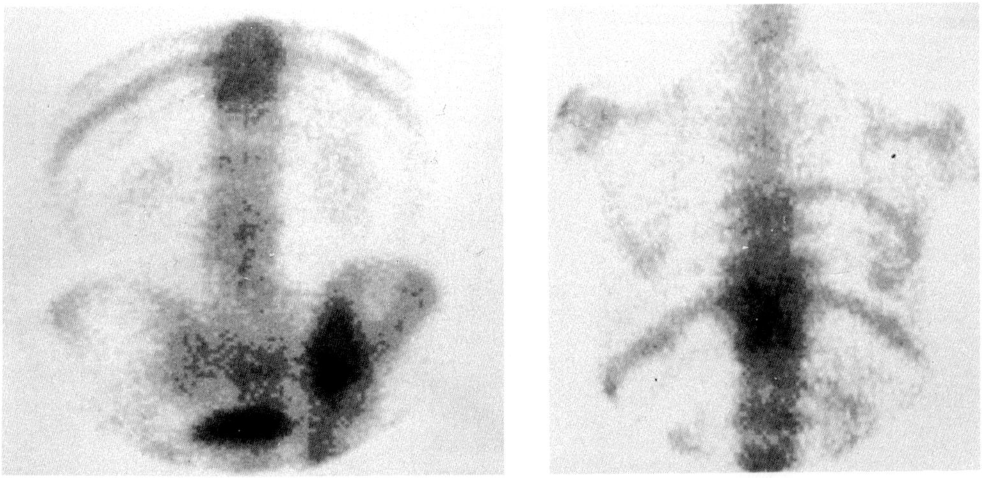

Figure 3.4

Bone scan appearances in a patient with widespread Paget's disease. The obvious rib involvement was not visible on radiographs

Table 3.4 Distribution of lesions in patients with familial expansile osteolysis compared with other patients with classical Paget's disease. Note the predilection of expansile osteolysis for appendicular sites.

Site	*Expansile osteolysis (n = 40)*		*Paget's disease (n = 197)*		*A/B*
	No of lesions	*% of lesions (A)*	*No of lesions*	*% of lesions (B)*	
Axial skeleton					
Pelvis and sacrum	0	0	263	20.6	0
Lumbar spine	1	1.0	226	17.7	0.06
Dorsal spine	0	0	232	18.1	0
Skull and face	0	0	83	6.5	0
Scapulae	2	2.1	48	3.8	0.55
Appendicular skeleton					
Femora and patellae	10	10.4	143	11.2	0.93
Tibiae	31	32.3	53	4.1	7.88
Humeri	9	9.3	41	3.2	2.91
Foot	12	12.5	39	3.1	4.03
Hand and wrist	7	7.3	6	0.5	14.6
Radii and ulnae	14	15.6	16	1.3	12.0
Fibulae	10	10.4	6	0.5	20.8

with a less florid family history have more extensive disease than otherwise, but this is largely due to a difference in the number of lesions rather than their extent (Table 1.3). The distribution of lesions is similar to patients with no family history (Table 3.5), except that there is a modest predilection for axial sites of involvement ($p<0.05$) and, in the appendicular skeleton, lesions are more frequently seen in the upper limbs ($p<0.05$).

Sex differences and distribution

There is little difference between sexes in the activity or the extent of disease in symptomatic patients (Table 3.6). There are, however, some interesting sex differences reported in the skeletal distribution of Paget's disease, when assessed by radiography or scintigraphy (Guyer, 1981; Salson, 1981; Harinck et al, 1986). In pagetic patients, sites reported to be more commonly affected by males include the ilium, sacrum, thoracic spine and scapula (Table 3.7). In our own patients, we have not found any sex difference in the frequency with which these sites are affected (Table 3.8). Other sites reported to occur with increased frequency in males include the lumbar spine, cervical spine, sternum ribs, clavicles, calcaneum and patella, but larger surveys would be required to prove this. In our own patients we find that the sternum and ribs are more frequently involved in men than women. In contrast, Paget's disease appears to occur less frequently in males in the face, skull (Table 3.8) and in one series also in the tibiae (Harinck et al, 1986). Since these are sites where deformity is frequently noted, and women have a higher social disadvantage by such deformities, it is possible that this represents in part a bias in presentation.

In terms of skeletal involvement, one series has shown that, at presentation, men have a greater proportion of their skeleton involved (approximately 20 per cent), than women (15 per cent) (Salson, 1981). Similarly, the number of skeletal foci is greater in men than in women. Others have found the reverse (6.5 vs 4.8 in the series of Harinck et al, 1986) whereas we find no difference (Table 3.6).

Table 3.5 Scintigraphic distribution of lesions in patients with or without a known family history of Paget's disease.

Site	Family history (n = 27)		No family history (n = 170)		A/B
	No of lesions	% of lesions (A)	No of lesions	% of lesions (B)	
Pelvis	36	12.1	172	17.4	0.70*
Lumbar spine	56	18.9	170	17.2	1.10
Femora	26	8.8	102	10.3	0.85
Thoracic spine	62	20.9	170	17.2	1.21
Skull	17	5.8	66	6.7	0.87
Sacrum	12	4.0	43	4.4	0.91
Tibiae	11	3.7	42	4.3	0.86
Scapulae	14	4.7	34	3.4	1.38
Humeri	12	4.0	29	2.9	1.38
Cervical spine	16	5.4	29	2.9	1.86
Sternum	5	1.7	22	2.2	0.77
Ribs	12	4.0	33	3.3	1.21
Os calces	4	1.3	15	1.5	0.87
Feet (excluding os calcis)	2	0.7	18	1.8	0.39
Elsewhere	12	4.0	45	4.5	0.89

*Significantly lower frequency ($p < 0.05$) in patients with a positive family history.

Table 3.6 Disease activity and extent assessed by biochemical and scintigraphic measurements according to sex. Values are the mean ± SEM (computed from log-transformed values in the case of alkaline phosphate and hydroxyproline). The higher apparent hydroxyproline excretion in women is due to the lower urinary creatinine concentrations.

	Men	Women	p
Number of patients	79	118	—
Total number of sites	526	762	—
Alkaline phosphatase (IU/l)	324 (295–355)	295 (275–316)	NS
Hydroxyproline (mmol/mol creatinine)	58.9 (53.7–64.6)	75.9 (70.8–81.3)	<0.05
Mean number of sites	6.65 ± 0.66	6.46 ± 0.64	NS
Percentage of skeleton affected	14.4 ± 1.3	14.2 ± 1.2	NS
Scintigraphic index	46.3 ± 4.2	46.8 ± 4.2	NS

NS: not significant.

Monostotic Paget's disease

Paget's disease most commonly affects several sites. However, in approximately 10–20 per cent of symptomatic patients the combination of scintigraphic and radiographic investigation reveals the presence of only one affected site. Estimates vary from 5 to 40 per cent of patients presenting to medical attention (Suchett-Kaye, 1970; Rauis, 1974; Shirazi et al, 1974; Salson, 1981; Merrick and Merrick, 1985; Harinck et al, 1986). In one

Table 3.7 Number and proportion of patients with positive scintigraphic findings at the sites shown (from Salson, 1981).

Site	Men		Women		p<
	No	%	No	%	
Pelvis	74	80	49	64	0.05
Sacrum	49	53	25	32	0.01
Thoracic spine	53	57	23	30	0.001
Scapula	29	31	11	14	0.01

Table 3.8 Scintigraphic distribution of Paget's disease in men and women.

Site	*Men*				*Women*			
	Patients (n = 79)		*Lesions (n = 525)*		*Patients (n = 118)*		*Lesions (n = 762)*	
	No	*%*	*No*	*%*	*No*	*%*	*No*	*%*
Pelvis	55	69.6	85	16.2	84	71.2	123	16.1
Femora	44	55.7	58	11.0	53	44.9	70	9.2
Lumbar spine	41	51.9	86	16.4	60	50.8	140	18.5
Dorsal spine	37	46.8	88	16.8	47	39.8	144	18.9
Sacrum	25	31.6	25	4.8	30	25.4	30	3.9
Skull	23	29.1*	23	4.4	52	44.1	52	6.8
Tibiae	23	29.1	23	4.4	27	22.9	30	3.9
Scapulae	17	21.5	19	3.6	21	17.8	29	3.8
Sternum	17	21.5†	17	3.2†	10	8.5	10	1.3
Cervical spine	14	17.7	20	3.8	18	15.2	25	3.3
Humeri	11	13.9	13	2.5	22	18.6	28	3.7
Ribs	9	11.4	26	5.0†	12	10.2	19	2.5
Os calces	9	11.4	9	1.7	8	6.8	10	1.3
Radii	6	7.6	8	1.5	2	1.7	3	0.4
Feet	5	6.3	6	1.1	10	8.5	14	1.8
Patellae	4	5.1	6	1.1	8	6.8	9	1.2
Clavicles	4	5.1	5	0.9	6	5.1	9	1.2
Face	2	2.5	2	0.4	6	5.1	6	0.8
Fibulae	2	2.5	2	0.4	4	3.4	4	0.5
Hands	2	2.5	2	0.4	4	3.4	4	0.5
Ulnae	2	2.5	2	0.4	3	2.5	3	0.4

*Significantly lower prevalence in men ($p<0.05$).
†Significantly higher prevalence in men ($p<0.05$).

centre, the frequency with which monostotic disease is detected has increased from 24 to 33 per cent over two years (Vellenga et al, 1984b; Harinck et al, 1986). Where surveys have been taken for reasons not related to Paget's disease the prevalence of monostotic disease is more frequent (Merrick and Merrick, 1985). These observations suggest that the prevalence of monostotic disease could be appreciably higher in the general community than in the referral population.

The most common sites for monostotic disease are the ilium, tibia and femur (Table 3.9). The frequency with which the tibia is affected by monostotic disease is 5-fold greater than that expected from the usual distribution of pagetic lesions in polyostotic disease. In contrast, there is a significantly lower incidence of vertebral lesions than expected (Table 3.9). It seems probable that these differences in apparent distribution are due to the greater likelihood of tibial lesions giving rise to symptoms than a single lesion at the spine. It is of interest that monostotic Paget's disease occurs twice as often in women than in men.

For these reasons, it is probably misleading to consider monostotic disease as a separate entity. In addition, the frequency distribution of the number of pagetic lesions is unimodal and log-normal (Figure 3.5; Vellenga et al, 1984b), in keeping with the distribution of alkaline phosphatase and hydroxyproline (Chapter 4). This suggests that the patients with Paget's disease comprise a single population so far as the number of pagetic foci is concerned.

Table 3.9 Frequency and sites of monostotic Paget's disease from two series, at Sheffield (unpublished) and at Lyon (Salson, 1981). The last column shows the distribution expected from the frequency of involvement of the sites in polyostotic disease.

Site	*Sheffield (n = 197)*		*Lyon (n = 170)*		*Combined (n = 367)*			
	No of patients	*% Total*	*No of patients*	*% Total*	*No of patients*	*% Total*	*% Monostotic lesions*	*Expected distribution*
Pelvis	11	5.6	8	4.7	19	5.2	37	16
Femur	4	2.0	6	3.5	10	2.7	19	10
Tibia	3	1.5	8	4.7	11	3.0	21	4
Skull	3	1.5	5	2.9	8	2.2	15	6
Vertebra	1	0.5	1	0.6	2	0.5	4	39
Patella	1	0.5	0	0.0	1	0.3	2	3
Humerus	0	0.0	1	0.6	1	0.3	2	1
Men	6	7.6	12	12.9	18	10.5		
Women	17	14.4	17	22.1	34	17.4		
Both	23	11.7	29	17.1	52	14.2		

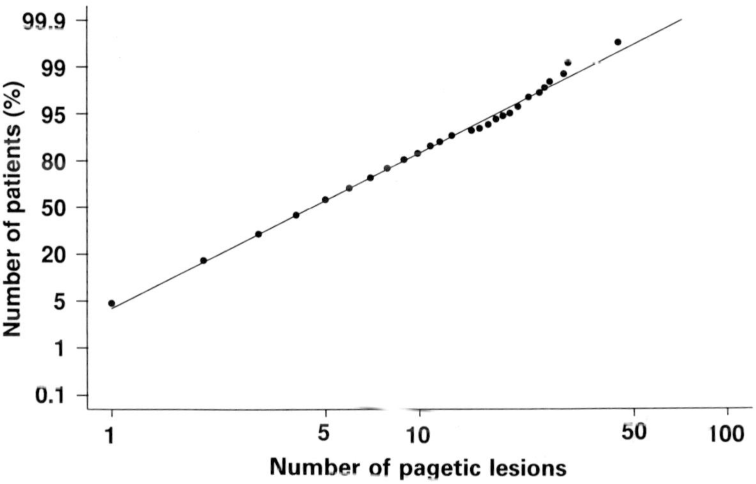

Figure 3.5

Cumulative frequency distribution of the number of pagetic lesions found in a series of 197 patients. The number of skeletal lesions is shown on a logarithmic scale and the number of patients on a probability scale.

Radiographic features

The radiographic features of Paget's disease are very distinctive but the disorder produces a large number of different appearances (Steinbach, 1961; Wilner and Sherman, 1966; Barry, 1969; Greenfield, 1980). Various radiographic stages of Paget's disease have been proposed (Khairi et al, 1974b), but most frequently mixed lesions of osteosclerosis and osteolysis are observed.

In keeping with the histopathological features described in Chapter 2, the early phase is of osteolytic activity, sometimes seen clearly in the skull as osteoporosis circumscripta or as a v-shaped advancing front in a long bone. A second 'combined' phase shows evidence of patchy osteolysis and sclerosis. This second phase is the most common radiographic finding. A later and third phase is that of predominant bone sclerosis. The gross appearances of affected bones may vary enormously. Changes may be striking, with thickening of the cortices and enlargement of the long bones, not only in width but also in length.

The most sinister radiographic feature is the appearance of sarcoma, which is reviewed in Chapter 5.

Although the earliest radiographic features are said to be osteoporosis circumscripta, there is some evidence that an earlier stage might be an increase in trabecular markings. We have described such lesions, positive on scintigraphy, in familial Paget's disease at the tibia (Osterberg et al, 1988), a site of predilection for later florid disease.

The common radiographic features include bony enlargement, cortical thickening, intracortical resorption with a loss of corticomedullary junction and accentuation of trabecular markings. None of these features is specific to Paget's disease, but the combination is virtually diagnostic. The combination of these several features is of importance in the differential diagnosis of osteosclerotic and osteolytic lesions (Chapter 6) and in assessment of the likelihood of mixed pathology (such as carcinoma of the prostate and Paget's disease).

The relative contribution of features may differ somewhat at different skeletal sites. In addition, the clinical complications of deformity and enlargement are site-dependent, and for this reason the sites are reviewed separately. There is not, however, a close relationship between radiographic appearances and bone pain attributable to pagetic lesions, except that more extensive disease is more likely to give rise to symptoms (Harinck et al, 1986). It has been said that sclerotic disease is more likely to be asymptomatic, but this is not the general view (Khairi et al, 1974b).

Pelvic girdle

The pelvis is the most common site affected (Table 3.10), and evidence for involvement is found in approximately two-thirds of patients. There is some evidence, which was reviewed in Chapter 1, that pelvic involvement is decreasing in frequency. The ischium, ilium and pubis are affected with equal frequency in large surveys (Dickson et al, 1945; Landler and Hadjipavlou, 1986a). The disorder is said to have a predilection for the right side in men but not in women (Salson, 1981), but we find no significant difference between sides and sex at the pelvis or elsewhere (Table 3.11).

Sclerosis is a common feature and the classical resorption front does occur but is rarely observed (Figure 3.6). More frequently, apparent radiographic osteolysis of the wing of the ilium is observed, largely due to surrounding areas of osteosclerosis at the iliac crest (Figure 3.7). An early radiographic manifestation is thickening and sclerosis of the iliopectineal line (Figure 3.8). This has been termed the rim or brim sign, but is not entirely specific for Paget's disease.

The extent of pelvic involvement varies. When the disorder affects an entire hemipelvis, the enlargement of the pubis and ischium and cortical thickening provide a sharp contrast with the unaffected side (Figure 3.9). In some patients

Table 3.10 Scintigraphic distribution of lesions in Paget's disease.

Site	*Patients (n = 197)*		*Lesions (n = 1287)*		*Lesions/ patient*
	No	*%*	*No*	*%*	
Pelvis	139	70.6	208	16.1	1.5
Lumbar spine	101	51.3	226	17.5	2.2
Femora	97	49.2	128	9.9	1.3
Dorsal spine	84	42.6	232	18.0	2.8
Skull	75	38.1	75	5.9	1.0
Sacrum	55	27.9	55	4.3	1.0
Tibiae	50	25.4	53	4.1	1.1
Scapulae	38	19.3	48	3.7	1.3
Humeri	33	17.0	41	3.2	1.2
Cervical spine	32	16.2	45	3.5	1.4
Sternum	27	13.7	27	2.1	1.0
Ribs	21	10.6	45	3.5	2.1
Os calces	17	8.6	19	1.5	1.1
Feet	15	7.6	20	1.6	1.3
Patellae	12	6.2	15	1.2	1.3
Clavicles	10	5.1	14	1.1	1.4
Face	8	4.1	8	0.6	1.0
Radii	8	4.1	11	0.8	1.4
Fibulae	6	3.0	6	0.5	1.0
Hands	6	3.0	6	0.5	1.0
Ulnae	5	2.5	5	0.4	1.0

focal lesions may resemble osteitis condensans ilii or sclerosing osteomyelitis (Burgener and Perry, 1978).

Pelvic deformity can be marked (Figure 3.10). Abnormalities include minor or major degrees of protrusio acetabuli. Protrusio is difficult to quantitate due to the distortion of anatomical landmarks, bilateral disease, the obliteration of reference points (such as the tear drop of the acetabulum; Figure 3.8) and a variable increase in the width of the acetabular wall. Medial enlargement of the acetabular wall may cause convexities of the pelvic brim and give a false impression of protrusio (Figure 3.11). Not surprisingly, uniform narrowing of the joint space with medial migration of the femoral head is common. This may or may not be associated with degenerative arthritis.

Whereas narrowing of the joint space at the hips is common (Graham and Harris, 1971; Goldman et al, 1977), the radiographic appearances differ somewhat from degenerative joint disease. Most patients show medial or concentric

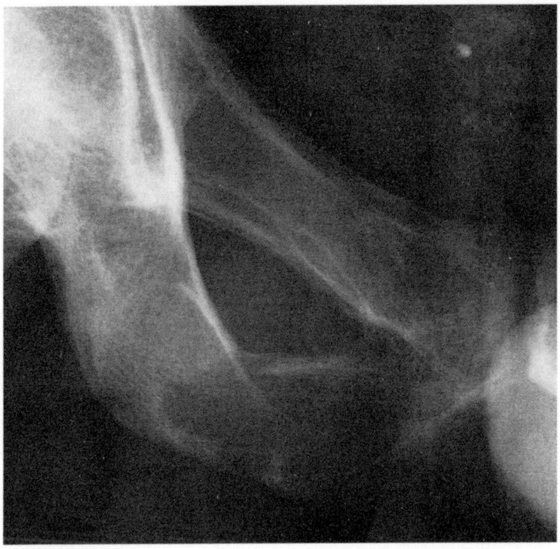

Figure 3.6

Radiograph of the pubis and ischium. Note the presence of a resorption front.

Table 3.11 Pattern of distribution of Paget's disease according to sex and site of involvement. The sites are chosen for presentation since smaller series have suggested a predilection for one side in all patients or patients of either sex. In this series there is no predilection for laterality in men, women or both.

Site	*Sex*	*Right only*	*Left only*	*Both*
Pelvis	Male	7	18	30
	Female	21	24	39
	M + F	28	42	69
Ilium	Male	7	17	30
	Female	21	24	37
	M + F	28	41	67
Femur	Male	14	16	14
	Female	15	21	17
	M + F	29	37	31
Tibia	Male	9	10	2
	Female	9	11	5
	M + F	18	21	7
Humerus	Male	4	5	2
	Female	9	7	6
	M + F	13	12	8

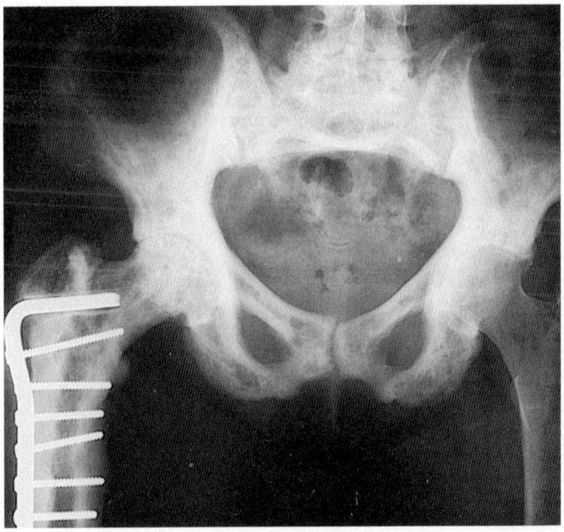

Figure 3.7

Radiograph of pelvis affected by Paget's disease. Note the apparent osteolysis of the iliac wing due to the surrounding osteosclerosis.

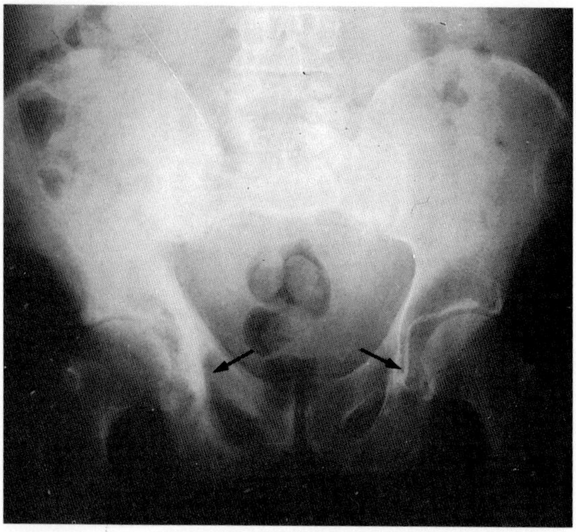

Figure 3.8

Cortical thickening of the pelvic brim due to Paget's disease of the right hemipelvis. Note the sclerosis of the iliopectineal line and obliteration of the 'tear drop' (arrows). The normal contralateral hip is shown for comparison.

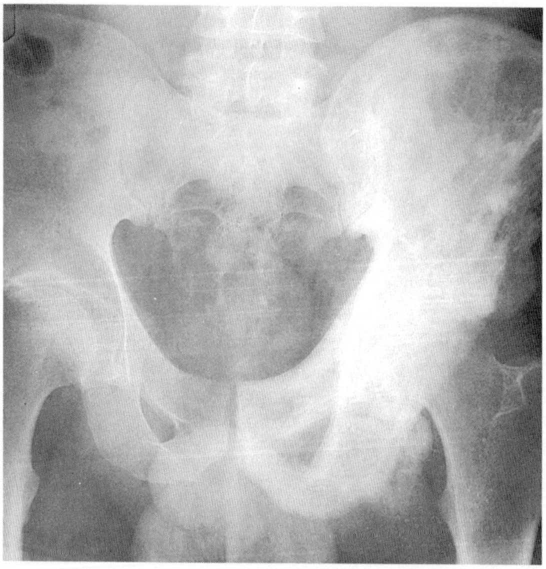

Figure 3.9

Radiograph of the pelvis. The affected hemipelvis is distinctive by the marked enlargement of the ilium and ischium. Note also the concentric narrowing of the left hip joint space.

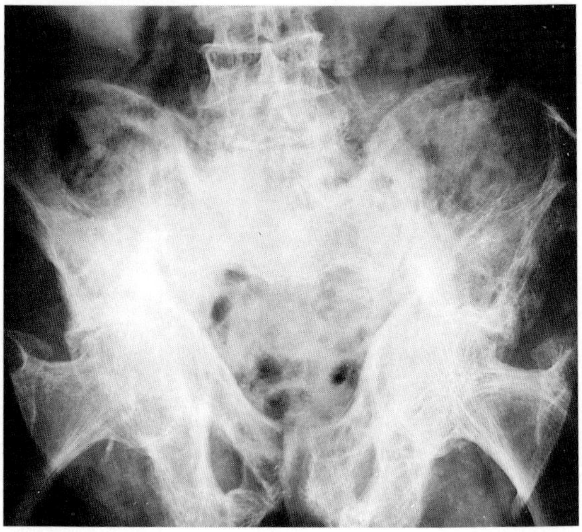

Figure 3.10

Radiograph of the pelvis showing a triradiate deformity.

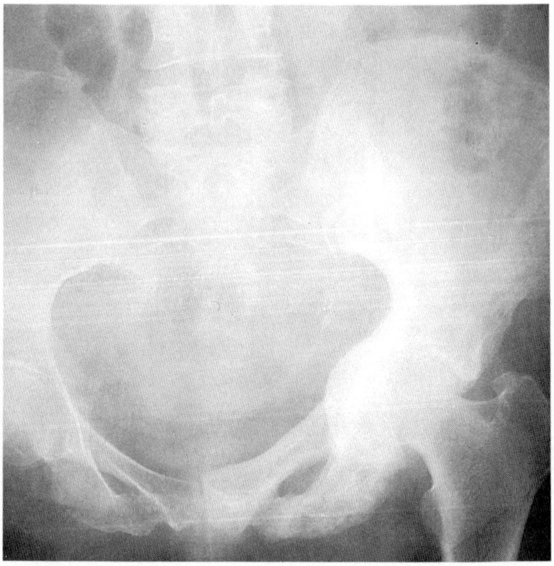

Figure 3.11

Radiograph of pelvis. The increase in the width of the acetabular wall gives a misleading impression of protrusio.

Principal radiographic features of Paget's disease affecting the hip.

Hypertrophy of medial acetabular wall
Hypertrophy of acetabular margins
Protrusia acetabuli
Concentric or medial narrowing of hip joint space
Coxa vara
Coxa plane and ovalization of femoral head
Osteoarthrosis

narrowing of the joint space. In contrast, osteoarthritis more frequently causes narrowing of the superior aspect (Roper, 1971b; Figures 3.12 and 3.13). In addition, osteophytosis is not a prominent feature (Graham and Harris, 1971) which has led some to question whether osteoarthrosis is a true feature of Paget's disease (Guyer and Sheperd, 1980). Coxa vara commonly occurs and in some patients progressive erosion of the femoral head occurs (Figure 3.14). Not surprisingly, radiographic abnormalities of the hip are commonly associated with symptoms.

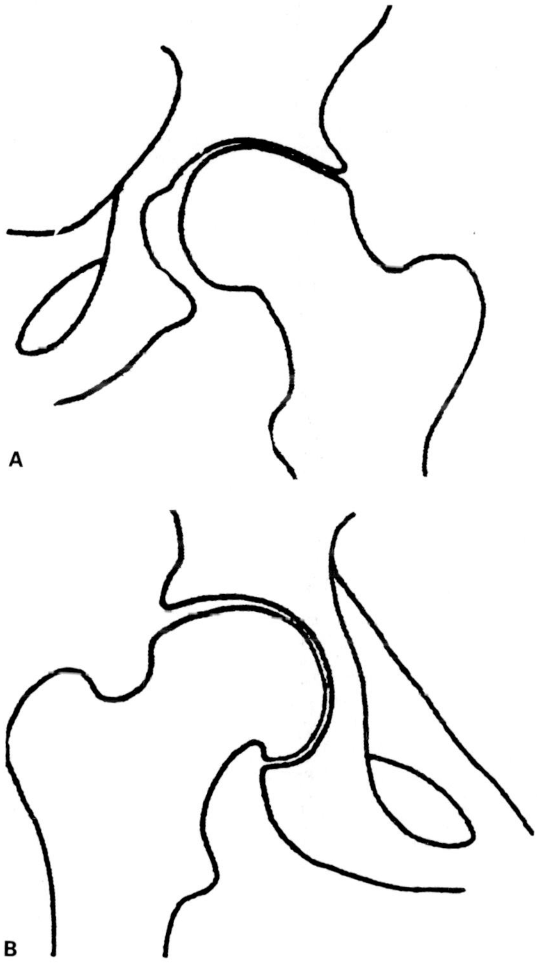

Figure 3.12

Tracings of the hips showing asymmetric (A) and concentric (B) narrowing of hip joint space. The latter is common in Paget's disease, whereas the former is more characteristic of osteoarthrosis.

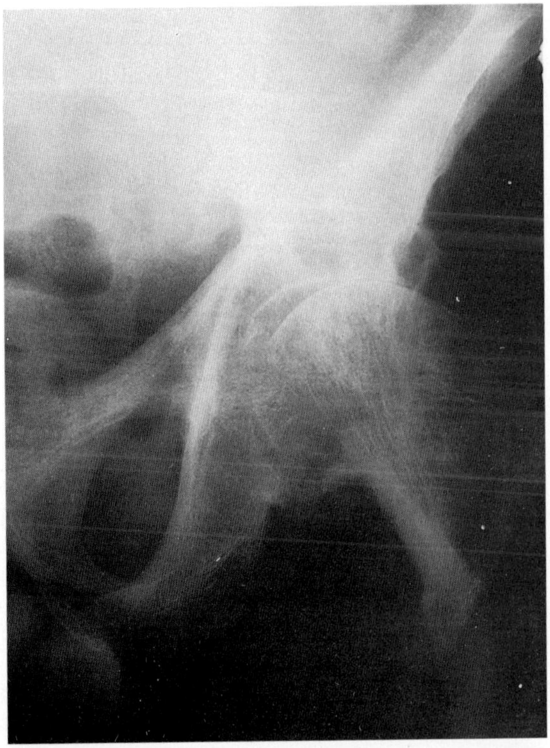

Figure 3.13

Radiographs of the hip affected by Paget's disease. There was narrowing of the superior joint space more characteristic of osteoarthrosis. Compare with Figure 3.9.

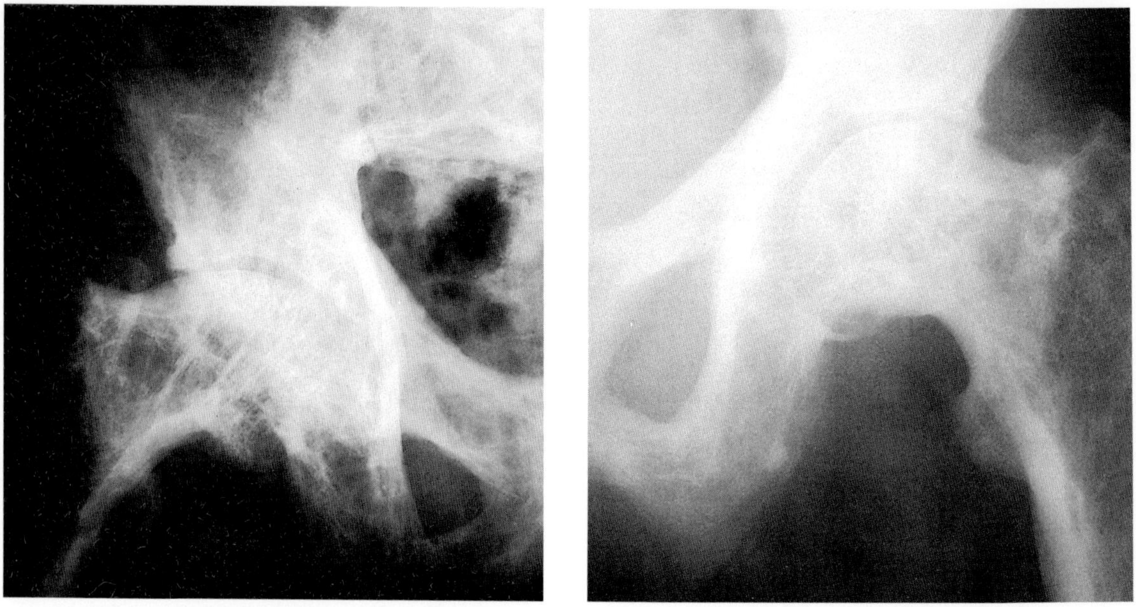

Figure 3.14

Paget's disease affecting the hip joint. Both radiographs show Paget's disease on either side of the joint space and the flattening of the head of the femur (coxa plana).

The spine

Paget's disease is found with high frequency in the spine and is present at one or more sites in the majority of patients (Table 3.10). Its spinal distribution is striking, and is more commonly found in the lumbar than cervical spine (Dickson et al, 1945; Guyer, 1981; Ziegler et al, 1985; Table 3.12). Indeed, the risk of Paget's disease increases progressively in a caudal direction from the cervical to the lower lumbar region. In one series, C1 and C2 were the most commonly affected cervical site (Guyer, 1981). In keeping with the general pattern of distribution, the number of vertebrae affected at different sites in individuals increases progressively from cervical spine caudally to the lumbar spine (Guyer and Sheperd, 1980; Table 3.13). Thus, in the cervical spine the disorder is commonly monostotic whereas it is rarely so in the thoracic or lumbar spine. The average number of vertebrae involved is four, but at any one level is one in the cervical spine, three in the thoracic spine and two at the lumbar spine (Table 3.14). The higher frequency of disease observed at lower (caudal) spinal sites may be related to the progressive increase in the size of vertebral bodies, and there is a close correspondence between disease frequency and vertebral-body volume (Table 3.13).

As in the case of pelvic disease, a classic resorption front is not commonly seen. Since a vertebral body is small compared with the other common sites of involvement, it is more likely to be completely involved at the time of presentation. A further reason may relate to the difficulty of radiographic assessment of the area. The most common radiographic finding is of thickened margins of the vertebral bodies and coarse central trabecular pattern. The rim of thickened cortex may be striking to give rise to a 'picture frame' (Figure 3.15) or 'rugger jersey' spine appearance (Figure 3.16). A striated appearance

Table 3.12 Pattern of vertebral involvement with Paget's disease in 170 patients from Lyon (Salson, 1981) and 197 patients from Sheffield (unpublished).

Site	*% patients*		
	Lyon	*Sheffield*	*Combined (± SEM)*
Lumbar spine	58	51	54 ± 3
Thoracic spine	44	43	44 ± 3
Cervical spine	14	17	15 ± 2
Thoracic + lumbar + cervical	7	8	8 ± 1
Thoracic + lumbar only	26	24	25 ± 2
Cervical only	1	4	3 ± 1
Thoracic only	5	8	7 ± 1
Lumbar only	16	17	16 ± 2

Table 3.13 Vertebral distribution of Paget's disease assessed by scintigraphy in 197 patients. C1 is not shown since this vertebra was not readily assessed by scintigraphy in the presence of Paget's disease at the base of the skull. Skeletal volume is shown as the volume of the vertebral body relative to D4.

Site	*No*	*% patients*	*% lesions*	*Relative skeletal volume*
C2	1	0.51	0.1	
C3	2	1.0	0.2	
C4	11	5.6	0.9	
C5	8	4.1	0.6	
C6	12	6.1	0.9	
C7	11	5.6	0.9	
D1	18	9.1	1.4	
D2	13	6.6	1.0	
D3	14	7.1	1.1	
D4	13	6.6	1.0	1.0
D5	18	9.1	1.4	1.1
D6	19	9.6	1.5	1.4
D7	22	11.2	1.7	1.5
D8	26	13.2	2.0	1.7
D9	18	9.1	1.4	1.9
D10	19	9.6	1.5	2.1
D11	22	11.2	1.7	2.3
D12	30	15.2	2.3	2.3
L1	41	20.8	3.2	2.7
L2	43	21.8	3.3	3.1
L3	49	24.9	3.8	3.3
L4	49	24.9	3.8	3.3
L5	44	22.3	3.3	3.1

Table 3.14 Pattern of vertebral Paget's disease in 197 patients assessed by scintigraphy.

Site	*No of patients*	*No of lesions*	*Lesions/ patient*
Cervical spine†	32	45	1.4
Thoracic spine	84	232	2.8
Lumbar spine	101	226	2.2
Cervical spine only	8	10	1.3
Thoracic spine only	16	21	1.3
Lumbar spine only	34	55	1.6
Any spinal site*	130	503	3.9

*Excluding the sacrum.
†Excluding C1.

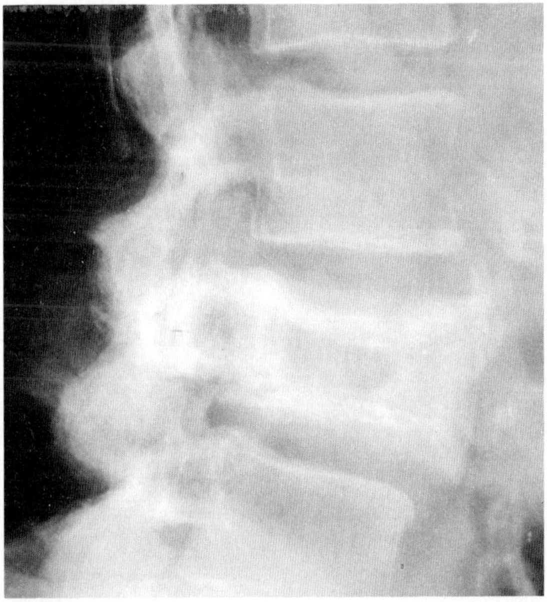

Figure 3.15

Paget's disease of the lumbar spine which shows an expanded body and involvement of the neural arches. There is marked sclerosis of the end-plates giving rise to a 'picture frame' appearance.

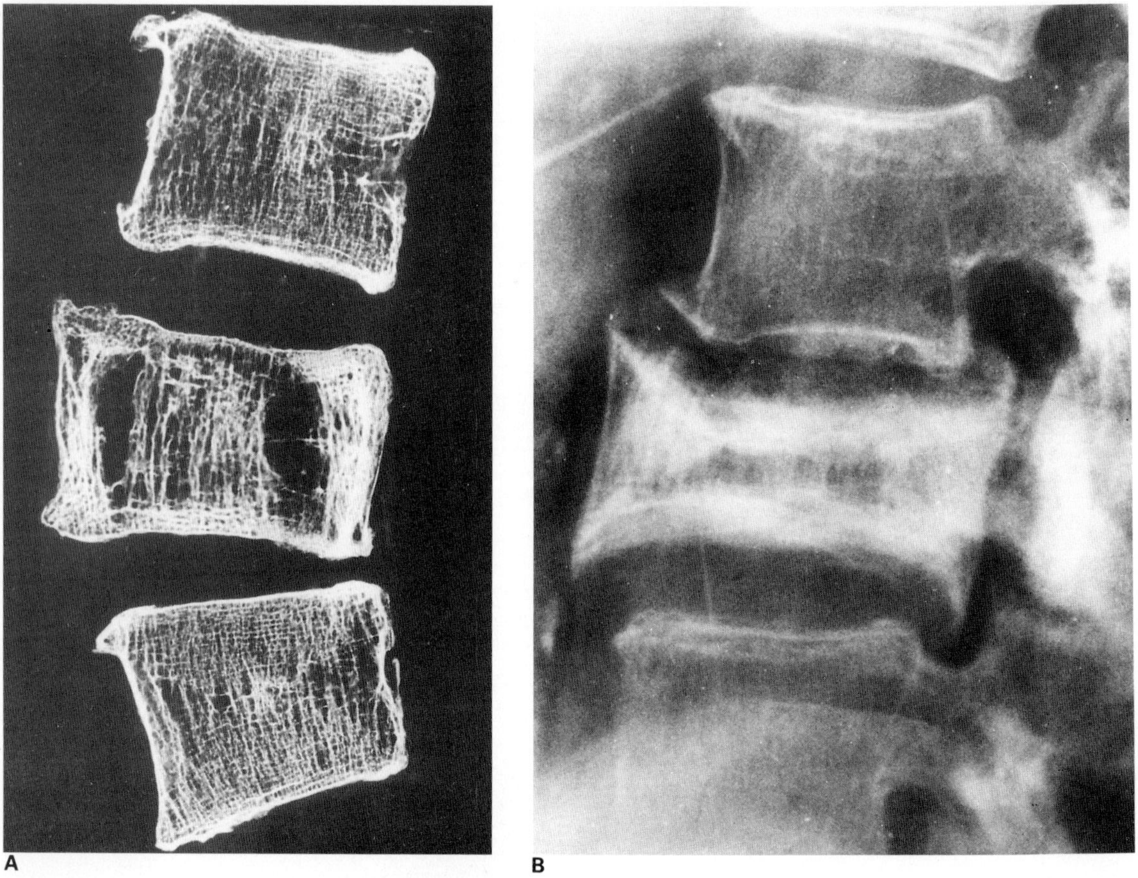

Figure 3.16

Radiographs of pagetic vertebrae from two patients, one in vitro (A) and the other in vivo (B). In both there is apparent cortical thickening and bony enlargement, but the distinction between cortical and trabecular bone is blurred due to marked intercortical resorption.

of the vertebral body can be marked with preferential accentuation of vertical trabecular markings (Figure 3.17). It can usually be differentiated from haemangioma by the thickened cortex and increased size of the vertebral body (Chapter 6). Dense osteosclerosis may occasionally be seen (Figure 3.18) and may present problems in differential diagnosis from other causes of ivory vertebrae (Chapter 6), particularly if bony enlargement is absent or not marked.

Enlargement of the vertebral bodies is commonly observed and may be predominantly anterior, posterior or lateral (Figure 3.19). Most frequently it is symmetrical and visible on anteroposterior and lateral radiographs. An increase in vertebral height is not seen so that when expansion is marked it may give the appearance of a flattened vertebra (Figure 3.20). Occasionally the increase in diameter of the vertebral bodies due to periosteal neostosis is not associated with

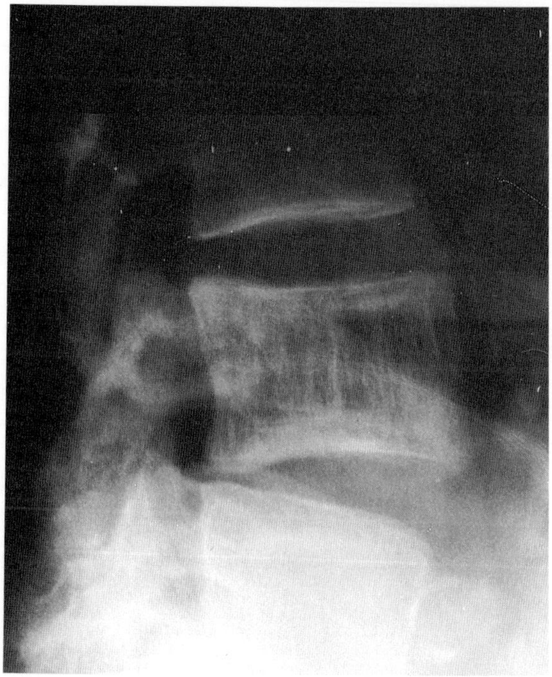

Figure 3.17 (left)

Lateral radiograph of the lumbar spine. The vertical trabecular markings are accentuated due to Paget's disease at L4. Note also pagetic involvement of the neural arch and spinous process.

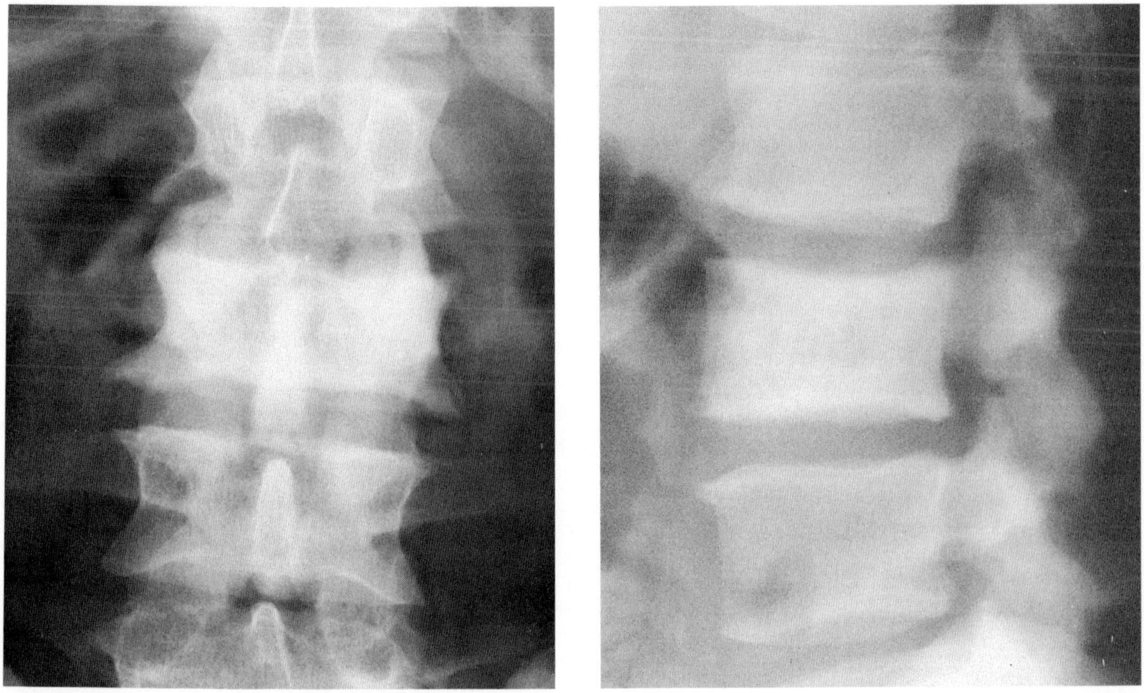

Figure 3.18

Solitary ivory vertebra due to Paget's disease.

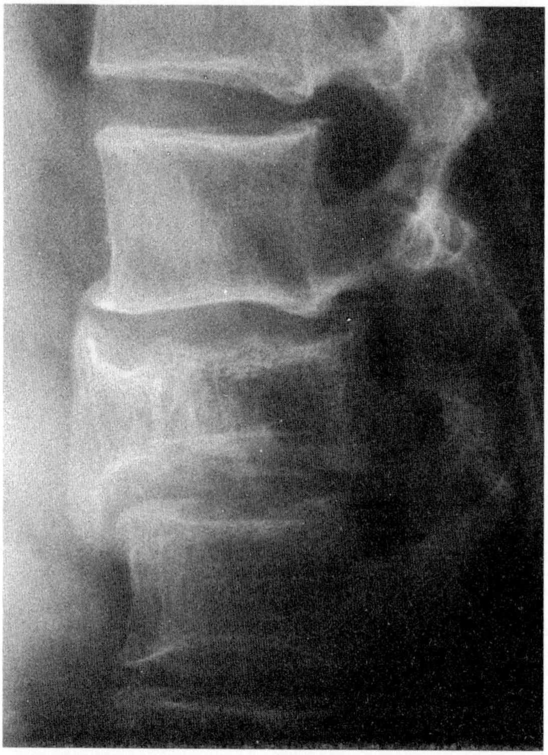

Figure 3.19

Lateral radiograph of lumbar spine showing vertebral enlargement. Note the marked increase in diameter with no increase in vertebral height.

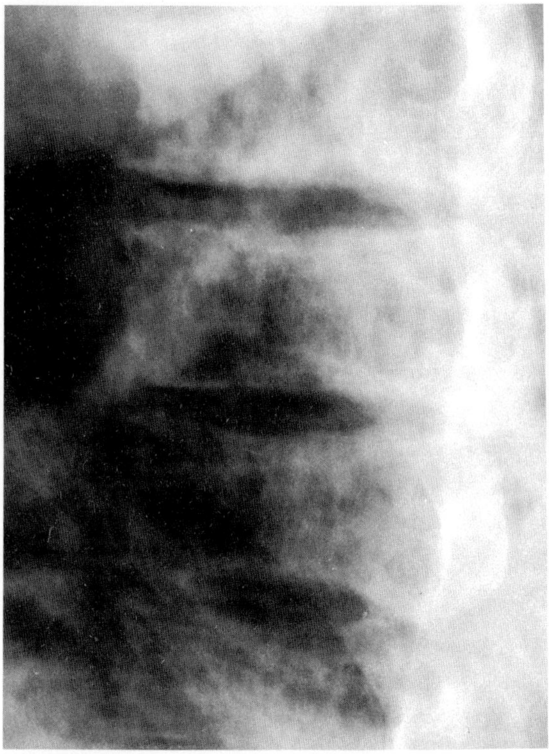

Figure 3.20

Lateral radiograph of the spine. All the vertebrae are enlarged without change in height so that the vertebrae appear to be flattened.

cortical thickening, which gives rise to a 'bone within a bone' appearance due to the preservation of the pre-existing cortex (Figure 3.21). Enlargement of the vertebral bodies is usual but not invariable (Figure 3.22) and, particularly if monostotic, can give rise to diagnostic difficulties (Chapter 6).

Vertebral compression fractures are very common and in one series accounted for the vast majority of pagetic fractures (Dickson et al, 1945). They are found with equal frequency in the lumbar and thoracic spine. Common findings are 'cod-fish' vertebral deformities and anterior wedging. Complete collapse occurs more commonly than in involutional osteoporosis. Fractures may induce marked spinal angulation or displacement (Figure 3.23). This is most likely to give rise to neurological syndromes in the dorsal spine (Chapter 5).

Although a resorption front is not observed in the pagetic spine, the vertebral bodies may appear osteopaenic, but this involves the entire vertebral body. This appearance is commonly associated with vertebral collapse (Figure 3.24). Minor degrees of vertebral collapse are rarely observed in sclerotic vertebrae and the question arises whether diffuse vertebral osteopaenia causes the fracture. An alternative possibility is that osteopaenia is secondary to the collapse (Maldague and Malghem, 1987), representing an

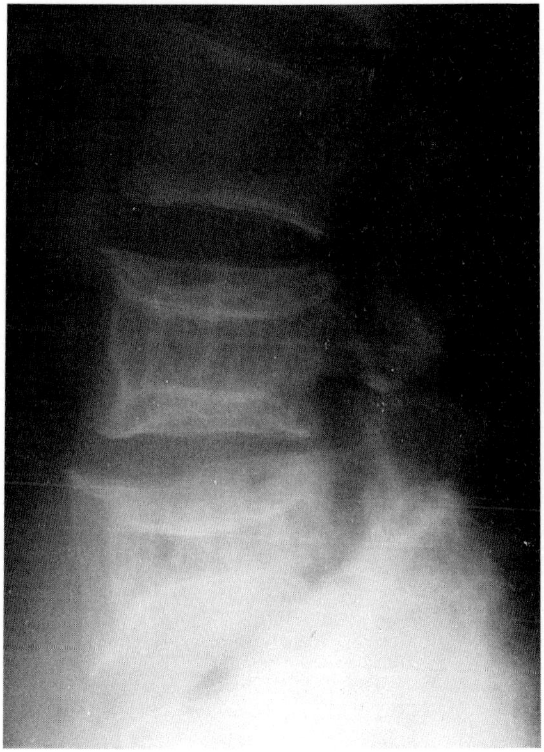

Figure 3.21

Radiograph of lumbar spine. Note the marked 'bone within bone' appearance at L3 and L4, but the obvious increase in trabecular markings. Despite the appearance vertebral height was not apparently increased.

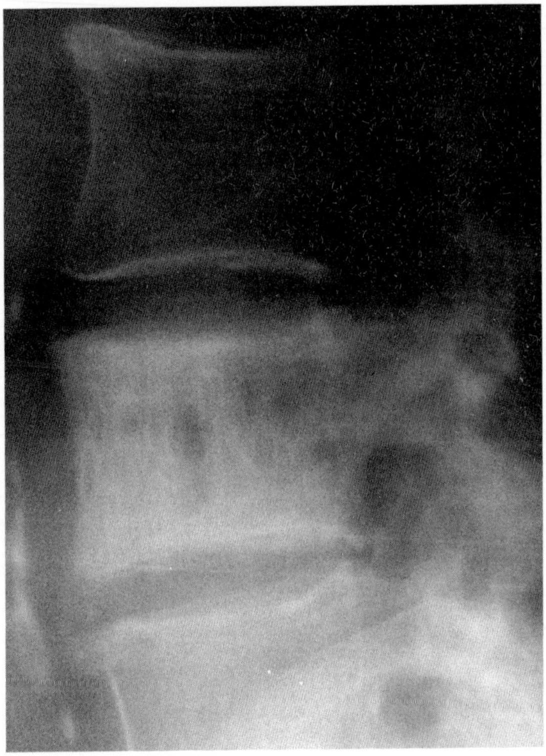

Figure 3.22

Lateral radiograph of the lumbar spine. The vertebra was shown to be pagetic, but is normal in shape and not enlarged.

exaggerated response to fracture. Both notions may be correct (Figure 3.25).

Paget's disease of the spine is not confined to the vertebral bodies. Marked thickening and sclerosis of the neural arches may occur. Osteosclerosis of the pedicles gives rise to a distinctive radiographic appearance on anteroposterior radiographs which we term the 'polo' sign (Figure 3.26). A similar appearance is seen on anteroposterior radiographs of the coracoid process (Figure 3.27). When the pedicles are markedly sclerotic they may appear rather like osteoblastic secondary lesions (Figure 3.28).

Degenerative changes may obscure the radiographic features of Paget's disease. The intervertebral discs of contiguously involved vertebral bodies may be replaced by bone with resultant fusion. It is generally accepted that Paget's disease does not extend across joints, but an exception may be the spine in the presence of marked degenerative disease and bony contact between vertebral elements (Figure 3.29). Occasionally, uncalcified or partially calcified osteoid may be found in the paraspinal region and give rise to a paravertebral shadow (Figures 3.30 and 3.31). Such extraskeletal extension has been infrequently described at other sites (Resnick et al, 1982; Monson et al, 1989) and the mechanism is not known. In the few cases that we have observed it is associated with vertebral collapse

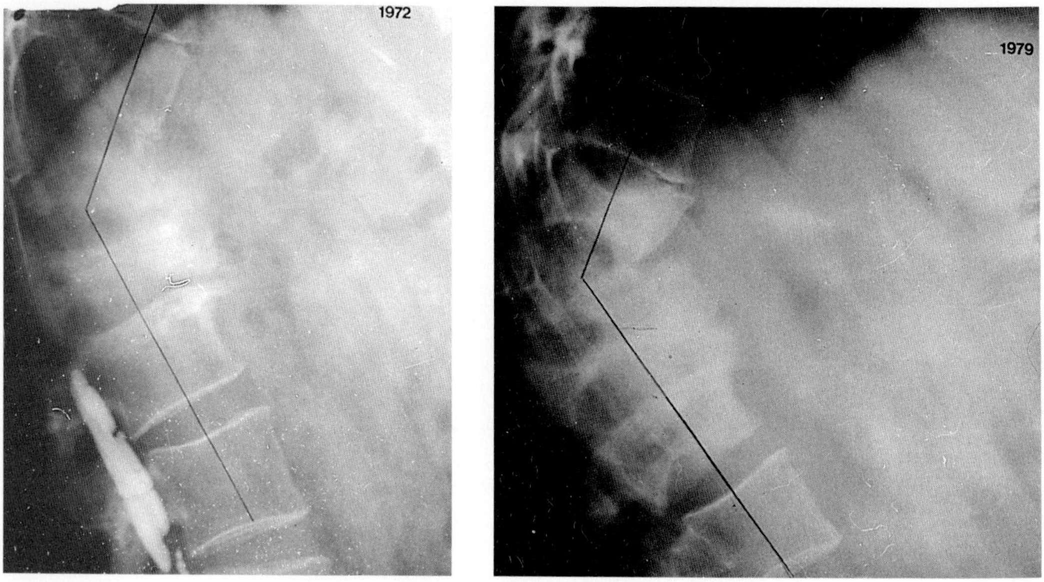

Figure 3.23

Paget's disease of the spine showing progressive dorsal angulation due to vertebral fracture over a period of 7 years.

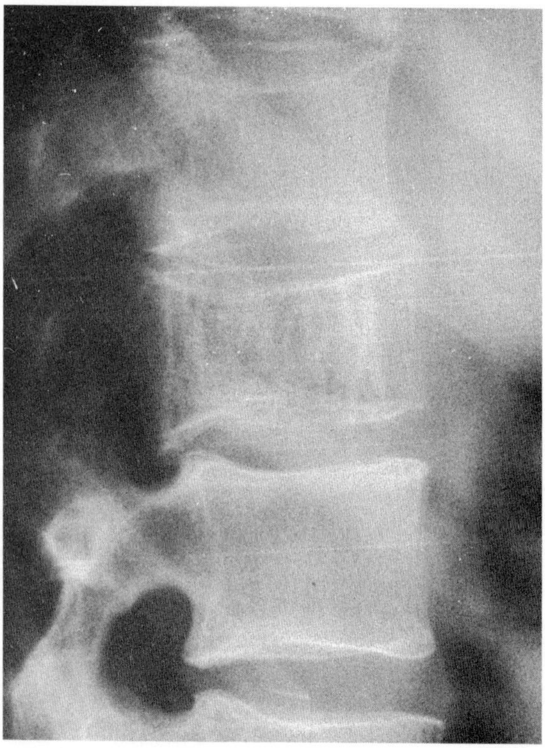

Figure 3.24

Lateral radiograph of thoracic spine. The osteopaenic vertebra is due to Paget's disease which affects the body and vertebral laminae. Note also the accentuation of vertical trabeculae.

and osteoarthritic changes. It is possible that this could be associated with extrusion of marrow elements into paravertebral sites or marked focal osteophytic hypertrophy. It is also possible that minor degrees of paravertebral osteoidosis may be a mechanism for extension of the disorder between vertebral bodies.

As for the hip, marked osteoarthrosis does occur but osteophytosis is said not to be a prominent feature despite the gross changes in bony shape, at least at the lumbar spine (Guyer and Sheperd, 1980). The presence of Paget's disease does appear, however, to be associated with osteophytosis at affected sites in some patients (Figures 3.32 and 3.33).

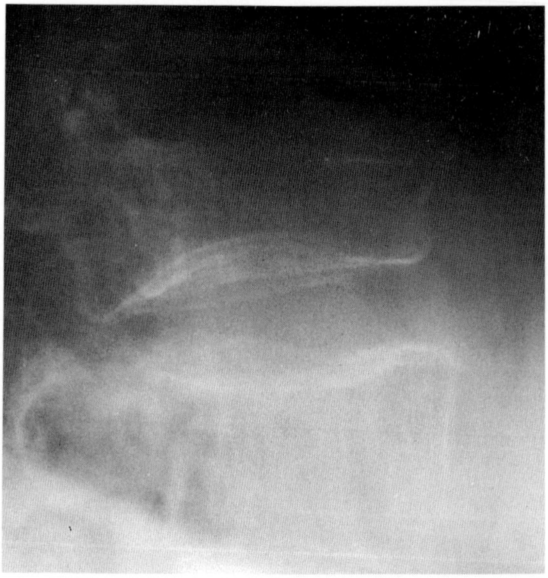

Figure 3.25 (left)

Anterior crush fracture of L1 associated with Paget's disease. Note absence of osteosclerosis, somewhat more evident at L2.

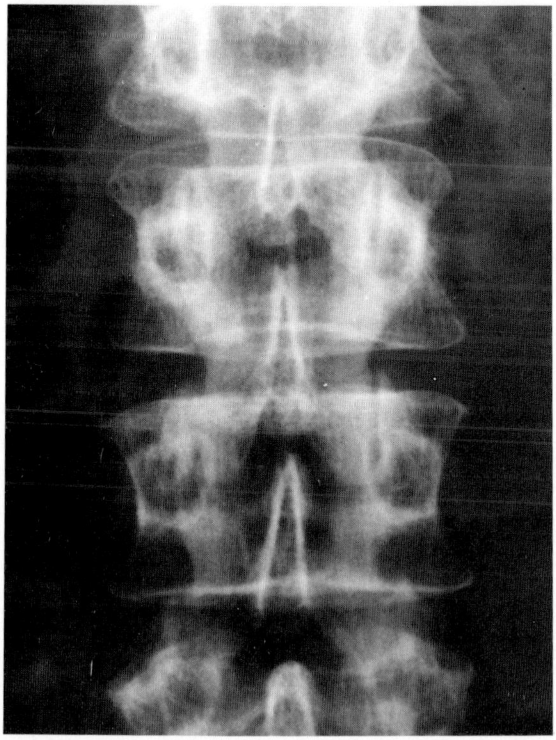

Figure 3.26

Osteosclerosis of the pedicles giving rise to a sclerotic ring – the 'polo' sign.

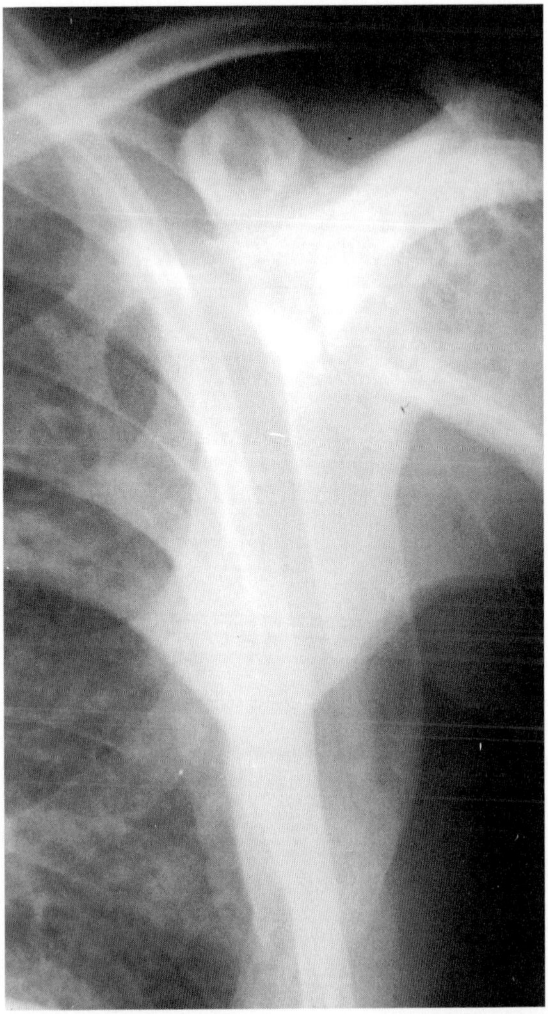

Figure 3.27

Paget's disease of the scapula and humerus. The pagetic coracoid process shows as a dense sclerotic ring – the 'polo' sign when viewed end on.

In some patients a clinical syndrome resembling ankylosing spondylitis may be associated with Paget's disease (Khairi et al, 1973; Mazieres et al, 1978). The features of the syndrome include limitation of chest expansion, reduction of spinal flexion, peripheral joint disease, ossification of spinal ligaments, extensive osteophytosis and obliterated sacro-iliac joints. In Singer's experience (1977a), determination of HLA leukocyte antigens in four patients did not reveal the B27 antigen, whereas this is found in about 90 per cent of patients with ankylosing spondylitis.

Bony overgrowth of the vertebral bodies or neural arches may encroach upon the intervertebral foramen, interfere with the blood supply to the

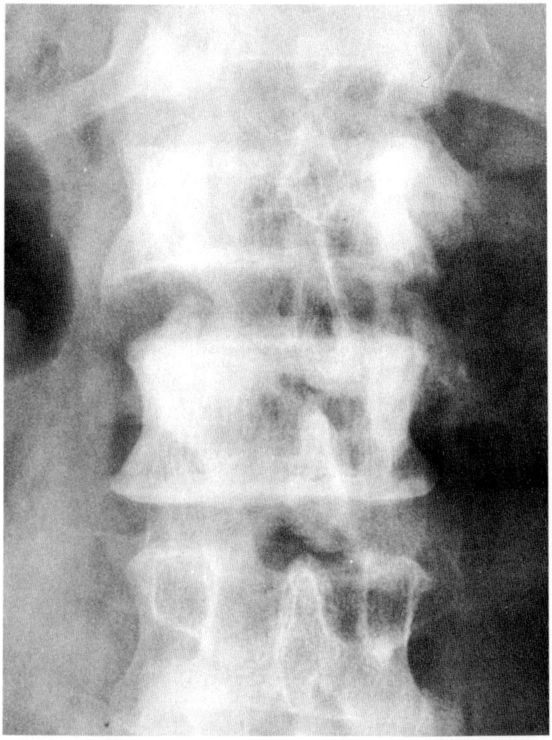

Figure 3.28

Anteroposterior radiograph of lumbar spine showing irregular osteosclerosis of the pedicles of L1, 2 and 3 having a superficial resemblance to metastatic disease. The pedicles of L4 are normal.

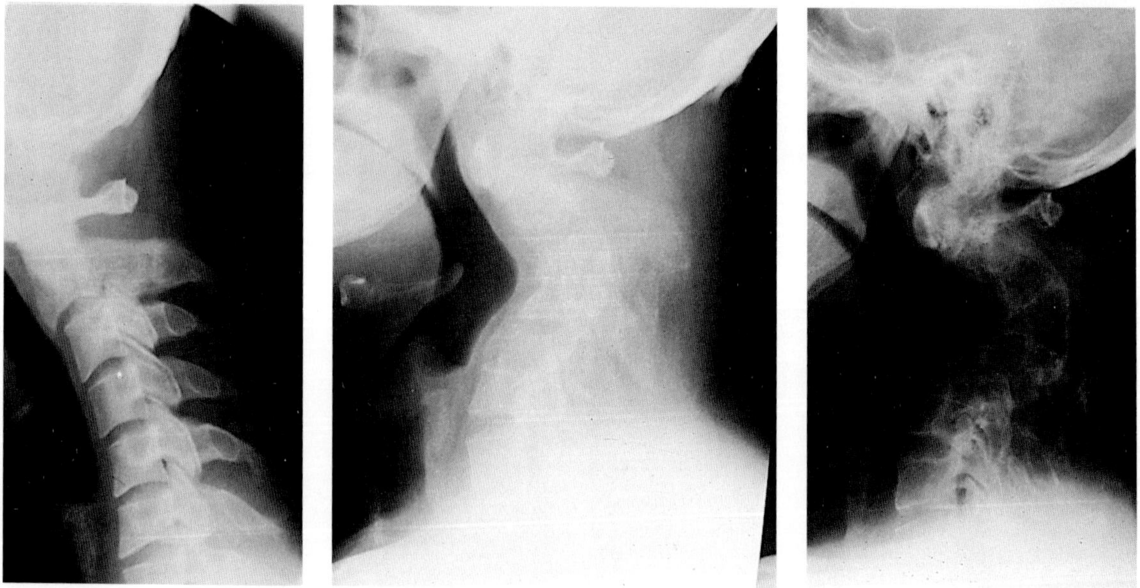

A B C

Figure 3.29

Serial radiographs to show the progression of Paget's disease over an interval of 13 (B) and 20 years (C). Note the apparent extension from C2 in a caudal direction. (From Bowie and Kanis, 1977.)

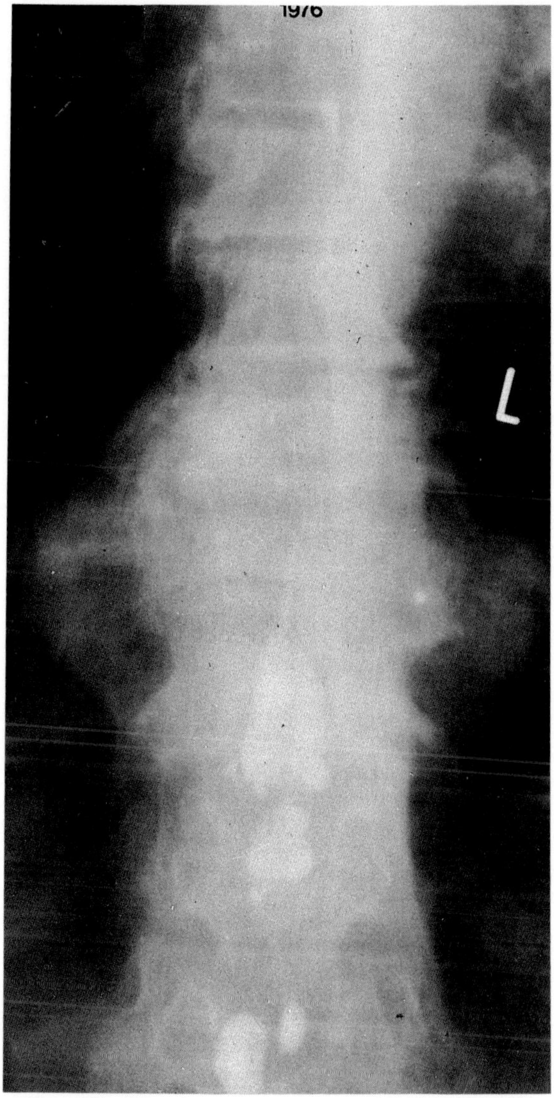

Figure 3.30 (left)

Anteroposterior radiograph of the thoracic spine in a patient with Paget's disease of T9, T10 and T11. Expansion and collapse of T10 was associated with a paravertebral shadow and a slowly progressive paraparesis. The shadow, due to partially calcified osteoid, may be mistaken for sarcoma.

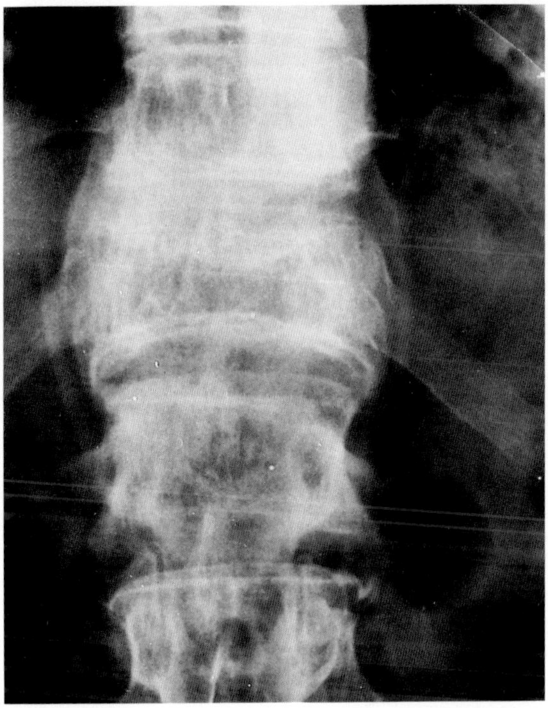

Figure 3.31

Paravertebral calcification in a patient with Paget's disease of the thoracic spine.

spinal cord or lead to narrowing of the spinal canal (Figure 3.34), giving rise to neurological syndromes (Chapter 5). Neurological complications are fortunately comparatively rare given the frequency of spinal involvement. In addition, the distribution of Paget's disease in the spine does not bear a close relationship to the frequency or the severity of neurological sequelae that may arise. For example, the cervical spine, although rarely involved, is comparatively frequently associated with serious complications due to vertebral collapse, enlargement or dislocation.

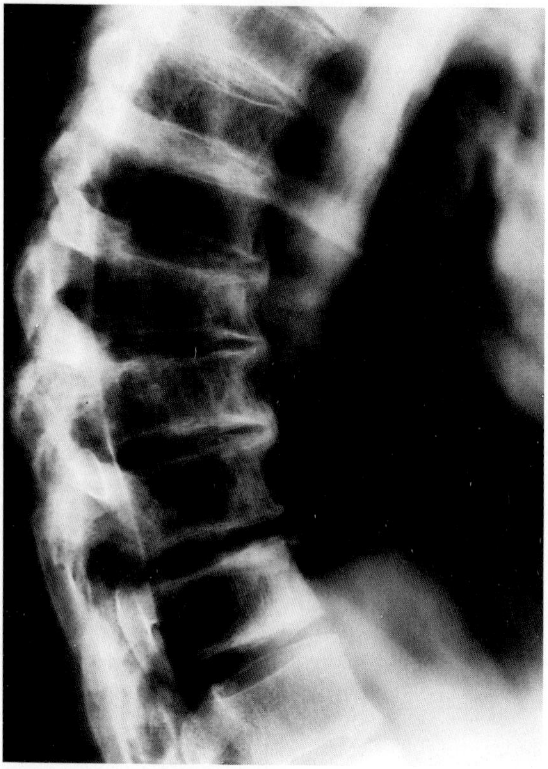

Figure 3.32

Lateral radiograph of the thoracic spine in a patient with Paget's disease. Osteophytes are prominent and appear to have caused fusion between affected vertebral bodies. Osteophytes were not present in those vertebral bodies not affected by Paget's disease.

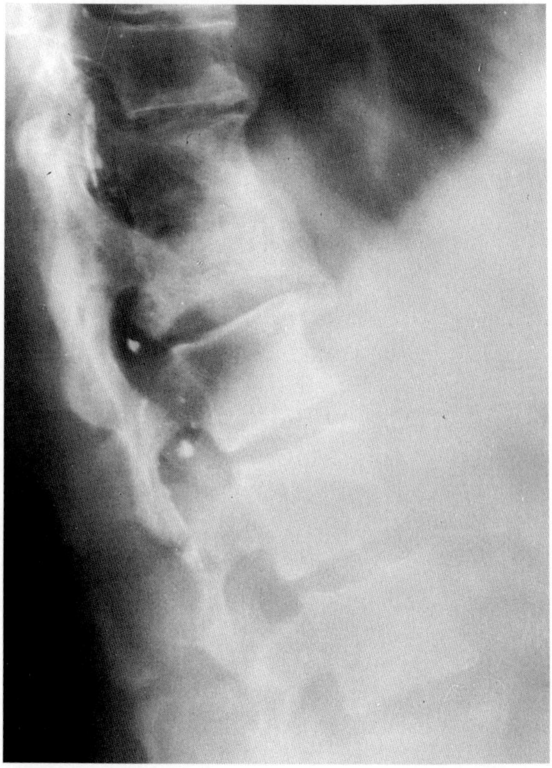

Figure 3.33

Lateral X-ray photograph showing Paget's disease of two thoracic vertebrae. Note the presence of osteophytes causing bony contact with adjacent vertebrae, but their absence elsewhere in the spine.

Table 3.15 Biochemical and scintigraphic findings in Paget's disease (mean ± SEM) in patients divided according to the presence of absence of skull involvement.

	Skull affected (75 patients)	*Skull spared (122 patients)*	*p<*
Sex (F:M)	2.43	1.18	0.05
Age at onset (years)	61.25 ± 1.5	61.5 ± 1.2	NS
Age at diagnosis (years)	70.6 ± 1.0	70.0 ± 0.8	NS
Alkaline phosphatase* (IU/l)	484 (429–546)	231 (219–244)	0.0001
Hydroxyproline (mmol/mol creatinine)*	105.7 (95.3–117.2)	52.3 (50.0–54.8)	0.0001
Number of affected sites	10.25 ± 1.0	4.2 ± 0.3	0.0001
Skeleton affected (%)	22.6 ± 1.7	9.1 ± 0.55	0.0001
Scintigraphic index	72.8 ± 6.3	30.5 ± 1.8	0.0001

*Mean and SEM computed after log-transformation.
NS: not significant.

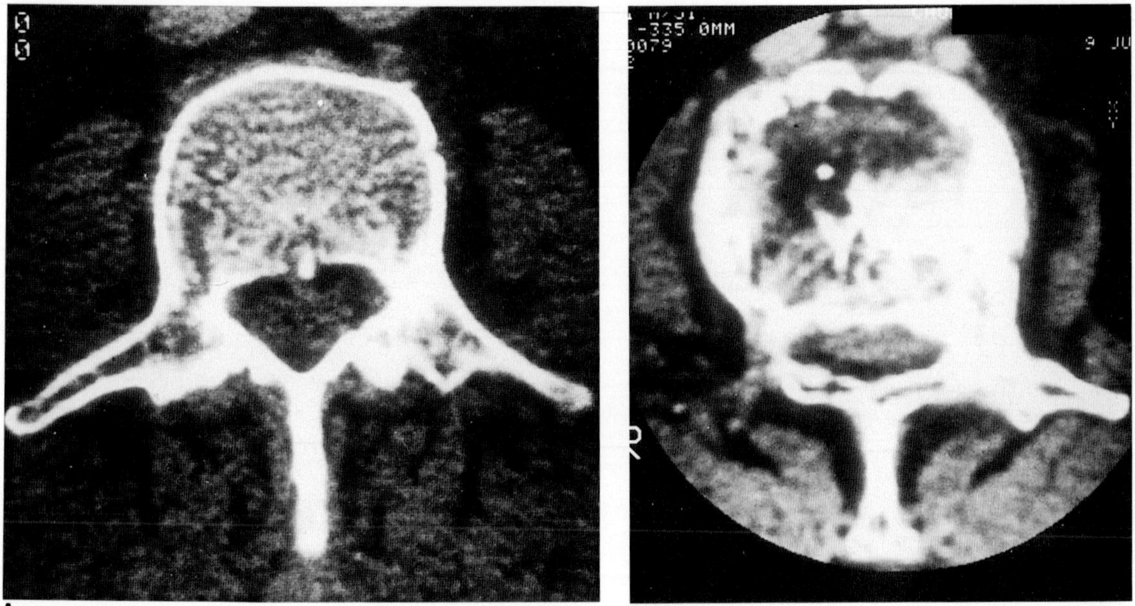

A B

Figure 3.34

Computerized axial tomogram of third lumbar vertebra in a patient with neurological complications (B). (A) shows a normal vertebra. Note the narrowing of the vertebral canal and marked sclerosis of cortical bone.

Skull and face

Involvement of the skull is less common than vertebral or pelvic disease (Table 3.10). When the skull is affected, patients have more extensive disease elsewhere (Harinck et al, 1986; Table 3.15). This does not necessarily mean that it occurs later in the natural history of the disorder since new foci of bone disease (rather than disease extension) rarely, if ever, occur. Two series have shown that skull disease is markedly more frequent in women, unlike the more normal male predominance for other lesions (Table 3.8; Harinck et al, 1986).

The disorder begins as a rarified area termed osteoporosis circumscripta. It is most frequent at the frontal or occipital regions and may advance to involve the whole of the cranial vault (Figure 3.35). On X-ray examination the outer table is commonly obliterated by the advancing resorption front, and the inner table is characteristically spared (Figure 3.36). Occasionally, the bone scan does not show increased uptake, suggesting the predominance of bone resorption. More frequently, increased scan uptake is observed indicating that radiographic osteopaenia is associated with increased bone formation (Figure 3.37). There is normally, but not invariably, a sharp demarcation line between the normal bone and osteolytic front. When present, this enables the rate of progression to be measured (Figure 3.35). The rate conforms to that documented in the long bones (generally 1 cm per annum; Stuart, 1977).

The later stage of the disorder is associated with patchy osteosclerosis. In contrast to osteoporosis circumscripta, osteosclerosis appears more predominantly on the inner table

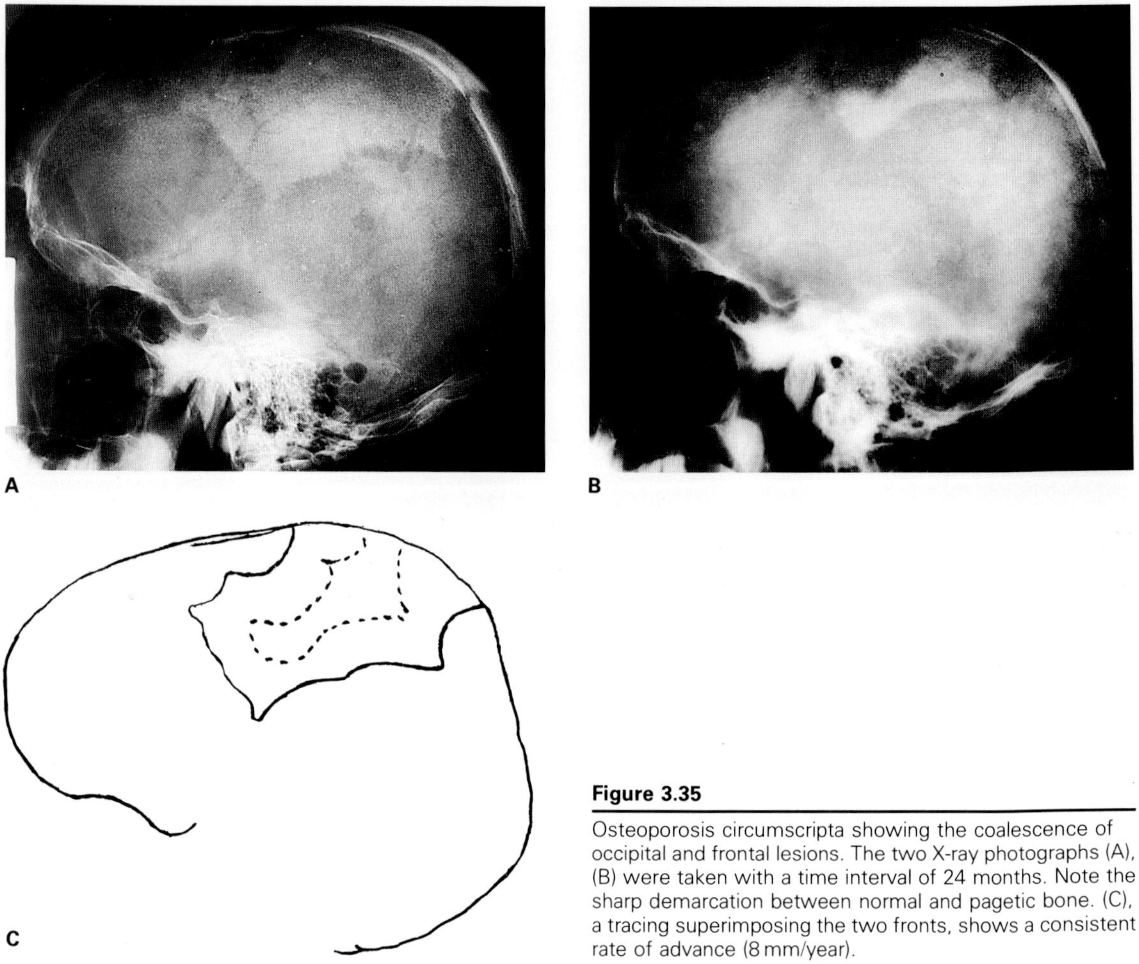

Figure 3.35

Osteoporosis circumscripta showing the coalescence of occipital and frontal lesions. The two X-ray photographs (A), (B) were taken with a time interval of 24 months. Note the sharp demarcation between normal and pagetic bone. (C), a tracing superimposing the two fronts, shows a consistent rate of advance (8 mm/year).

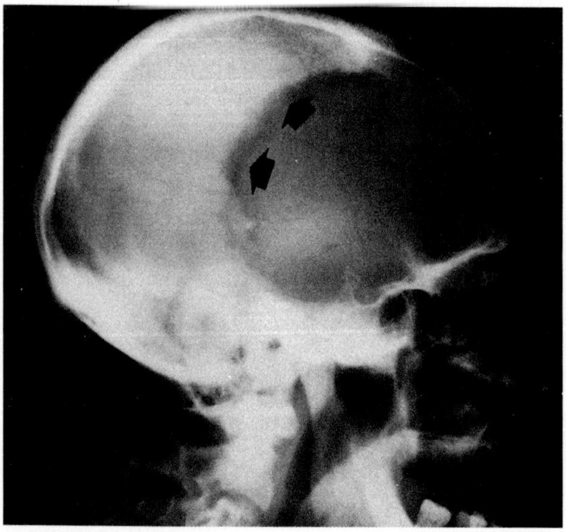

Figure 3.36

Marked osteoporosis circumscripta of the skull giving an 'oil stain' appearance. Note the preferential resorption of the outer table of the skull.

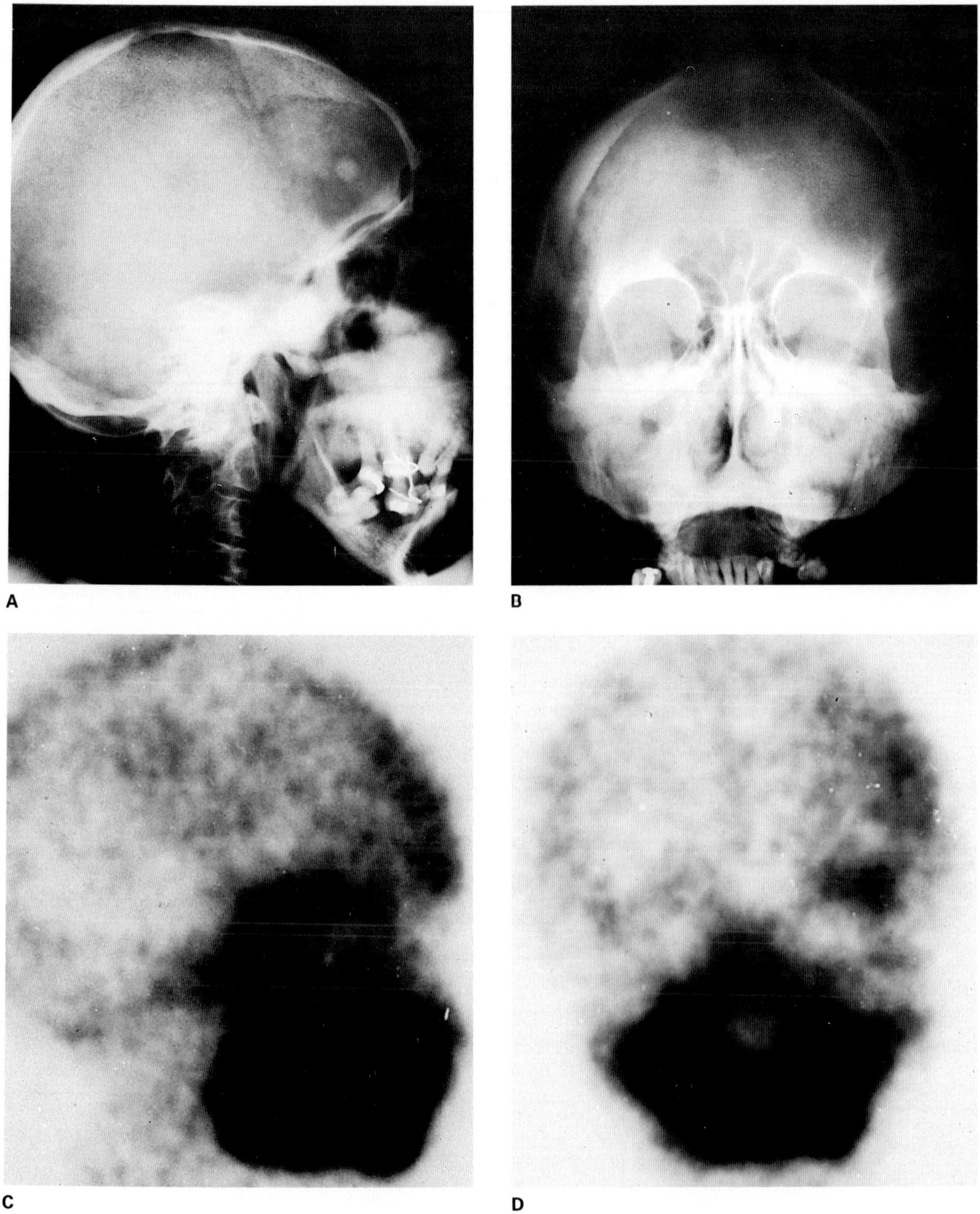

Figure 3.37

Radiograph (A) (B) and bone scan (C) (D) of a patient with osteoporosis circumscripta. The osteoporosis is associated with increased scintigraphic uptake. The patient also has dense maxillary disease.

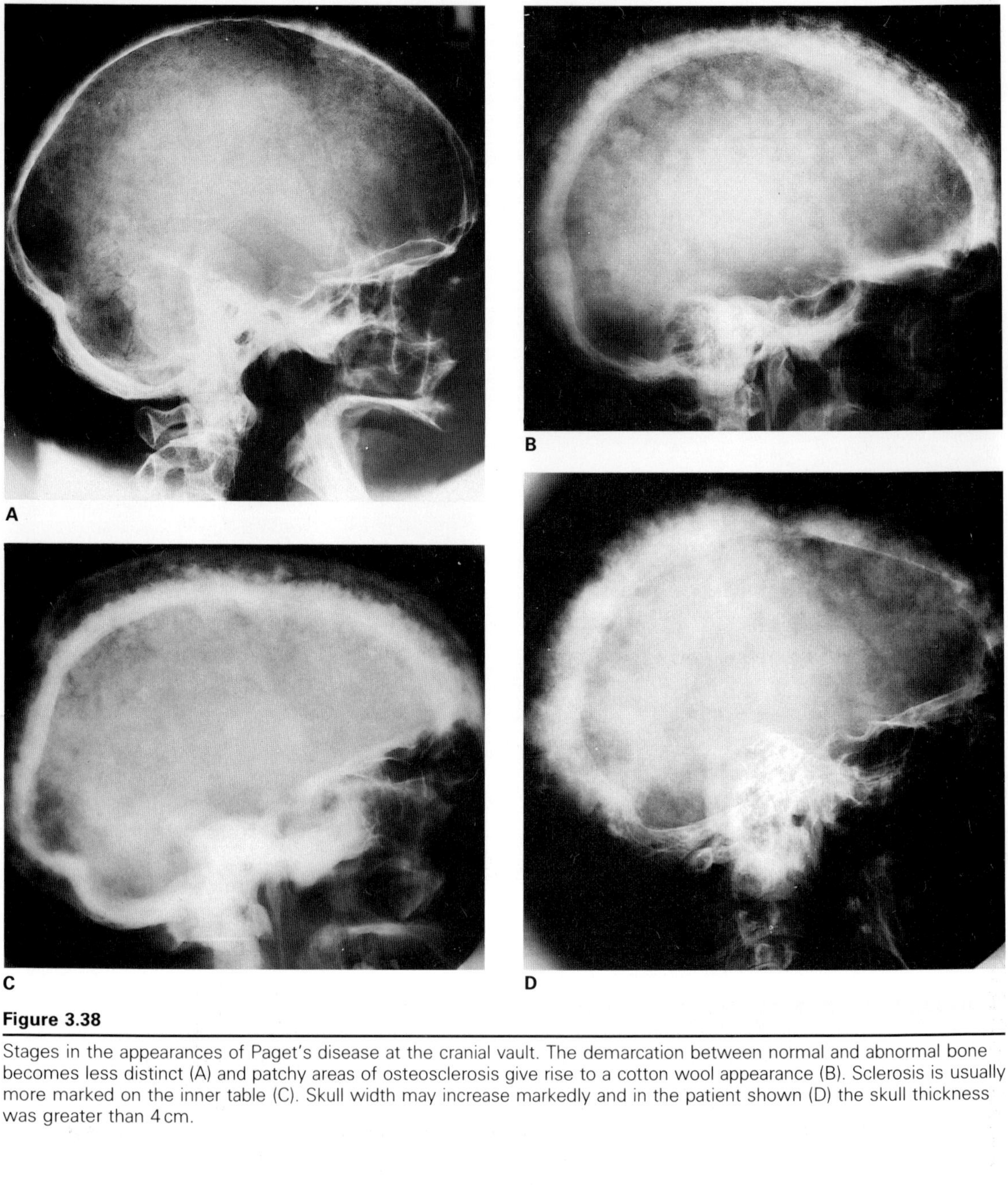

A B C D

Figure 3.38

Stages in the appearances of Paget's disease at the cranial vault. The demarcation between normal and abnormal bone becomes less distinct (A) and patchy areas of osteosclerosis give rise to a cotton wool appearance (B). Sclerosis is usually more marked on the inner table (C). Skull width may increase markedly and in the patient shown (D) the skull thickness was greater than 4 cm.

(Figure 3.38), resulting in thickening. Irregular areas of sclerosis in the thickened diploe give a characteristic cotton wool appearance or discrete islands of osteosclerosis which may bridge the inner and outer tables (Figure 3.39). In surveys of symptomatic Paget's disease sclerotic lesions are observed twice as frequently as osteoporosis circumscripta (Meunier et al, 1987). Cranial invol-

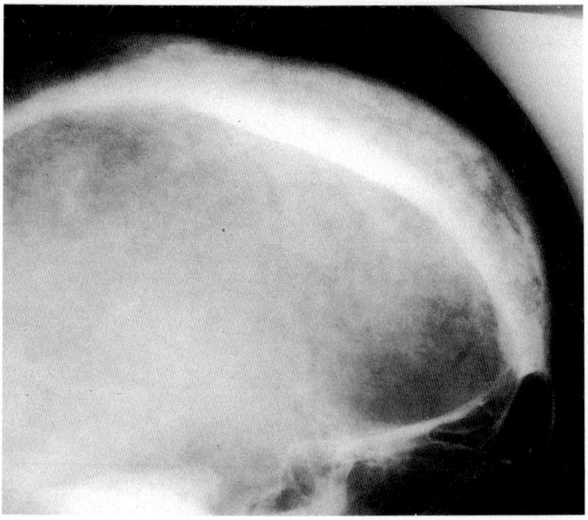

Figure 3.39

Radiographic detail of the cranial vault to show bridging of inner and outer tables with sclerotic lesions.

vement may occasionally result in internal or external asymmetric thickening of the vault (Figure 3.40).

Involvement of the base of the skull may be associated with platybasia, basilar invagination, brain stem compression and cranial nerve palsies (Chapter 5). The petrous temporal bones are frequently involved and contribute to the aetiology of deafness. Various radiographic criteria have been utilized to diagnose platybasia (Table 3.16), but in many cases the diagnosis is obvious (Figure 3.41) and there is no close relationship between the degree of platybasia and neurological complaints.

Involvement of the facial bones is less common than skull lesions, and when confined to these sites may give rise to diagnostic difficulties. Maxillary Paget's disease is more common than mandibular. In one series the upper jaw was affected in 64 per cent of cases, the lower in 18 per cent and the remainder had involvement of both (Smith and Eveson, 1981).

Maxillary and mandibular disease may give rise to marked cosmetic deformity due to symmetric (Figure 3.42) or asymmetric (Figures 3.43 and

Table 3.16 Some indices of basilar impression from radiography of the skull.

Method	*Measurement*	*Criteria for basilar impression*
Boogard's line	Line between the glabella (niason) and posterior lip of foramen magnum	Tip of odontoid peg above line
Bull's angle	Angle (β) between the plane of first cervical vertebra and plane of hard palate	$\beta > 19°$
Chamberlain's line	Line between posterior lip of hard palate and posterior lip of foramen magnum	Odontoid peg above line
Fischgold's line	Line between mastoid tips (tomography required)	Tip of odontoid peg >2 mm above line
McGregor's line	Line between upper surface of posterior edge of hard palate and most caudal point of occipital curve	Tip of odontoid peg >4.5 mm above line

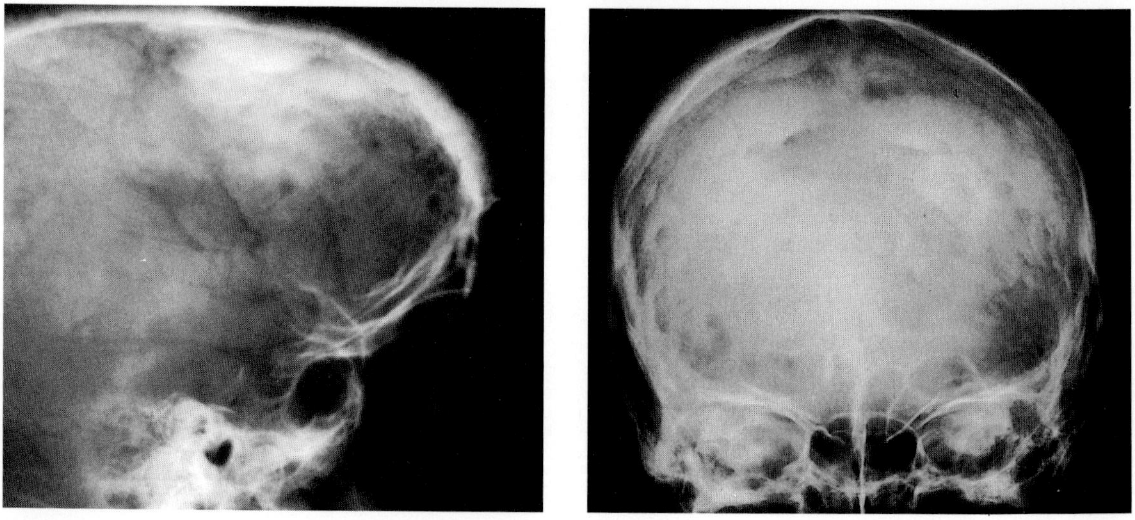

Figure 3.40

Paget's disease of the skull with irregular hyperostosis similar in appearance to craniometaphyseal dysplasia.

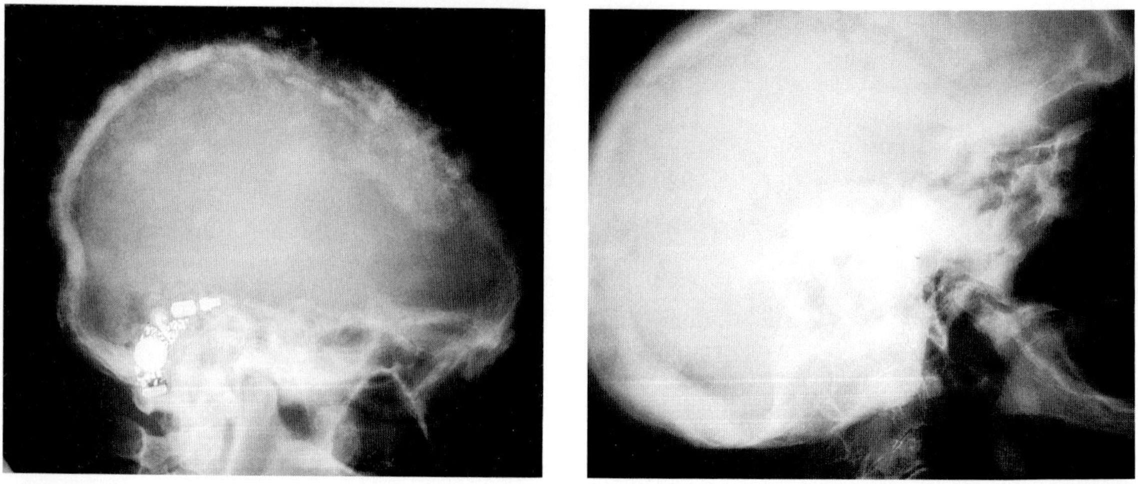

Figure 3.41

Platybasia due to Paget's disease.

3.44) enlargement. Maxillary disease is commonly associated with radiodense lesions and the perinasal sinuses may be obliterated (Figure 3.45). The alveolar ridges may widen and exacerbate dental problems due to loosening or migration of teeth (Figure 3.43). When Paget's disease affects the jaw it is usually extensive, occurring throughout both sides of the jaw. It may give rise to marked enlargement.

Not surprisingly, the teeth may be involved in Paget's disease. Early radiographic changes include an osteopaenic phase at the apices which

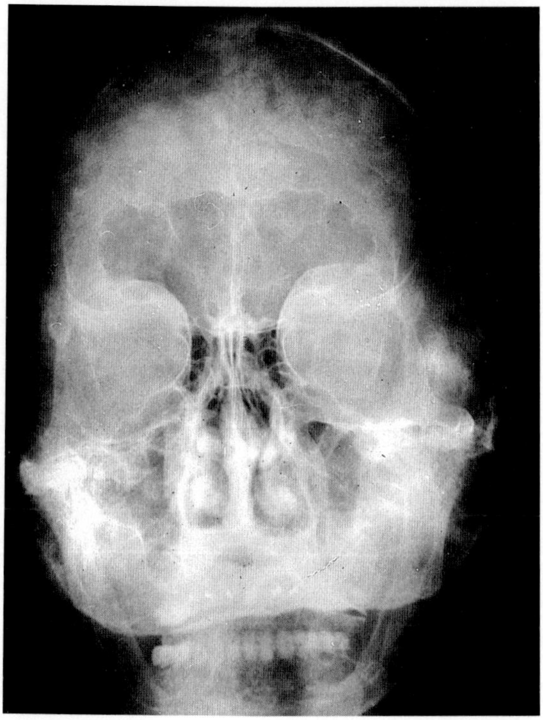

Figure 3.42

Anteroposterior radiograph of skull and facial bones of a female showing marked bilateral maxillary hypertrophy.

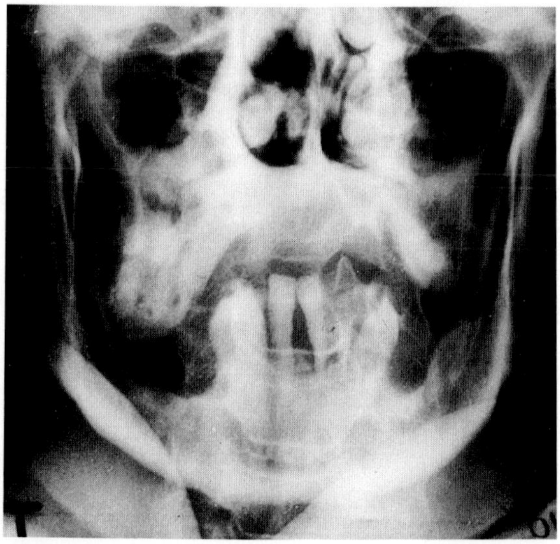

Figure 3.43

Radiograph to show hypertrophy of the maxillary alveolar ridges more marked on the left- than on the right-hand side.

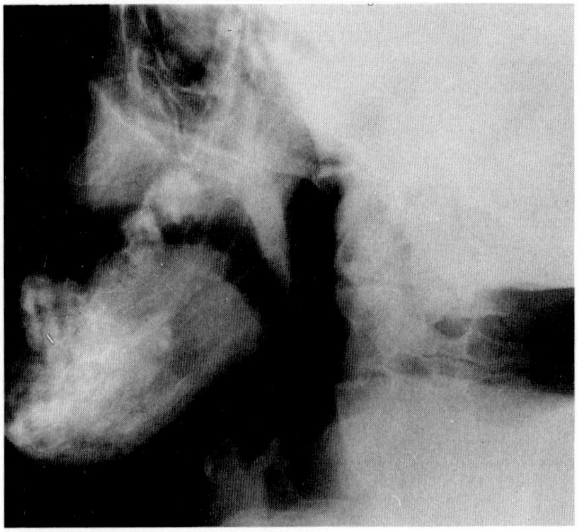

Figure 3.44

Prognathism due to mandibular enlargement from Paget's disease.

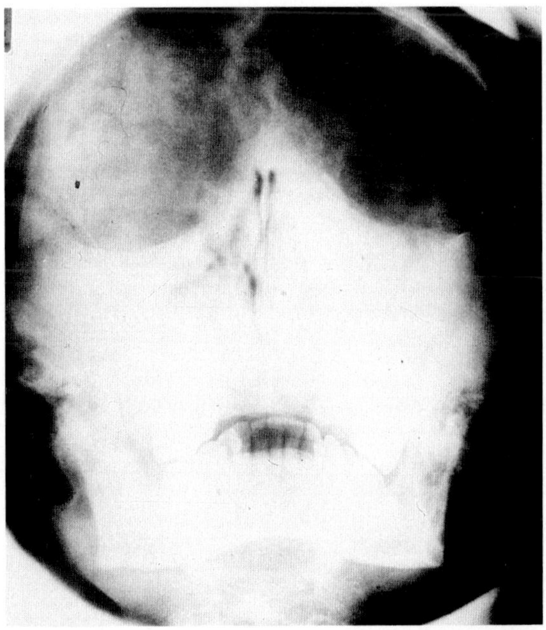

Figure 3.45

Dense maxillary sclerosis and obliteration of the paranasal sinuses due to Paget's disease.

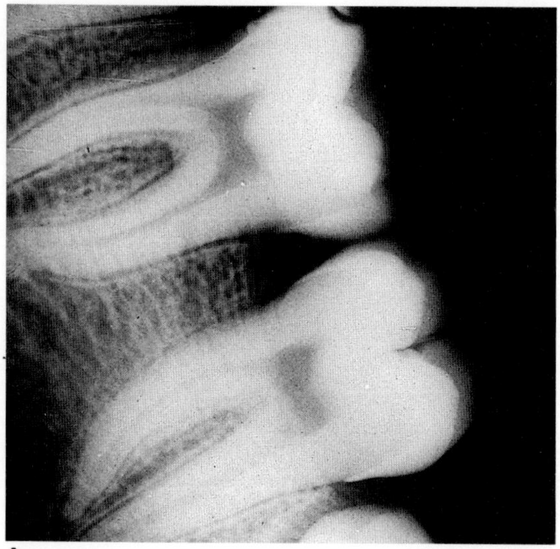

A

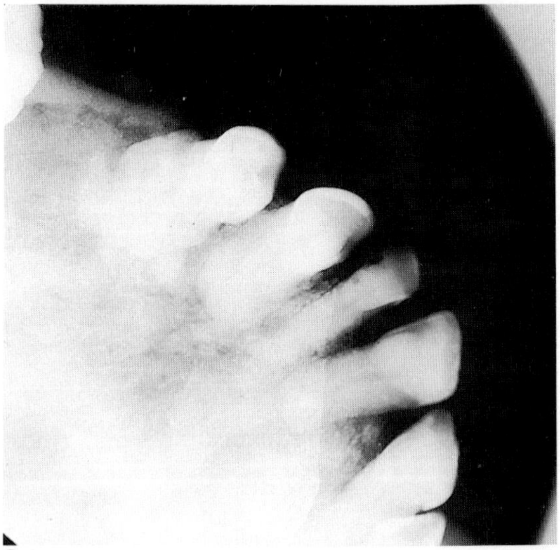

B

Figure 3.46

Radiographs of normal (A) and pagetic teeth (B). The pagetic teeth show marked hypercementosis. The trabecular architecture of the alveolar bone is anarchic and the lamina dura is lost.

may resemble granulomata in radiographic appearance. Trabecular markings may be accentuated and a cotton wool appearance of the alveolar bones is a later phase. The lamina dura is generally lost. The most striking radiographic appearance is hypercementosis (Figure 3.46), and the cementum shows the characteristic mosaic appearance on histological examination (Plate 12).

Table 3.17 Frequency of long-bone involvement assessed by scintigraphy in 197 patients with a total of 1287 lesions.

Long bone	*No of patients*	*% all patients*	*No of lesions*	*% all lesions*	*% skeletal weight*
Femora	97	49.2	128	9.9	10
Tibiae	50	25.4	53	4.1	8
Humeri	33	16.8	41	3.2	6
Clavicles	10	5.1	14	1.1	1
Radii	8	4.1	11	0.9	4
Fibulae	6	3.0	6	0.5	4
Ulnae	5	2.5	5	0.4	4

Long bones

The frequency of long-bone involvement is shown in Table 3.17. The femur is the most commonly involved long bone. As might be expected from a random distribution of foci, the frequency decreases in proportion to the long-bone volume (Dickson et al, 1945; Table 3.17). An exception may be the clavicle which is more frequently involved than might be predicted on this basis and often bilateral. It is of interest that, in some series, Paget's disease of the humerus is seen significantly more frequently on the right than the left and the same may be true of the femur (Schmorl, 1932; Guyer, 1981; Meunier et al, 1987; Shirazi et al, 1974; Ziegler et al, 1985). This

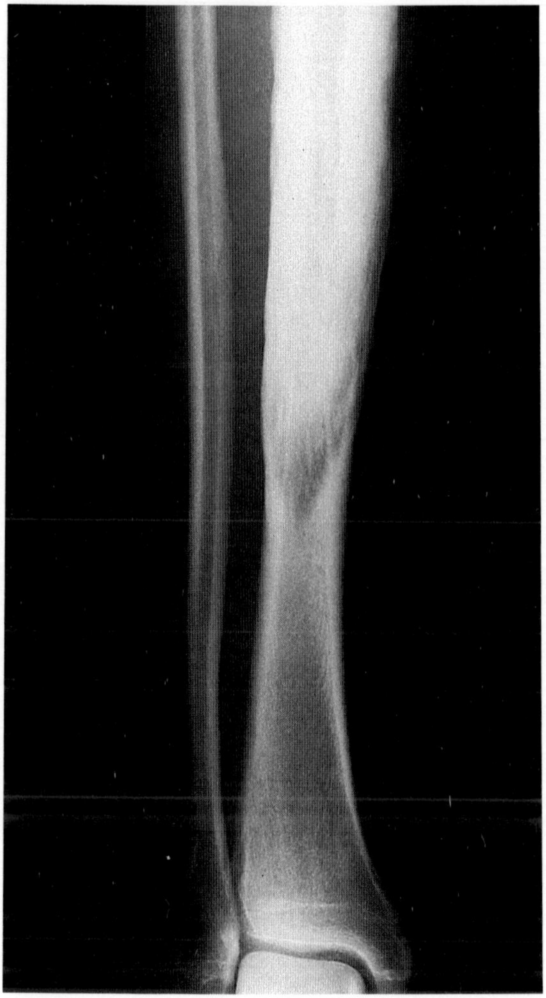

Figure 3.47

Anteroposterior radiograph showing characteristic v-shaped resorption front at the mid-tibial region. The bone below is normal. Note that the proximal tibia has become markedly sclerotic several centimetres behind the resorption front.

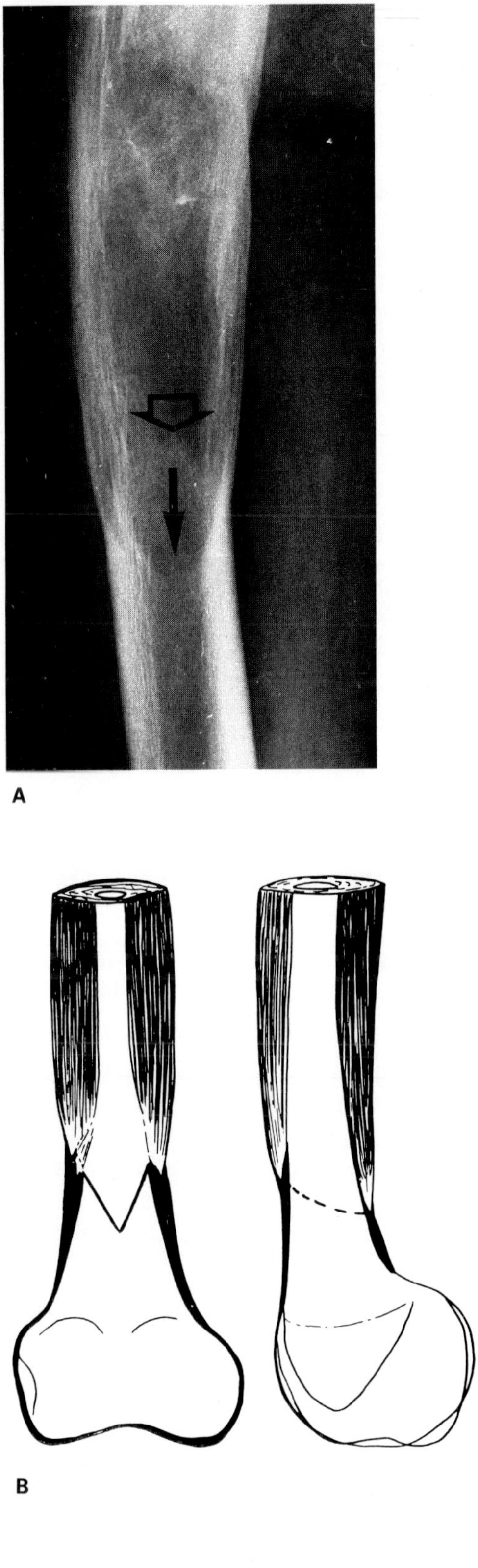

Figure 3.48

Features of the resorption front. The radiograph (A) of the femoral diaphysis shows the sharp distinction between the resorption front and normal bone distally. Note also the marked intracortical resorption and diaphyseal expansion. The double shadows (arrowhead) indicate the asymmetric advance as depicted in the line drawings (B) (From Maldague and Malghem, 1989.)

suggests that the distribution is not entirely random, at least in its laterality. In our own series of patients, however, we find no evidence for laterality at these (Table 3.11) or any other site.

The classic radiographic feature of early Paget's disease is the advancing resorption front variously described as a v-shaped lesion, the arrow sign, blade of grass appearance, etc (Ravault et al, 1970; Figures 3.47 and 3.48). The appearance is due to the asymmetry of cortical extension of the disease. In the tibia, the advancing tip is most commonly found on the anterior aspect, whereas in the femur it is on the posterior cortex (Maldague and Malghem, 1987). Thus, the v-sign is visible on anteroposterior radiographs of tibial films, but appears as an oblique line on lateral views (Figures 3.47 and 3.49).

The osteolytic lesion commonly begins as a single focus at the end of a long bone or at an apophysis such as the greater trochanter or tibial tubercle. In the femur, tibia and humerus the site is much more commonly proximal than distal. Occasionally a central or several multicentric foci are observed, but this is most unusual (Guyer, 1981; Schubert et al, 1984). The rate of advance in individuals is very reproducible so that it can be used to monitor treatment (Doyle et al, 1974a; Stuart, 1977; Maldague and Malghem, 1987) or to estimate the duration of the disease. The rates of advance vary somewhat between patients, ranging from 7.5 to 15 mm/year (Figures 3.49 and 3.50). In younger patients the rate of advance is more rapid and we have observed rates of up to 20 mm/year. In osteosclerotic disease, the rate of advance is slower (Stuart, 1977). In some patients extension of disease does not appear to occur at all (Woodhouse et al, 1977b).

The resorption front often, but not invariably, involves both cortical and trabecular bone. Early resorption fronts may be limited to intracortical, endosteal or subperiosteal bone and are not necessarily associated with changes in skeletal contour. Radiographically, they may appear as small linear cortical clefts parallel to the long axis of the bone (Figure 3.51). Such lesions are generally visible on bone scans (Vellenga et al, 1984b, 1985a) indicating that bone formation is occurring. As discussed in Chapter 2, the reasons for the radiographic osteolysis are related to the increase in bone turnover. Within the area of translucency behind the resorption front the remaining trabeculae may either be accentuated or lose their definition. The area of translucency may be extensive so that as the advance occurs, the whole of the affected bone remains osteopaenic (Figure 3.50). More commonly, patchy areas of sclerosis or lysis are visible with variable degrees of accentuation of cortical and trabecular architecture. There may be loss of differentiation of the inner cortical margin (Figure 3.50) or accentuation with intracortical striation (due to tunnelling resorption).

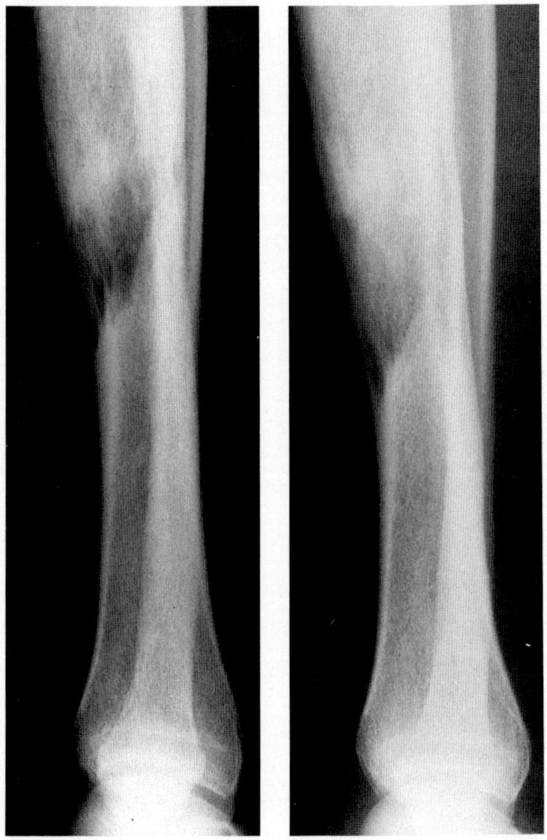
A B

Figure 3.49

Lateral radiograph of tibia to show the advance of the resorption front. (B) taken 42 months after (A) shows an advance of 12 mm/year.

As cortical extension proceeds, the outer diameter of the long bone may remain unchanged

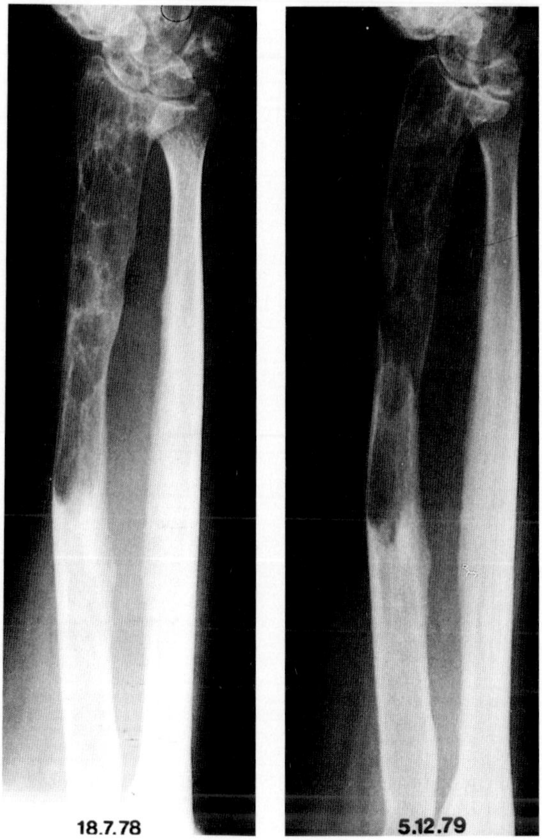

Figure 3.50

Radiographs of the forearm showing progressive involvement of the radius. The rate of advance was 15 mm/year.

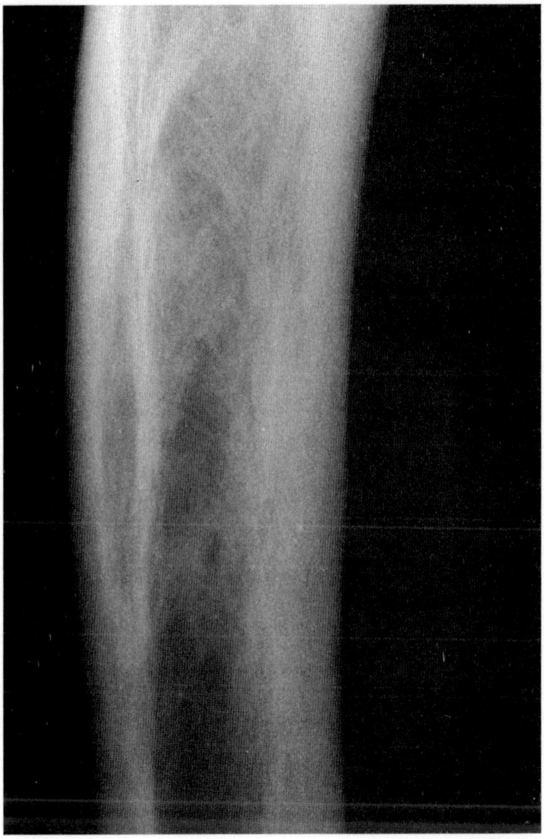

Figure 3.51

Intracortical resorption cleft of the tibia.

(Figure 3.52) or be associated with net periosteal apposition (Figure 3.53). Commonly, the external diameter increases in size, but some time later, to give a secondary expanding resorption front several centimetres distant from the resorbing front (Figure 3.54). Sometimes marked periosteal apposition occurs at the site of the primary resorption front and is associated with endosteal net resorption. This gives rise to a cystic or club-shaped appearance and is a particular feature in younger patients (Figure 3.53). Such patients are at high risk from fracture when this affects weight-bearing bones such as the tibia or femur. More characteristically, an increase in circumference of bones is associated with focal areas of osteosclerosis and cortical thickening. The various permutations of periosteal and endosteal changes have been discussed in Chapter 2.

A resorption front confined to trabecular bone may not be visible on radiographic examination but probably does occur. The finding of pagetic lesions with trabecular thickening but without visible changes in cortical bone supports this view.

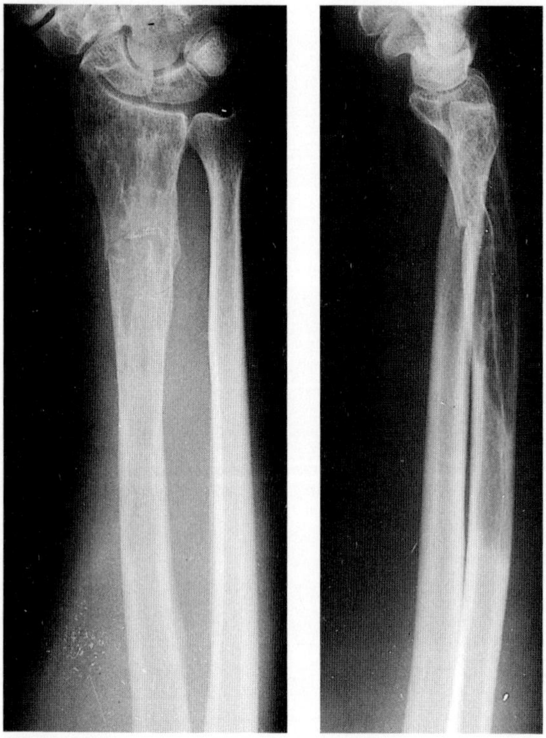

A B

Figure 3.52

Anteroposterior (A) and lateral (B) radiograph of the forearm. Note the presence of two resorption fronts visible on the lateral film. Note also that the width of the affected bone is not increased, but that the apparent cortical width has decreased.

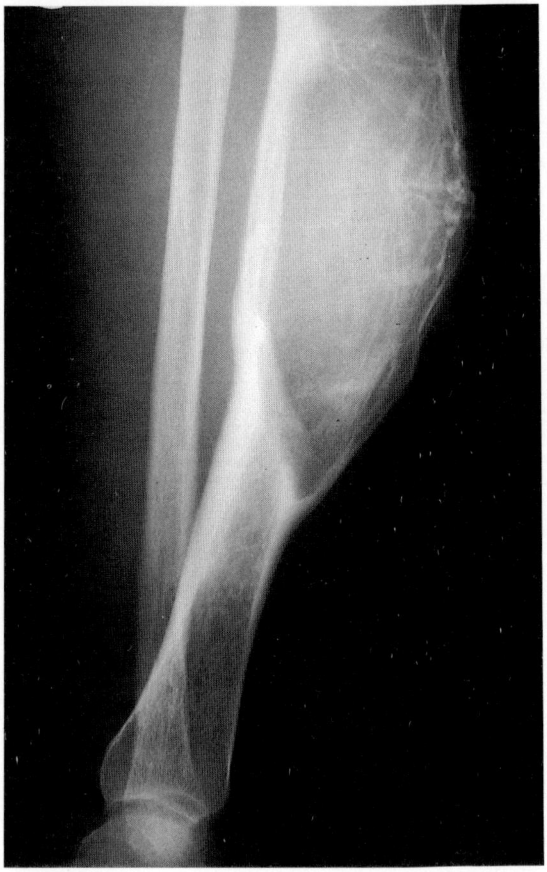

Figure 3.53

Lateral radiograph of the tibia to show the resorption front. Note the net periosteal apposition which is occurring at the front to cause bony enlargement (compare Figure 3.50). A fissure fracture is seen at the most convex aspect of the deformed tibia. There is marked thickening of the concave (posterior) cortex.

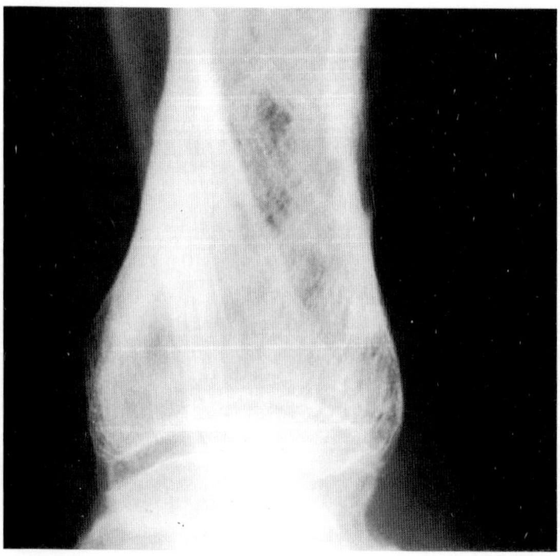

Figure 3.54

Lateral radiograph showing the lower tibia entirely affected by Paget's disease. Bony expansion is occurring in a distal direction with a secondary extending front.

The long bones may increase in length, and this increases the mechanical difficulties in weight-bearing joints. Progressive deformity with anterior bowing of the tibia and lateral bowing of the femur are characteristic. This has been attributed to 'softening of the bones', but this explanation seems somewhat naive. It seems more likely that progressive deformity is related to abnormalities in periosteal and endocortical modelling and remodelling, and an inadequate response to mechanical forces (Chapter 2).

Fissure fractures are characteristic of long-bone involvement (Figure 3.55). They are usually multiple, lying side by side, but may show various degrees of healing. They are generally indolent and appearances remain unchanged for many years. They occur in approximately 5 per cent of patients. Common sites include the femur, tibia and humerus, more frequently in the proximal half of the diaphysis. Histological studies suggest that these are true fractures (Schmorl, 1932) and therefore quite distinct from Looser's zones. In addition, fissure fractures are only seen in pagetic bone which makes their distinction from Looser's zones straightforward. They are characteristically present on the convex surface in patients with significant deformity (Hosking, 1977) lying perpendicular to the long axis of bone (Chapter 5). Since bowing of the tibia is commonly anterior and that of the femur lateral, fissure fractures are best viewed on lateral and anterior films respectively (Figure 3.56).

The cause of fissure fractures is unknown. In some patients deformity is associated with the preferential buttressing of the concave cortex, and with endosteal resorption and thinning of the convex cortex. When this occurs, the likelihood of stress fractures may be increased due to the cortical thinning (see Figure 3.53). Fissure fractures are not always associated with bowing deformity and do not always occur through osteopaenic bone. Indeed, the bone may be markedly osteosclerotic. In such cases it is possible that turnover rates are low, increasing the risk of fatigue damage.

Fissure fractures may give rise to complete fractures. This occurs more frequently at the femur and the tibia than at the humerus. They may also extend through the width of the cortex and further extension may be associated with a visible increase in the size of the crack, particularly on weight-bearing X-rays (Figure 3.57). A minority of fissure fractures extend and are obvious potential sites for fracture (Figure 3.58). Most fissure fractures remain for many years and the majority are asymptomatic. Callus formation may be seen which walls off the boundary where fissures breach the external or internal cortical surface. This may give rise to a scalloped radiographic appearance on these surfaces leaving the unhealed fracture in situ (Figure 3.59). Careful radiographic positioning is required since small degrees of rotation may give the impression of walling off (Figure 3.60) and with larger degrees they may not be visible at all (Figure 3.56).

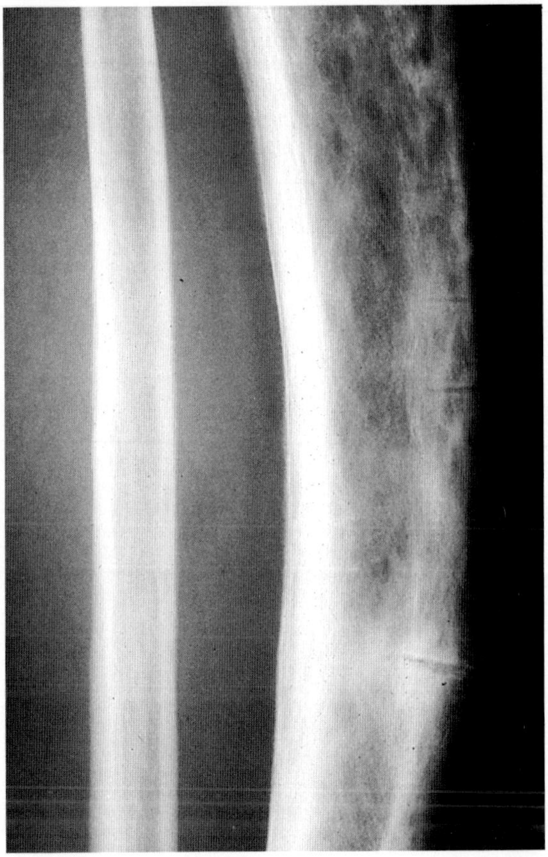

Figure 3.55

Characteristic fissure fracture on the anterior aspect of the tibia.

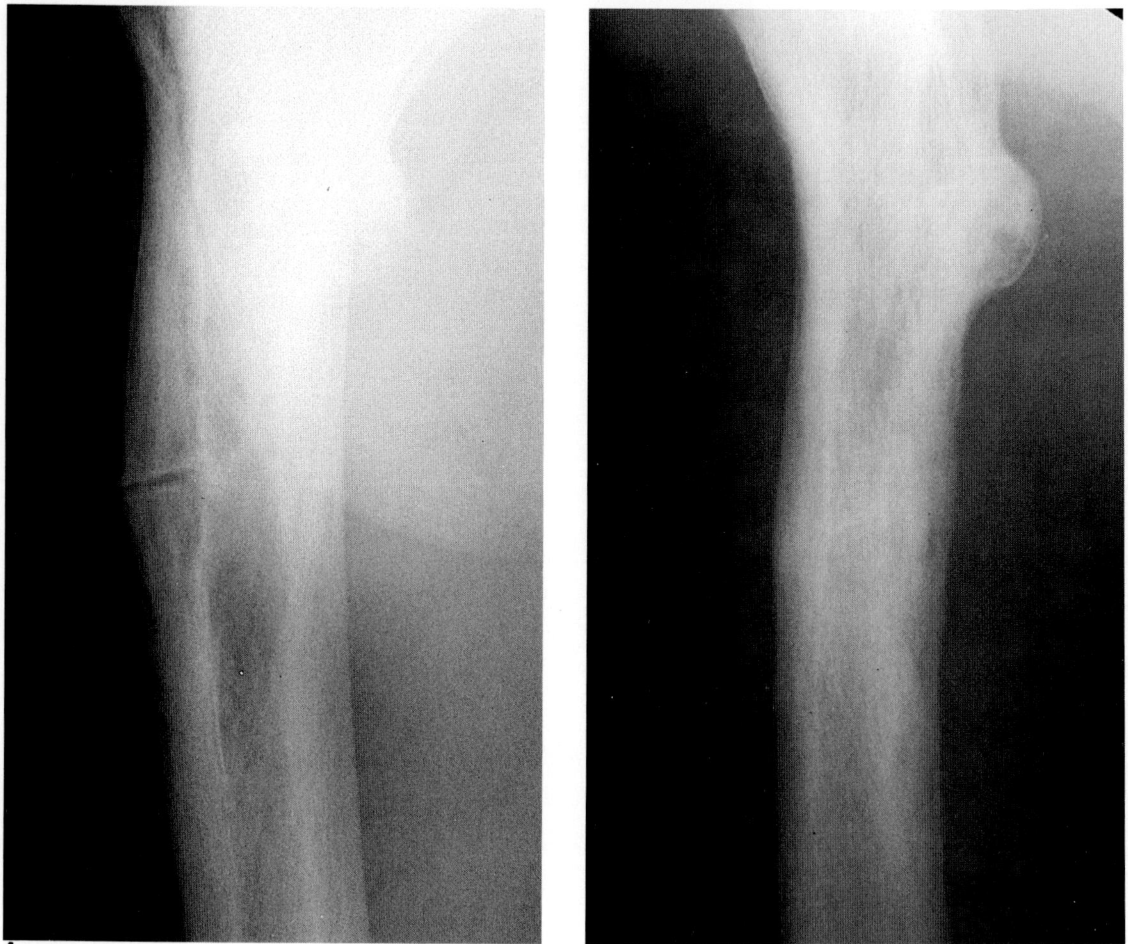

A B

Figure 3.56

Anteroposterior (A) and lateral (B) radiographs of the proximal femur. A fissure fracture is evident on (A) but is not visible on the lateral view (B).

Soft-tissue lesions like those occurring at paraspinal sites have occasionally been described adjacent to long bones (Resnick et al, 1982).

Sarcoma

The radiographic features of sarcoma are reviewed in Chapter 5.

Natural history of radiographic change

Radiographic population surveys show that the extent of skeletal involvement increases with age in both men and women (Guyer, 1981; Figures 3.61 and 3.62). In sequential studies, extensions of existing pagetic foci are well documented, but they rarely extend across joints (Doyle et al,

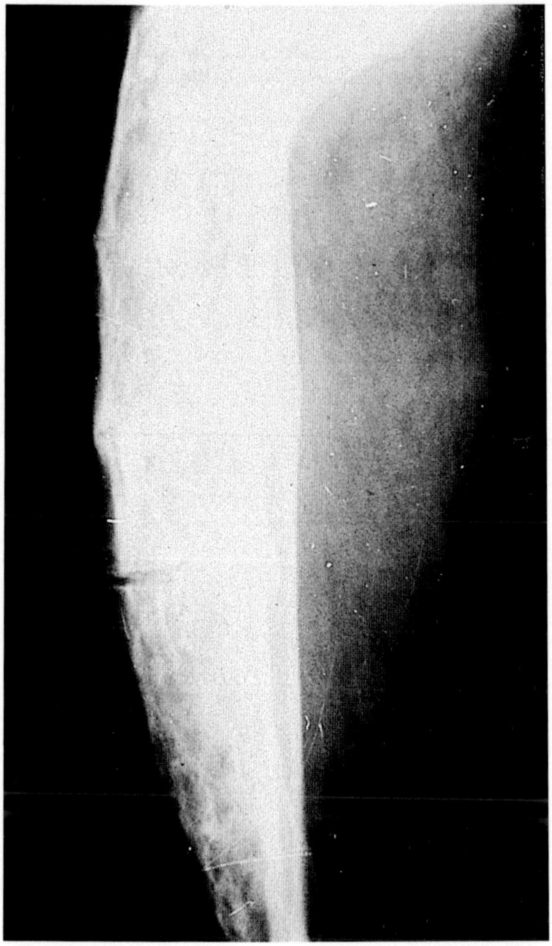

Figure 3.57

Lateral radiograph of tibia showing several asymptomatic fissure fractures. The patient developed pain at the site of a fissure fracture which has extended and is distracted on weight bearing.

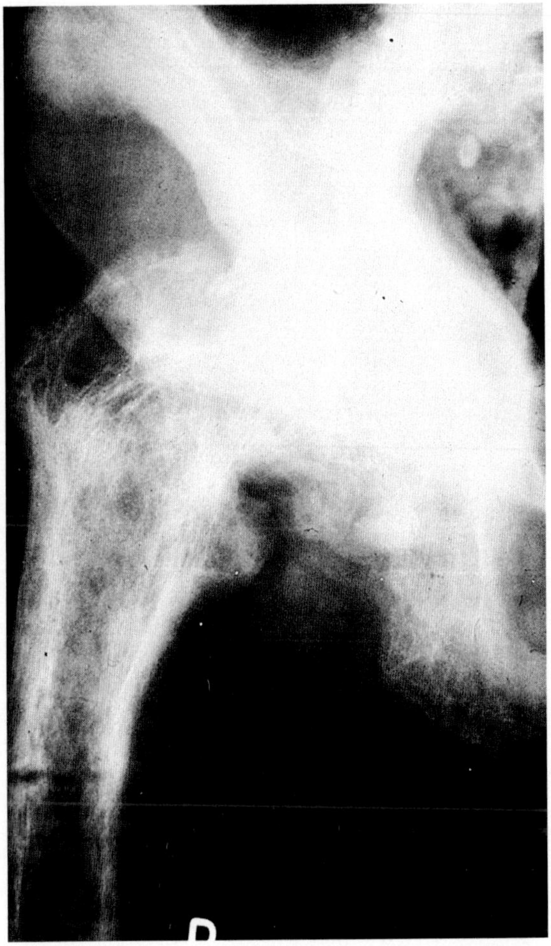

Figure 3.58

Radiograph of proximal femur. The fissure fracture has extended to involve the majority of the cortical circumference.

1974a; Guyer and Clough, 1978). Thus when a bone is completely affected the disorder becomes limited in its further extension. Long-term studies also show a progressive increase in serum alkaline phosphatase (Woodard, 1959). The rate of advance of Paget's disease is more rapid in young patients and less marked in the presence of marked osteosclerosis.

Despite much evidence for disease extension, it is remarkable how infrequently new foci of Paget's disease have been observed. Indeed, claims suggesting the appearance of new foci have not used radiography and scintigraphy concurrently and so, in view of the false-positive rates for both, they must be interpreted cautiously (Brailsford, 1954; Woodhouse et al, 1977a). In addition, pagetic foci may be visible only on microscopy without scan or X-ray abnormalities. This notion is supported by the finding that the frequency distribution of pagetic foci does not

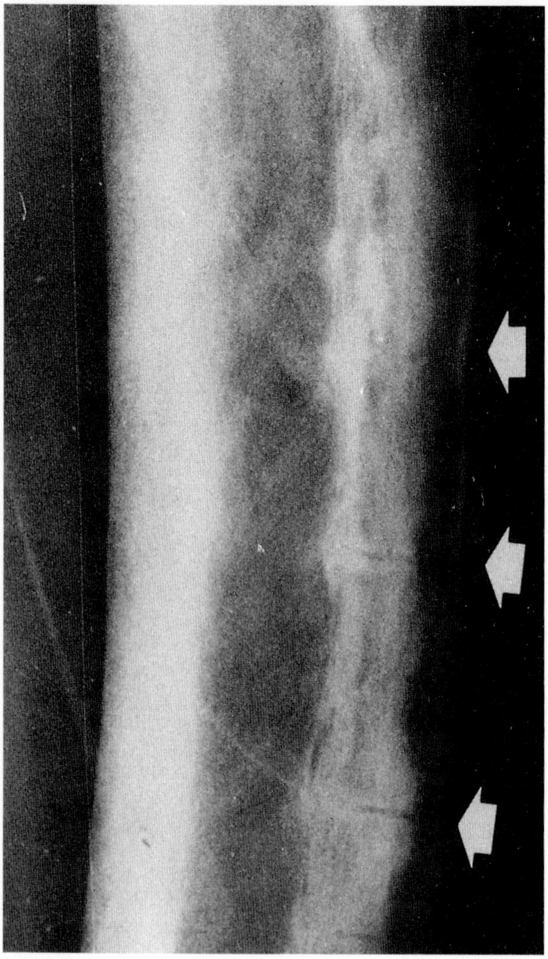

Figure 3.59

Multiple fissure fractures on the convex surface of a deformed pagetic femur. Callus formation is present on their inner aspect giving a scalloped appearance. The outer cortical aspect of the fracture appears to be buried in new periosteal bone. (From Maldague and Malghem, 1989.)

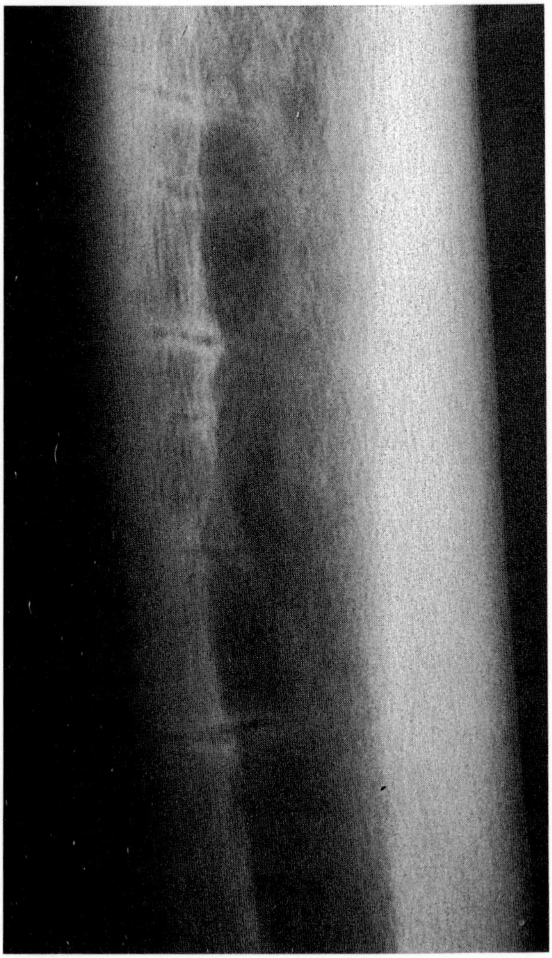

Figure 3.60

Multiple fissure fractures on the lateral aspect of the femoral shaft. The fissure fractures appear to be walled off on their outer cortical edge but this is due to rotation of the femur indicated by the fissure lines within the medullary area of the radiograph.

change with age (Harinck et al, 1986). In our own patients the extent of disease involvement increased as expected with age (Figure 3.62). The proportion of the skeleton affected is less than that reported by Guyer (1981; Figure 3.61) due perhaps in part to the more complete radiographic survey in our patients. In addition, the proportion of the skeleton affected in pagetic populations is not normally distributed, and the mean values presented here are after log-transformation. Apart from the absolute value, the data between the two surveys are comparable. Both show an apparent doubling of extent of the disease over 40–50 years. In contrast, there is

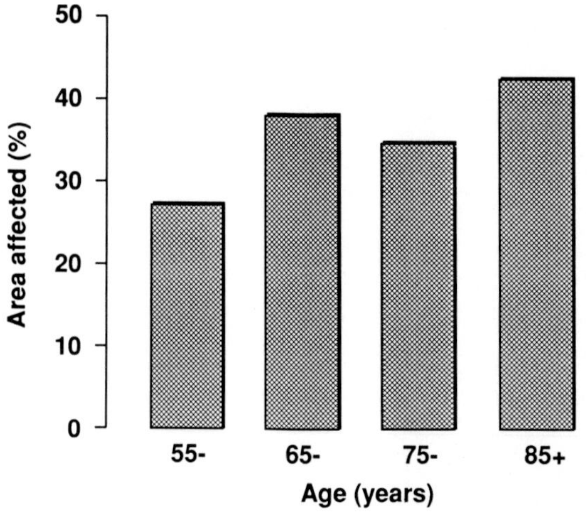

Figure 3.61

Extent of skeletal involvement in Paget's disease with age in 400 skeletal surveys.

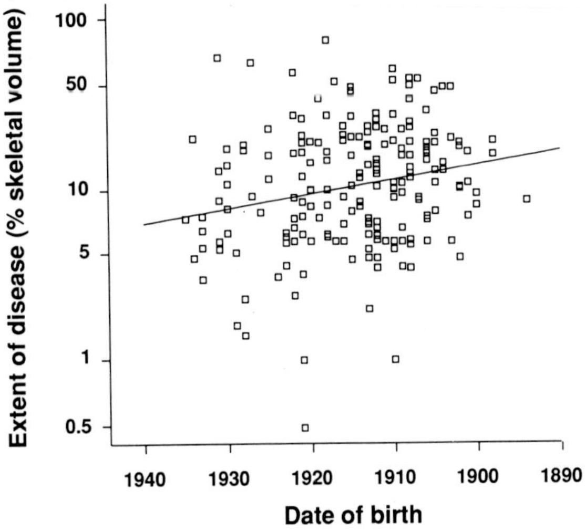

Figure 3.62

Relationship between extent of disease involvement and date of birth. There is a weak ($r = -0.21$) but significant correlation between the two variables ($p < 0.004$). The regression line suggests a two-fold increase in extent of disease over 50 years (6.3 to 15.8 per cent).

no significant correlation between the number of skeletal lesions with age. Indeed, the number of lesions appears to decrease somewhat, although not significantly, with age (Figure 3.63).

These observations suggest that although the extent of disease increases in the population, this is associated with an increase not in the number of lesions with age, but in the extent of each lesion. As discussed in Chapter 1, the pattern of disease also appears to be changing with less frequent disease at the pelvis, sacrum and upper femora, but more frequent involvement elsewhere.

These observations suggest that new foci of disease rarely occur once the disorder is established. The reasons for this may be, in part, related to the long latent period between the onset of Paget's disease and its clinical presentation. If new foci do not develop by the time patients present, this has some bearing on aetiological considerations. It suggests that abnormal osteoclasts have a relatively circumscribed domain, and at the onset of the disorder some seeding process occurred, but that reseeding is infrequent or non-existent.

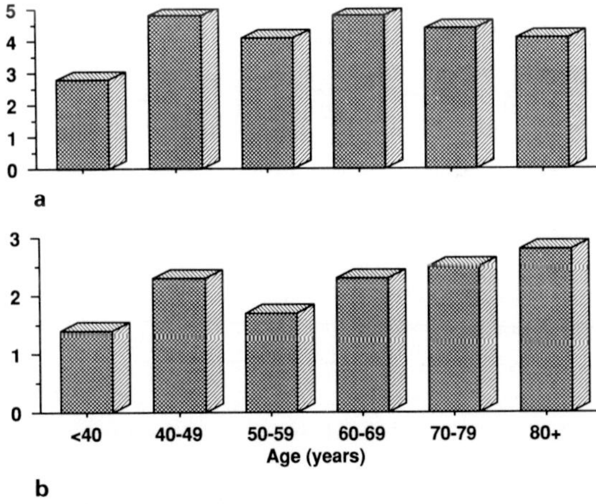

Figure 3.63

(A) The number of pagetic foci and (B) the extent of skeletal involvement (mean) in 195 patients divided by age. Note that the number of skeletal lesions does not increase with age after the age of 40, although each lesion affects a greater proportion of the skeleton with increasing age. Two young patients were omitted from the analysis, each with more than 20 lesions. If these are included, the mean number of lesions increases to 6.0 in the age group less than 40.

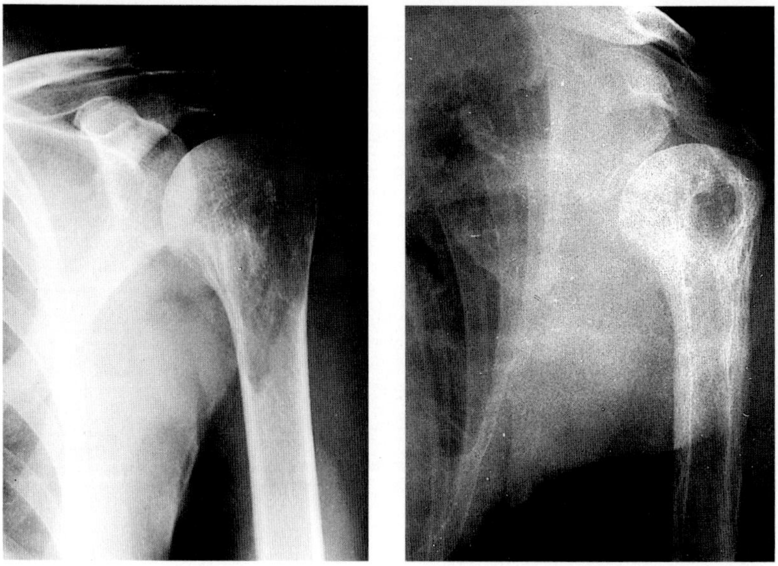

Figure 3.64

Radiographs of the humerus in a patient with Paget's disease. There is a well demarcated resorption front and osteopenia confined to the proximal humerus. Five years later (right) the proximal half of the humerus is involved and cortical thickening is apparent.

Paget's disease may extend across joints, particularly at the spine (Figure 3.29). It seems probable that this occurs in the presence of bony contact, either due to osteoarthrosis or to paravertebral osteoid. Extension of pagetic lesions into bone grafts or after arthodesis has also been described (Hartman and Dohn, 1966; Klenerman, 1966; Jaffe, 1977; Stevens, 1981).

Sequential changes in the extent of disease can be monitored by radiography. Changes over several years can be shown readily (Figure 3.64), but the demonstration of changes in the appearance of bone within lesions requires some knowledge of the natural history of radiographic appearances. This requires great attention to detail in minimizing the errors of repositioning. In the long bones small errors in rotation may have dramatic effects on the radiographic appearances (Figure 3.65). On the basis of careful radiographic studies, several groups have indicated changes which may be ascribed variously to the natural history of the disorder or to a treatment-dependent effect. These changes are discussed in greater detail in Chapter 8.

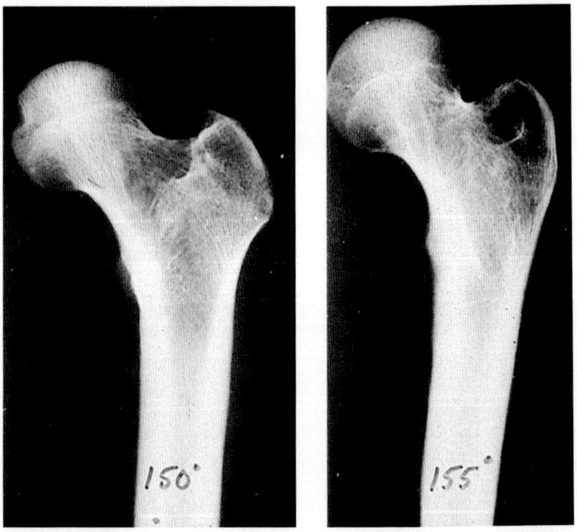

Figure 3.65

Radiograph of femoral head to show the effect of a 5-degree rotation on X-ray appearances. Note the apparent change in the density trabecular markings and medullary width.

Scintigraphy

Recent advances in bone imaging have greatly aided the identification of Paget's disease. Bone scanning agents such as ^{18}F- and ^{99m}Tc-labelled polyphosphonates or diphosphonates reveal areas of increased skeletal vascularity and turnover (Khairi et al, 1974b; Shirazi et al, 1974; Fogelman et al, 1981a). As reviewed, bone scanning is more sensitive than radiography in the detection of early disease, but unlike radiography cannot assess deformity, changes in shape nor detect the presence of fissure fractures. It is also less specific than radiography. It is of particular value in assessing the extent of disease activity (Figure 3.66).

Bone-scan appearances of Paget's disease are usually characteristic, showing markedly increased uptake of tracer which is usually evenly distributed throughout the affected sites including the resorption front. When the whole bone is affected, the visual appearance can be striking (Figure 3.67). In the mandible, this has been termed the 'black beard sign' (Mailander, 1986; Figure 3.68). In many instances the uptake in pagetic bone is sufficiently intense to differentiate this from uptake due to compression fractures, joint disease, etc. A monostotic lesion may be more difficult to interpret, but metastatic bone disease commonly shows heterogeneity of uptake and multi-centric foci within the same bone (Chapter 6).

Sarcoma in pagetic bone may affect the scan appearance. Whereas ^{99m}Tc-diphosphonate uptake is increased in osteosarcoma, the uptake is generally less intense than at pagetic sites. Thus the presence of sarcoma may cause decreased uptake at this site (see Chapter 5). In contrast, uptake of ^{67}gallium citrate is enhanced (Yeh et al, 1982) and gallium scans may be a useful adjunct to diagnosis and to monitor progress. Pagetic lesions are also enhanced (Waxman et al, 1980) and it is of interest that gallium appears to localize preferentially on osteoclasts (Mills et al, 1988a), inhibit bone resorption and is now being tested as a drug in Paget's disease (Bockman et al, 1989).

Scintigraphy is a useful initial screening test in the investigation of patients, principally because it provides adequate visualization of the whole skeleton without the necessity for multiple radiographs (Figure 3.66). Thereafter, we commonly

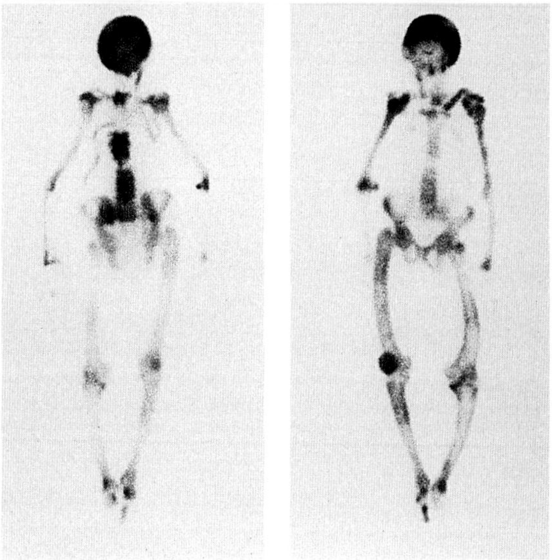

Figure 3.66

Radionuclide scan appearances in a patient with extensive uptake at the thoracic and lumbar spine and skull. Uptake is not increased at the tibia despite the bowing deformity due to Paget's disease. Note also the patchy uptake at the deformed pagetic femur. The patient had received diphosphonate treatment.

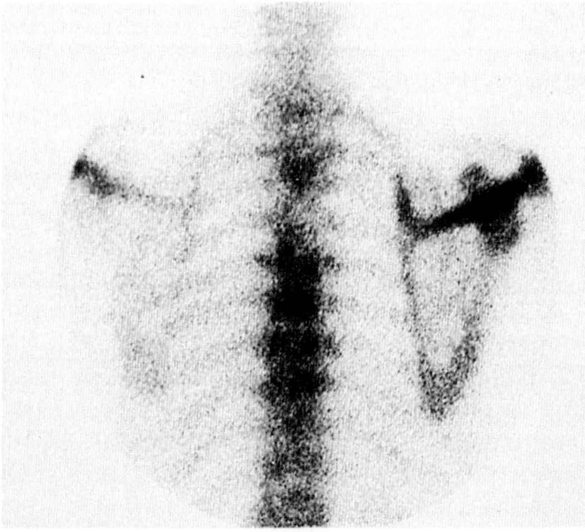

Figure 3.67

Increased scintigraphic uptake at the scapula due to Paget's disease contouring the whole bone.

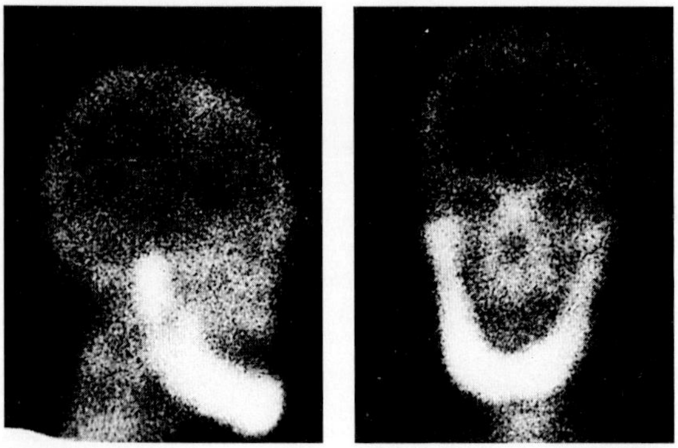

Figure 3.68

Bone scan showing marked increase in scintigraphic uptake of the jaw due to Paget's disease – the so-called 'black beard sign'.

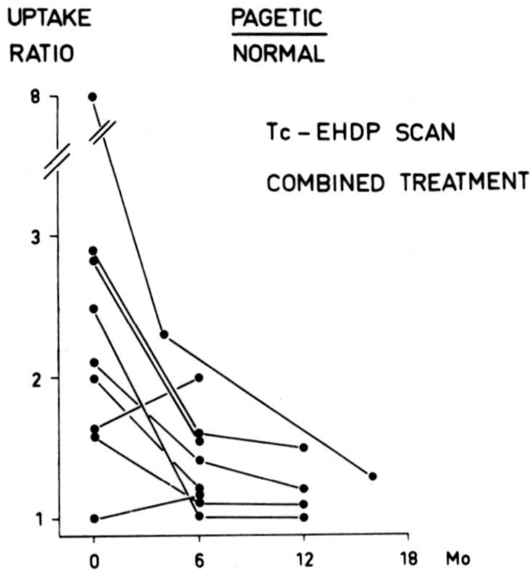

Figure 3.69

Uptake of ^{99m}Tc-etidronate assessed over a region of pagetic involvement expressed as a ratio to the uptake over an equal area on the contralateral unaffected site. The uptake ratio can be utilized to monitor treatment. The nine patients shown above received a combination of etidronate and calcitonin which decreased the uptake ratio towards normal. (From Bijvoet et al, 1977.)

X-ray affected sites to look for evidence of lysis, stress fracture, joint involvement and deformity, since their presence may influence subsequent treatment. Scintigraphy can also be used to monitor treatment, particularly in patients with less extensive disease in whom biochemical indices of disease activity lie within the laboratory reference range.

Scintigraphic appearances may change with time as the disease progresses. There is not invariably an increase in the extent or intensity of uptake and decreased uptake may also occur in apparently untreated patients without any perceptible change in radiographic appearance (Merrick and Merrick, 1985). New scintigraphic foci, rather than extension, have been reported occasionally (Merrick and Merrick, 1985; Vellenga et al, 1981, 1982), but may not represent new foci of disease. Prior treatment, particularly with diphosphonates, may have marked effects on the distribution of scan uptake due to variable degrees of relapse within foci (Figure 3.66). Also some sites may relapse whereas others remain quiescent. There is generally a good correlation between relapse judged by scintigraphy and other estimates of disease activity, but because relapse may be heterogeneous, particularly after diphosphonate treatment, there are many exceptions to this generalization.

Several methods have been devised to quantitate scintigraphy which generally depend either on the uptake of tracer at specific sites or on the extent of pagetic involvement. The former have been widely used to evaluate the effects of treatment. Semiquantitative methods have been utilized (for example Vellenga et al, 1984a, 1985b) which score the intensity of focal uptake (Table 3.18). Alternatively, scan uptake can be measured by quantitating uptake in defined areas of interest. This presents many technical difficulties, but is more readily standardized in Paget's disease affecting the appendicular skeleton, where uptake at one site can be compared utilizing the unaffected side as a control (Figure 3.69). There are small differences in the skeletal uptake of various scanning agents. As in the case of radiography, care is required to obtain reproducible results.

Table 3.18 Scintigraphic system used to score pagetic lesions. A scintigraphic index for each lesion is multiplied by the fraction of the skeleton affected. The sum of all scores for all lesions provides a semiquantitative scintigraphic index.

Score	*Pagetic site*	*Adjacent normal bone*
1	As normal	Well visualized
2	Barely distinguished	Well visualized
3	Slightly increased	Well visualized
4	Moderately increased	Well visualized
5	Marked uptake	Poorly visualized
6	Marked uptake	Not visualized

The extent of disease as assessed by scintigraphy generally bears a close relationship to biochemical estimates of disease activity such as serum activity of alkaline phosphatase and urinary hydroxyproline excretion (Chapter 4; Khairi et al, 1973; Henley et al, 1979; Salson, 1981; Harinck et al, 1986). Since there is a close relationship between the extent of skeletal involvement and the number of pagetic foci, the latter also correlates with biochemical indices of disease activity (Figure 3.70).

There is a very close relationship between scintigraphic index and the extent of disease activity (Figure 3.71). Indeed, use of the index (to describe the focal degree of uptake as well as its extent) contributes little to the scintigraphic assessment of anatomical extent alone (<8 per cent). This supports the view that bone-cell activity is relatively constant in the untreated disorder and that the biochemical indices reflect more the extent of activity rather than variable degrees of activity.

There has been some interest in the measurement of whole-body retention of diphosphonates as an integrated index of metabolic activity (Smith et al, 1984b). In the case of Paget's disease there is a very striking correlation between whole-body retention and biochemical estimates of disease activity (Chapter 4), suggesting that this technique does not offer advantages over routine biochemistry for monitoring the disorder.

Since the diphosphonates are used with increasing frequency in the management of Paget's disease, the question arises as to whether apparent improvements in scintigraphy are related to a decrease in metabolic activity or a skeletal saturation with the therapeutically-administered diphosphonate. The latter would

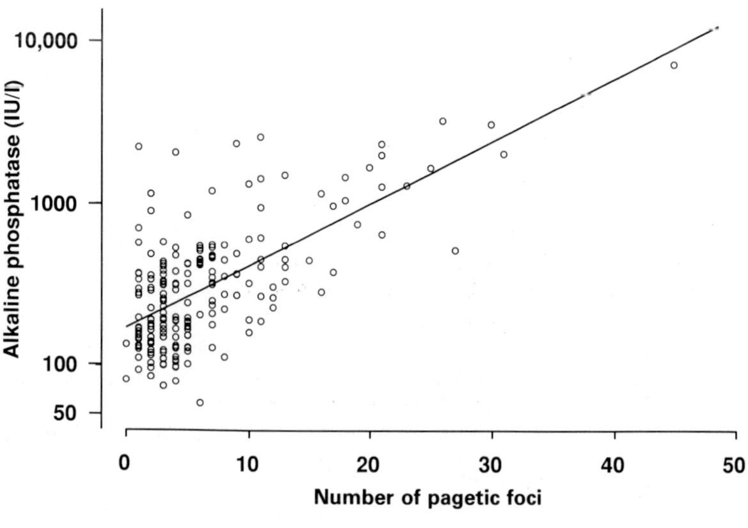

Figure 3.70

Relationship between the number of sites affected by Paget's disease and serum activity of alkaline phosphatase ($r = 0.66$).

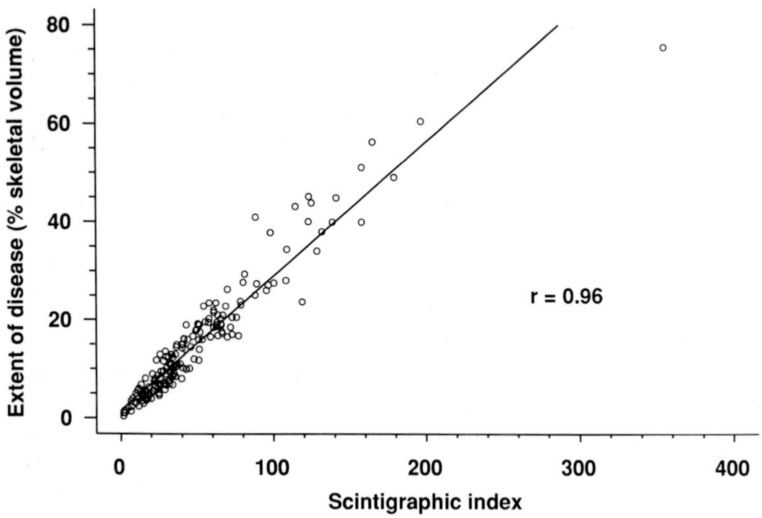

Figure 3.71

Relationship between scintigraphic index and extent of skeletal involvement. Note that 92 per cent of the variance in the relationship (r^2) is accounted for by the extent of the disease.

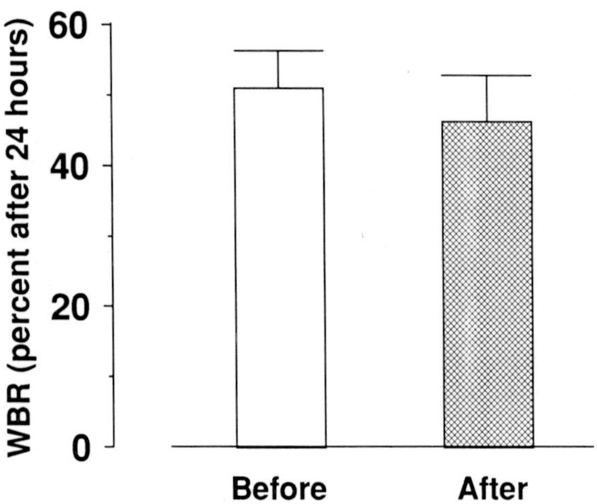

Figure 3.72

Effect of diphosphonate treatment on whole-body retention (WBR) of diphosphonate. Ten patients were given 1500 mg of clodronate iv over 5 days. Mean diphosphonate retention (51.1 ± SEM 5.3) did not change significantly after treatment (46.3 ± 6.6).

artificially suppress apparent activity. This seems to be unlikely for two reasons. In the first place, the relationship between disease activity measured independently by biochemical tests and scintigraphy does not alter during the course of diphosphonate treatment (Smith et al, 1984b). Second, the whole-body retention of diphosphonates is not decreased when patients are loaded with very large intravenous doses of diphosphonates over a short period of time before any changes in bone formation or blood flow are apparent (Figure 3.72). The doses of diphosphonate given under these circumstances are equivalent to those normally given during several weeks of treatment. Theoretical calculations suggest that it would take 13–130 years to saturate all skeletal sites, depending on the dose of diphosphonate used.

Other radiographic techniques

Nuclear magnetic resonance has not yet been widely applied in the evaluation of Paget's disease, except for sarcomatous transformation (Chapter 5). It is likely to be of value at sites where soft tissues may be disrupted by the disorder such as the skull and spine (Tjon-A-Tham et al, 1985).

A variety of other techniques have been developed for skeletal assessment. These include computed axial tomography, single and dual photon absorptiometry, dual-energy X-ray absorptiometry and ultrasound attenuation of bone. CT scanning is particularly useful for the visualization and assessment of neurological syndromes (Figure 3.73 and see also Figure 3.34), spinal and cranial stenosis, facet arthropathy (Zlatkin et al, 1986) and bone tumours (Seret et al, 1987; Figure 3.74). Subtraction of sequential CAT images may be used to follow the natural history or treatment of the disorder (Bone et al, 1989; see further Chapter 8).

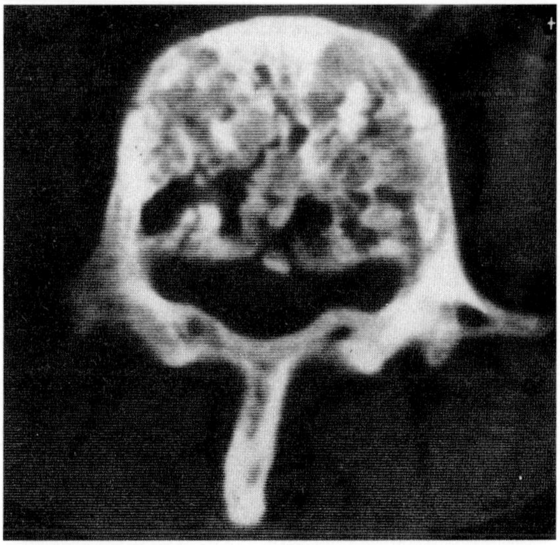

Figure 3.73

Computerized axial tomogram at L3 showing marked narrowing of the vertebral canal, increased cortical thickness and dedifferentiation of the cortico-trabecular bone interface. (From Maldague and Malghem, 1989.)

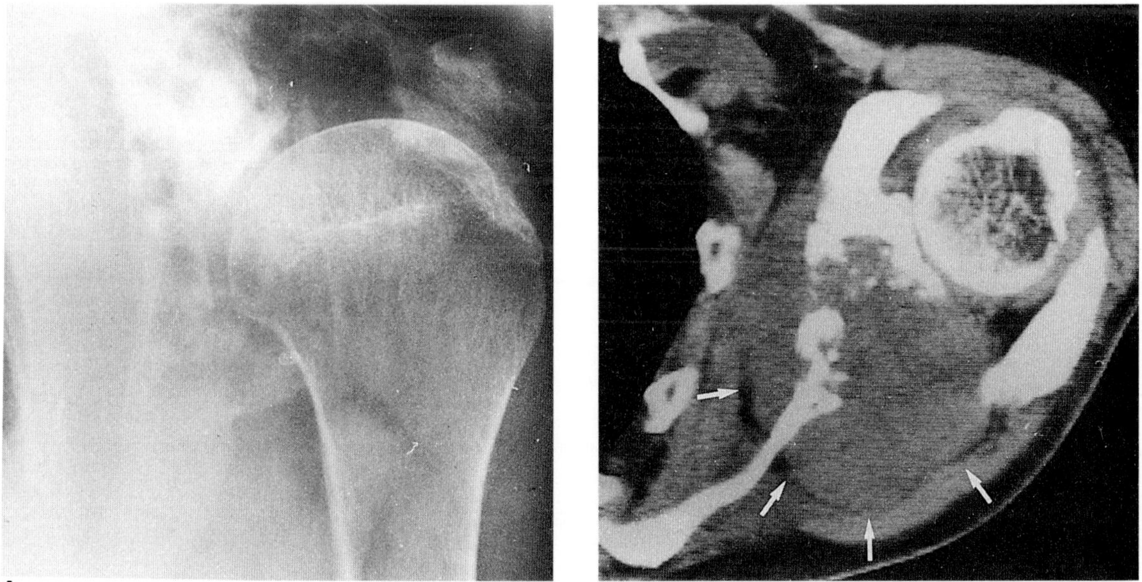

A B

Figure 3.74

Sarcomatous change in Paget's disease of the scapula. The marked soft-tissue extension is more evident on computerized axial tomography (B). (From Maldague and Malghem, 1989.)

Skeletal blood flow

Increased vascularity of bone is a marked feature of Paget's disease, and several techniques have been developed to assess this in man. The early phase of the bone scan is dependent on blood flow and may change rapidly following treatment (Boudreau et al, 1983). The uptake of ^{18}F has been specifically applied in Paget's disease. Following its intravenous injection, radiofluorine is rapidly taken up into hard tissue and provides an index of skeletal blood flow when allowance is made for renal clearance. Such techniques demonstrate that resting total skeletal blood flow is markedly increased. In health, up to 6 per cent of blood flow is delivered to the skeleton, whereas this can be increased to up to 40 per cent in patients with extensive disease. As expected, there are significant correlations between bone blood flow and biochemical indices of disease activity (Wooton et al, 1978; Figure 3.75). The technique has also been used to monitor treatment. It is of particular interest that treatment for only 7 days with calcitonin is capable of inducing falls in skeletal blood flow in excess of any change in serum activity of alkaline phosphatase (Wooton et al, 1981). This has some relevance to therapeutics where the rapid control of bone blood flow may be desirable as an adjunct to orthopaedic surgery.

Thermography

An increase in temperature of the skin overlying the site of involvement can be detected in many patients with Paget's disease. This has been attributed to an increase in bone blood supply, but skin blood flow is also increased. The extent to which these are independent is unknown. Thermography, particularly of the tibia, has been utilized to assess response to treatment and skin temperature decreases, for example, during treatment with calcitonin (Ring et al, 1977; Plate 13). It is of interest that those patients with tibial Paget's disease and the more marked thermographic appearances complain of pain more frequently than others.

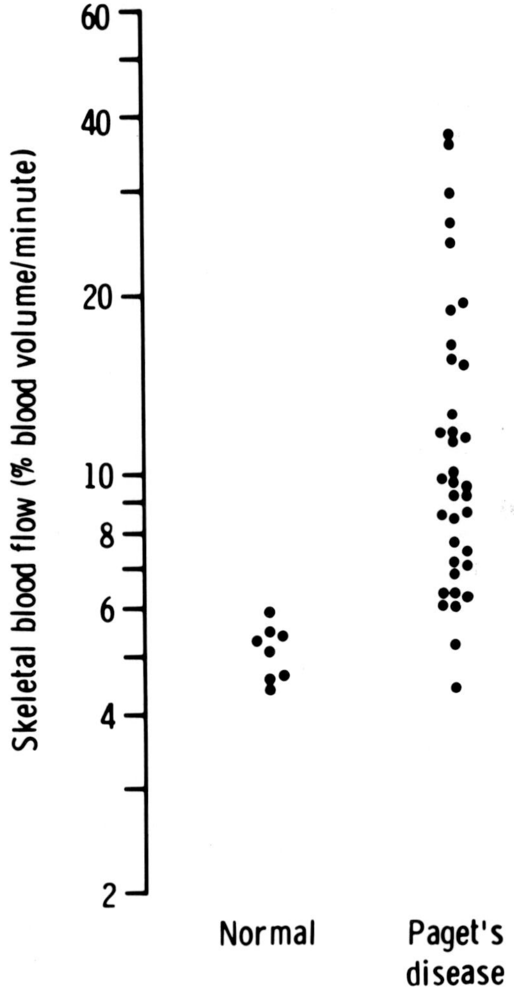

Figure 3.75

Skeletal blood flow measurements in normal subjects and in untreated patients with Paget's disease. Note the logarithmic scale. (From Wooton et al, 1981.)

CHAPTER 4

Biochemical and endocrine aspects of Paget's disease

Indirect markers of skeletal metabolism provide a valuable tool for the diagnosis and assessment of patients, and also for the evaluation of treatment. In contrast to focal assessment of disease by bone histology, scintigraphy and radiography, biochemical markers of disease activity provide an integrated index, if not of the activity of the underlying disorder, then of its extent. Because bone is composed of an organic matrix and a mineral phase, and because all elements of bone turnover are augmented in Paget's disease, disease activity has been assessed in terms of calcium metabolism, collagen turnover and indices of the functional activity of bone cells themselves.

Extracellular calcium metabolism

Although the rates of bone resorption and deposition may be increased many fold, it is remarkable that in Paget's disease there is little disturbance in plasma calcium and phosphate metabolism (Harinck et al, 1986; Nagant de Deuxchaisnes and Krane, 1964). Kinetic studies using radioisotopes of calcium indicate an increase in the readily exchangeable pool of calcium and computed measurements of mineral accretion and resorption rates are both increased (Figure 4.1) (Nagant de Deuxchaisnes and Krane, 1964; Harris and Heaney, 1969a,b,c; Hosking et al, 1981; Harinck et al, 1986).

Focal impairment of skeletal balance does occur, accounting for the areas of osteolysis and osteosclerosis, but integrated rates of bone formation and resorption are generally, but not always, matched. Traditional balance studies (Nagant de Deuxchaisnes and Krane, 1964; Heaney, 1969a,b,c; Bell et al, 1970; Shai et al, 1971; Woodhouse et al, 1971; Kanis et al, 1975) indicate that calcium balance is close to zero and that it seldom fluctuates by more than 5 mmol/day. This would suggest that total skeletal, and therefore total body calcium is close to normal. Such a conclusion is supported by estimates of total body calcium which are similar to normal subjects (Spinks et al, 1982).

Serum calcium values are determined in part by the rates of flux of calcium to and from the extracellular fluid. Major sites of exchange are the gut, kidney and bone which are influenced by the major calcium-regulating hormones, parathyroid hormone, calcitriol and possibly also calcitonin. With some exceptions, discussed later, calcium and phosphate values in serum are usually normal, as are urinary measurements (Table 4.1). This reflects the close matching of calcium accretion and resorption rates in bone, and the integrity of normal homeostatic mechanisms (Figure 4.2).

Fasting urine samples commonly show an increase in the calcium/creatinine ratio, even though the daily excretion rate of calcium is normal (Figure 4.3). High fasting urinary excretion

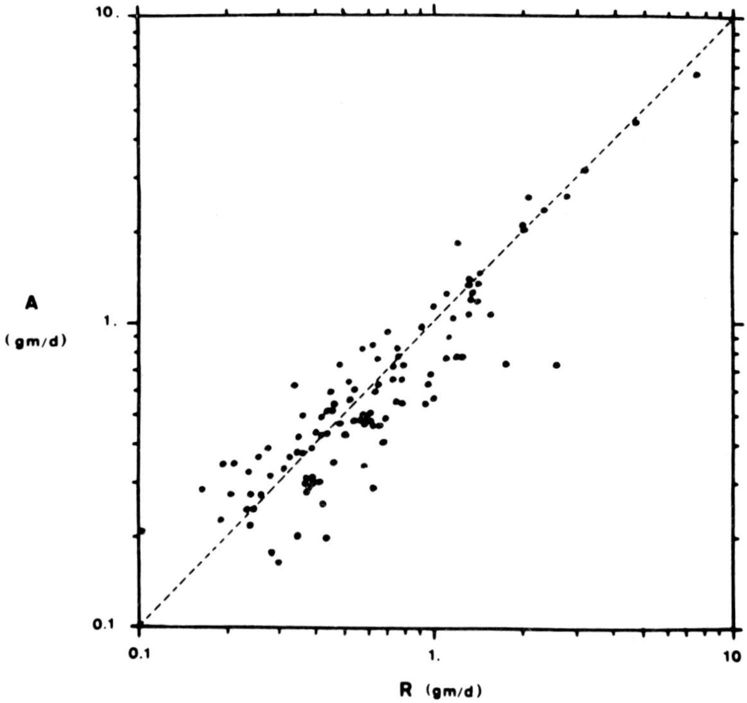

Figure 4.1

The relationship between the rate of mineral accretion (A) and resorption (R) in patients with a variety of metabolic bone disorders including Paget's disease (the higher values). Note the logarithmic scales for accretion and resorption and the close correlation between these measurements even when resorption rates are increased 20-fold. The dotted line represents the line of identity. (From Harris and Heaney, 1969a.)

Table 4.1 Clinical details and biochemical measurements (mean ± SEM) in untreated patients with Paget's disease stratified according to serum activity of alkaline phosphatase. Patients were allocated to the high disease activity group when serum alkaline phosphatase exceeded 285 IU (50 per cent of patients).

	Disease activity		*p*	*Reference range*
	High	*Low*		
Sex (M:F)	42:57	37:61	NS	
Age at diagnosis (years)	67.9 ± 1.1	68.2 ± 1.0	NS	
Family history of Paget's disease	19	8	<0.05	
Number of pagetic lesions	9.2 ± 0.8	3.8 ± 0.3	<0.0001	
Alkaline phosphatase (IU/l)	599 (549–642)†	156 (151–161)†	—	30–105
Urinary hydroxyproline (mmol/mol creatinine)	111.3 (103.5–119.6)†	41.9 (40.2–43.7)†	<0.0001	<40
Urinary calcium (mol/mol creatinine)	0.31 ± 0.02	0.29 ± 0.02	NS	<0.4
Serum calcium (mmol/l)	2.42 ± 0.01	2.43 ± 0.01	NS	2.41 ± 0.15*
Serum phosphate (mmol/l)	1.15 ± 0.01	1.14 ± 0.01	NS	0.6–1.5
Serum PTH (pmol/l)	57.4 ± 2.1	51.1 ± 2.1	NS	<100
Serum pCol1c (μg/l)	109 (94–127)	189 (149–240)	<0.001	
ESR (mm/hour)	15.6 ± 1.3	14.8 ± 1.5	NS	
Serum urate (μmol/l)	367 ± 17	369 ± 21	NS	M<500 F<440

*Age- and sex-matched values from hospital controls.
†SEM computed from log-transformed data.
NS: not significant.

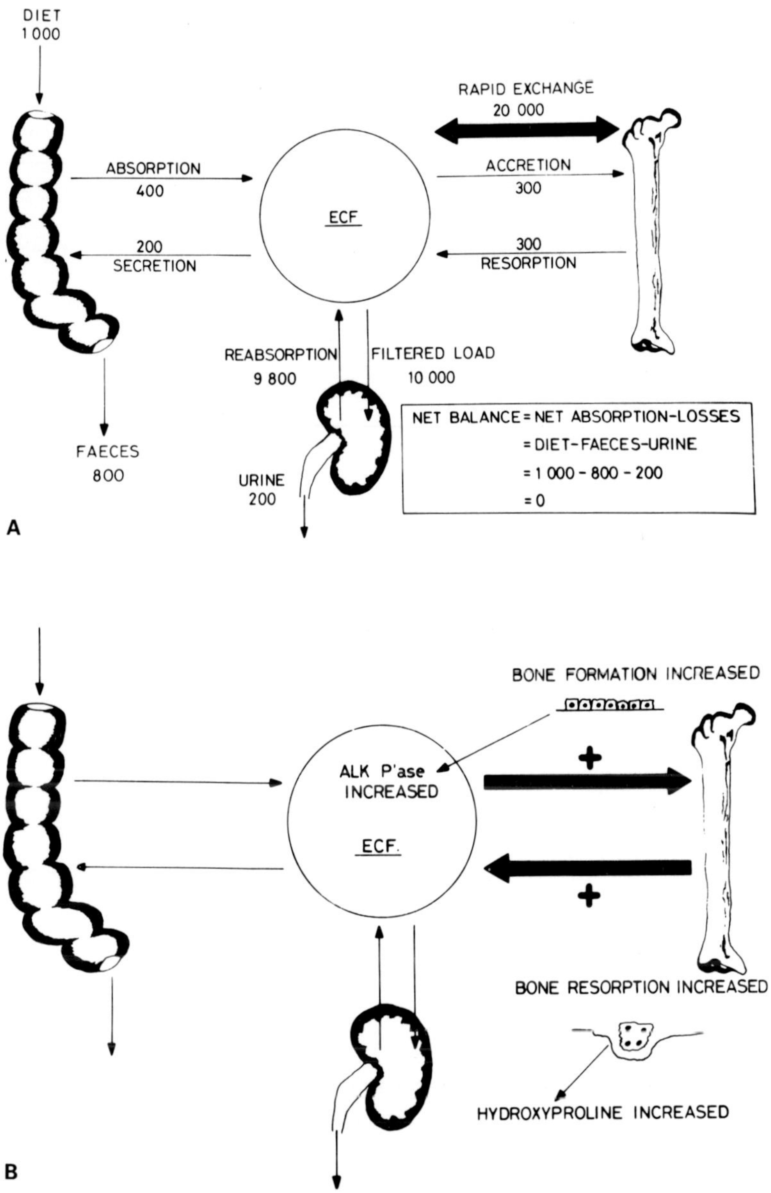

Figure 4.2

(A) shows the major fluxes of calcium (mg/day) in the normal adult. (B) shows the changes in Paget's disease of bone. Bone formation and resorption are increased but there are no major changes in flux across gut or kidney, nor changes in plasma calcium.

rates are found in one-third of the patients when compared with age-matched hospital controls. In the post-absorptive (that is, fasting) state the contribution of the gut to calcium excretion is minimized, and the ratio of calcium to creatinine excretion more closely reflects the net flux of calcium from bone to the extracellular fluid (Kanis et al, 1980). Thus, increased fasting calcium excretion suggests increased bone resorption, suppressed formation or both. It is possible that the high fasting calcium excretion in Paget's disease might be a consequence of overnight immobilization. Bone formation is inhibited and resorption is characteristically increased during

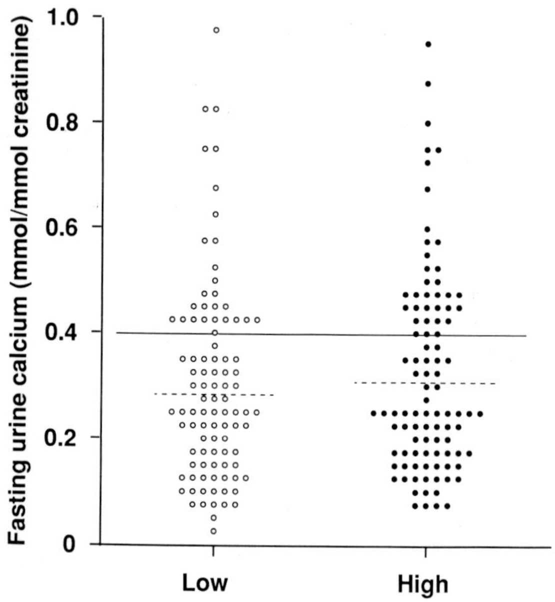

Figure 4.3

Fasting urinary excretion of calcium (expressed as a ratio of urinary creatinine excretion) in 197 patients with Paget's disease. The patient population was split into half according to their serum activity of alkaline phosphatase. There was no difference in mean excretion (dotted lines) between the two groups, nor in the prevalence of fasting hypercalciuria (>40 mmol/mmol; 27 vs 31 per cent in the low- and high-activity group respectively).

immobilization. Because pagetic bone is responsive to immobilization, and because of the accelerated bone turnover, the demands on extracellular calcium homeostasis may be amplified. The lack of difference in fasting calciuria between patients with extensive or more modest disease suggests that this view may be an oversimplification (Table 4.1 and Figure 4.3).

Immobilization hypercalciuria, and more rarely hypercalcaemia, occur in Paget's disease with prolonged immobilization for similar reasons as those discussed above (Nagant de Deuxchaisnes and Krane, 1964; Lawrence et al, 1973; Figure 4.4). Bone resorption is accelerated and the amount of bone formed at each remodelling site is decreased (Minaire et al, 1987), and the pagetic process amplifies the effects of these changes on serum calcium homeostasis. Accelerated bone resorption normally occurs around fracture sites and this too is amplified in Paget's disease (see Chapter 5). For this reason hypercalcaemia has been reported after fracture even in the absence of immobilization.

Immobilization hypercalcaemia is more marked in the presence of primary hyperparathyroidism. Since primary hyperparathyroidism and Paget's disease are relatively common disorders, the two may often occur by chance. In our own experience the majority of pagetic patients with hypercalcaemia have been found to have primary hyperparathyroidism on further investigation. It has been claimed that both renal calculi and primary hyperparathyroidism are found more frequently in patients with Paget's disease (Posen et al, 1978; Hamdy, 1981; Harinck et al, 1986), but the data are inconclusive (Nagant de Deuxchaisnes et al, 1964) and the associations may be no higher than one might expect by chance for common conditions.

Parathyroid function

In patient populations mean serum values for PTH are normal (Kanis et al, 1977; Harinck et al, 1986) but several recent studies suggest that a significant minority of patients have elevated values of PTH despite normal plasma concentrations of calcium (Chapuy et al, 1981; Russell et al, 1981; Siris et al, 1989). The prevalence of hyperparathyroidism in the presence of normocalcaemia ranges from 5 to 25 per cent of patients, and a combined estimate is 12 per cent (Chapuy et al, 1981; Russell et al, 1981; Salson, 1981; Harinck et al, 1986).

The reason why some patients have high values of PTH is not known. It is possible that some patients have parathyroid adenomas, but remain normocalcaemic because the increased fluxes across bone can offset the tendency to hypercalcaemia. An alternative and perhaps more likely explanation is that increased PTH secretion is secondary to hypocalcaemia induced by a slightly greater rate of mineral deposition compared with the rate of mineral resorption. Two

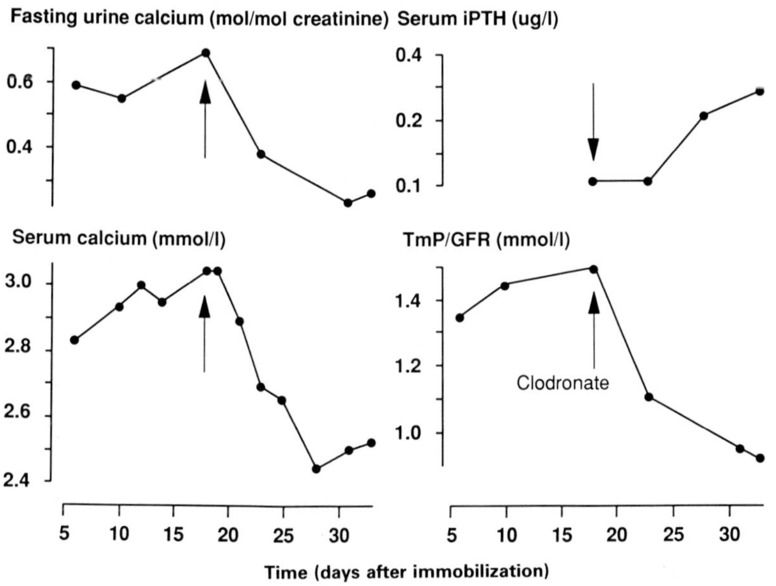

Figure 4.4

Effect of immobilization and fracture on serum calcium in a patient with Paget's disease. The increase in serum calcium was associated with an increase in net bone resorption, as judged by fasting urinary calcium. The rise in estimated renal phosphate threshold was presumed to be a consequence of the calcium-induced suppression of parathyroid hormone (iPTH). These abnormalities reversed with treatment with an inhibitor of bone resorption (clodronate 800 mg daily).

series have shown that patients with the higher PTH values have lower values for serum calcium (Chapuy et al, 1981; Siris et al, 1989). These abnormalities are all consistent with mild secondary hyperparathyroidism arising from an increase in net calcium losses from the extracellular fluid compartment to bone. The notion is attractive in that it can explain the mild increase in bone turnover noted in pagetic patients and uninvolved skeletal sites (Meunier et al, 1980).

In our own studies we had found a high prevalence of hyperparathyroidism (25 per cent), a finding confined to patients with the more extensive disease (Figure 4.5). If the stimulus to hypersecretion of PTH was hypocalcaemia due to increased delivery of calcium to bone, then hypocalcaemia and a low fasting urinary excretion rate for calcium would be expected consequences. We found no such differences when patients were divided into those with high or low disease activity. In addition, we found no difference in serum calcium between patients with high and normal values for PTH (Figure 4.6). In contrast, the estimated renal tubular resorption of

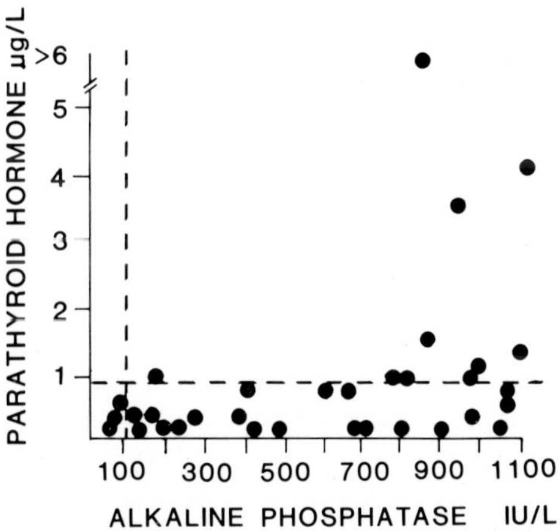

Figure 4.5

Relationship between serum activity of alkaline phosphatase and immunoreactive parathyroid hormone in 33 untreated patients with Paget's disease. Dotted lines denote the upper limit of the reference range. Note that high values of parathyroid hormone were confined to patients with the most marked disease activity. (From Russell et al, 1981.)

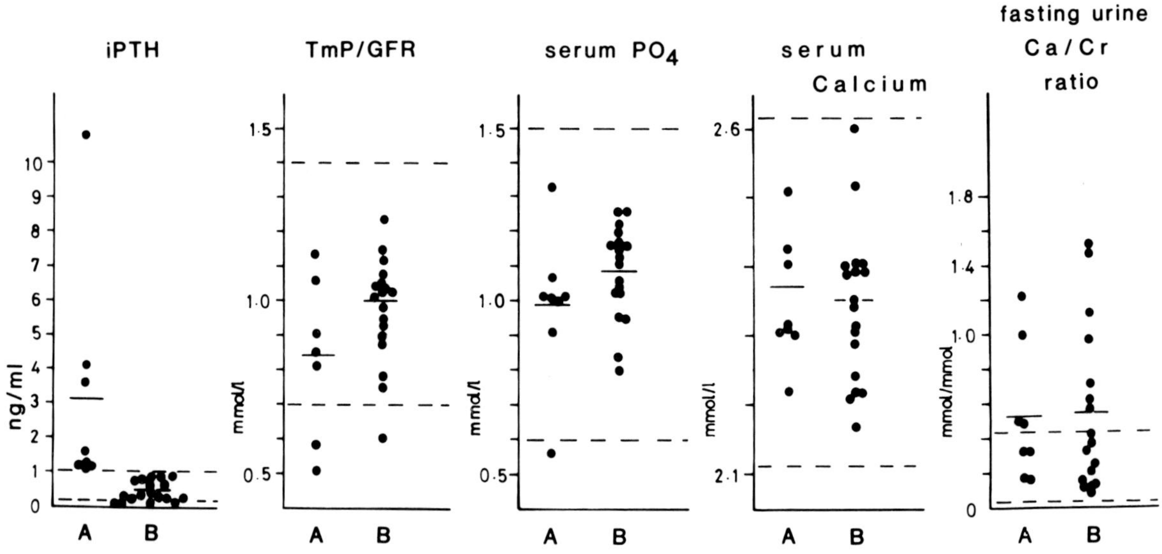

Figure 4.6

Biochemical measurements in untreated patients with Paget's disease divided by their serum values for immunoassayable PTH. Patients with iPTH values greater than normal (A) had lower serum phosphate concentrations (PO_4) and renal tubular reabsorption of phosphate (TmP/GFR), than patients with normal values for PTH (B). There were no differences in serum or fasting urinary calcium.

phosphate is lower in the patients with hyperparathyroidism, indicating that PTH is exerting biological effects, at least on the kidney. This suggests that the notion that hypocalcaemia is the stimulus to hyperparathyroidism is an oversimplification.

Irrespective of the cause of hyperparathyroidism, one consequence seems to be accelerated turnover at non-pagetic sites (Chapter 2). The consequence of mild secondary hyperparathyroidism on disease activity is not known, but it is clear that Paget's disease can be expressed in the absence of PTH and has, for example, been reported in a patient with hypoparathyroidism (Genuth and Kline, 1972).

A recent survey of ours has shown no difference in basal values of PTH between patients with high and low disease activity. Moreover, PTH values were consistently within the normal range (Table 4.1). The assay measured intact PTH, whereas other studies have used region-specific assays. Since we find no differences in serum calcium and phosphate, TmP/GFR or calcium excretion, this suggests that hyperparathyroidism is uncommon in our current population.

Calcitonin

Serum values for calcitonin appear to be normal in Paget's disease (Kanis et al, 1977; Figure 4.7). Studies of its endogenous secretion rate suggest that its rate of production and metabolic clearance are also normal (Kanis et al, 1982; Figure 4.8). For these reasons Paget's disease is not due to calcitonin deficiency. It is of interest that calcitonin is one of the major drugs used to treat

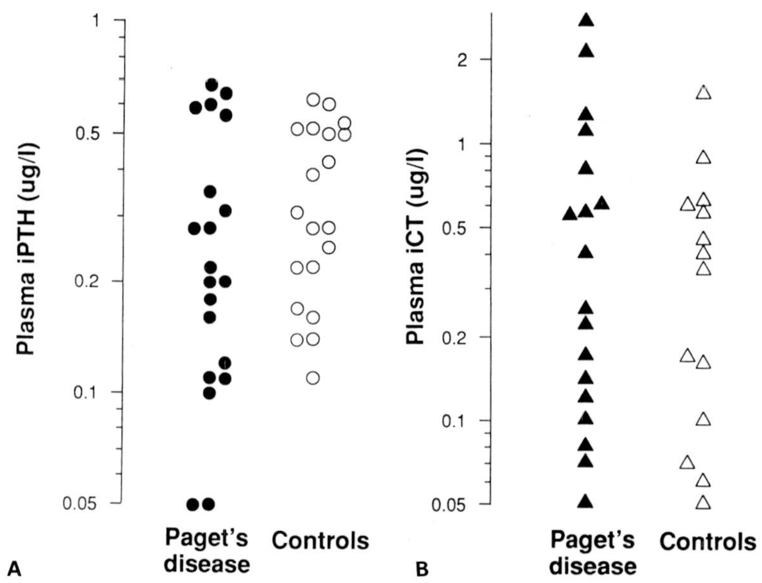

Figure 4.7

Plasma levels of parathyroid hormone (A) and calcitonin (B) in control subjects and patients with Paget's disease. (After Kanis et al, 1977.)

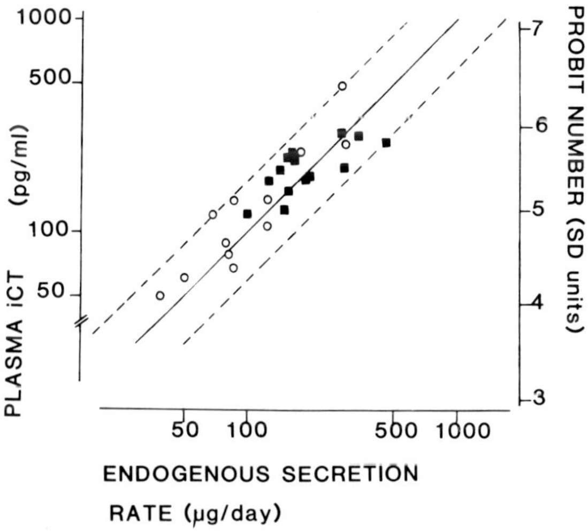

Figure 4.8

Relationship between metabolic clearance rate (MCR), plasma calcitonin (iCT) and endogenous secretion rate for calcitonin. The diagonal lines denote the normal range (± 2SD). There is no difference in endogenous secretion and plasma values between normal subjects (○) and patients with Paget's disease (■). (From Kanis et al, 1982.)

Paget's disease, and the question arises whether pagetic bone cells might have impaired sensitivity to endogenous calcitonin. The acute responses of patients and normal subjects to low doses of calcitonin suggest that this is not so (Chapter 7), but the acute calcitonin test measures a hypocalcaemic response to calcitonin and is at best an indirect test of the sensitivity of osteoclasts to calcitonin.

The daily doses of calcitonin used in therapeutics for Paget's disease are generally 50 IU or greater. This compares with a daily secretion rate of 13 units or less (Kanis et al, 1982). It is now clear that relatively low doses of calcitonin, close to the endogenous production rate, are capable of decreasing bone turnover, for example in osteoporosis (Reginster et al, 1987; Overgaard et al, 1989). These doses are, however, inadequate to suppress bone turnover in patients with Paget's disease except those with near normal disease activity (Chapter 7). These considerations suggest that the therapeutic effects of calcitonin in Paget's disease are pharmacological.

Vitamin D

In the absence of co-existing vitamin D deficiency, serum values for calcifediol (25-hydroxyvitamin D; 25-OHD) and calcitriol (1,25-dihydroxyvitamin D; 1,25$(OH)_2D_3$) are normal (Guilland-Cumming et al, 1985; Harinck et al, 1986; Lawson-Matthew et al, 1988). It is of interest that low values of 24,25$(OH)_2D_3$ have been reported principally in patients with increased disease activity (Guilland-Cumming et al, 1985; Figure 4.9). As with PTH, this is probably a consequence of the disorder rather than a causal factor, and indeed treatment with 24,25$(OH)_2D_3$ (secalciferol) and the restoration of serum values to normal has no effect whatsoever on disease activity (Haining et al, 1987).

In contrast to the modest changes in calcium metabolism found in untreated patients, treatment of Paget's disease can induce marked transient changes, both in extracellular calcium homeostasis and in the major calcium-regulating hormones (these are reviewed in detail in Chapter 7).

Other hormones

A number of other hormones are known to alter the activation of bone remodelling. These include the thyroid hormones, gonadal steroids, adrenal corticosteroids and growth hormone. No abnormalities in growth hormone, cortisol or in thyroid hormones have been observed in patients with Paget's disease; neither do values change with treatment of the disorder (Walton, 1978). There are some analogies between the hyper-remodelling of Paget's disease and abnormal skeletal metabolism in other disorders such as hyperparathyroidism and thyrotoxicosis in which increased bone remodelling also occurs. Few of the histological features of pagetic bone are specific to Paget's disease and many may merely reflect the vastly accelerated rate of bone remodelling. The focal nature of the disorder demands a focal cause, but it is possible that bone cells might be more susceptible to physiological modulators of skeletal turnover of which an increasing array are being identified (Canalis et al, 1989). As for the major calcium-regulating hormones there is no convincing evidence for abnormalities in the secretion of hormones thus far examined.

Alkaline phosphatase

Plasma alkaline phosphatase is the most frequently used and probably the most useful biochemical marker for Paget's disease. The alkaline phosphatase is thought to be derived from osteoblasts, but the mechanism for its release into the extracellular fluid is uncertain. It is possible that alkaline phosphatase is released by dying osteoblasts at the end of their life span, or that there is constant shedding of alkaline phosphatase attached to plasma membranes throughout the life-time of active osteoblasts. There is some experimental evidence from studies of bone cells in tissue culture that such phenomena can occur.

The function of alkaline phosphatase is also unclear (Whyte, 1989). It is an ectoenzyme, since the catalytic sites face towards the exterior of the cells. A suggested function is that it is involved in calcium and phosphate transport. A possible extracellular substrate is inorganic pyrophosphate, a known inhibitor of calcification. Studies in hypophosphatasia, for example, have shown high plasma values of pyrophosphate, which may be the result of the decreased amounts of alkaline phosphatase normally present on cell surfaces (Whyte, 1989).

In health about half of the alkaline phosphatase measurable in plasma is derived from bone, the rest coming mainly from the liver. The bone and liver enzymes differ only in their post-translational modification. There may also be contributions to the plasma from the intestine and other tissues, including the placenta in pregnancy. These different isoenzymes may be measured by semiquantitative techniques based on electrophoresis, chemical or heat inactivation or immunological methods, but the separation of

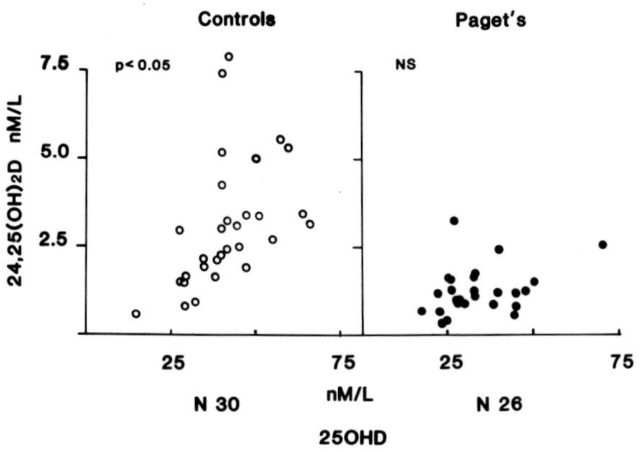

Figure 4.9

Relationship between serum 25-hydroxyvitamin D (25OHD) and 24,25-dihydroxyvitamin D (24,25(OH)$_2$D$_3$) in healthy subjects (left) and patients with Paget's disease. Note the correlation between values for the two metabolites in control subjects. In patients with Paget's disease values for 24,25-dihydroxyvitamin D are significantly lower for the prevailing level of 25OHD.

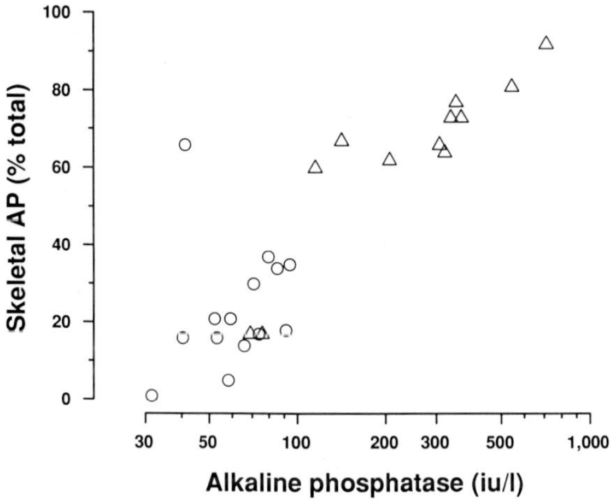

Figure 4.10

Relationship between total and skeletally-derived alkaline phosphatase in normal subjects (○) and patients with Paget's disease (△). Note that the contribution of non-skeletal sources to total phosphatase activity decreases with increasing disease activity. (Parvainen, McCloskey and Kanis, unpublished work.)

skeletally-derived phosphatase is imperfect. Complete resolution of the isoenzymes by anion exchange high pressure liquid chromatography has recently been described (Parvainen et al, 1988).

In Paget's disease the increment in total activity of alkaline phosphatase is attributable to an increase in the bone isoenzyme (Figure 4.10). As the extent of disease activity increases the proportion of skeletally-derived phosphatase in the circulation increases (Table 4.2) and, for this reason, it is only rarely necessary to undertake isoenzyme studies in Paget's disease. Moreover, other methods exist to exclude significant contributions from extraskeletal tissues such as the liver, for example by measurement of 5′-nucleotidase or gammaglutamyl transferase.

The turnover of bone alkaline phosphatase in the circulation is rapid and the half-time lies between 1 and 2 days (Figure 4.11). This suggests that changes in serum alkaline phosphatase should reflect fairly accurately the changes in osteoblast release of the enzyme (Walton et al, 1975; Posen and Grunstein, 1982). This has important implications for the assessment of responses to treatment, since failure of alkaline phosphatase to change within the first few weeks of treatment with any agent cannot be attributed

Table 4.2 Skeletal contribution to total alkaline phosphatase in health and that expected in Paget's disease of bone.

	Total alkaline phosphatase (IU/l)	*Bone-derived fraction (IU/l)*	*% bone-derived*
Healthy controls	63	25	40
Paget's disease	100	62	62
	200	162	81
	500	462	92
	1000	962	96
	500	4962	99

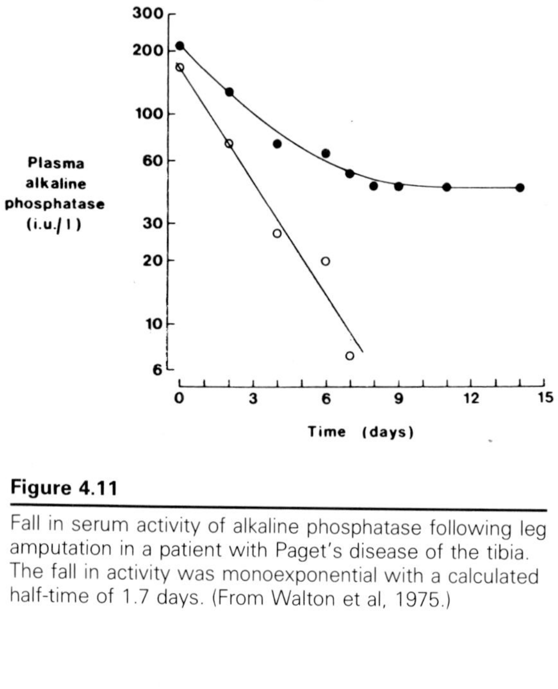

Figure 4.11

Fall in serum activity of alkaline phosphatase following leg amputation in a patient with Paget's disease of the tibia. The fall in activity was monoexponential with a calculated half-time of 1.7 days. (From Walton et al, 1975.)

to a long circulating time for the enzyme, but rather to the delayed responses of the osteoblastic cell population.

Serum activity of alkaline phosphatase measured at intervals in untreated patients remains relatively constant, but population studies in patients indicate that alkaline phosphatase values slowly increase over several years (Woodard, 1959) as does the extent of radiographic abnormalities (Guyer, 1981; Chapter 3), reflecting the progressive nature of the disease. There is a significant correlation between alkaline phosphatase measurements and the extent of skeletal involvement measured by techniques such as radiography, scintigraphy or calcium tracer kinetics (Khairi et al, 1973; Franck et al, 1974; Khairi et al, 1974; Meunier et al, 1987; Figure 4.12). There is also a very close correlation between alkaline phosphatase and urinary hydroxyproline, reflecting the close association between bone formation and bone resorption rates (Franck et al, 1974; Walton et al, 1977a; Figure 4.13).

In metabolic bone disorders serum activity of alkaline phosphatase provides an index of the number of functional osteoblasts. Indirect evidence (Chapter 2) suggests that the functional capacity of osteoblasts is normal, at least in their capacity for matrix synthesis and mineralization. It is of interest in this respect that the relationship between serum alkaline phosphatase and urinary hydroxyproline is similar but not identical in Paget's disease to that observed in primary hyperparathyroidism, a disorder also characterized by increased bone turnover. In hyperparathyroidism the urinary excretion rate of hydroxyproline is greater than in Paget's disease for any given activity of alkaline phosphatase, but the differences are small (unpublished observations). This suggests that the factors which determine the shedding of alkaline phosphatase to the extracellular fluid in Paget's disease are also likely to be normal.

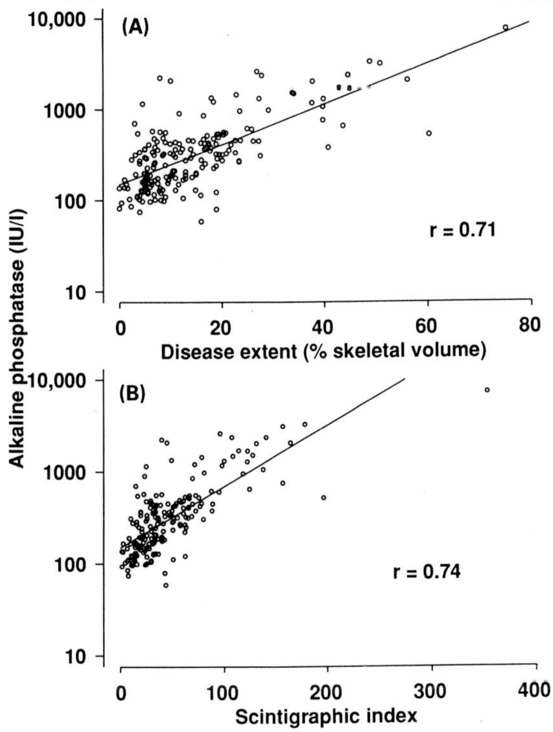

Figure 4.12

Relationship between serum activity of alkaline phosphatase with (A) the extent and (B) degree of scintigraphic uptake in untreated patients (previously unpublished).

In patients who develop osteosarcoma at sites of Paget's disease the alkaline phosphatase may rise sharply and fail to be suppressed with treatment.

When large populations of patients with Paget's disease (or normal subjects) are examined, the distribution of values for alkaline phosphatase are skewed rather than Gaussian. Analysis of the distribution of alkaline phosphatase (Figure 4.14) suggests that patients with all grades of severity of the disease show a unimodal log-normal distribution, thereby suggesting a single disease population, at least as defined by their activity of alkaline phosphatase (Walton et al, 1977a; Harinck et al, 1986). This accords with the known distribution of the extent of skeletal involvement and the number of pagetic lesions which also has a unimodal log-normal distribution (Chapter 3; Figure 4.12).

An interesting observation is that up to 10 per cent of patients with symptomatic Paget's disease have values of alkaline phosphatase which lie within the laboratory reference range. The reference range in the elderly is higher than that normally quoted, and up to 20 per cent of patients have normal values when age-adjusted ranges are used. It is therefore important not to exclude the diagnosis of Paget's disease on the basis of an apparently normal value for alkaline phosphatase. In such patients, who commonly have

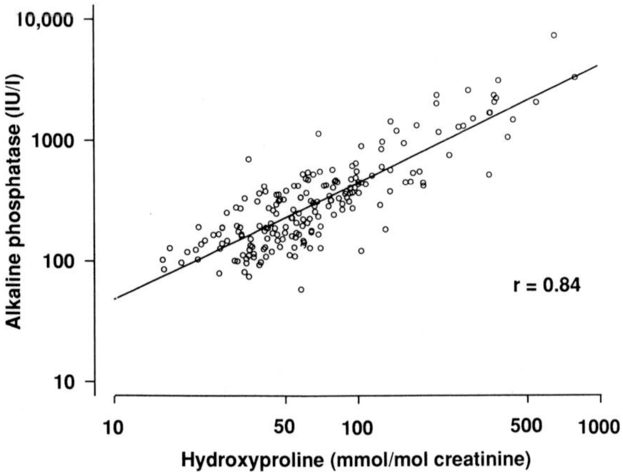

Figure 4.13

Relationship between serum alkaline phosphatase and fasting urinary hydroxyproline excretion (expressed as hydroxyproline/creatinine ratio) in a series of 197 untreated patients with Paget's disease. Note the close relationship between the two measurements over a 100-fold range of values (log scale). Upper limit of normal is 105 IU/l for alkaline phosphatase and 40 μmol/mmol for hydroxyproline/creatinine.

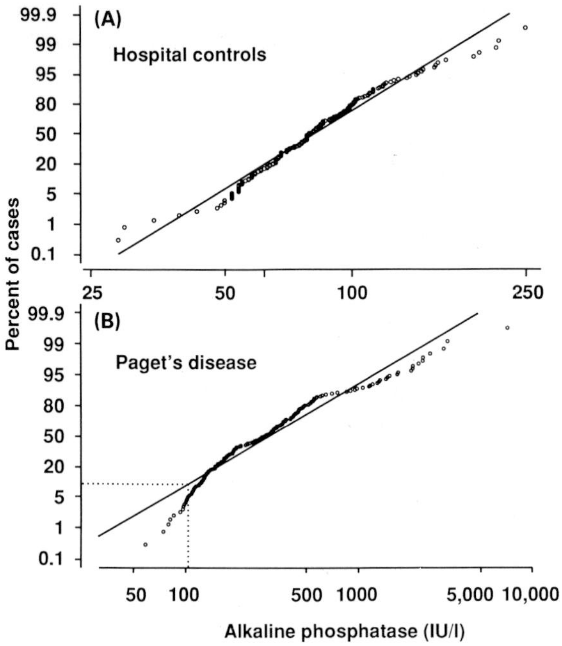

Figure 4.14

Probability plot to show the distribution of plasma alkaline phosphatase (IU/l) in a series of 197 hospital controls (A) and untreated patients with Paget's disease (B). The distributions of values conform to that expected of a unimodal logarithmic distribution (solid line) suggesting that the patients belong to a single population ranging from the most mildly affected to the most severely affected patients. The upper limit of the normal range is shown as a dotted line. Note that 8 per cent of patients have a value for alkaline phosphatase which lies within the laboratory reference range. This value would increase if age and sex-matched reference ranges were utilized.

monostotic Paget's disease, the alkaline phosphatase usually falls after appropriate medical treatment, suggesting that the initial value, despite being in the laboratory reference range, was abnormally high for that individual.

There is a considerable day-to-day fluctuation in serum activity of alkaline phosphatase in patients with Paget's disease (Woodard, 1959; Gray et al, 1987). The long-term within-patient coefficient of variation in our laboratory is approximately 10 per cent. This has important implications for the assessment of response to treatment and also for the definition of relapse. This is discussed in detail in Chapter 8, but for practical purposes we interpret a change in activity of alkaline phosphatase of greater than 25 per cent as indicative of response or relapse, since the probability of this happening by chance is very low.

Hydroxyproline

Measurements of hydroxyproline in urine provide the other major biochemical marker used to monitor Paget's disease. The most abundant natural isomer of hydroxyproline is 4-hydroxyproline, and this is produced as a translational hydroxylation of proline by the enzyme prolyl-hydroxylase during collagen biosynthesis (Prockop et al, 1979). Approximately 11 per cent of the amino-acid composition of collagen is hydroxyproline, but it also occurs in certain other proteins, notably the C1q component of complement and the acetylcholine-receptor protein. Collagen is the major protein of bone and skin, and most hydroxyproline of endogenous origin that is excreted in urine (perhaps 90 per cent) probably comes from the turnover of collagen in these tissues. When bone turnover is increased, the relative skeletal contribution to total excretion is correspondingly increased.

Hydroxyproline is not re-utilized for new protein biosynthesis and up to 90 per cent of the free amino acid undergoes oxidative degradation via glutamate. The remainder is excreted in urine, but only 1 or 2 per cent of hydroxyproline in urine is present as the free amino acid and the rest is in peptide form (Krane et al, 1970). Approximately 90 per cent is in the form of small (dialysable) peptides which by virtue of their structure are known to be derived from collagen degradation. The remaining 10 per cent occurs in larger peptides of a molecular weight of 5–10 000 daltons or greater, which on the basis of labelling with ^{14}C-glycine in patients in vivo (Nagant de Deuxchaisnes and Krane, 1964) and other evidence are thought to arise during bone formation rather than degradation (Haddad et al, 1970a; Krane, 1980). These components may be derived from the N and C terminal pro-peptide extensions

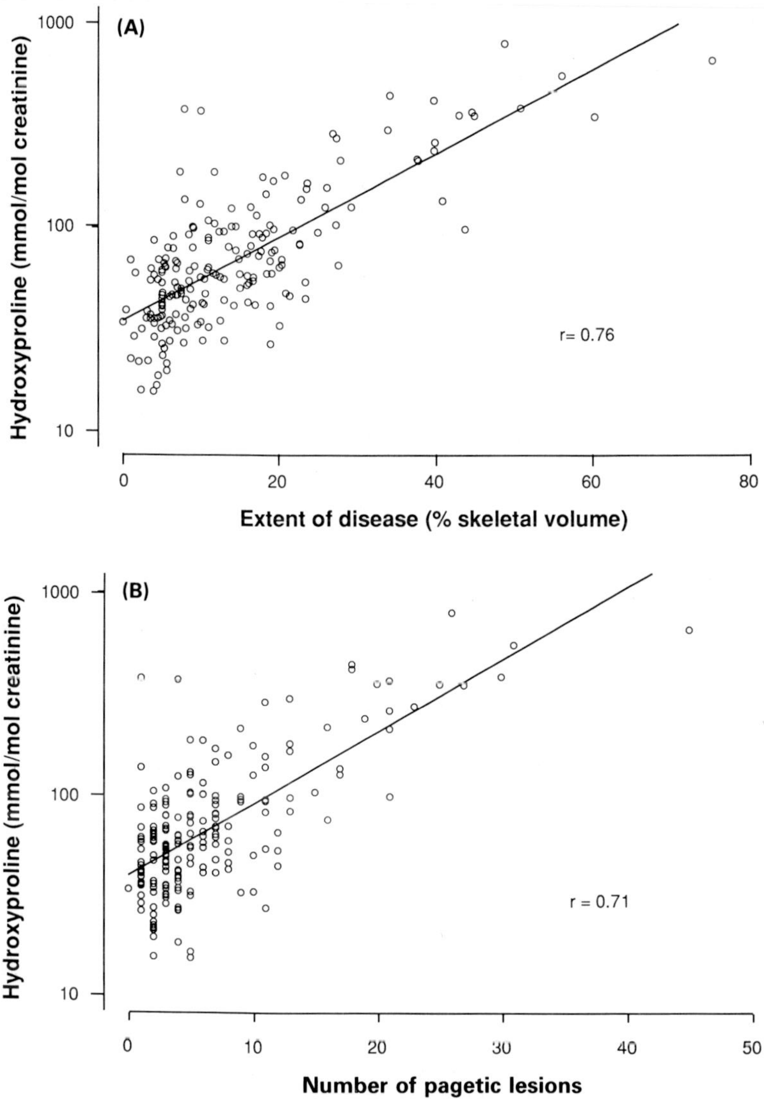

Figure 4.15

Relationship between urinary excretion of hydroxyproline (μmol/mmol creatinine) and (A) the scintigraphic assessment of disease extent and (B) the number of pagetic lesions.

which are cleaved from procollagen during its processing to mature collagen (see Figure 2.1).

As for alkaline phosphatase, there is a close relationship between the urinary excretion of peptide-bound hydroxyproline and the extent of bone involvement in Paget's disease (Franck et al, 1974; Meunier et al, 1987; Figure 4.15). The close correlation between serum activity of alkaline phosphatase and hydroxyproline (Figure 4.13) indicates that either can be used to predict the extent of disease activity (Table 4.3).

A major difficulty in the use of hydroxyproline is that it is a rather laborious chemical measurement and is generally less widely available than the measurement of alkaline phosphatase. It also discriminates patients with and without Paget's disease less well than does plasma alkaline phosphatase. Thus, up to 20 per cent of patients with Paget's disease have hydroxyproline excretion rates within the normal range, approximately double the number of false negatives seen in the case of alkaline phosphatase (Walton et al, 1977a;

Table 4.3 Relationship between serum activity of alkaline phosphatase and other indices of the extent of skeletal involvement in Paget's disease of bone. Data derived from 197 untreated patients assessed by scintigraphy.

Alkaline phosphatase (IU/l)	*Skeletal involvement (%)*	*Number of skeletal foci*	*Urine hydroxyproline (mmol/mol creatinine)*
50*	0	0	21
100	3.4	1.1	25
150	5.3	3.0	36
200	6.9	3.8	46
300	9.3	7.2	60
400	10.7	10	76
500	12.4	12	89
750	15.6	17	132
1000	18.8	20	185
1500	25.3	24	260
2000	29.3	27	315
2500	32.8	29	385
3000	38.1	32	455
4000	45.8	35	570
5000	53.1	37	675
10000	69.0	46	1250
15000*	100.0	52	1660

*Values derived from extrapolation.

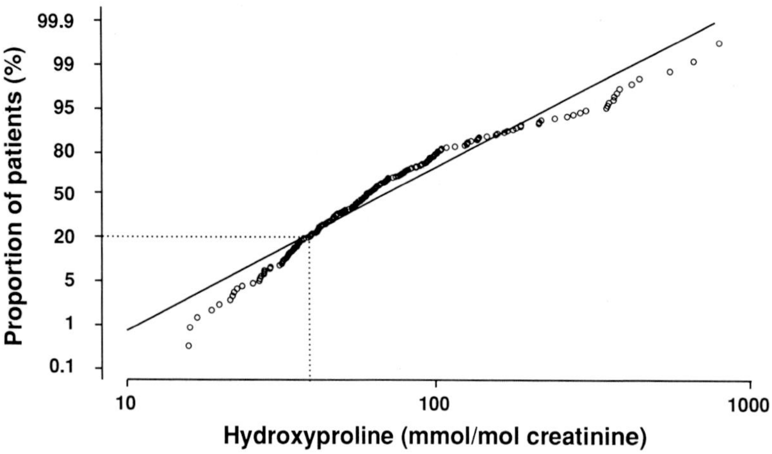

Figure 4.16

Distribution of urinary hydroxyproline excretion (μmol/mmol creatinine) in 197 untreated patients with Paget's disease. The values are plotted on a probability scale. The distribution conforms to that expected of a unimodal logarithmic distribution (solid line). The upper limit of normal (40 μmol/mol) is shown as a dotted line. Note that 20 per cent of patients have a value which lies within the laboratory reference range.

Figure 4.16). Similarly, the coefficient of variation within patients is twice that of the serum activity of alkaline phosphatase, rendering this measurement less useful than phosphatase in assessing response to and relapse from treatment (Gray et al, 1987).

An inconvenience in the use of hydroxyproline assays is that there are significant dietary sources of hydroxyproline in food products derived from animal sources. It is traditional to measure hydroxyproline, therefore, only after restricting the collagen and gelatin intake of patients. This makes it necessary to avoid meats, gravies, ice-creams and several other food products. In practice, this dietary restriction is less necessary in most patients with Paget's disease than in other

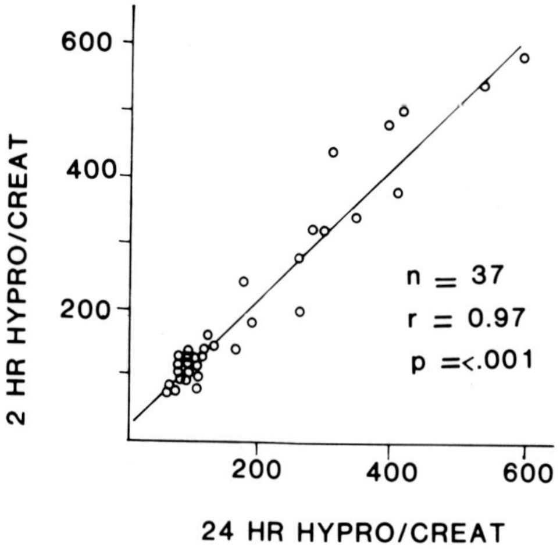

Figure 4.17

Relationship between peptide-bound hydroxyproline (mmol/mol creatinine) in early morning fasting urinary specimens and corresponding 24-hour samples on an unrestricted diet.

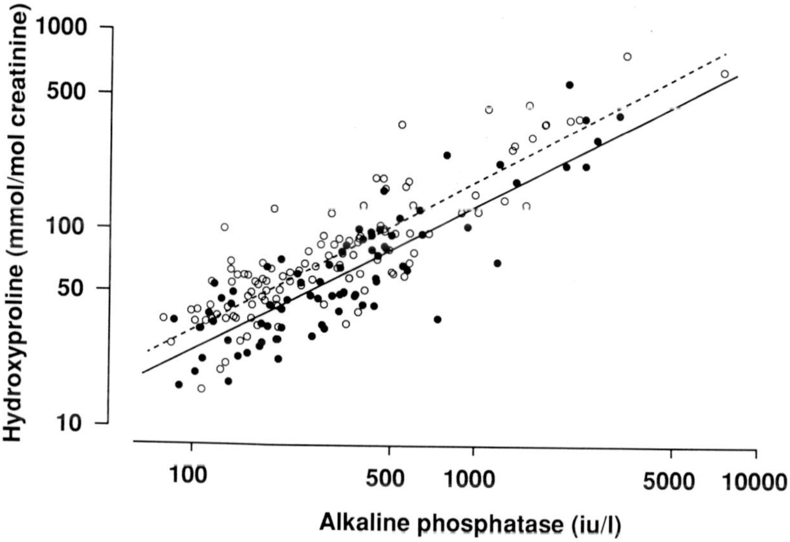

Figure 4.18

Relationship between urinary excretion of hydroxyproline (mmol/mol creatinine) and serum activity of alkaline phosphatase (IU/l) in untreated men (●) and women (○) with Paget's disease. Note the significant correlation between the two indices of disease but the higher apparent hydroxyproline excretion in women for any given activity of alkaline phosphatase.

bone disorders, since urinary hydroxyproline is so markedly elevated that variations in dietary intake make relatively little difference.

Another way of simplifying the procedure is to make use of the early morning urine taken after an overnight fast. In Paget's disease there is a very close relationship between fasting values for hydroxyproline (expressed as a ratio to creatinine) taken without dietary restriction and the corresponding daily excretion rate (Figure 4.17). The use of fasting spot urines also avoids the need for timed collections since hydroxyproline concentrations are expressed as a ratio of creatinine concentrations. In our laboratory the upper limit of normal is <40 mmol/mol creatinine. A minor drawback with the use of a hydroxyproline/

creatinine ratio is related to variations in creatinine output which in turn depend upon muscle mass. Thus, for any given activity of alkaline phosphatase, the apparent hydroxyproline excretion is slightly higher in women than in men due to a lower muscle mass and lower excretion rates for creatinine (Figure 4.18).

The measurement of urinary hydroxyproline is a particularly useful way to monitor acute changes in bone resorption in Paget's disease. Changes can be seen within a few hours of administration of agents such as calcitonin and within days with the diphosphonates. In contrast, the activity of alkaline phosphatase changes more slowly.

Other biochemical markers of bone metabolism

Since bone turnover may be so markedly elevated in Paget's disease, this disorder has been extremely useful in evaluating the potential of other indices of skeletal metabolism. Those evaluted in Paget's disease are shown in Table 4.4.

Collagen products

Although the urinary excretion of peptide-bound hydroxyproline is the most practical and extensively used method of measuring changes in turnover of bone collagen, there are several other ways of detecting changes in collagen metabolism (Russell et al, 1981; Krane and Simon, 1987).

Hydroxylysine is another hydroxylated amino acid produced by the post-translational modification of lysine residues in the alpha chain of collagen. It is less abundant than hydroxyproline and accounts for 0.4 per cent of the amino-acid composition of bone collagen, but may be less completely metabolized (Segrest and Cunningham, 1970). Some of the hydroxylysine residues are glycosylated, but the extent and nature of this glycosylation differs in various tissues. Beta-1-galactosyl-o-hydroxylysine appears to be a more specific marker for bone collagen whereas glucosyl-galactosyl-o-hydroxylysine is more abundant in skin (Segrest and Cunningham, 1970). Thus, in bone the ratio of glycosyl-galactosyl-hydroxylysine to galactosyl-hydroxylysine is approximately 0.5, whereas in the skin this ratio exceeds 2 (Pinnell et al, 1971; Krane et al, 1977). In patients with severe Paget's disease the urinary ratio approaches 0.5, indicating a bony source (Figure 4.19). The ratio rises following suppression of disease activity with diphosphonates.

The collagen of bone is predominantly type I, so that each molecule is made up of a triple helix containing two alpha 1 and one alpha 2 chains. In Paget's disease the collagen in bone is also predominantly type I (Cheung et al, 1980), although it seems likely that the highly fibrous stroma in the marrow cavity in active Paget's disease contains type III collagen. During the maturation of procollagen, both amino- and carboxyterminal fragments are removed and

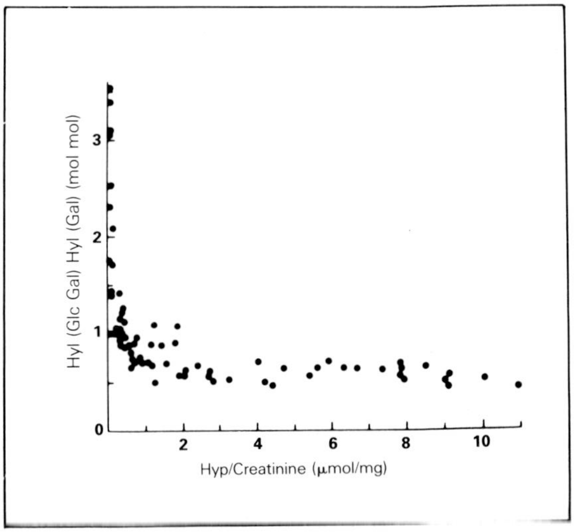

Figure 4.19

Excretion of peptide-bound glycoslyated hydroxylysine in urine. The ratio of glucosyl galactolyl hydroxylysine to galactosyl hydroxylysine is plotted against hydroxyproline excretion in patients with Paget's disease. In extensive disease the ratio decreases to approach a value of 0.5. (Adapted from Krane et al, 1977.)

Table 4.4 Biochemical markers used to assess the activity of Paget's disease.

Measurement	*Source*	*Changes in Paget's disease*
Formation		
Alkaline phosphatase	Liver/bone/gut	Increased
Skeletal alkaline phosphatase	Bone: osteoblasts	Increased
Osteocalcin	Bone: osteoblasts	Increased
Non-dialysable hydroxyproline	Post-translational maturation of collagen increased	
Procollagen type I	Bone:osteoblasts	Increased
Procollagen type III	? fibrous tissue	Increased
α_2HS glycoprotein	Liver: incorporated into bone	Decreased
Resorption		
Hydroxyproline (dialysable)	Collagen degradation	Increased
Hydroxylysine and its glycosides	Collagen degradation	Increased
Glucosylgalactosyl/galactosyl hydroxylysine	Skin/bone collagen	Decreased
Acid phosphatase	? osteoclasts	Increased
3-hydroxy-lysyl-pyridinolone	Collagen crosslinks	Increased
Proline iminopeptidase	? osteoclasts ? osteoblasts	Increased
Urinary or serum free GLA	Osteocalcin degradation	Increased

radioimmunoassays raised against the triple-chain carboxyterminal extension of procollagen type I (pCol1c) and the aminoterminal extension of type III (pCol111n) have been developed.

Such clinical data as are available suggest that pCol1c values correlate with histological indices of bone formation in Paget's disease (Table 4.1) and in a variety of metabolic bone disorders (Parfitt et al, 1987). In Paget's disease values for pCol1c and pCol111n are both increased (Taubman et al, 1976; Krane et al, 1980; Wilder-Smith et al, 1987). During the treatment of Paget's disease with inhibitors of bone resorption, decreases in both peptides are observed (Wilder-Smith et al, 1987). In our own hands the procollagen peptides are less sensitive and specific as a marker of turnover than alkaline phosphatase (unpublished).

Other potential markers for collagens of skeletal origin are the 3-hydroxy pyridinium residues which are the major cross-links of mature collagen. Unlike hydroxyproline, they are not thought to be metabolized. The major compound, hydroxylysyl pyridinolene is derived from three residues of hydroxylysine, whereas the less abundant lysyl pyridinolene is derived from two hydroxylysine residues and one lysine residue (Eyre et al, 1984). The latter is not present in cartilage and may be useful to assess bone resorption. Serum values fall after treatment with diphosphonates (P. Delmas, personal communication), but their clinical value is not yet known.

Osteocalcin

Osteocalcin, also known as bone gamma-carboxyglutamic-acid-containing protein (BGP) is a vitamin K-dependent protein that binds calcium and has a high affinity for hydroxyapatite. It is the most abundant non-collagenous protein in bone, and is thought to be synthesized exclusively by osteoblasts (Price et al, 1979). It is also found in serum and for these reasons there has been considerable interest in its assay as a possible means for the diagnosis or evaluation of patients with metabolic bone disorders, particularly in osteoporosis (Brown et al, 1984).

Serum concentrations of BGP are increased in untreated patients with Paget's disease (Price et al, 1980; Coulton et al, 1988) and serum values correlate significantly with activity of both alkaline phosphatase and urinary hydroxyproline (Price et al, 1980). Its promise as a more sensitive and specific marker has not been upheld in the sense that it is both less specific and less sensitive than either hydroxyproline or alkaline phosphatase (Figure 4.20; Delmas et al, 1986; Coulton et al, 1988). Moreover, when bone turnover is decreased with the use of therapeutic agents such as the diphosphonates, changes in osteocalcin levels are inconsistent, and do not follow those for alkaline phosphatase (Papapoulos et al, 1987; Coulton et al, 1988; Figure 4.21). This might suggest that BGP does not reflect the same aspect of osteoblast function as reflected by alkaline phosphatase. It is relevant that neither osteoblast function nor skeletal matrix is normal in Paget's disease, and there are several possible explanations for these disparate responses between alkaline phosphatase and osteocalcin (Coulton et al, 1988). Irrespective of the reasons, serum measurements of osteocalcin do not provide a sensitive or specific index of disease activity, nor a means to monitor treatment (Figure 4.22). Serum osteocalcin circulates in heterogeneous form, presumably due to the appearance of cleavage fragments. Recent work suggests the presence of a cleavage fragment specific for Paget's disease (Taylor et al, 1989). If this is sufficiently sensitive its assay would provide a useful marker for the disease.

Like many small proteins, BGP is cleared and degraded by the kidney. Estimation of the total urinary excretion of glutamic acid (GLA) has not shown increased values in the urine of patients with Paget's disease (Gundberg et al, 1983). Since BGP is incorporated into bone matrix, it is subject to osteoclastic destruction. As such it is likely to be degraded to small peptides and amino acids. For this reason there has been recent interest in the measurement of free GLA in serum as a possible index of bone resorption. Unfortunately, values are not markedly increased in Paget's disease, perhaps due to adsorption of free GLA on to bone after osteoclastic resorption (Delmas, personal communication).

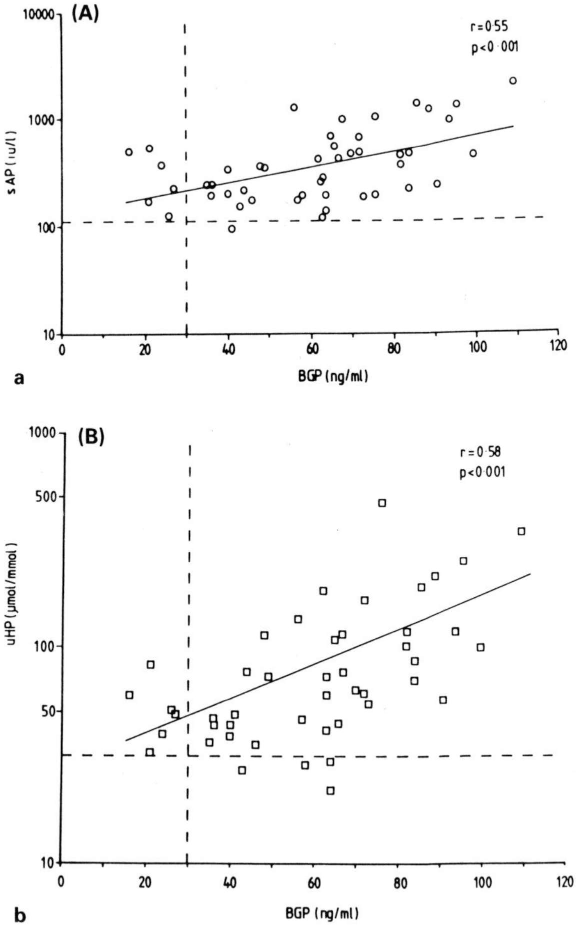

Figure 4.20

Relationship between serum osteocalcin and serum activity of alkaline phosphatase (A) and urinary hydroxyproline (B) in untreated Paget's disease. Note the significant correlation between the two but that more patients have a normal value for osteocalcin than is the case for alkaline phosphatase or hydroxyproline. (From Coulton et al, 1988.)

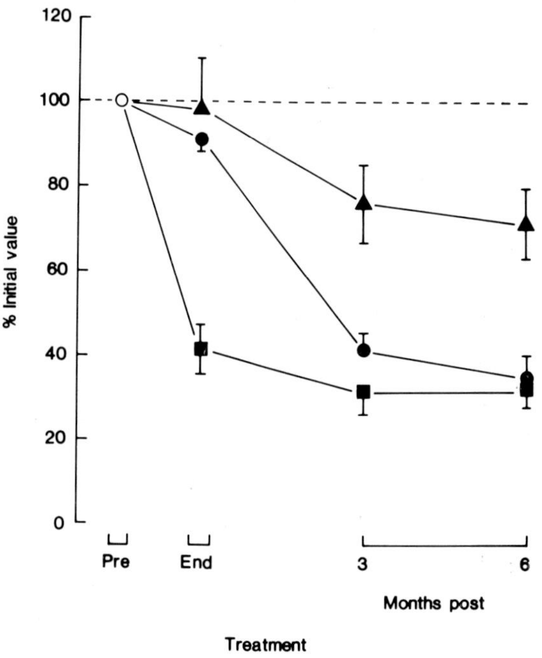

Figure 4.21

Changes in mean serum and urine measurements (± SEM) in six patients given etidronate (20 mg/kg per day) for 1 month. Note the early decrease in hydroxyproline excretion (■) followed by the later fall in alkaline phosphatase (●). In contrast, the changes in serum osteocalcin are less marked (▲) and follow neither hydroxyproline nor phosphatase values.

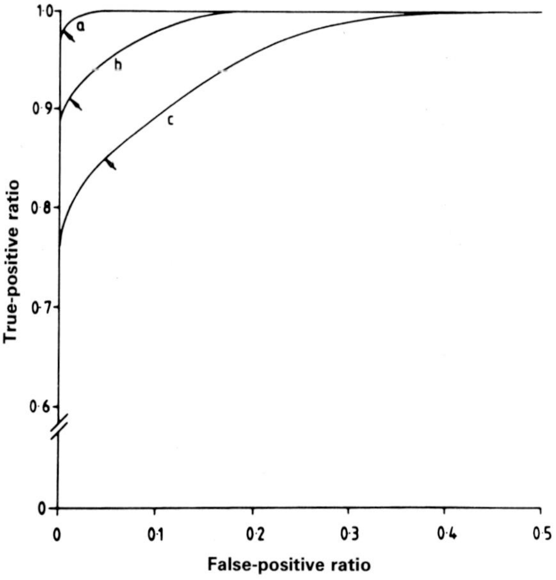

Figure 4.22

Receiver operating characteristic curves using three biochemical indices of disease activity in normal subjects and control subjects. The sensitivity (true-positive ratio) is plotted against 1-specificity (false-positive ratio) at varying cut-off points for alkaline phosphatase (a), urinary hydroxyproline (b) and osteocalcin (c). Arrows denote the sensitivity and specificity at the upper end of the laboratory reference range. Note that serum activity of alkaline phosphatase has the most marked sensitivity and specificity. (From Coulton et al, 1988.)

Alpha$_2$ HS-glycoprotein

Alpha$_2$ HS-glycoprotein is an acute-phase protein produced by the liver. Relatively large amounts are found in bone, and it has been clearly shown that this protein is selectively taken up by bone from plasma for reasons that are still unknown (Ashton et al, 1976). Serum values of the glycoprotein are reduced in patients with Paget's disease (Ashton and Smith, 1980), which presumably reflects the enhanced uptake of the protein into newly formed bone. The concentrations of alpha$_2$ HS rise during effective treatment of Paget's disease (Figure 4.23; Ashton and Smith, 1980; Russell et al, 1981). Although this may provide a biochemical probe for rates of matrix synthesis, the sensitivity and specificity of this assay is too low to make it of great clinical value.

Acid phosphatase

Serum acid phosphatase is raised in some patients with Paget's disease (Harinck et al, 1986), and significant correlations have been noted between serum acid and alkaline phosphatase

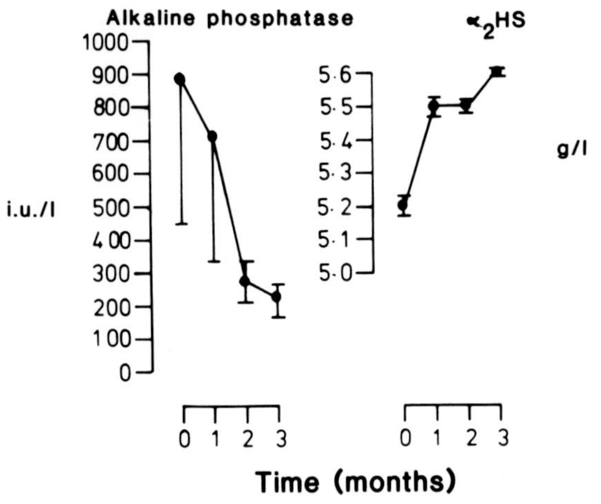

Figure 4.23

Changes in serum alkaline phosphatase and alpha$_2$ HS-glycoprotein before and during treatment with the diphosphonate clodronate.

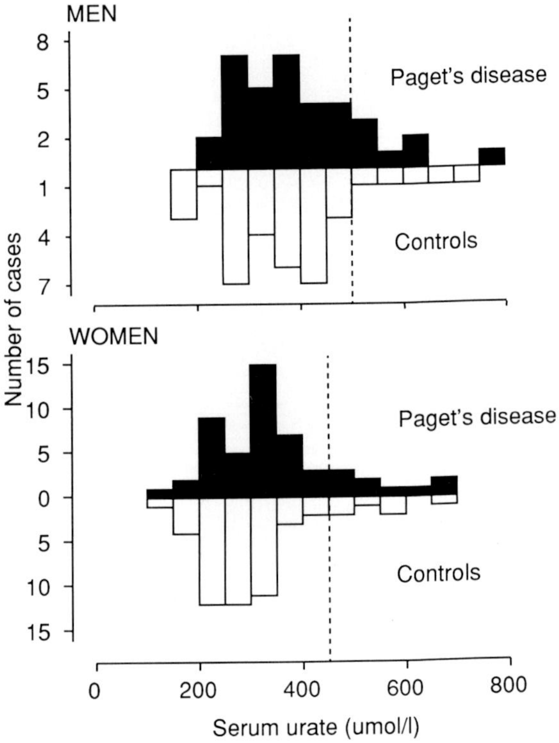

Figure 4.24

Distribution of serum urate in men (top) and women (bottom) with Paget's disease and in age- and sex-matched hospital controls (open bars). Hospital controls were obtained randomly but excluded patients with abnormal serum creatinine values and increased activities of alkaline phosphatase.

(Woodard, 1959). Osteoclasts are rich in acid phosphatase, and this is assumed to be the source. Serum values are not markedly increased and acid phosphatase activity has, therefore, neither the specificity nor the sensitivity for routine clinical use.

Proline iminopeptidase

Proline iminopeptidase was originally studied because it was thought to be involved in the degradation of collagen. The source of the enzyme is unknown, but probably includes the liver. Serum values are high in Paget's disease and decrease on treatment (Whitley et al, 1976), but it offers no advantages as a clinical aid over alkaline phosphatase or hydroxyproline.

Uric acid

Serum uric acid concentrations are often said to be increased. The prevalence of hyperuricaemia in the published literature is 21 per cent and ranges from 13 to 42 per cent of patients (Franck et al, 1974; Simon et al, 1975; Altman and Collins, 1980; Arlot and Meunier, 1981; Salson, 1981; Harinck et al, 1986). In one series, values of serum urate correlated with estimates of disease activity (Franck et al, 1974). A possible explanation relates to the increased turnover of nucleic acids in bone cells, and this may also explain an increase in the urinary excretion of pseudouridine, presumably derived from RNA (Fennelly and Hogan, 1972). A decrease in urate excretion occurs with treatment of the disorder, which supports this view (Arlot and Meunier, 1981).

As recognized by Sir James Paget, there does seem to be an association between Paget's disease and gout (Altman and Collins, 1980; Lluberas-Acosta et al, 1986; see Chapter 5), but in our experience it is rare. In our patients, serum urate values are indeed higher than the laboratory reference range. But when patients are age- and sex-matched, we find no difference in the distribution of serum urate between patients with Paget's disease and hospital controls (Figure 4.24). This suggests that reports of a high prevalence of hyperuricaemia may be due to the use of an inadequate control population. Moreover, we find no relationship between serum uric acid concentrations and biochemical estimates of disease activity (Table 4.1).

CHAPTER 5

Clinical features and complications

The variable effects on skeletal shape and size and the widespread distribution of Paget's disease result in a plethora of clinical features. It is to the great credit of Sir James Paget (1882; 1889) that his accurate accounts of the severe form of the disease are as appropriate now as they were over 100 years ago. It is important to recognize, however, that only a small proportion of patients with Paget's disease come to medical or surgical attention.

The proportion of the pagetic population with symptoms is difficult to establish. A widely quoted figure is 5 per cent but estimates vary from less than 1 per cent to as much as 30 per cent (Collins, 1956; Smith, 1979; Ziegler et al, 1985). The difficulty relates to uncertainties about the prevalence of the disorder and its natural history. Our own referral pattern at Sheffield is consistent with a prevalence of symptomatic disease of between 4 and 5 per cent. No prospective studies have been undertaken to examine this question nor to determine how frequently complications of clinical significance will develop in asymptomatic patients. In one hospital series (Galbraith et al, 1977) asymptomatic patients discovered by chance were not younger than their symptomatic counterparts. This does not suggest a high rate of conversion from asymptomatic to symptomatic disease. This is an important area for future investigation because of the improved results of treatment in recent years.

Most patients who come to medical attention have more than one lesion, but symptomatic disease is found in only about one-third of lesions (Meunier et al, 1987). As would be expected, patients with monostotic disease are less likely to be symptomatic since the prevalence of monostotic disease is higher in the general hospital

Clinical features and complications of Paget's disease.

Common
- Bone pain – pagetic
  - – articular
- Fracture – long bones, vertebral bodies
- Neurological – deafness
- Deformity and enlargement of bones

Uncommon
- Pain – fissure fracture
- Spinal neurological syndromes
- Hypercalcaemia and calcuria of immobilization or fracture
- Cardiovascular disease
- Vascular bleeding from bone during surgery
- Extraskeletal calcification and urolithiasis

Rare
- Gout
- Epidural haematoma
- Osteosarcoma and other bone tumours
- Cranial nerve lesions (except VIII)
- Brain stem and cerebellar syndromes
- Hypercalcaemia
- Extramedullary haematopoiesis

Significance uncertain
- Pseudogout
- Angioid streaks
- Hyperparathyroidism
- Chondrocalcinosis

community than in the pagetic population (Shirazi et al, 1974; Merrick and Merrick, 1985). The presentation of patients is however similar, irrespective of the number of lesions (Table 5.1).

The common problems encountered are bone pain, skeletal deformity and fracture (Table 5.1), but many other features and complications are found (see page 110). Apart from fracture, the onset is insidious and 30 per cent of patients have had symptoms at presentation for more than 10 years (Figure 5.1). A minority of patients have symptoms for 30 years or more before presenting for medical advice. A significant minority (7 per cent) have symptoms which were present before the age of 40.

Pain

Pain is the most common presenting complaint (Table 5.1), and is certainly multi-factorial in origin (see below). It is most common in the long bones such as the tibia and femur, but it can arise in any bone, including the skull.

In clinical practice it may be very difficult to distinguish bone pain arising from Paget's disease from that arising due to unrelated disorders. There are, however, several related sources of pain associated with Paget's disease.

It seems likely that Paget's disease itself produces bone pain. It is often described as a boring or nagging pain, which keeps patients awake at night and is not necessarily aggravated by weight bearing. Pain attributed to pagetic lesions, rather than their complications, is the most common presentation accounting for 50 per cent of hospital-based referrals (Franck et al, 1974; Nagant de Deuxchaisnes and Krane, 1964; Altman and Collins, 1980; Winfield and Stamp, 1984).

Some causes of pain in Paget's disease.

Pagetic bone pain
Fissure fracture and complete fracture
Pagetic arthropathy
Osteoarthrosis
Neurological compression syndromes
Vascular steal syndromes
Sarcoma

Table 5.1 Presenting fractures of Paget's disease in a consecutive series of 197 patients referred to Sheffield. There is no difference in the pattern of presentation between patients with monostotic and polyostotic disease.

	All patients		*Monostotic disease*	
	No of patients	*%*	*No of patients*	*%*
Pain	169	86	19	83
Deformity	34	17	4	17
Asymptomatic	24	12	20	12
Neurological	33	17	2	9
Cranial nerve lesions	21	11	2	9
Spinal cord/nerve root	10	5	0	0
Peripheral nerve lesions	2	1	0	0
Fracture	21	11	2	9
Other	5	3	0	0
Tumour	1	1	0	0

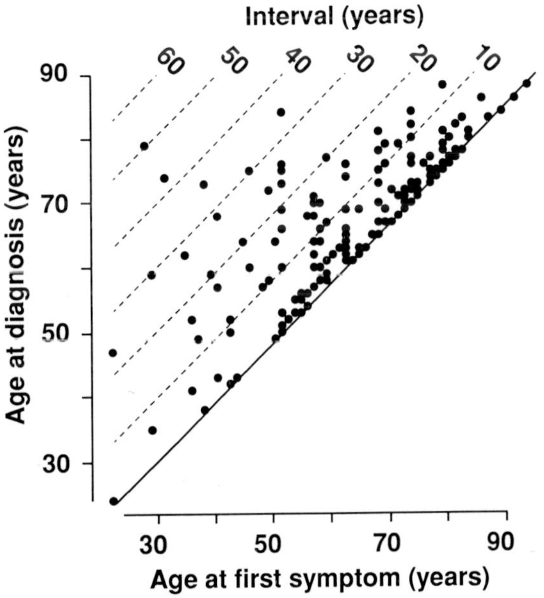

Figure 5.1

The relationship between the age at the onset of symptoms, the age at diagnosis and the duration of symptoms before diagnosis in symptomatic Paget's disease.

The mechanism for pagetic pain is not known. Some have found that those patients with the more sclerotic lesions on X-ray examination do not have symptoms (Khairi et al, 1973), but most experience would suggest little relationship between radiographic appearances and symptoms. Neither is there a close relationship between the extent of disease in any one lesion and bone pain. Patients may be asymptomatic even in the presence of very extensive disease. Nevertheless, the probability of symptomatic disease increases as might be expected with the extent of focal lesions (Harinck et al, 1986; Table 5.2).

It has been suggested that pagetic pain is due to the increased vascular supply of bone or periosteal stretching. Whereas bone pain is not significantly associated with periosteal neostosis (Khairi et al, 1973) superficial bone tenderness is not infrequent. In some cases this may be due to co-existing fissure fracture, but in others no fractures are evident, even on close examination.

It is of interest that thermographic studies of the tibia suggest that pain is significantly more frequent in those patients with the higher skin temperature (Ring et al, 1977; Figure 5.2). The early literature suggests that decompression of bones by drilling also relieves pain (Barry, 1969) which would support a vascular rather than a periosteal origin. Such a notion is consistent with the finding of raised intramedullary pressure in affected bones (Arlet and Mazieres, 1975).

Skin temperature may be markedly increased in association with dilatation of superficial veins (Altman and Collins, 1980; Hamdy, 1981). These are striking physical findings, but are seldom a cause for complaint. Occasionally a bruit or, more commonly, breath sounds can be transmitted and heard on auscultation over a hot bone and may be heard by the patient with extensive cranial disease.

Microfractures may cause pain, particularly on weight bearing or on percussion over the affected site. This is by no means invariable and many patients with alarming multiple fissure fractures do not complain of pain. The occurrence of new pain, particularly on weight bearing in a patient with fissure fracture, commonly heralds an impending complete fracture.

A major cause for pain is joint disease. The relationship of this type of pain to weight bearing or joint movement may be one way of excluding pain of pagetic origin (Table 5.3). This is not a reliable guide however, and patients who have symptoms or radiographic features of joint disease may respond to effective treatment of their Paget's disease. Pain arising from joints is particularly difficult to evaluate at the spine, hip and knee. At accessible sites, injection of local anaesthetic into and around the joint may enable the distinction to be made between pagetic and joint pain (Stevens, 1981). Many, including ourselves, prefer to give a trial of medical treatment, and we have been impressed by the number of patients in whom surgical referral for hip replacement has been totally avoided. Pain arising from malignant transformation and from neurological syndromes is discussed later in this chapter.

Table 5.2 Prevalence of bone pain (excluding osteoarthritic pain) and the extent of pagetic involvement. Extensive involvement signifies more than 50 per cent of the bone involved except for the hemipelvis (>75 per cent). Extensive disease was significantly associated with bone pain. (From Harinck et al, 1986.)

Site	*Limited disease*		*Extensive disease*		*p>*
	No of bones	*% with pain*	*No of bones*	*% with pain*	
Long bones	90	8	101	61	0.001
Skull	24	12	27	37	0.05
Hemipelvis	32	6	117	24	0.01

Bone enlargement and deformity

Though not an invariable finding, bones affected by Paget's disease often enlarge (Chapter 3) and are a presenting complaint in one-fifth of patients (Table 5.1). Clinically obvious bone enlargement is seen, particularly in the limbs (Figure 5.3) and also in the skull (Figure 5.4) and facial bones (Figure 5.5). Bone enlargement contributes signi-

Table 5.3 Characteristics of pagetic pain and joint pain (from Ibbertson et al, 1979). In practice the distinction is problematic.

Bone pain	*Joint pain*
With pressure	With movement
At rest	With active movement
Relieved by movement	Relieved by rest
Mainly at night	Mainly by day

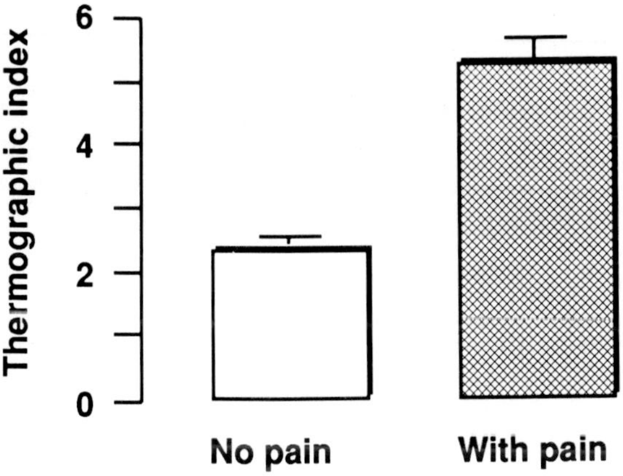

Figure 5.2

Quantitative thermography (mean ± SEM) in patients with Paget's disease of the tibia. Patients with bone pain had significantly higher skin temperature than those without. (Data plotted from Ring et al, 1977.)

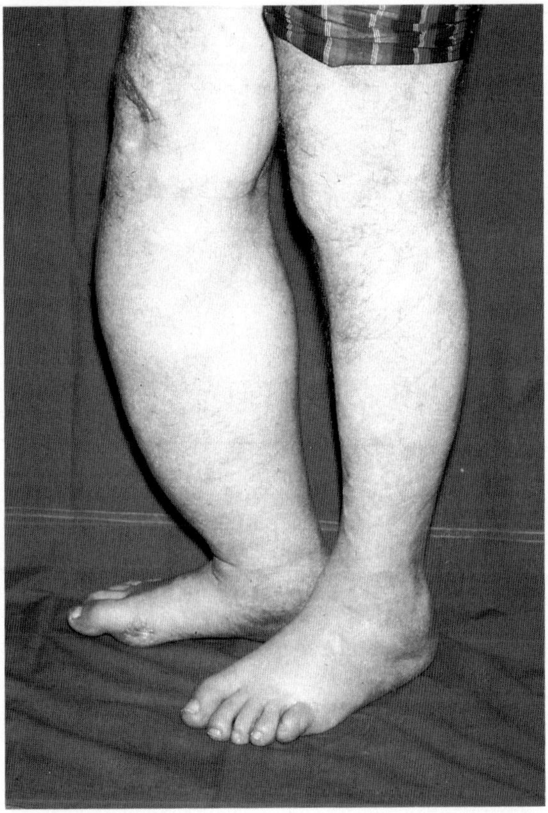

Figure 5.3

Marked enlargement of the tibia due to Paget's disease.

ficantly to the neurological complications of Paget's disease and more uncertainly to joint disease.

The most frequent deformity of long bones is bowing, which is characteristically lateral in the case of the femur and anterior in the case of the tibia (Figure 5.6). When marked, the legs may cross even on abduction of the hip so that walking is virtually impossible (Figure 5.7). Lateral bowing of the tibia also occurs and the knee joint may be externally rotated. Leg length does not usually increase at the tibia, and indeed at the femur, the interepiphyseal length is more often reduced because of the curvature, despite the increase in bone length. The incidence of fissure fractures is significantly greater in patients with marked bowing (Hosking, 1977; Redden et al, 1981). When bowing is severe, the overlying skin blood flow may be compromised and the skin becomes atrophic (Plate 14). Minor skin injuries are slow to heal and some require grafting. In some patients, skin over a bony site, particularly at the tibia, ulcerates even without marked deformity and without evidence of perfusion problems at the contralateral side (Plate 15). These ulcers rarely heal completely and skin grafts are not usually

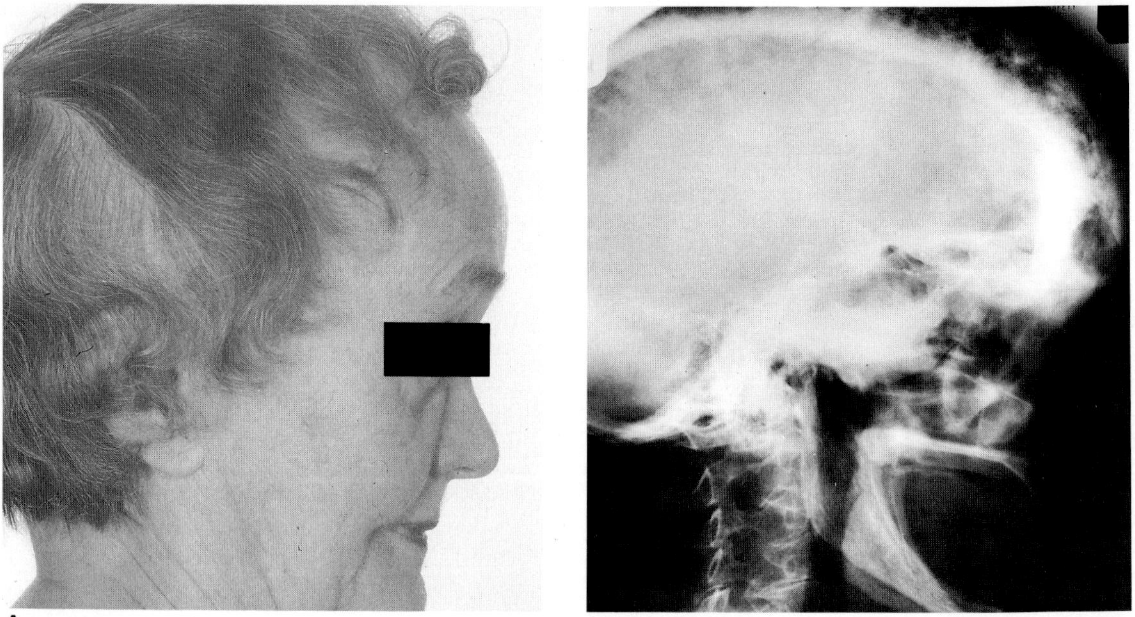

A

B

Figure 5.4

Clinical photograph (A) and associated radiograph (B) in a patient with pagetic involvement of the cranium. There is anterior bossing of the forehead due to calvarial thickening. Note also platybasia which was asymptomatic.

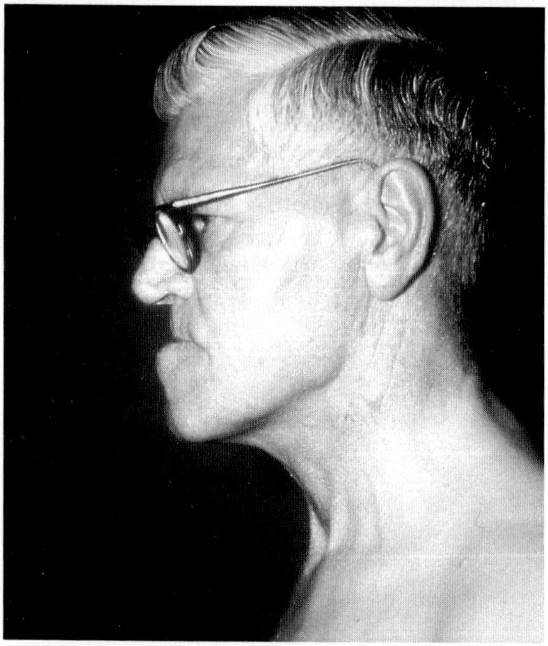

Figure 5.5

Paget's disease of the lower jaw giving rise to prognathism and dental malocclusion.

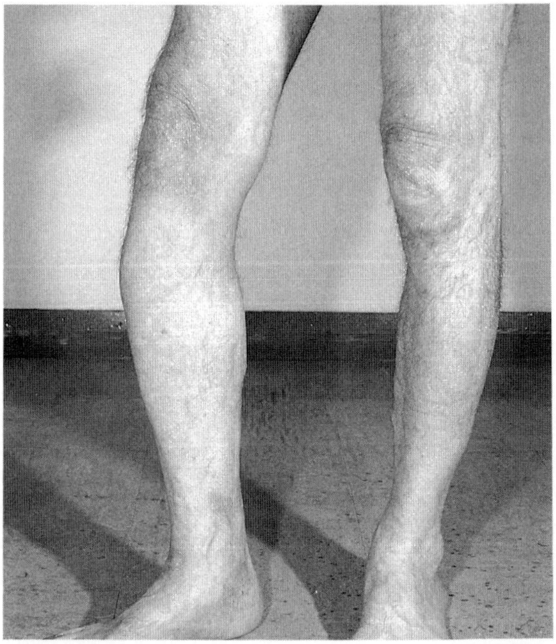

Figure 5.6

Moderate anterior bowing deformity at the right tibia in a patient with Paget's disease.

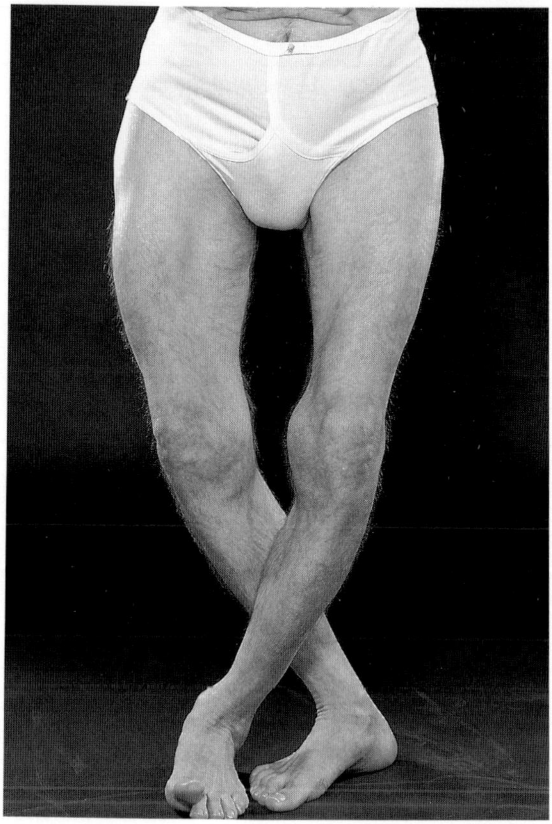

Figure 5.7

Clinical photograph of a patient with marked lateral bowing of the tibiae and femora in whom walking was impeded by his crossed legs.

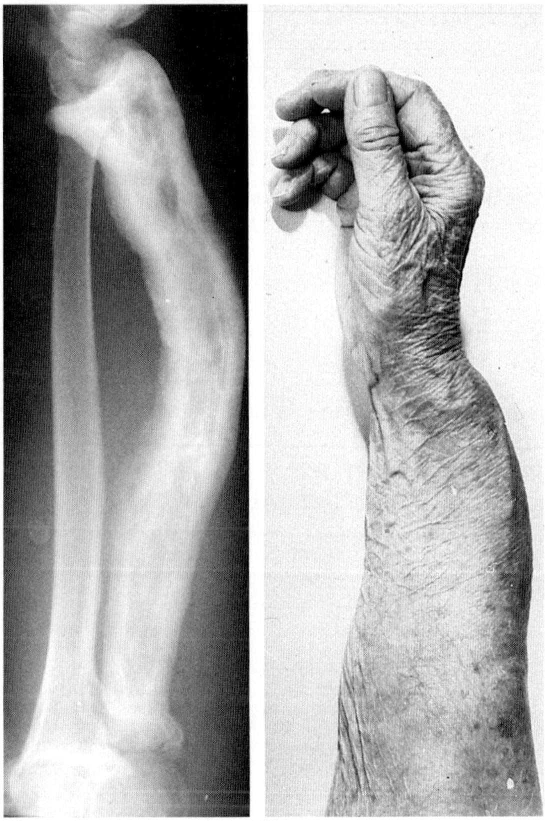

A B

Figure 5.8

(A) Anteroposterior radiograph and (B) clinical photograph of the forearm. Note the marked bony enlargement, increase in length and deformity of the radius which caused supination of the wrist.

viable. Rarely, hypertrichosis occurs over the vascular bone.

Characteristic deformities occur at the radius, skull, face and clavicles (Figures 5.4 and 5.8). Deformity of the jaws may be marked, causing dental and cosmetic problems (Figure 5.5 and Plate 16). Skull deformity may be quite asymmetric, even when the whole vault is affected. This gives rise to bony protuberances.

Both tibial and facial deformities are seen more frequently in women than in men, but this may be because the cosmetic results of deformity cause more concern amongst women and because of their longer life-expectancy. The bony enlargement and deformity is a helpful feature in the differential diagnosis, in that it distinguishes Paget's disease from osteosclerosis due to other causes (Chapter 6).

Fractures

Three types of fractures are common, namely fissure fractures, fractures of long bones and vertebral compression fractures (Table 5.4). Avulsion fractures may also occur through pathological bone but are less common.

Table 5.4 Sites of previous fracture in 367 patients with Paget's disease (from Dickson et al, 1945).

Site	*Prevalence (%)*
Thoracic spine	6.5
Lumbar spine	6.5
Femur	2.4
Tibia	2.4
Humerus	0.5

Fissure fractures

Fissure fracture is a frequent complication and affects almost exclusively long bones, most commonly the femur, tibia and humerus. Occasionally, they are seen at other sites such as the pelvic brim. In surveys of symptomatic patients they occur in 8–31 per cent of patients (Traver and Clarence, 1936; Nagant de Deuxchaisnes and Krane, 1964; Barry, 1969; Nagant de Deuxchaisnes, 1985).

The radiographic features of fissure fractures and their distinction from Looser's zones have been described in Chapter 3. An important predisposing factor associated with fissure fractures is a bowing deformity of long bone (Hosking, 1977; Redden et al, 1981; Figure 5.9). It has been suggested that fissure fracture is a feature of the early osteolytic phase of the disease, but most

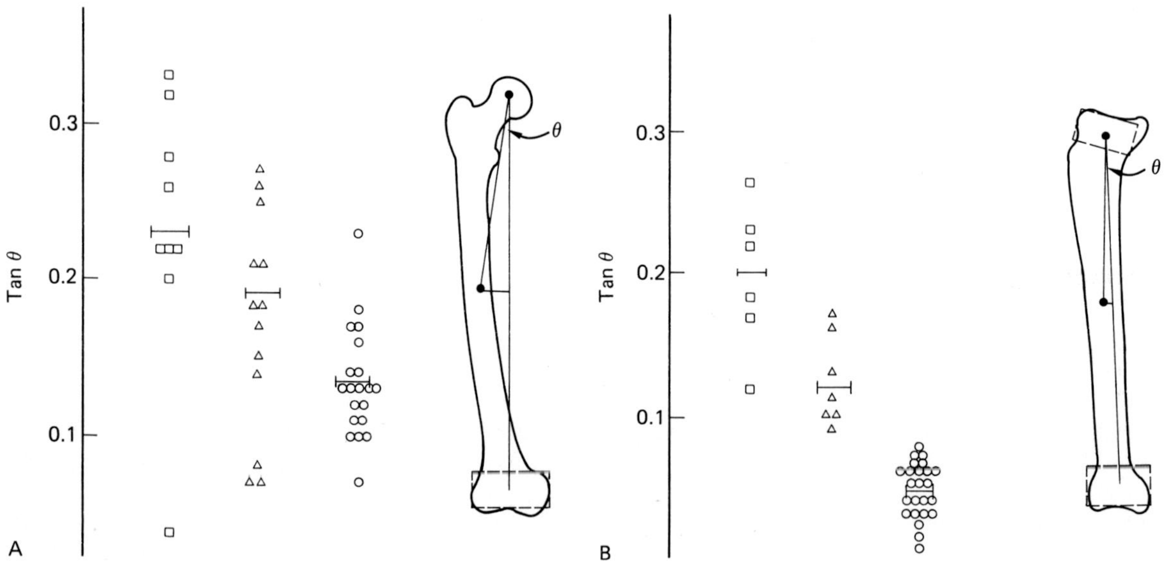

Figure 5.9

Relationship of fissure fractures and deformity. Bowing deformity was associated as shown at the femur (A) and tibia (B) in pagetic patients with (□) and without (△) fissure fractures and in uninvolved bone (○). (From Redden et al, 1981.)

clinical observations indicate that fissure fractures occur with equal frequency in patients with radiographic sclerosis or a mixed picture at the time of diagnosis (Figures 5.10 and 5.11). In addition, there is no biochemical evidence of a predominance of lysis since the expected relationship between hydroxyproline and alkaline phosphatase is preserved and fractures are found irrespective of whether local bone turnover is active or quiescent (Redden et al, 1981).

Although fissure fractures may be painful, they are more often asymptomatic. Where pain develops this may herald complete fracture, but many patients have indolent pain, particularly on weight bearing, which is associated with local tenderness and is attributed to underlying fissure fractures. These pose very difficult problems in management (Chapter 8).

Complete fractures of long bones

Complete fractures of long bones occur most commonly in the femur, followed by the tibia and forearm. These sites together account for 70–90 per cent of pathological fractures of long bones (Dickson, 1945; Rauis, 1974; Louyot et al, 1975).

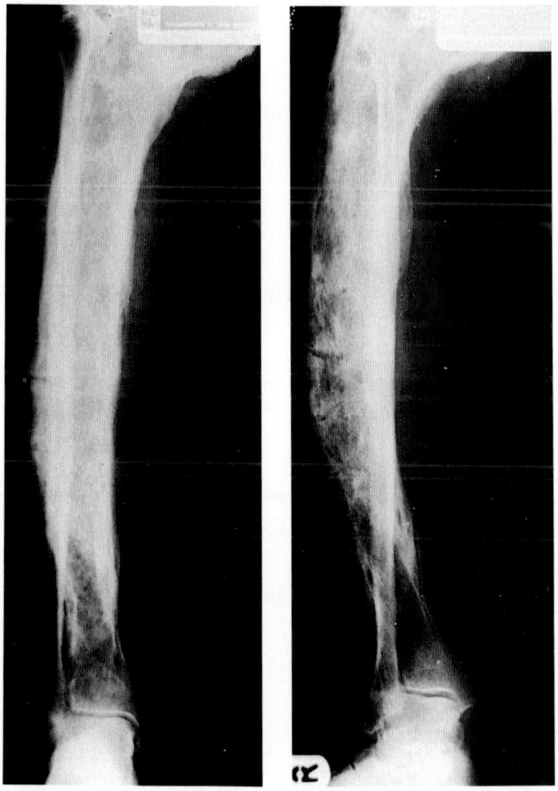

Figure 5.10

Multiple fissure fractures of the tibia in a patient with anterior bowing. The patient had no symptoms.

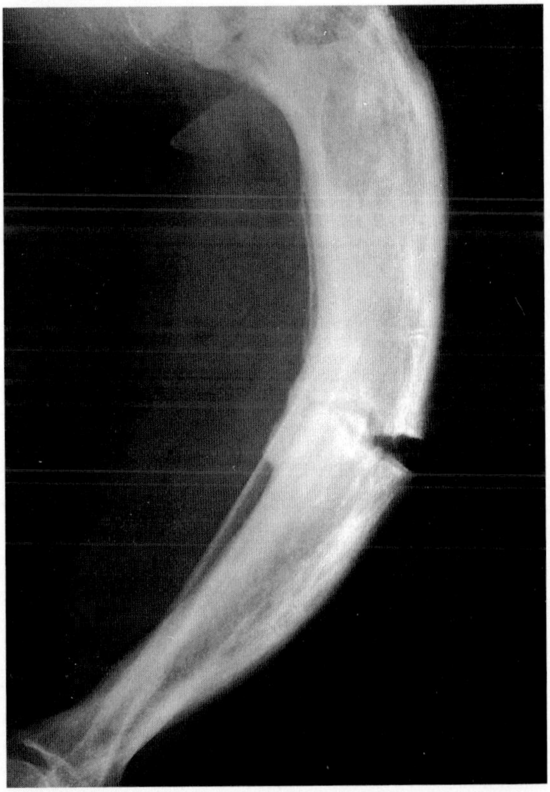

Figure 5.11

Complete fracture in a markedly bowed tibia. The patient had asymptomatic fissure fractures until two weeks beforehand when she developed pain on weight bearing.

Fracture is the most common presentation of Paget's disease to orthopaedic surgeons and, in a review of fractured femurs, the presentation with fracture led to the first diagnosis of Paget's disease in more than three-quarters of patients (Grundy, 1970). In our own practice, fractures (excluding vertebral fractures) occurred in 11 per cent of patients (Table 5.1) comparable to other series (Galbraith et al, 1977). The risk of fracture varies in proportion to the extent of bone involvement (Grundy, 1970; Harinck et al, 1986). Half the patients with femoral fractures have involvement of the entire femur. The risk of fracture does not depend on the radiographic appearance. A possible exception is in patients with rapidly advancing osteolytic disease of the tibia who appear to be at particular risk (Figure 5.12).

The overall risk of fracture in the pagetic population is disputed. The reasons for the controversy relate to the uncertain effects of treatment on fracture frequency (Chapter 8). No prospective data are available and retrospective analyses give differing estimates of incidence which vary from 1.5 to 6.6 fractures per 100

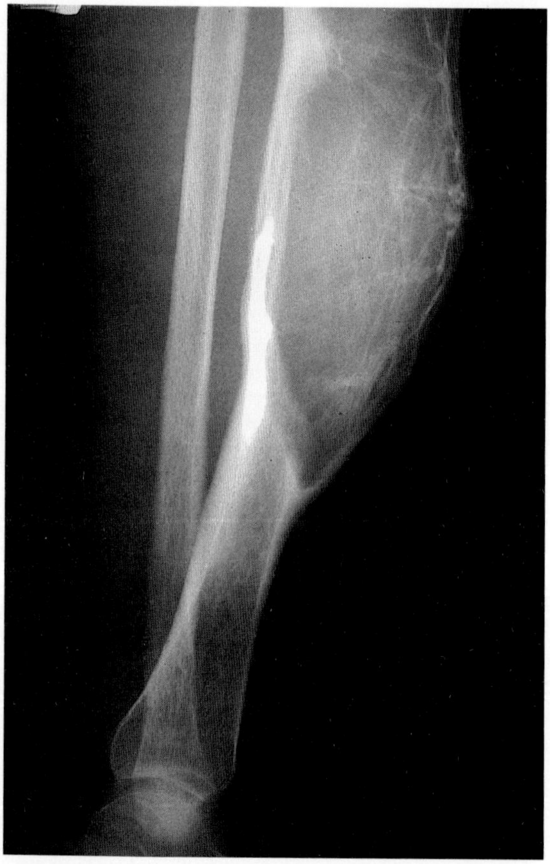

Figure 5.12

Progressive osteolytic Paget's disease of the tibia in a young man. The fissure fracture at the tibial convexity became complete 3 months later.

Table 5.5 Sites of fractures of the femur in Paget's disease of bone. Note the comparative rarity of cervical fracture. Combined data of Barry (1969), Grundy (1970) and Dove (1980).

Site of fracture	*No of fractures*	*%*
Femoral neck	50	14.5
Trochanteric	42	12.2
Subtrochanteric	97	28.1
Upper third of shaft	60	17.4
Middle third of shaft	64	18.5
Lower third of shaft	32	9.3

Table 5.6 Distribution of femoral fractures (as a percentage) in patients with Paget's disease and control patients in Sheffield. The controls are all patients admitted with femoral fracture to Royal Hallamshire Hospital between April 1988 and March 1989. There was a highly significant difference in the distribution of fractures ($\chi^2 = 36$; $p<0.001$) between patients with and without Paget's disease.

	Pagetic ($n = 15$)	*Controls ($n = 533$)*
Neck of femur	20	81
Subtrochanteric	33	10
Shaft	47	9

patient years (Nagant de Deuxchaisnes and Krane, 1964; Altman and Collins, 1980; Johnston et al, 1983; Nagant de Deuxchaisnes et al, 1985).

Fractures commonly follow trivial injury. In about half the patients with long-bone fracture no history of significant trauma is given, and in a further 25 per cent the trauma is minimal. In the case of femoral fractures in particular, they may be preceded by pain and represent the extension of fissure fractures (Grundy, 1970; Figure 5.11). Several studies indicate that the distribution of femoral fracture is quite different from that in elderly patients without Paget's disease (Barry, 1969; Grundy, 1970; Dove, 1980; Table 5.5). In Paget's disease subtrochanteric fractures and fractures of the shaft are the most common and femoral neck fractures are comparatively rare. In contrast, fractures of the femoral neck are the most common in the elderly without Paget's disease (Table 5.6).

Unlike fractures of normal bones, complete fractures through pagetic long bones are generally transverse rather than spiral (Figure 5.13), the so-called 'chalk stick' or 'banana' fracture.

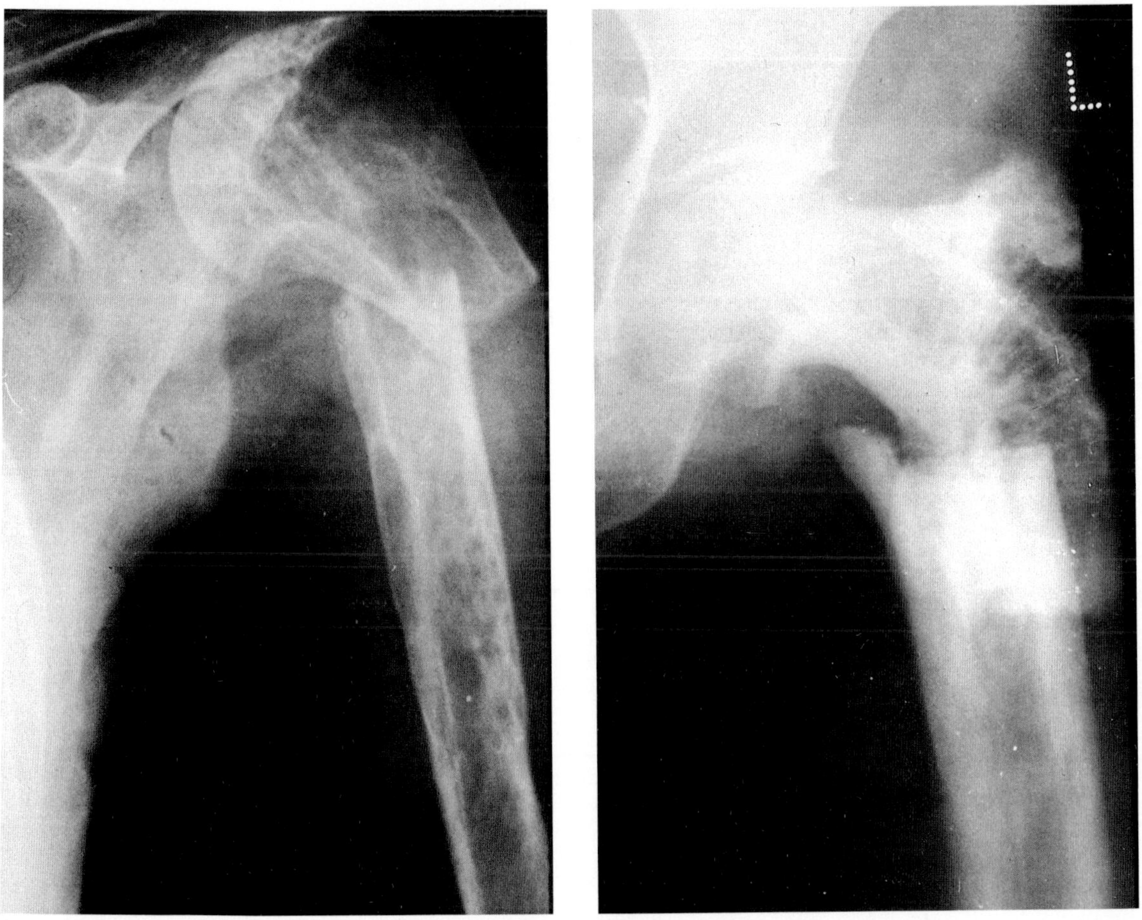

A B

Figure 5.13

Fractures of the humerus (A) and femur (B) which are transverse and typical of fractures through pagetic bone.

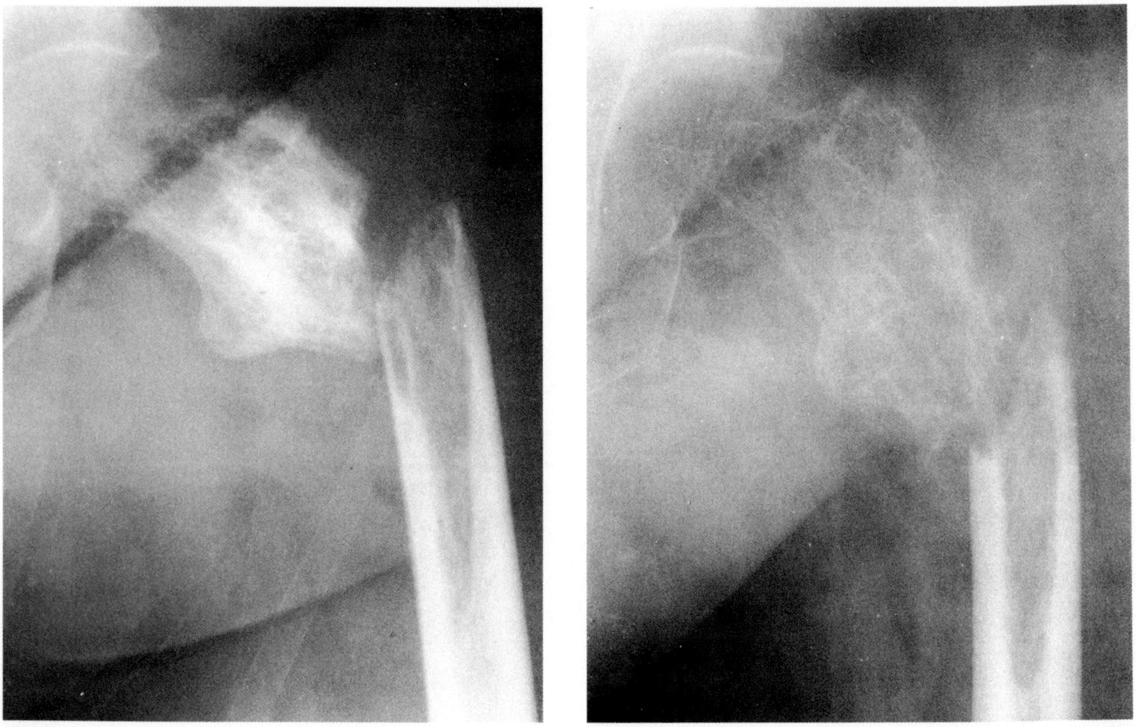

A B

Figure 5.14

Effect of immobilization after fracture in Paget's disease. (A) shows a recent fracture with characteristically mixed patchy osteosclerosis and radiolucency. Two months later (B), marked rarefaction of bone occurred due to immobilization amplified by the high pre-existing bone turnover. A biopsy was taken which excluded sarcoma. (From Maldague and Malghem, 1989.)

There is commonly a small lip of bone on the concave end of the fracture line. These observations are consistent with the view that many fractures represent extensions of incomplete fractures. In addition, the prevalence of multiple fissure fracture in patients with a complete fracture is high (33 per cent in the series of Grundy, 1980), indicating a greatly increased risk of complete fracture in patients with fissure.

A number of complications of fracture arise with increased frequency at pagetic sites, many of which are discussed elsewhere, including the management of fracture (Chapter 8). Indeed, the increased risk of complications often dictates the management. Radiographic rarefaction secondary to fracture may be very marked (Figure 5.14) and should be distinguished from sarcomatous transformation which causes pathological fracture.

Complications of fracture arising with increased frequency in pagetic bone.

Excessive blood loss
Compartment syndromes and neurovascular complications
Delayed and non-union
Hardware failure
Increased deformity
Focal rarefaction of bone
Hypercalciuria and hypercalcaemia
Heterotopic ossification

Union of fracture

Many complete fractures appear to heal well either with closed or surgical reduction, but a high incidence of non-union has been reported by several authors (Nicholas and Killoran, 1965; Barry, 1969; Dove, 1980; Grundy, 1980). Dove (1980) found an overall incidence of 40 per cent in 150 femoral fractures. The rate of non-union was 75 per cent for cervical fractures and 36 per cent for sub-trochanteric and diaphyseal fractures. In addition, the early mortality was high (18 per cent at 3 months), in part related to the problems of conservative management. In other series the rate of non-union is lower (Rauis, 1974) but even when cervical fractures of the femur are excluded, the incidence of non-union is still appreciable (Table 5.7; Figure 5.15).

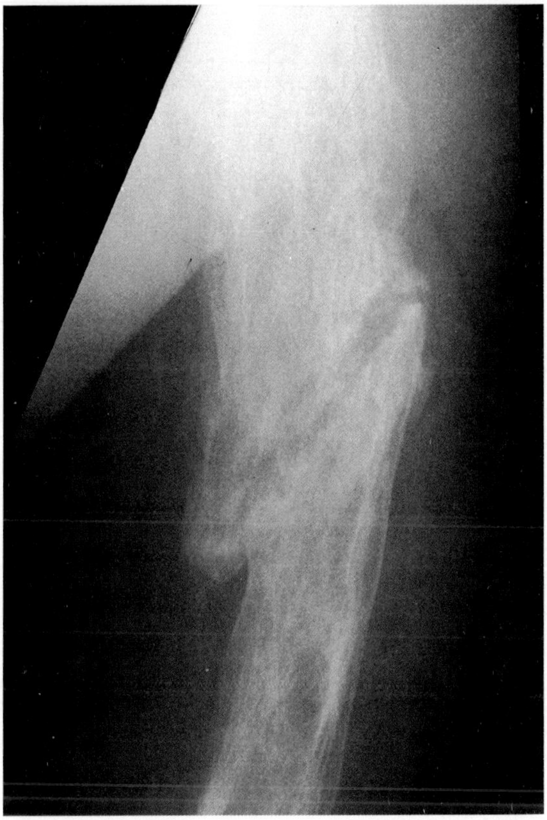

Figure 5.15

Non-union of fracture of the left humerus managed conservatively.

Other fractures

Fractures of long bones other than the femur, tibia and humerus are rare and account for 8 per cent of long-bone fractures (Louyot et al, 1975). Apart from the long bones and vertebral bodies, the most common sites for fracture are the patellae and pelvis. These sites account for 20 per cent of all extra-vertebral fractures in our own series. There is a high incidence of avulsion fracture at both sites.

Table 5.7 Incidence of non-union in femoral fractures. Combined data of Grundy (1970), Barry (1969) and Dove (1980). Non-union defined according to Dove (1980).

Site of fracture	*No of evaluable patients*	*No with non-union*	*% with non-union*
Femoral neck	39	28	72
Trochanteric	30	4	13
Subtrochanteric	94	20	21
Upper third of shaft	44	10	23
Middle third of shaft	55	14	25
Lower third of shaft	33	11	33
	295	87	29

The radiographic appearances of vertebral fractures are discussed in Chapter 3. Of particular importance is the frequency with which osteolysis is observed in fractured vertebral bodies and, in the absence of vertebral enlargement, may be mistaken for collapse due to involutional osteoporosis. Fractures may result in kyphosis and substantial loss of height. Back pain is common. Occasionally a single or multiple fracture gives rise to an angular deformity or displacement (see Chapter 3, Figure 3.23) which contributes to neurological complications.

Neurological syndromes

Neurological complications are common and are among the more serious clinical problems encountered (Table 5.8; Schmidek, 1977; Douglas et al, 1981a,b). They arise mainly from Paget's disease affecting the skull or vertebral column. Occasionally, bone enlargement may cause entrapment of peripheral nerves such as the median nerve at the wrist or common and lateral peroneal and posterior nerves of the leg.

Table 5.8 Neurological syndromes in Paget's disease.

Mechanism	*Symptoms*
Skull	
Deformity of skull base (basilar invagination)	Acute brain stem compression; long tract, cranial nerve syndromes; internal hydrocephalus; vascular compression
Narrowing of cranial nerve foramina	I, II, V, VII, VIII lower motor neurone cranial nerve palsies
Hyperaemia of skull vault	Dementia; vascular 'steal' from internal carotid system
Vertebrae	
Compression of spinal cord, nerve roots or cauda equina	Root pain; paraparesis, quadriparesis; cauda equina lesion
Compression or steal of vascular supply	Paraparesis; quadriparesis

Platybasia and cranial syndromes

Platybasia is invagination of the base of the skull which gives rise to impaction of the odontoid process on to the brain stem. A variety of neurological problems may result (Freidman et al, 1971; Schmidek, 1977) due to hydrocephalus, vascular steal or nerve entrapment. These include ataxia, muscle weakness due to long tract defects and disturbances of the control of respiration. Other features include vertebrobasilar insufficiency, cerebellar dysfunction and entrapment of the lower cranial nerves.

A variety of radiological criteria have been devised for the assessment of platybasia (see Table 3.16; Chapter 3). These are of some interest, but many patients with marked platybasia have few if any symptoms. The syndromes which arise include acute brainstem lesions with obstructive hydrocephalus and papilloedema (Bull et al, 1959; Taylor and Chakravorty, 1964). Less acute features may be associated with communicating hydrocephalus giving rise to varying degrees of ataxia with a broad-based gait, deterioration of mental function and incontinence (Culebras et al, 1974; Goldhammer et al, 1979; Martin et al, 1985). Occasionally, this may present with Parkinsonism (Botez et al, 1977). The syndrome is important to recognize since surgical shunting procedures may give dramatic results. The syndrome needs to be distinguished from symptoms due to the vascular steal syndrome.

Headache, confusion and agitation are common in the elderly, and have all been described in Paget's disease (Hamdy, 1981). The causal relationship is, however, not always certain. Pagetic bone pain or hydrocephalus may cause headache, but an alternative, though not mutually exclusive, possibility is a vascular steal syndrome. Patients with extensive skull involvement commonly have an increased blood flow through the external carotid arteries (Blotman et al, 1975) and tortuosity of the superficial temporal artery may be clinically obvious. This may give rise to a steal syndrome and also account for headache and other neurological syndromes (Ibbertson et al, 1979). Irrespective of the mechanism, we have seen the occasional patient with headache in whom there was a close relationship between biochemical indices of disease activity and headache over many years.

The incidence of epidural haematoma is low in

the elderly, thought to be due to the adherence of the dura to the inner table of the skull. The occasional report of epidural haematoma in elderly pagetic patients after trivial trauma (Drapkin, 1984; Itoyama et al, 1986) suggests that increased bone vascularity might increase the risk of this disorder.

Deafness

Deafness is by far the most common complication of Paget's disease of the skull and is found in 30–50 per cent of patients with skull involvement at presentation (Rozenkrantz et al, 1952; Nager, 1975; Hamdy, 1981). It has been suggested that Beethoven's deafness was due to Paget's disease (Naiken, 1971). Vestibular disturbances occur in a smaller proportion of patients (up to 25 per cent) and occasionally tinnitus may be incapacitating (Nager, 1975). It is important to recognize that deafness is common in old age, and it may sometimes be very difficult to determine to what extent deafness when present is attributable directly to Paget's disease.

The mechanism of hearing loss is multifactorial (Davies, 1968; Lindsay and Lehman, 1969; Nager, 1975). A predominant component is sensorineural hearing loss due to involvement of the petrous temporal bone and progressive involvement of the internal auditory canal. Sometimes invasion of the cochlea by pagetic bone occurs, but the labyrinthine capsule appears to be relatively resistant and its involvement by the pagetic process is a late feature (Proops et al, 1985). Conductive hearing loss may result from involvement of the ossicles of the middle ear, resulting in ankylosis and rigidity of the foot plate of the stapes (Waltner, 1965). Chronic otitis media may also occur due to narrowing of the eustachian tube or occlusion of the external auditory canal (Sparrow and Duval, 1967). Direct compression of the eighth nerve can be caused by basilar invagination with tension of the nerve, but is thought to be uncommon.

Other cranial nerve lesions

Four out of the 23 patients initially described by Paget became blind, but this frequency is atypical and blindness is rarely encountered. Narrowing of the optic foramen may produce papilloedema and optic atrophy. Vascular changes include retinal artery occlusion. Choroidoretinal changes such as angioid streaks are reviewed later. Diplopia occasionally arises due to pressure on occulomotor nerves. Cranial nerve defects of all types have been described and may give rise to anosmia, trigeminal neuralgia, facial palsy or bulbar palsy with dysphagia (Gardner and Dohn, 1966; Schmitt et al, 1968; Schmidek, 1977; Eretto et al, 1984).

Spinal disease

The spine is one of the common sites in the skeleton to be affected by Paget's disease (Chapter 3), and it is not surprising that pain and neurological complications have been widely described (Schmidek, 1977; Douglas et al, 1981; Hamdy, 1981; Altman et al, 1987).

Although spinal cord dysfunction is a serious complication, it is important to stress that it is exceptional. Most patients with Paget's disease of the spine have no symptoms. Even when radiographs are taken to investigate the cause of low back pain and sciatica, the finding of Paget's disease does not necessarily indicate that the symptoms and radiographic findings are causally related. Indeed, the experience of long-term medical treatment suggests that back pain attributable to Paget's disease occurs in a minority – at least as judged by response to treatment (Altman et al, 1987). Computerized axial tomography has shown a high prevalence of facet arthropathy. In many instances this is asymptomatic, but among symptomatic patients the radiographic abnormalities are generally more marked (Zlatkin et al, 1986; Table 5.9).

Neurological lesions most frequently arise when Paget's disease affects the thoracic spine, perhaps because the vertebral canal is narrowest at this region and most easily compressed by architectural abnormalities (Hartman and Dohn, 1966; Douglas et al, 1981b). The mechanism of spinal syndromes is heterogeneous. Cord and spinal compression are frequently associated with enlargement of the vertebrae and a decrease in the diameter of the spinal canal and nerve foramina (Klenerman, 1966; Direkze and Milnes,

Table 5.9 Relation between back pain (values expressed as percentages) and arthropathy of facetal joints affected by Paget's disease (Zlatkin et al, 1986).

Grade of facetal arthropathy	*Symptomatic (n = 21)*	*Asymptomatic (n = 15)*
Mild	5	33
Moderate	14	33
Severe	81	20

1970; Brown et al, 1971; Figure 5.16). Expansion of the pedicles and laminae also occurs and can be well visualized by axial tomography. Spinal syndromes may also arise due to pagetic extension into the ligamintum flavum or epidural fat (Clarke and Williams, 1975; Hadjipavlou et al, 1988).

In several patients with a typical clinical history no anatomical abnormalities have been shown on myelography (Sadar et al, 1972; Herzberg and Bayliss, 1980; Douglas et al, 1981). The lack of demonstrable cord compression in these cases suggests that ischaemia may be a major cause of neurological dysfunction, because the highly vascular pagetic bone diverts the blood supply from neural tissue. This notion is consistent with the known anatomical relationship between the blood supply of the cord and the vertebral bones (Crock and Yoshizawa, 1977). Mathe et al (1976) describe a delay in filling and emptying of the anterior spinal artery in patients with paraparesis, but with only partial obstruction on myelography.

The importance of a vascular steal syndrome is suggested by the very rapid response of many patients to medical treatment with agents such as calcitonin, which are known to decrease rapidly bone blood flow. Indeed, the results of medical treatment in slowly progressive paraparesis are at least as good as those obtained by surgery (Douglas et al, 1981; Chapter 8).

When disease of the thoracic spine is associated with compression of neural tissue, the Paget's disease characteristically involves a single dorsal vertebra. Pagetic involvement of the lumbar vertebrae with evidence of compression of the cauda equina and intermittent neurogenic claudication has also been described (Klenerman, 1966).

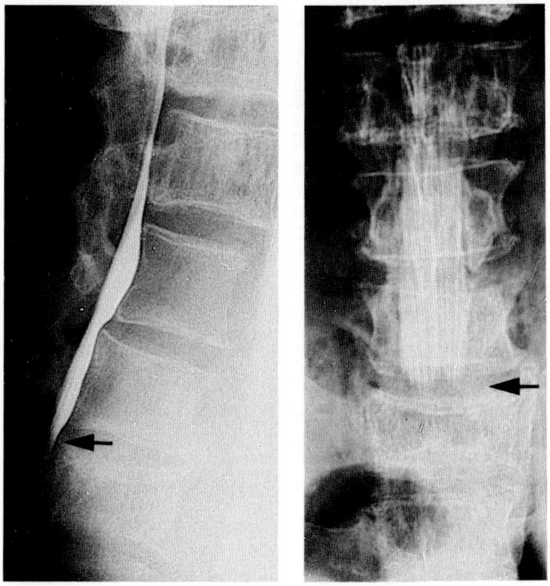

Figure 5.16

Myelogram in a patient presenting with calf pain on exercise. Two years later he developed back pain and a slowly developing paraparesis. The myelogram taken at this time shows complete obstruction at T12 (arrowed) and narrowing opposite the bodies of L3 and L4. The patient recovered with medical management. (From Douglas et al, 1981a).

Patients usually present with a slowly progressive impairment of spinal cord function with gradual onset of sensory and motor disease below the level of the lesion. Pain is a frequent complaint and may be secondary to local disc or articular problems, or may arise from the pagetic bone itself, from sarcomatous transformation, from vascular insufficiency or from root compression.

Joint disease

Pain arising from joints is a common accompaniment of Paget's disease. There are many causes of pain arising at joints (see page 125). Pain most often occurs when bones below and/or above the

Causes of pain arising at joints in Paget's disease.

Pagetic involvement below articular cartilage (pagetic arthropathy)
Osteoarthrosis
Deformity of bones above or below the joint
Bone pain referred to joints
Ankylosing spondylitis (HLA B27 negative)
Gout*
Chondrocalcinosis*
Periarthritis*

*Association of uncertain significance.

articular cartilage are affected (Franck et al, 1974). Sites which most commonly give rise to symptoms are the spine, hip and knee.

In most cases the disorder is not associated with striking radiographic features (Chapter 3). In the lumbar spine the frequency of spondylosis is not appreciably greater than in a control population (Guyer and Sheperd, 1980). Osteoarthrosis of the hip also occurs relatively infrequently (Graham and Harris, 1971; Roper, 1971b; Goldman et al, 1977) and focal degeneration of cartilage is uncommon. Pagetic tissue may involve the subchondral plate and give rise to uniform thinning of articular cartilage. Focal penetration of the subchondral plate may also occur (Milgram, 1977).

The mechanisms whereby joint pain arises are uncertain but are likely to be related to distortion of the joint by bony enlargement and deformity, and to the alteration of mechanical forces across the joint which arise from deformity of surrounding bones such as the neck of femur (coxa vara) and the innominate bone (protrusio acetabulae). Pain is said to arise more frequently in the presence of protrusio acetabulae or with the concurrent involvement of the head of femur and acetabulum than with femoral involvement alone (Singer, 1977). Hip pain is by no means invariable however, even in patients with significant narrowing of the joint space and marked protrusio.

The radiographic features of pagetic coxarthropathy are described in Chapter 3 and may be very florid, even when symptoms are not present. The natural history of Paget's disease of the hip has not been well studied, but in the few patients that we have managed conservatively, the disorder is relentlessly progressive irrespective of the medical management (Figure 5.17; see also Figure 8.8; Chapter 8).

The knee is a fairly common site of symptoms. It is most commonly associated with Paget's disease of the distal femur and is relatively uncommon with Paget's disease of the tibia in the absence of femoral involvement (Figure 5.18). Patellar disease rarely gives rise to symptoms.

At the spine, there is some relationship between the degree of facetal arthropathy and the presence of back pain (Table 5.9). Osteophyte formation, though not usually florid, may occasionally be very marked and give rise to ankylosis, particularly of the spine, but also at other sites.

Paget recognized an association of clinical gout with the disorder that others have also observed (Altman and Collins, 1980; Lluberas-Acosta et al, 1986; Figure 5.19), perhaps related to the high turnover of urate (Chapter 4). One survey found Paget's disease in 23 per cent of elderly patients with gout compared with a 2 per cent prevalence of Paget's disease in age-matched patients without gout. In a review of our most recent 200 cases we have only observed one patient with the clinical manifestations of gout so that, if the association is real, then its expression seems to vary between centres.

Chondrocalcinosis is also said to occur in Paget's disease more frequently but the evidence for this, reviewed later, is even less convincing than is the case for gout.

Oral and dental disease

When Paget's disease affects the jaw it is usually very extensive and gives rise to marked cosmetic and functional disability. It most frequently affects the maxilla alone, but in a substantial minority affects the mandible alone (20 per cent) or both (20 per cent; Smith and Eveson, 1981).

Alveolar ridges may widen and the palate flattens (Plate 16). In edentulous patients progressive disease may pose problems for the fitting of dentures due to the changing size of the alveolar ridges. Teeth may become loose or migrate. Hypercementosis of the teeth is a characteristic feature (Lucas, 1955; Cooke, 1956;

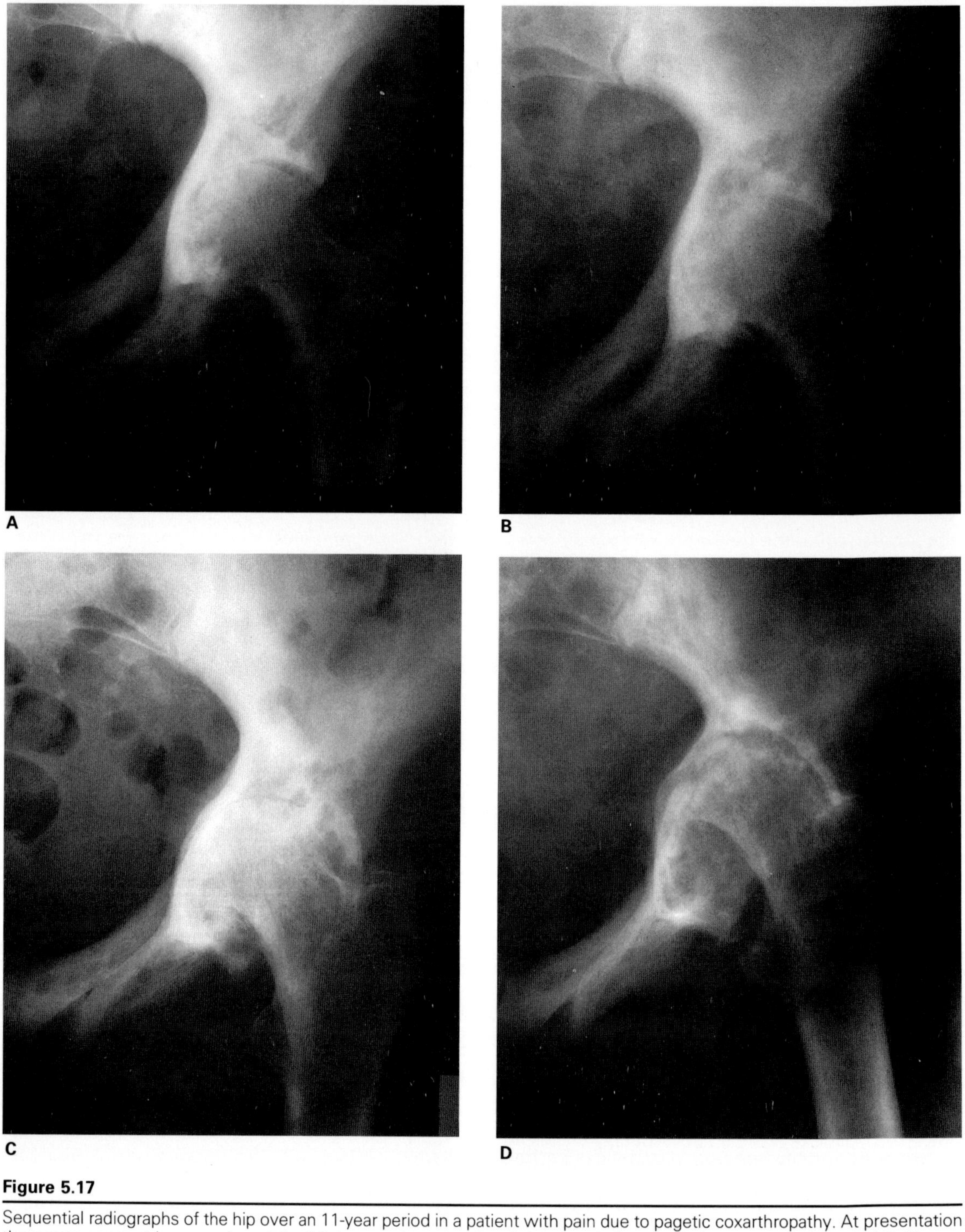

Figure 5.17

Sequential radiographs of the hip over an 11-year period in a patient with pain due to pagetic coxarthropathy. At presentation there was concentric narrowing of the joint space, hypertrophy of the acetabular margin but no osteophytosis (A). Three years later there had been some thinning of the acetabular wall (B) which after a further 4 years (C) encroached onto the pelvic brim. Four years later (D) the head of the femur had eroded with disruption of the acetabulum.

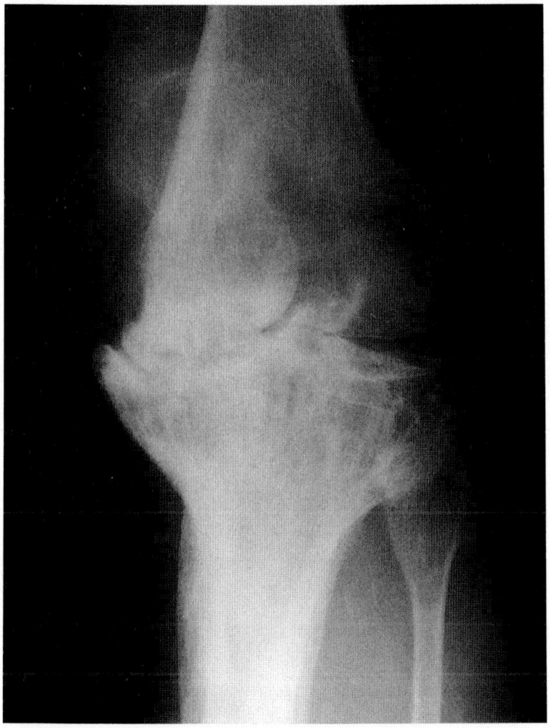

Figure 5.18

Marked osteoarthrosis at the knee joint associated with tibial Paget's disease. Osteoarthrosis at this site is more usually associated with Paget's disease of the femur.

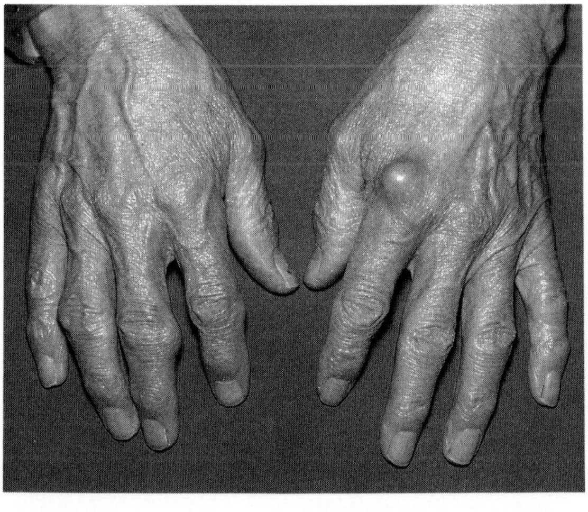

Figure 5.19

Gouty tophus associated with extensive Paget's disease.

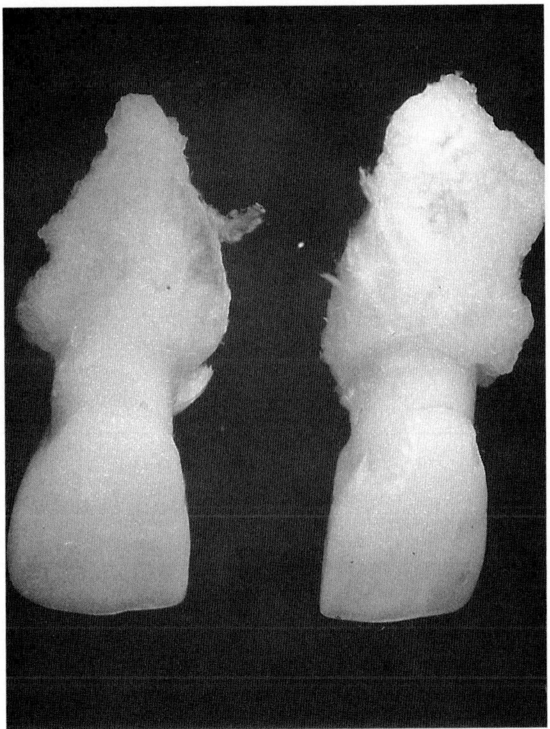

A

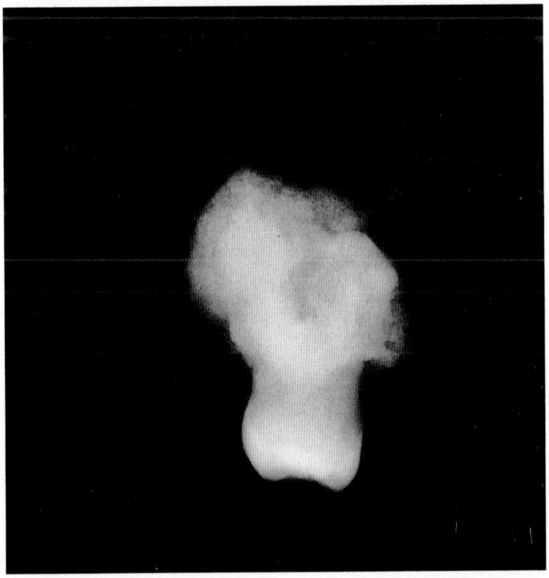

B

Figure 5.20

(A) Photograph and (B) radiograph of teeth affected by Paget's disease. The roots show marked hypercementosis and extraction was associated with the removal of surrounding alveolar bone.

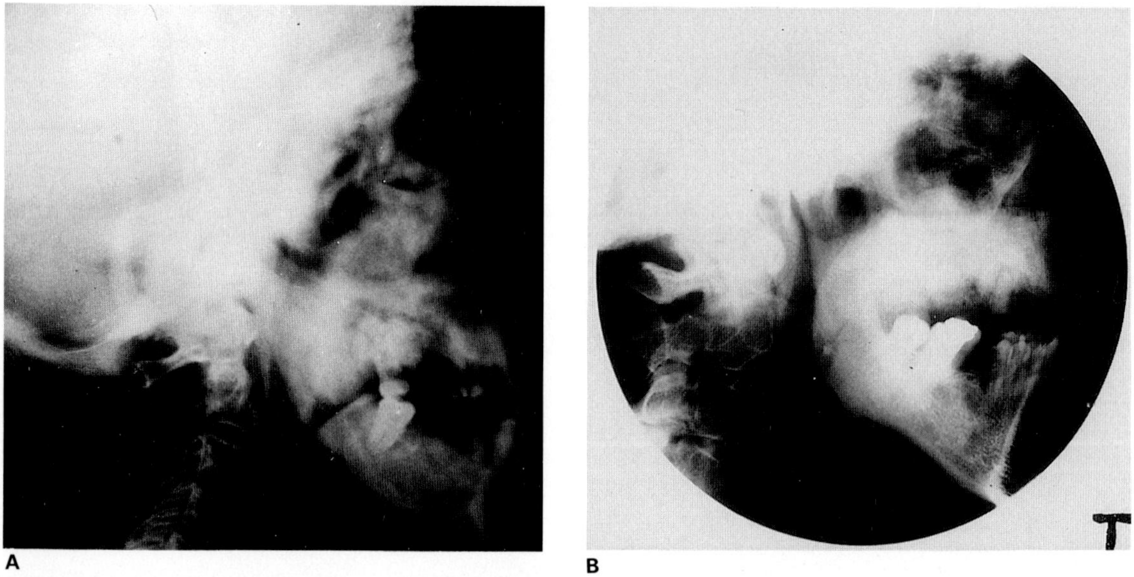

Figure 5.21

Sequential radiographs of the jaws in a patient (A) before and (B) after surgical extraction of teeth. Note the marked hypercementosis before surgery of the upper molar and the imperfect extraction of roots after surgery.

Figure 5.20) and may pose difficulties with tooth extraction (Figure 5.21) and significantly increases post-extraction morbidity (Sofaer, 1984). The radiographic features are described in Chapter 3.

Cardiovascular complications

Cardiac output may be increased in patients with Paget's disease (Howarth, 1953; Henley et al, 1979; Figure 5.22), associated with an increase in the capillary bed (Rhodes et al, 1972). It can give rise to high output failure, particularly in patients with extensive disease where 30 per cent or more of the skeleton is involved (Henley et al, 1979). This is thought to be due to the increase in skin and bone blood flow. Increased cutaneous blood flow may be very obvious clinically (Heistad et al, 1975). Features include an increase in skin temperature and dilation of superficial veins, particularly over the scalp. In addition, there may be prominence and tortuosity of the superficial temporal artery, presumably reflecting an increase in external carotid blood flow (Blotman et al, 1974, 1975).

Increased bone blood flow is undoubtedly of importance in the pathophysiology of several neurological syndromes. The highly vascular bone itself also increases the risk of substantial bleeding during surgery, and there is anecdotal evidence of massive blood loss during orthopaedic surgery (Barry, 1969; Bowie and Kanis, 1977; Stevens, 1981). Although few controlled trials have been undertaken (Goutallier et al, 1984), many surgeons now prefer to have their patients with Paget's disease medically treated before elective surgery.

There seems to be a reasonable degree of correlation between bone blood flow, cardiac

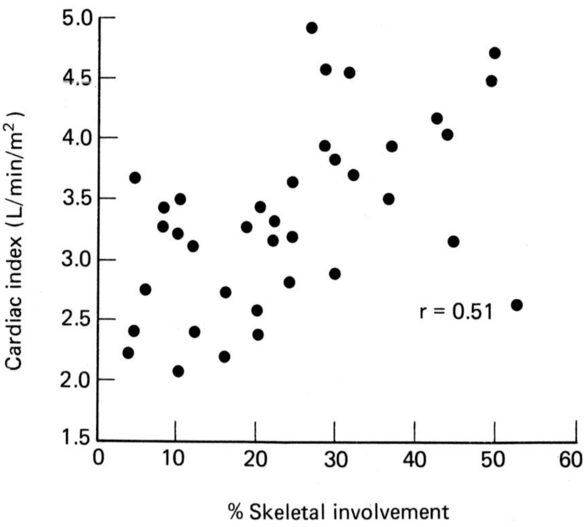

Figure 5.22

Relationship between cardiac index and extent of Paget's disease as judged by radiography. (From Henley et al, 1979.)

index and biochemical estimates of disease activity (Henley et al, 1979; Wooton et al, 1981). Others have not found the relationship to be so striking (Crosbie et al, 1975), perhaps due to a variable incidence of ischaemic heart disease and hypertension.

It seems likely that a high cardiac output would compromise cardiac function in the presence of ischaemic heart disease. In addition, there is evidence that left ventricular function is compromised in the presence of Paget's disease when disease extent involves 15 per cent or more of skeletal volume (Arnalich et al, 1984). It has been suggested that calcification of blood vessels is more common in Paget's disease (Acar et al, 1968; Barry, 1969; Hamdy, 1981). There is more convincing evidence for an association with aortic valvular calcification identified at autopsy (Strickberger et al, 1987). The prevalence was 4-fold greater in Paget's disease than in age- and sex-matched controls. A gradient of risk was also evident with the extent of Paget's disease (Figure 5.23). Mitral valve calcification was not observed

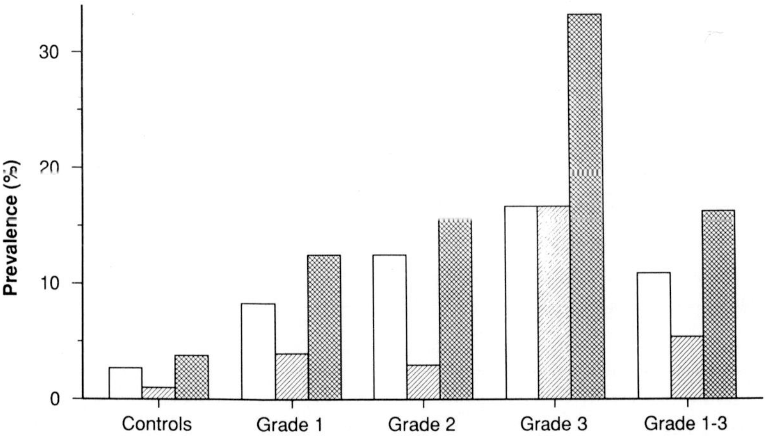

Figure 5.23

Prevalence of aortic calcification in an autopsy series of 77 subjects with Paget's disease and 184 age-, sex- and race-matched controls. Cases of Paget's disease were stratified according to the extent of disease, grade 3 being the most extensive. Aortic calcification was graded as moderate (open bars), severe (hatched) or either (cross-hatched). Note the higher prevalence of aortic calcification which increases with the extent of the disease. (Data from Strickberger et al, 1987.)

with greater frequency. It is possible that the vascular and valvular changes could be related to the increase in cardiac output and haemodynamic damage from increased aortic flow. Such changes could increase the risk of cardiovascular disease.

Whereas blood flow to the skin is usually increased over bony sites affected by Paget's disease, the circulation to the skin may be severely compromised. We have observed several patients with tibial lesions and chronic dependent ulcers overlying the anterior border of the tibia (Plate 15). They arise after trivial trauma and rarely heal. They are quite characteristic of the pagetic site since no evidence for skin atrophy or dependent ulceration or stasis is observed on the contralateral leg when this is unaffected by Paget's disease. The aetiology of this is presumably related to vascular stasis or steal.

Neoplastic disease

Sarcoma arising in pagetic bone is fortunately rare, but is a serious complication of the disorder. The abnormal bone remodelling characteristic of Paget's disease and the convincing evidence for neoplastic transformation has been cited as evidence that Paget's disease is a benign neoplasm (Rasmussen and Bordier, 1974), a suggestion supported by the cellular pleomorphism of bone cells. As a concept it does not, however, give any clues as to the multi-focal origin of Paget's disease itself.

The true incidence of sarcomatous transformation is unknown, largely because of uncertainties concerning the incidence of the uncomplicated disorder. The incidence in hospital series of patients ranges from 1–10 per cent (Porretta et al, 1957; Barry, 1969; Wick et al, 1981), but its incidence in the pagetic community at large is likely to be much less, probably in the order of 0.15 per cent (Price, 1962).

Osteosarcoma has a bimodal distribution with modes in youth and in old age. A component of the second mode is due to co-existing Paget's disease (MacKenzie et al, 1961; Price, 1962; Table 5.10). In approximately 25 per cent of patients with sarcoma over the age of 50, there is a reported association with Paget's disease (Sissons, 1966), but this could be an underestimate.

Table 5.10 Mortality from primary malignant tumours of bone in England and Wales 1951–3, categorized according to age (from MacKenzie et al, 1961).

	40–4	*45–9*	*50–4*	*55–9*	*60–4*	*40–64*
Total no of cases	30	33	55	52	76	246
No with Paget's disease	2	2	11	17	31	63
Percentage with Paget's disease	6	6	20	33	41	26

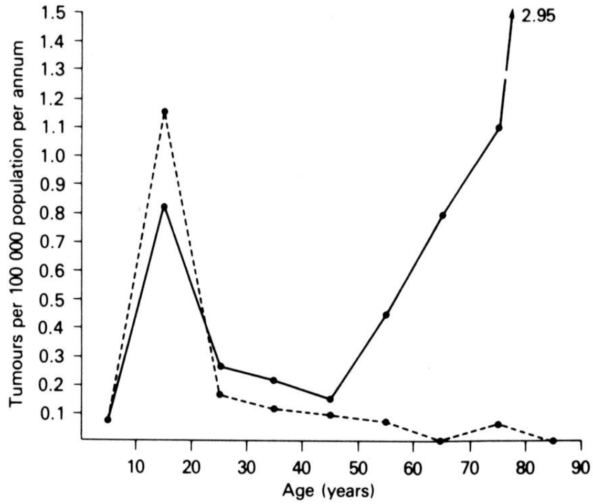

Figure 5.24

Incidence of osteogenic sarcoma in south-west England (solid line) and in Norway (dotted line). Note the bimodal incidence with age in the UK and the absence of a second mode in the elderly in Norway where Paget's disease is rare. (Adapted from Price, 1962.)

It is of interest that when sarcomas of the tibia, humerus and ilium are considered the association rises to 60 per cent and for the skull nearly all patients have co-existing Paget's disease (Porretta et al, 1957). It is of particular interest that an increase in the incidence of sarcoma in middle age is not observed in Norway (Price, 1962; Figure 5.24), where the prevalence of Paget's disease is extremely low. This suggests that Paget's disease may be under-reported in adults with sarcoma, and we have observed sarcoma in monostotic disease where the diagnosis of Paget's disease was unsuspected and only made at subsequent microscopy of tumour tissue. If Paget's disease accounts for most of the bone sarcomas in adults, it would be of interest to know whether a Lancashire focus for pagetic sarcoma exists as it appears to do for the uncomplicated disease.

It has been estimated that Paget's disease carries a 30-fold increase in the risk of bone sarcoma in adults (Price, 1962). In addition, sarcomatous change is more common in patients with widespread disease in whom the relative risk of sarcoma may be increased a further 5-fold. Sarcomata are twice as common in men than in women, similar to the sex distribution in non-pagetic sarcomata (Barry, 1969; Price and Goldie, 1969), and seem to arise exclusively at sites of pagetic involvement (Plates 17 and 18), although metastases have been found in normal bones. Claims for a multi-centric origin or neoplastic transformation in normal bone are likely to be due to early metastatic spread of the disorder to other skeletal sites (Porretta et al, 1957; Barry, 1961; Nagant de Deuxchaisnes and Krane, 1964).

Although sarcoma arises in pagetic tissue, the frequency with which this is found at various sites does not conform precisely to the frequency of pagetic involvement throughout the skeleton (Porretta et al, 1957; Barry, 1961). Instead it conforms more to the distribution of non-pagetic sarcoma. The pelvis and femora are common sites, followed by the humerus, face and skull (Villiaumey and Larget-Piet, 1974; Wick et al, 1981). Sarcoma thus appears to spare the vertebral column and to have a predilection for the humerus, femur and tibia greater than that expected from the distribution of disease (Table 5.11).

Table 5.11 Anatomical distribution of sarcoma complicating Paget's disease (combined data of Barry, 1961; Price and Goldie, 1969; Greditzer et al, 1983; Schajowicz et al, 1983; Smith et al, 1984a; Haibach et al, 1985; Seret et al, 1987).

Site	*No*	*%*	*Expected number of Pagetic lesions*	*Relative risk*
Pelvis and sacrum	134	26	390	1.39
Femur	125	25	280	1.81
Humerus	94	19	158	2.41
Face and skull	51	10	270	0.77
Tibia	47	9	116	1.64
Spine	15	3	300	0.20
Scapula	10	2	120	0.34
Clavicle	6	1	55	0.44
Other	26	5	370	0.28
TOTAL	508		2059	1.00

Several different histological types of sarcoma are described (McKenna et al, 1964; Barry, 1969; Greditzer et al, 1983), but the most common is osteosarcoma, characterized histologically by the abundance of osteoid tissue with varying degrees of calcification (Plates 19 and 20). Benign giant cells are commonly present and may occasionally be abundant. Fibrosarcoma is the next most common, which is found in about 20 per cent of cases. Both osteosarcoma and fibrosarcoma are more common in men. The remaining types of tumour are rare (15 per cent) and include chondrocarcinoma (Plate 21), reticulosarcoma and pleomorphic tumours.

Perhaps surprisingly, the incidence of giant-cell tumours is low, and they may be benign or malignant (Hutter et al, 1963; Brook, 1970; Bloch-Michel et al, 1975; Upchurch et al, 1983; Plate 22). Benign lesions of the jaw may be indistinguishable from reparative granulomata. The morphology of giant-cell tumour is similar to that in other patients, but it has a predilection for the skull and face rather than the long bones of the limbs. Thus, although benign giant-cell tumours carry a good prognosis, many surgical difficulties arise in their management in Paget's disease because of encroachment on vital tissues. They may also respond to radiotherapy. An interesting series has been reported in the USA, three cases of which occurred in the one family. Two further cases shared the same ancestry in that they came from Avellino, near Naples (Jacobs et al, 1979). These lesions responded to treatment with corticosteroids.

A common presentation of patients with sarcoma is pain at the site of the tumour, often unresponsive to analgesics. The development of a new pain in a patient with long-standing Paget's

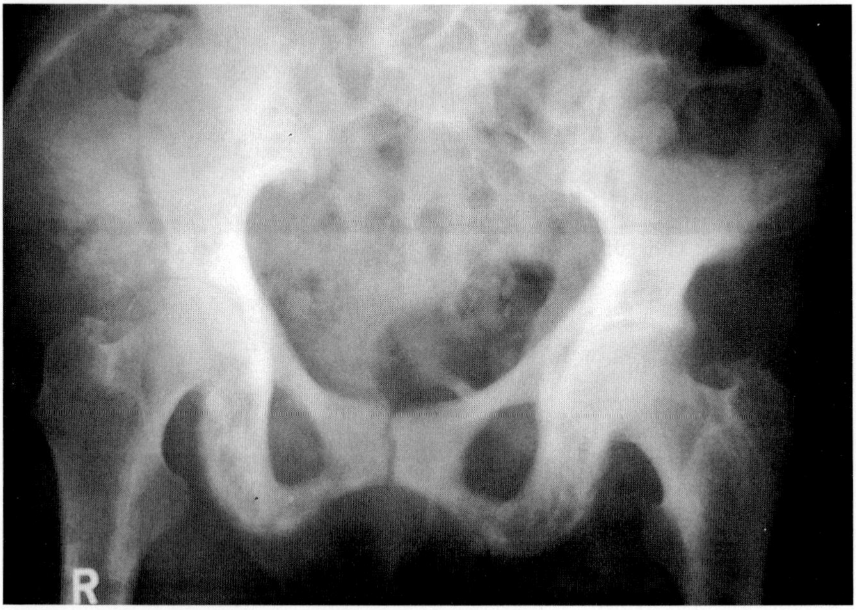

Figure 5.25

Pagetic sarcoma of the ilium presenting as fracture. Note the marked iliac hypertrophy.

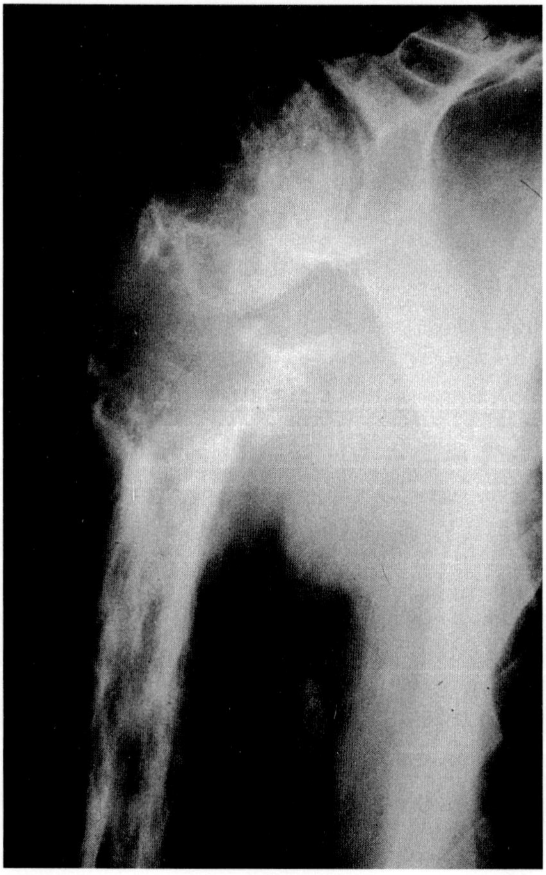

Figure 5.26

Fracture of the humeral neck associated with pagetic sarcoma.

disease not attributable to microfractures should arouse a high degree of suspicion. Patients may also present with pathological fracture (Figures 5.25 and 5.26). There may be swelling at the site of the tumour, which in some cases may enlarge very rapidly within a few weeks, but pain may precede any clinical or radiographic sign. Complaints arising from metastases (for example in other skeletal sites and lung) may also be found at presentation.

Unlike non-pagetic osteosarcoma, there is no predilection for the ends of the long bones. In addition, the earliest focus of transformation is commonly medullary rather than cortical. This means that the traditional radiographic features of osteosarcoma such as sun-ray spicules of new bone formation (Figure 5.27) and Codman's triangle due to periosteal elevation (Figure 5.28) are less frequently observed and found in one-

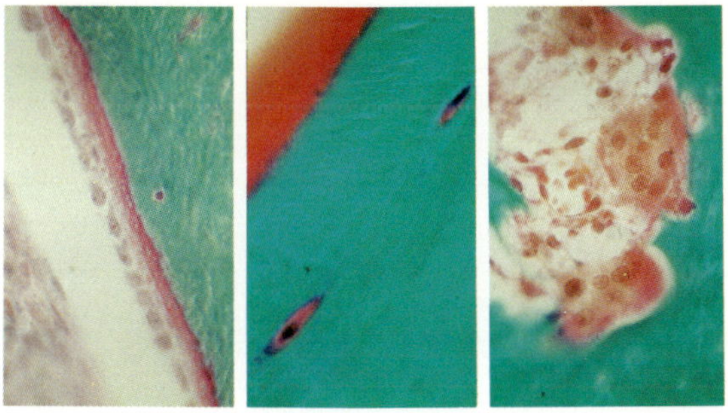

Plate 1

Bone cell types. Using Goldner's trichrome stain mineralized bone appears green and osteoid red. (Left) Osteoid synthesis by a sheet of osteoblasts (× 400). (Centre) Osteocytes buried within bone matrix (× 1000). (Right) Multinucleated osteoclasts creating a resorption cavity (× 400).

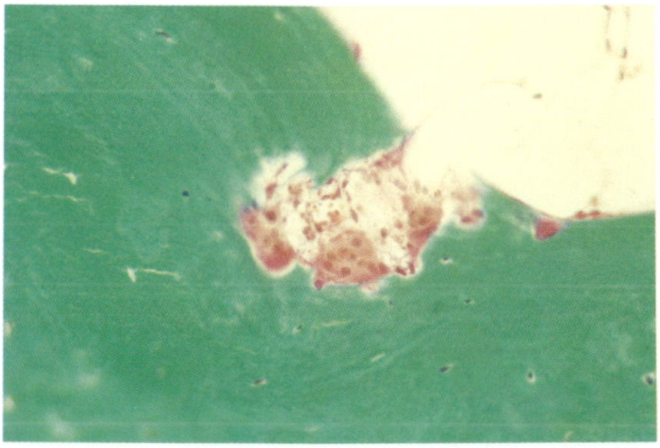

A

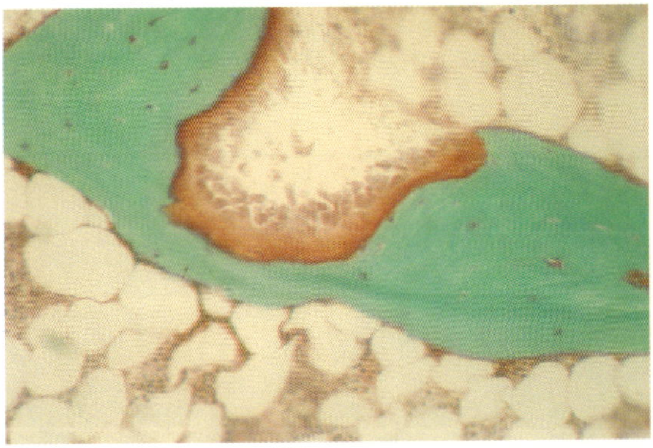

B

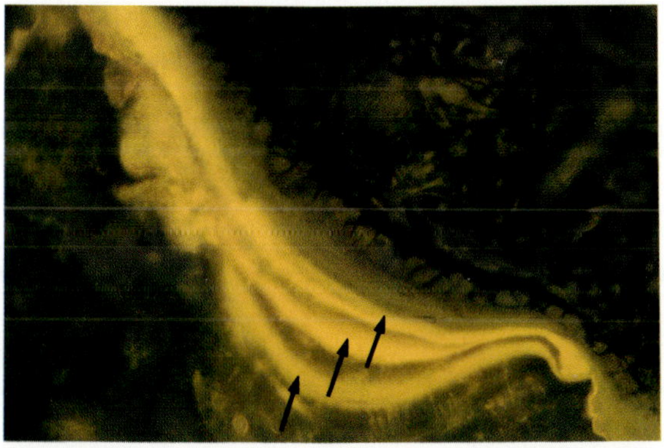

C

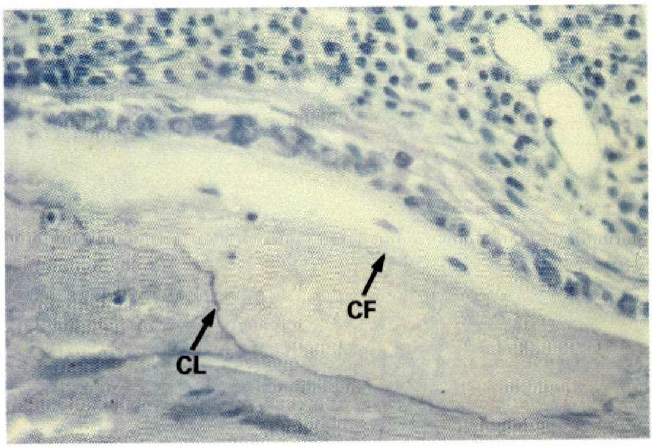

D

Plate 2

Steps in the remodelling sequence of trabecular bone. The activation of resorption comprises the formation of a team of osteoclasts (A) which are creating a resorption cavity within mineralized bone (× 200; stained green). At the completion of resorption, osteoblasts are attracted to the bed of the eroded surface (B, × 100) and are laying down an osteoid matrix (stained orange brown). As formation proceeds, mineralization occurs several days later (C) which is marked by tetracycline uptake at the site of mineralization (× 400). In this specimen three courses of tetracycline were given on separate occasions which are visible as three fluorescent bands under ultraviolet light (arrows). Note also the canalicular and osteocytic fluorescence. (D) (toluidine blue stain; × 400) shows a later stage of remodelling. The extent of previous resorption is shown by the cement line (CL) and the eroded cavity is now nearly completely infilled. The new bone matrix is partially mineralized and the site of mineralization is marked by the calcification front (CF).

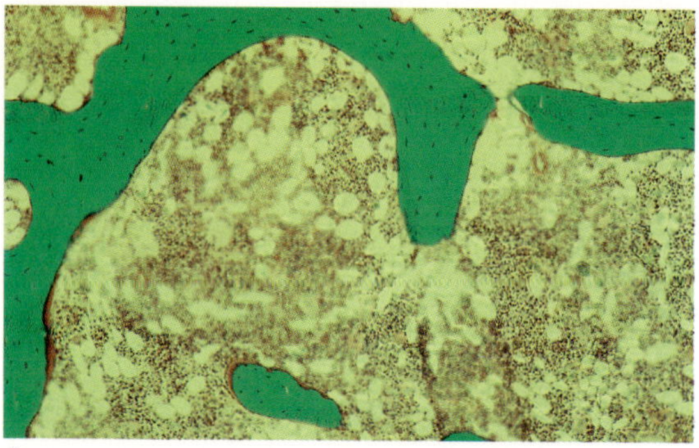

A

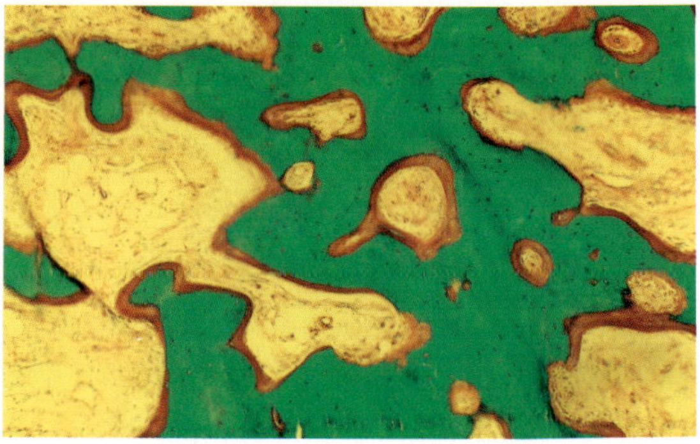

B

Plate 3

Comparison of normal (A) and pagetic bone (B) at the same magnification (× 100). Note that the trabecular bone surface in Paget's disease is nearly all covered by active events (osteoid formation stained orange), whereas this occupies the minority of the surface of normal bone.

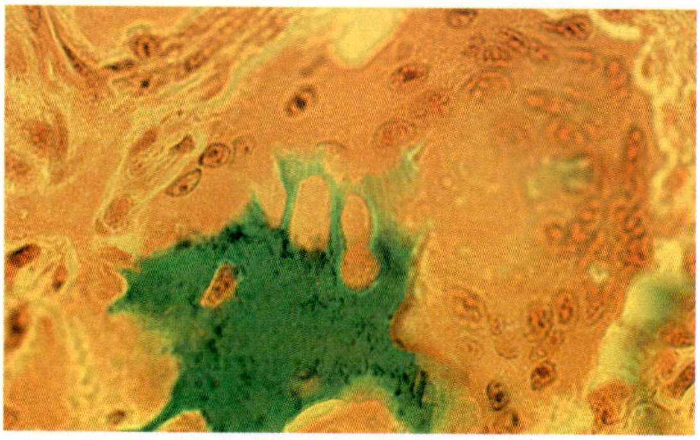

Plate 4

Giant osteoclast. Note that the osteoclast has almost engulfed a remnant of mineralized bone (stained green). Note also the marked marrow fibrosis (Goldner's trichrome; × 1000).

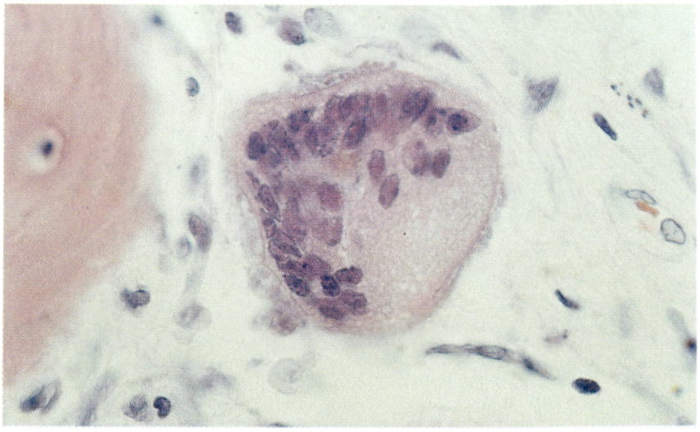

Plate 5

Pagetic osteoclast viewed by light microscopy showing a large number of nuclei. The nuclear staining is patchy with a central pallor and signifies the presence of large amounts of cytoplasmic inclusion material (haematoxylin and eosin; × 1000).

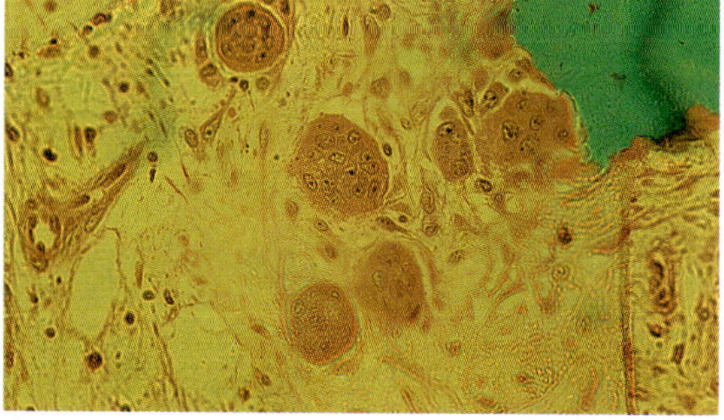

A

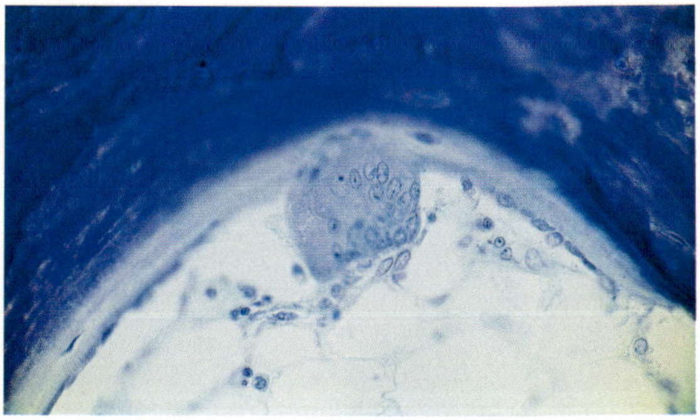

B

Plate 6

Pagetic giant osteoclasts. (A) (Goldner's stain × 200) shows abundant osteoclasts within the marrow stroma. (B) shows the resorption of osteoid by a giant osteoclast (toluidine blue; × 400).

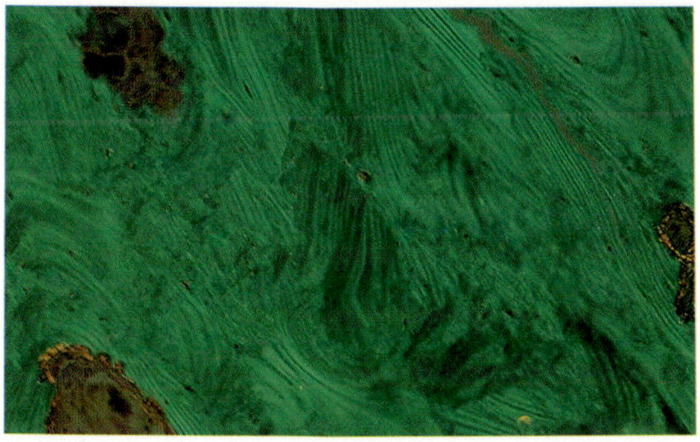
A

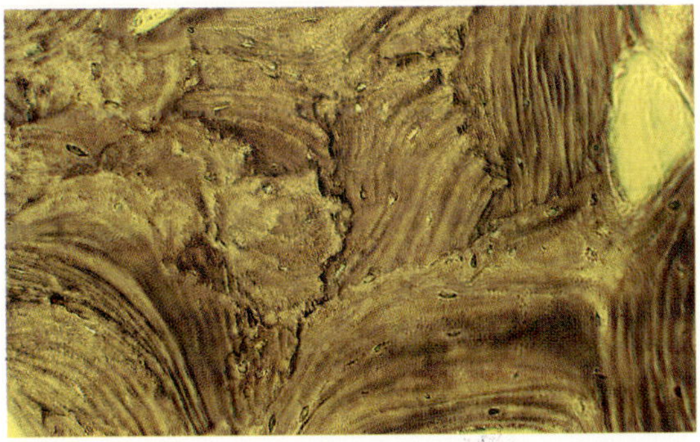
B

Plate 7

Mosaic appearance of pagetic bone. (A) (Goldner's trichrome; × 200) shows an admixture of woven and lamellar bone. The lamellar bone of each BSU is orientated differently to give a patchwork or mosaic appearance. (B) (same patient; toluidine blue; × 200) shows similar features but in addition the reversal lines are stained, accentuating the mosaic.

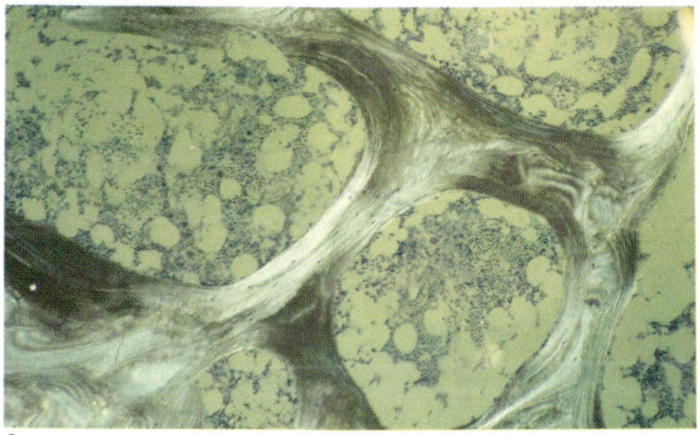
A

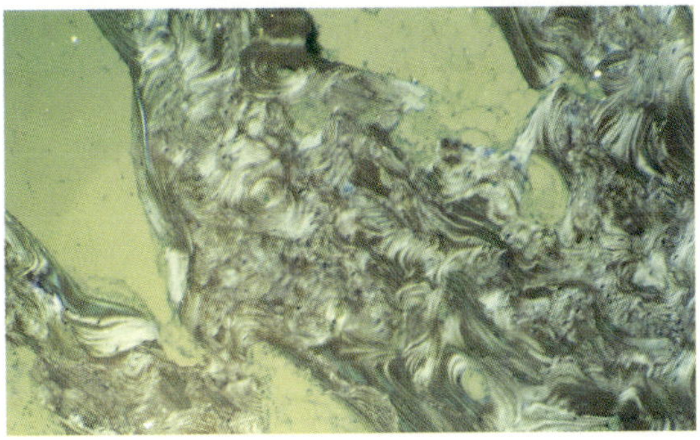
B

Plate 8

Sections of trabecular bone viewed under polarized light (× 100) showing the characteristics of normal lamellar bone (A) and woven bone (B) in Paget's disease. Note that the lamellar bone is laid down in the long axis of the trabeculae. In Paget's disease this orientation is lost.

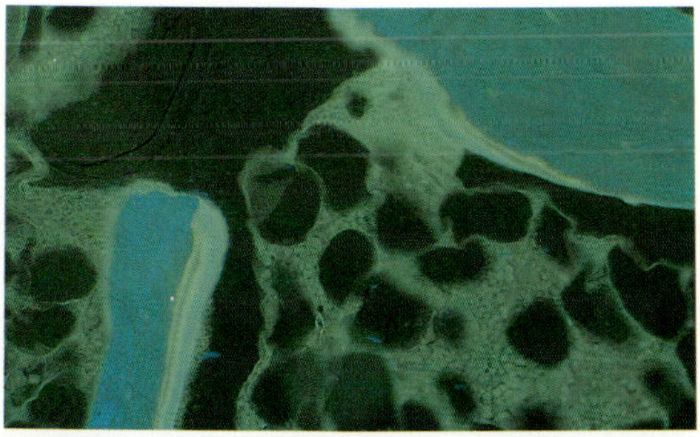
A

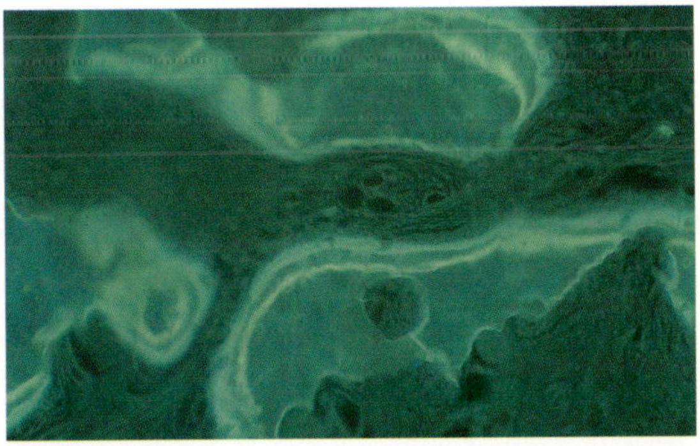
B

Plate 9

Tetracycline fluorescence after double labelling in a normal subject (A) and a patient with Paget's disease (B). The time interval between the two labels was the same (10 days) as is the magnification of the sections (× 100). Note the marked increase in mineral apposition rate (the label separation) in the pagetic biopsy and the larger surface occupied by mineralization (unstained undecalcified sections).

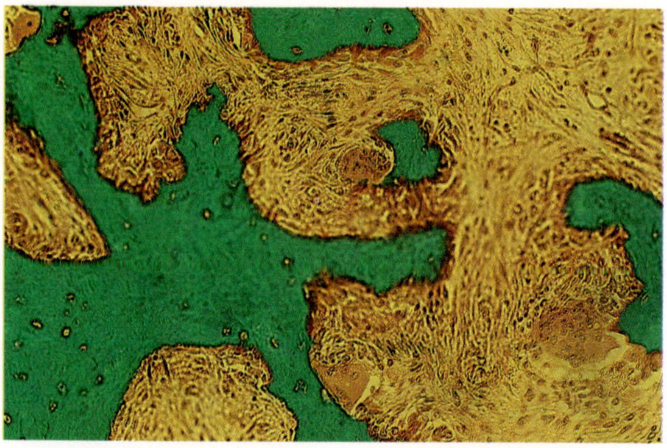

Plate 10

Section of trabecular bone in Paget's disease showing intense marrow fibrosis (Goldner's trichrome stain; × 66).

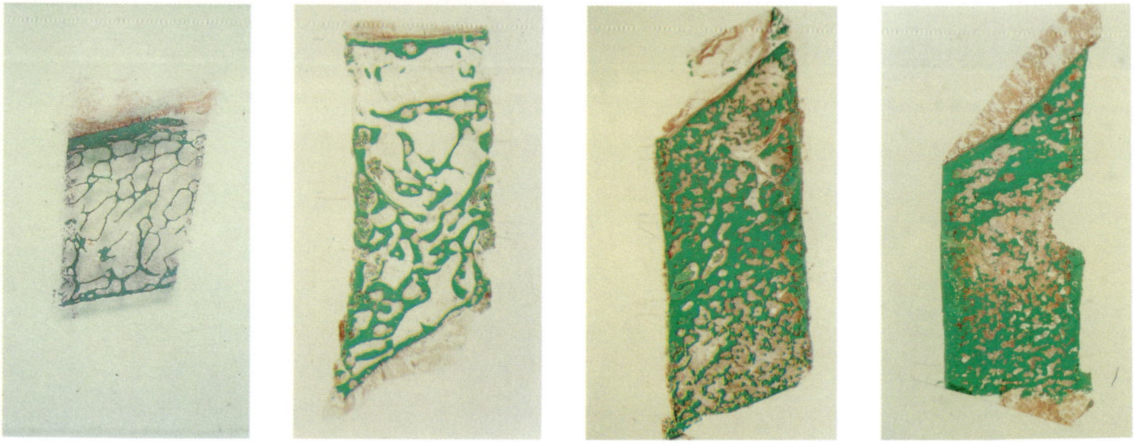

A B C D

Plate 11

Low-power microphotographs of transiliac biopsies in a normal subject (A) and patients with Paget's disease (B) (C) (D). Note the marked trabecular osteosclerosis (Goldner's trichrome stain; × 6). Sclerosis is predominantly due to trabecular thickening. When marked, the surface-to-volume ratio of trabecular bone decreases, and the differentiation from the cortex becomes indistinct.

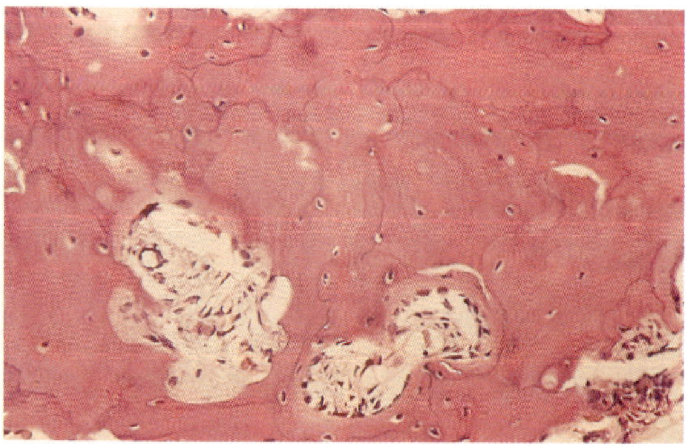

Plate 12

Histological section through pagetic cementum to show irregular resorption arrest lines (cement lines) characteristic of pagetic bone.

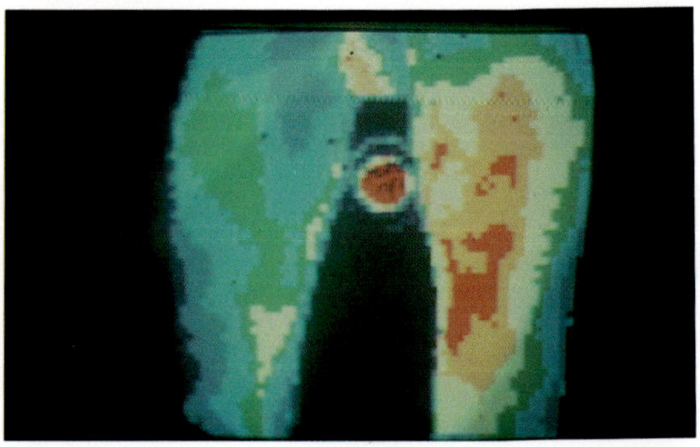

Plate 13

Thermogram of the thighs showing marked increase in skin temperature on the left due to an increase in capillary blood flow overlying Paget's disease. (From Kanis, 1984a.)

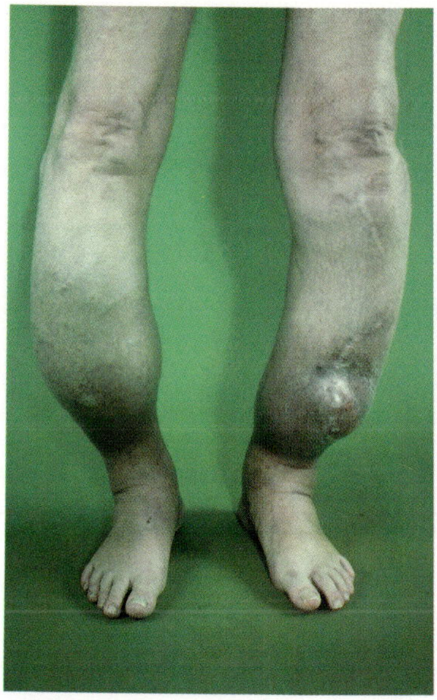

Plate 14

Marked deformity of both tibiae due to Paget's disease. Note the scars of the skin overlying the left tibia which are due to recurrent ulceration.

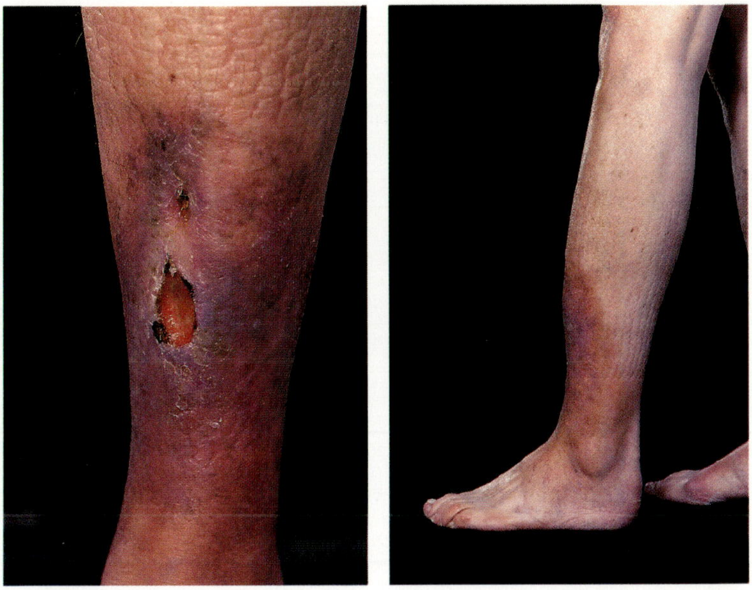

Plate 15

Persistent chronic ulcer overlying the anterior ridge of the tibia in a woman with Paget's disease of the tibia and a moderate anterior bowing deformity.

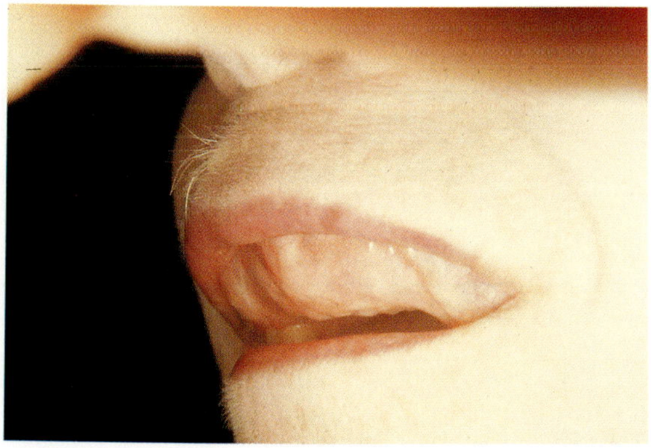

Plate 16

Facial deformity due to Paget's disease of the maxilla. Note the maxillary hypertrophy so that the alveolar ridge protrudes well below the lower hip.

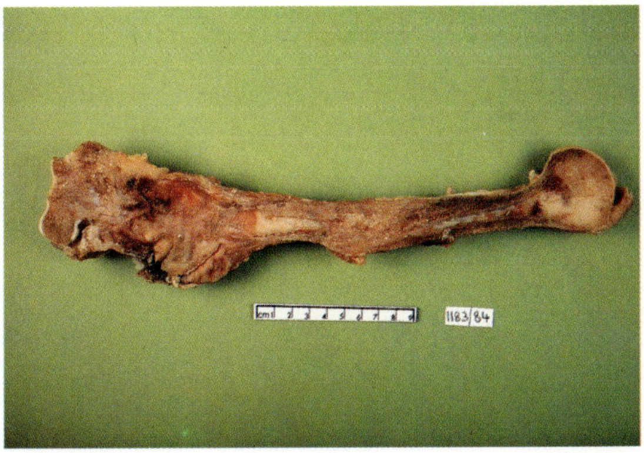

Plate 17

Gross specimen of bisected humerus extensively affected by Paget's disease. Sarcoma is present in the distal one-third arising from pagetic bone.

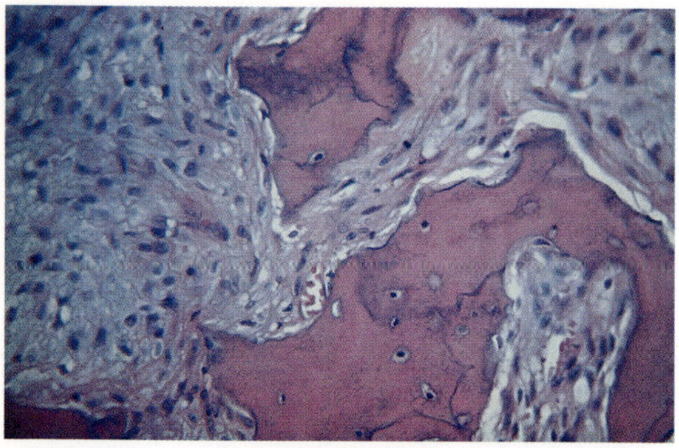

Plate 18

Sarcoma infiltrating bone showing the mosaic arrangement of cement lines indicative of pre-existing Paget's disease. Neoplastic bone formation is seen within the lesion, characteristic of osteosarcoma.

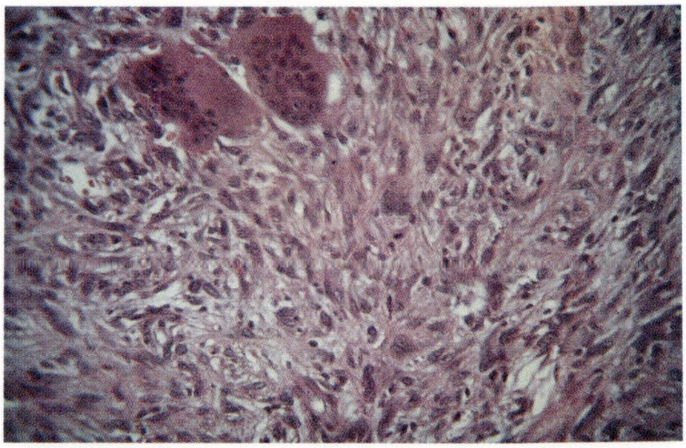

Plate 19

Sarcoma composed of spindle cells and benign multinucleate giant cells (malignant fibrous histiocytoma). This is one of the common histological patterns in sarcoma arising in pagetic bone.

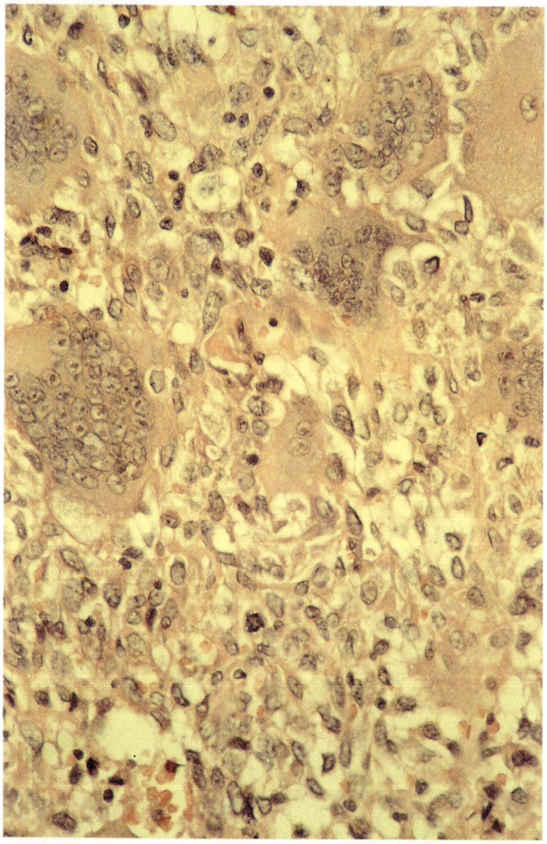

Plate 20

Area of high-grade osteosarcoma with hyperchromatic and pleomorphic cells with small areas of osteoid and large numbers of bizarre but benign multi-nucleated giant cells.

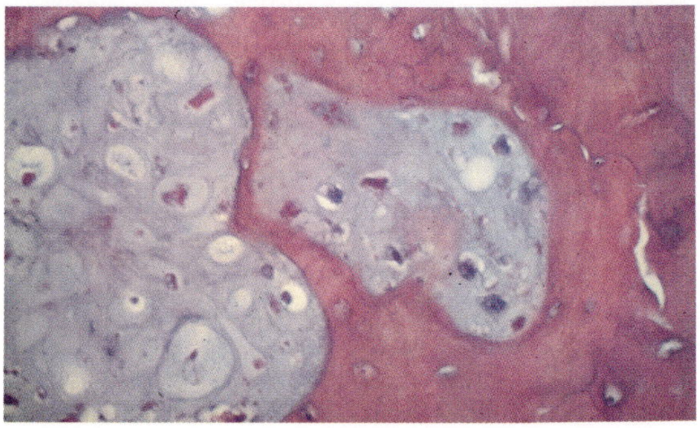

Plate 21

Chondrosarcoma infiltrating pagetic bone. This is a very uncommon form of pagetic sarcoma.

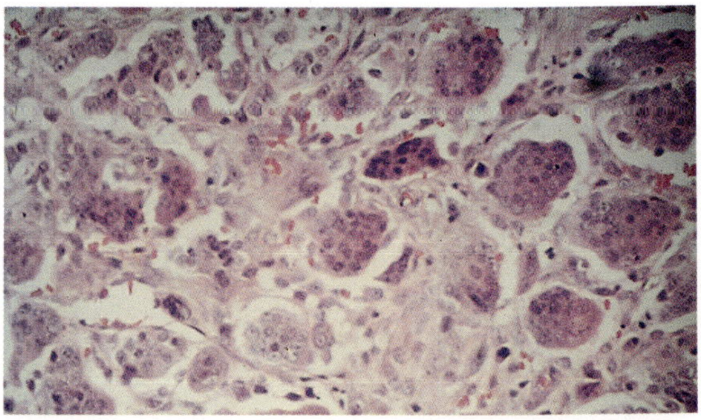

Plate 22

Tumour composed of a large proportion of benign multinucleate cells admixed with round and elongated stromal cells. This is a benign lesion closely resembling a giant cell tumour. This uncommon complication of Paget's disease must be distinguished from malignant fibrous histiocytoma.

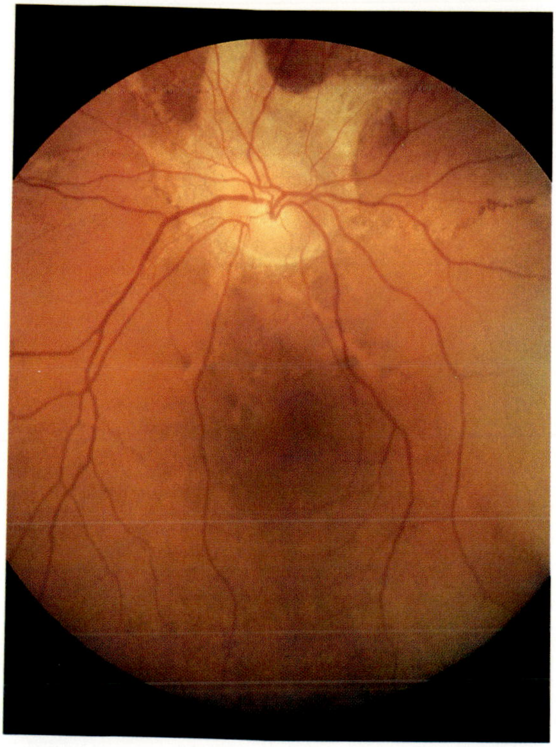

Plate 23

Fundal photograph of left eye. Angioid streaks are radiating from the optic disc.

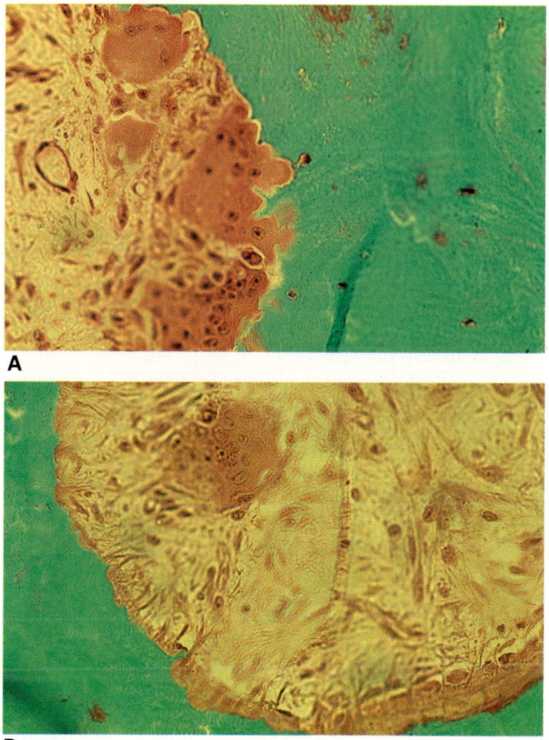

A

B

Plate 25

Early histological effects of diphosphonate treatment. (A) shows an untreated patient. Note the large number of osteoclasts which are adherent to the bone surface. Two weeks after the start of treatment with clodronate (B), osteoclasts are still present but detached from the bone surface (Goldner's trichrome stain ×1000).

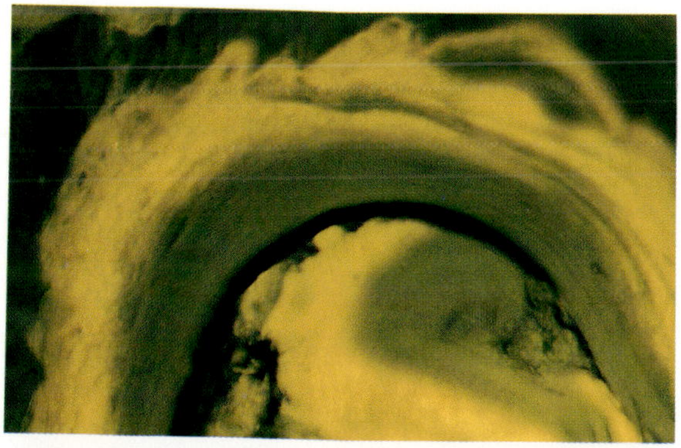

Plate 24

Microphotograph showing tetracycline fluorescence (×425) in osteomalacia co-existing with Paget's disease. Note the wide osteoid seam and the diffuse tetracycline uptake (yellow fluorescence) despite the lamellar bone formation (compare with Plate 2).

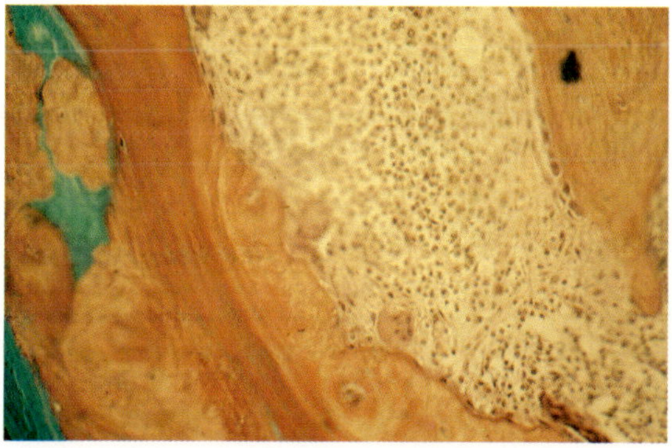

Plate 26

Effect of etidronate (20 mg/kg per day) for one year in a patient with Paget's disease and renal failure. Note that mineralized bone (stained green) has been almost entirely replaced by unmineralized osteoid. Note also the active bone turnover (resorption and formation) on osteoid surfaces.

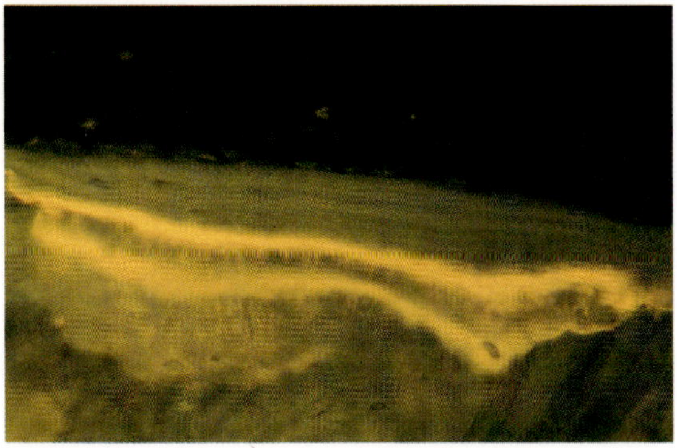

A

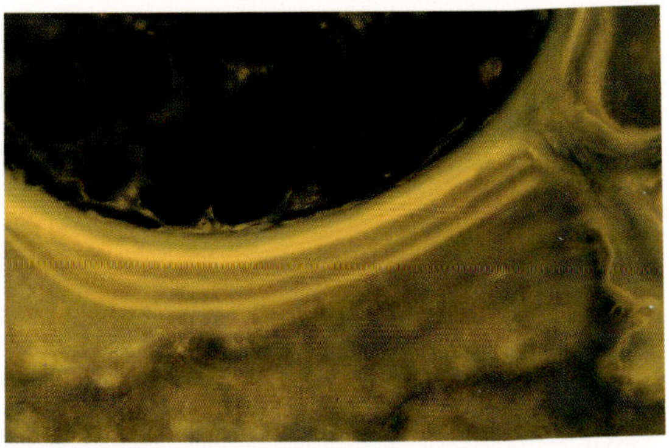

B

Plate 27

Comparative effects of intravenous etidronate (A) and clodronate (300 mg daily for 5 days) (B) on triple tetracycline uptake (see Figure 7.33 for explanation). In the case of clodronate, three equidistant fluorescent bands are observed, indicating that the rates of mineralization before and after treatment remained unchanged. In the case of etidronate the third label is lost and the osteoid seam width has increased due to continued bone formation without mineralization.

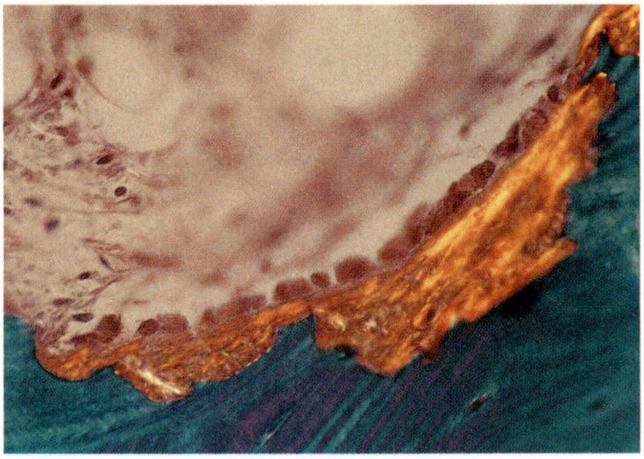

A

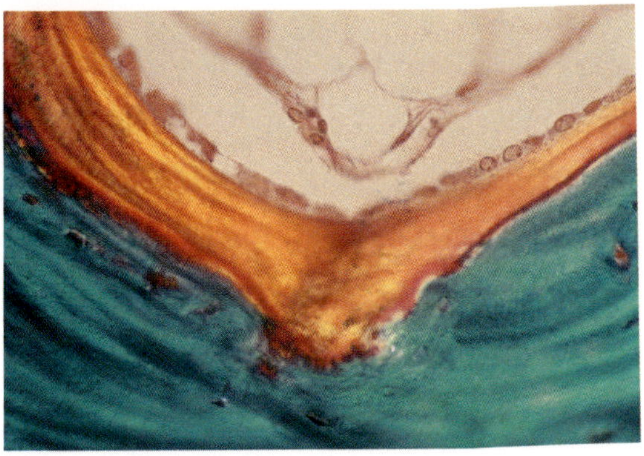

B

Plate 28

Section from transiliac bone biopsy before and after treatment with etidronate. Before treatment (A) a mosaic appearance is seen in mineralized bone, the bed of the resorption cavity (the reversal surface) is scalloped and the new bone formed is woven. (B) After long-term treatment with etidronate (5 mg/kg per day) new bone formed is lamellar and the reversal surface is smooth. Mild focal osteomalacia is also present (Goldner's trichrome stain × 425).

Plate 29

Acute effects of etidronate on bone. The biopsy was taken two weeks after the start of treatment with high intravenous doses of etidronate. Note the new bone formed was lamellar though unmineralized (toluidine blue; polarized light × 15).

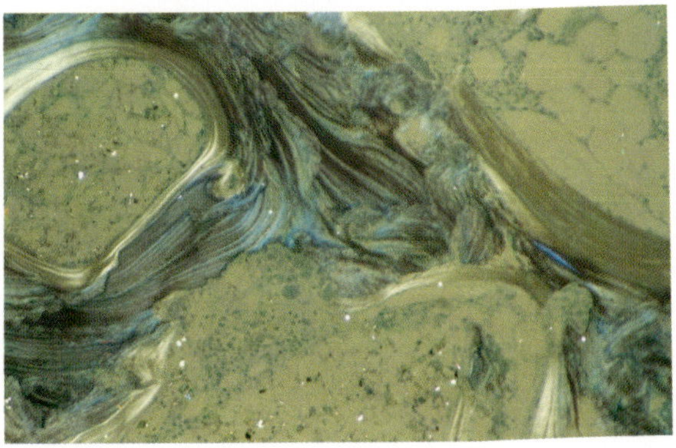

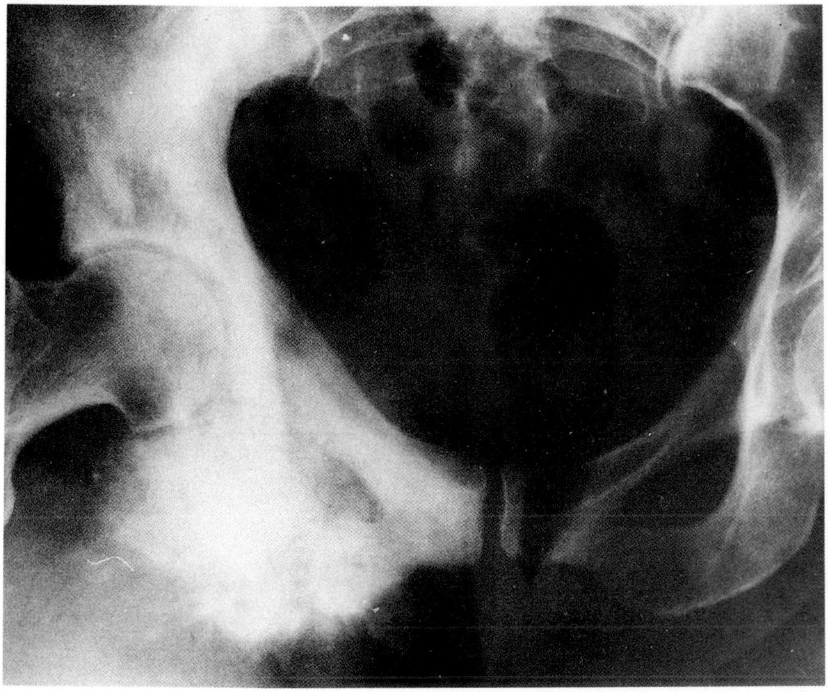

Figure 5.27

Sarcomatous transformation of Paget's disease of the hemipelvis showing marked bone formation and sun-ray spicules at its outer border. The displacement of the anal gas shadow indicates marked pelvic extension. (From Maldague and Malghem, 1989.)

third or less of patients (Barry, 1969; Ross et al, 1973). The most helpful radiographic feature is osteolysis within the bone with the ablation of the coarse trabecular pattern characteristic of uncomplicated Paget's disease (Figure 5.29; Porretta et al, 1957; Smith et al, 1984a).

Other less common features include a soft-tissue mass, which is evident clinically or radiographically in about half the patients (Figures 5.30 and 5.31), pathological fracture, new bone formation or the presence of distant metastases. The diagnosis is usually confirmed by an open or needle biopsy. Occasionally, sarcoma may present as a sclerotic area of bone (Figure 5.32). The bone scan may be unhelpful. Scintigraphic uptake is usually increased, but this may be less than the surrounding Paget's disease, and show an area of relatively reduced uptake which may extend into the surrounding tissues (Figure 5.30). The rarefaction on X-ray examination after fracture may be marked and should not be confused with sarcoma (Figure 5.14). Nor should the benign paraspinal mass be confused with sarcoma (Figure 5.33). Biochemical measurements are not particularly helpful. Serum activity of alkaline phosphatase may rise briskly, sometimes to very high levels, and is unresponsive to medical management of Paget's disease.

The prognosis of Paget's sarcoma is abysmal and the disorder is rapidly progressive (Porretta et al, 1957; Barry, 1961; Seret et al, 1987). The tumours rapidly metastasize to other skeletal sites and to the lung (Figure 5.34). There is about a 50 per cent 6-month survival, and less than 10 per cent of patients survive more than 5 years, irrespective of the type of sarcoma (Wick et al, 1981). Malignant giant-cell tumours carry a similarly poor prognosis.

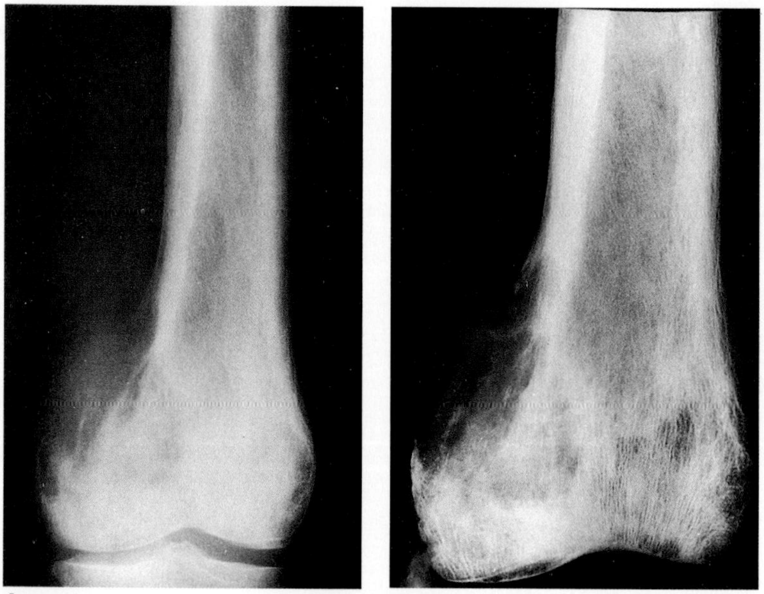

A B

Figure 5.28

Radiographs (A) in vivo and (B) in vitro of the distal femur. Both show characteristic features of Paget's disease, but an added supracondylar lesion associated with marked osteolysis and periosteal elevation due to sarcoma. (From Maldague and Malghem, 1989.)

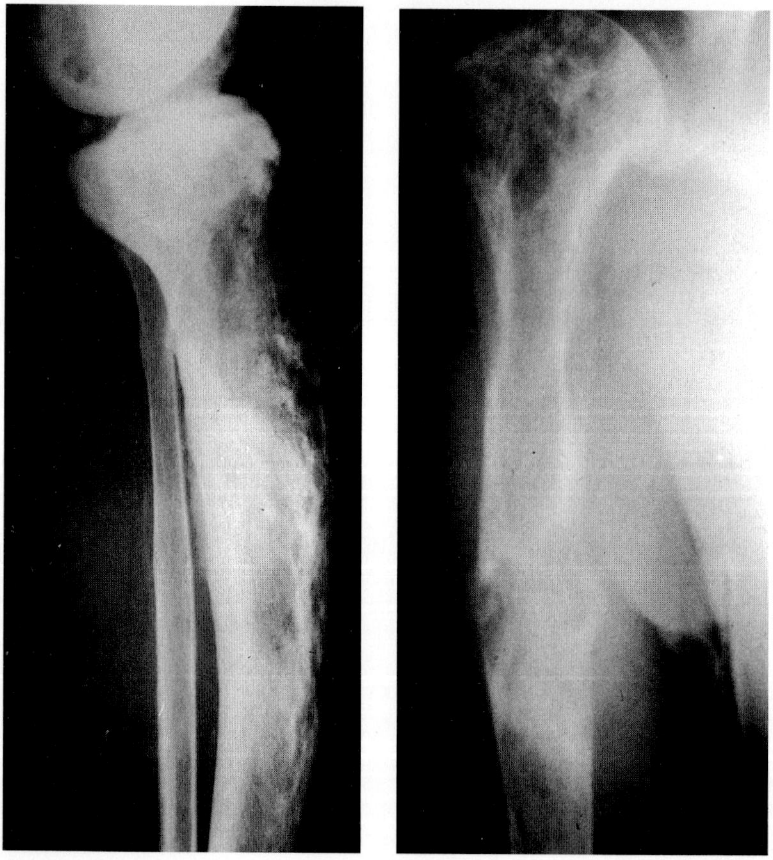

A B

Figure 5.29

Radiographs showing osteogenic sarcoma at the midshaft of the humerus (A) and proximal tibia (B). Note the focal osteolysis and disruption of pagetic architecture.

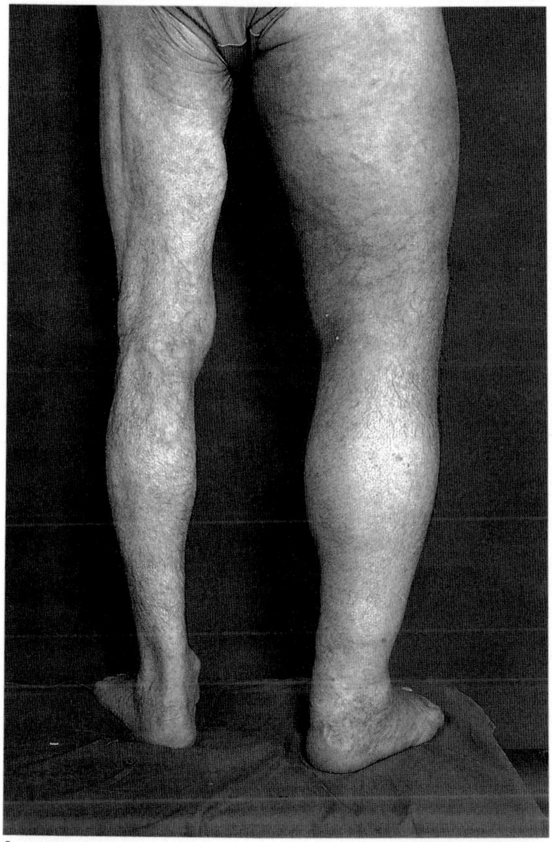

A

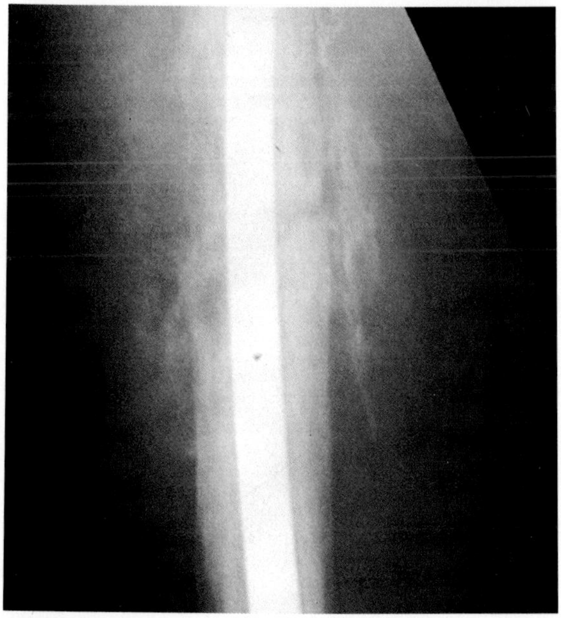

B

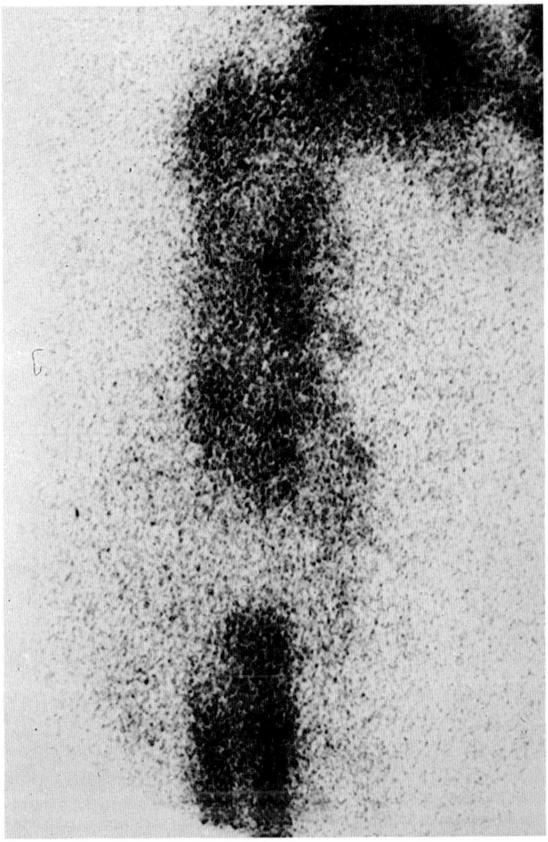

C

Figure 5.30

(A) Clinical photograph, (B) radiograph and (C) bone scan in a patient with sarcoma of the femur. The thigh is markedly enlarged. The pagetic femur shows intense scintigraphic uptake. Uptake is less in the mid-shaft due to the presence of sarcoma.

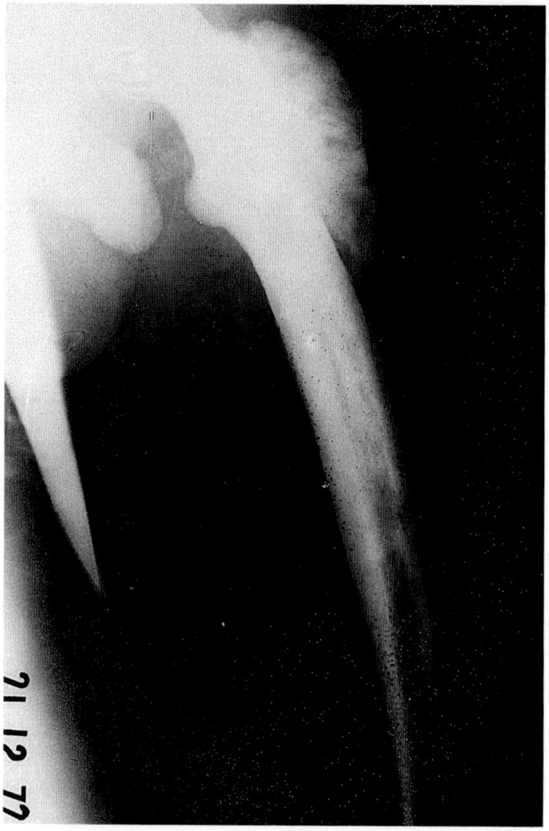

Figure 5.31

Radiograph showing osteosarcoma arising in the femur. Note the marked periosteal outgrowth.

Other tumours

Many other types of neoplasia have been described in patients with Paget's disease (Singer et al, 1977; Fromm et al, 1980). These include multiple myelomatosis, lymphatic leukaemia, Hodgkin's disease, reticulum cell sarcoma and carcinomas of the breast, rectum, kidney, bronchus and prostate. There is no evidence to suggest that the incidence of these tumours in Paget's disease is greater than that expected in the elderly population.

Since pagetic bone is highly vascular it has been suggested that metastases from non-skeletal tumours might have a predilection for those skeletal sites affected by Paget's disease. A number of case reports support this view of locus minoris resistentiae but the evidence is not convincing (Levine et al, 1986). On the other hand, skeletal metastases within pagetic sites may be underdiagnosed (Nichols et al, 1987) and the question must remain open.

Hypercalcaemia and hyperparathyroidism

As reviewed previously (Chapter 4) hypercalcaemia is a rare complication of Paget's disease and occurs during (and remarkably also following) immobilization. It arises particularly in patients with widespread disease after immobilization or fracture (Nagant de Deuxchaisnes and Krane, 1964; Nathen et al, 1973: Fuss et al, 1978; Bannister et al, 1986).

On the other hand, most patients with hypercalcaemia in Paget's disease have other disorders accounting for their hypercalcaemia. Secondary hyperparathyroidism is common (Chapter 4) but it has been suggested that the incidence of primary hyperparathyroidism is also high in Paget's disease (Posen et al, 1978). In this series, 9 patients out of 173 (5.2 per cent) had primary hyperparathyroidism, but this does not match the general experience.

Extraskeletal calcification

The evidence has been reviewed earlier concerning the association of Paget's disease with aortic valve calcification and vascular calcification. There are a number of additional studies on populations or reports of individual cases which suggest an increased frequency of nephrolithiasis (O'Reilly and Race, 1933; Nagant de Deuxchaisnes and Krane, 1964; Barry, 1969; Fromm et al, 1980; Harinck et al, 1986), chondrocalcinosis (Singer, 1977), salivary stones (Rozenkrantz et al, 1952) and cutaneous calcification (Singer, 1977).

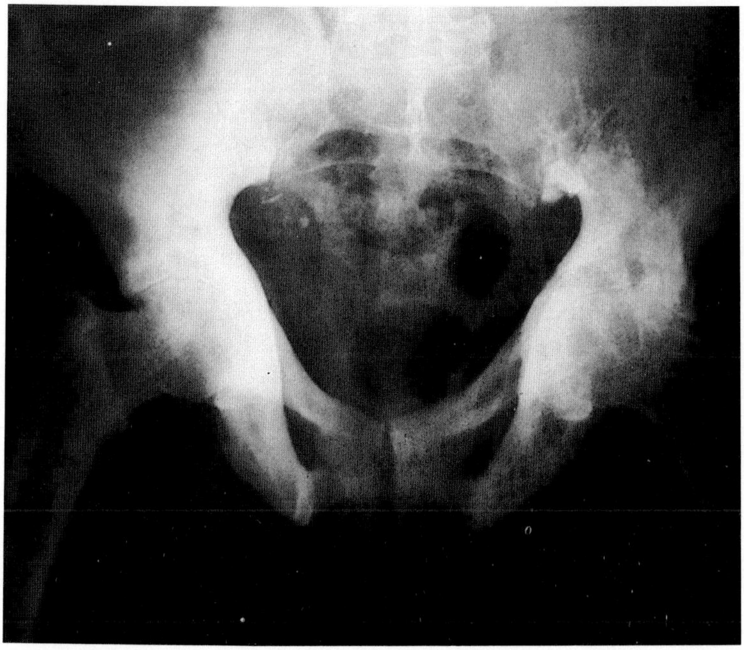

Figure 5.32

Sarcoma of the left hemipelvis evident as increased bone sclerosis.

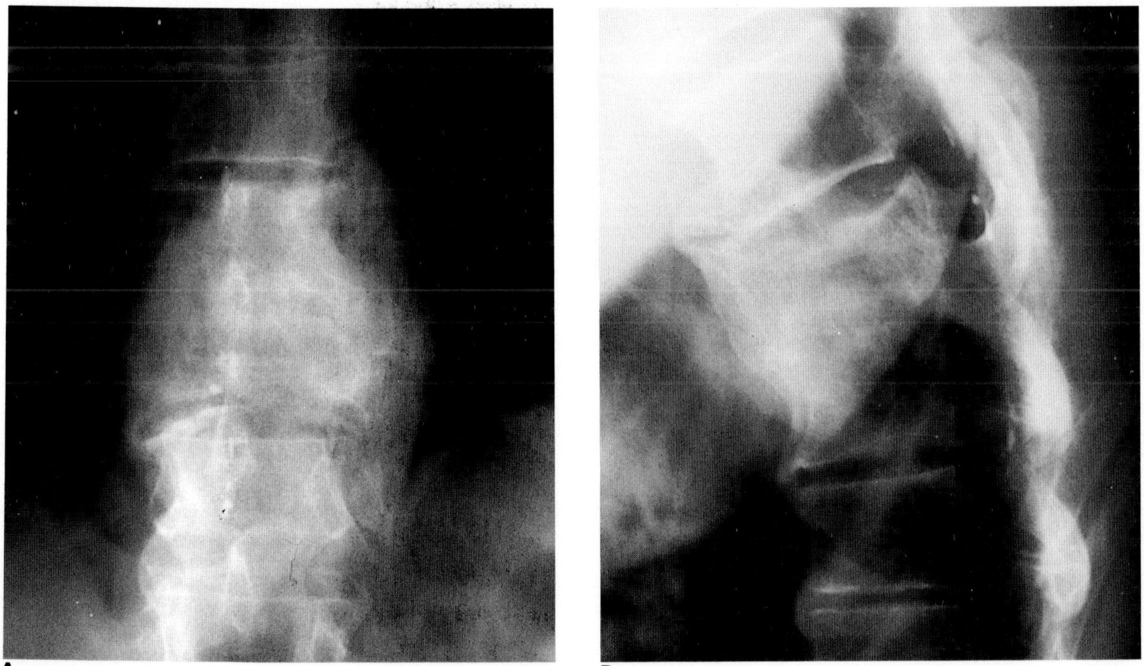

A B

Figure 5.33

(A) Anteroposterior and (B) lateral radiographs of thoracic spine showing marked osteoarthrosis and vertebral collapse. The AP view shows paravertebral calcification which may be mistaken for sarcoma (see also Figures 3.30 and 3.31).

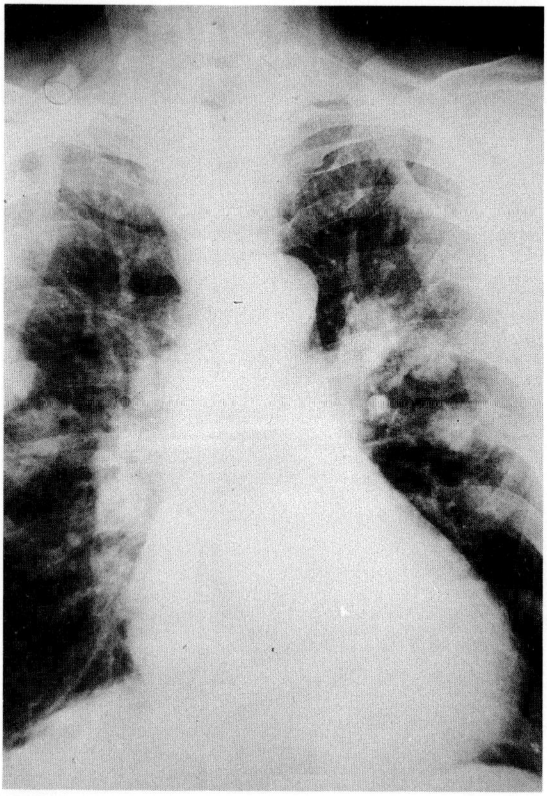

Figure 5.34

Cannon-ball metastases of the lungs due to osteosarcoma.

These findings might suggest a predilection for extraskeletal calcification, perhaps related to large fluctuations in calcium homeostasis, high rates of blood flow or to abnormal collagen metabolism. In some instances, any association is likely to be coincidental and, for example, no marked difference in the prevalence of chondrocalcinosis has been observed when pagetic and control populations are compared (Boussina et al, 1975).

Collagen metabolism

Angioid streaks are seen in the fundi of a majority of patients with polyostotic Paget's disease (Paton, 1972), but an increased frequency has been questioned (Lievre, 1974). Angioid streaks are due to degenerative breaks and fissures in Brusch's membrane (lamina elastica) which expose the vascular choroid, giving the fissure a red colour (Plate 23). They are often of no clinical significance but may progress to macular degeneration and choroidal atrophy. Pseudoxanthoma elasticum has also been reported with Paget's disease (Singer, 1977), a disorder also associated with angioid streaks. This and the evidence for extraskeletal calcification has raised the question whether there might be some generalized disorder of connective tissue. Skin biopsies from patients with Paget's disease have suggested a decreased amount of polymeric collagen in pagetic skin (Francis and Smith, 1974), but the authors themselves think the evidence is unconvincing and might be secondary to an unidentified primary disorder (Smith, 1979). In addition, it is difficult to see how generalized changes in bone-matrix production or collagen assembly could result in focally increased bone resorption.

Other disorders

Extramedullary haematopoiesis has been reported in the dorsal paraspinal region and in the pelvis (Kadir et al, 1977). It may arise as a result of pathological fracture, perhaps associated with intense marrow fibrosis. Unlike other causes of extramedullary haematopoiesis, the patients themselves are not anaemic.

The literature contains very many case reports describing Paget's disease in association with other disorders. The associations with vitiligo, pernicious anaemia and autoimmune thyroiditis have led to the view that Paget's disease is a disorder of autoimmunity. These and many other associations (Buxbaum and Kammerman, 1984) are likely to be fortuitous, but cannot be placed into proper perspective until studies documenting the medical associations of large populations are available together with appropriate controls.

CHAPTER 6

Differential diagnosis

The clinical diagnosis of Paget's disease is frequently straightforward, and is usually confirmed by the finding of abnormal biochemical indices of disease activity associated with characteristic radiographic and scintigraphic abnormalities. Nevertheless, difficulties occasionally arise in the interpretation of symptoms and laboratory investigations. These are reviewed below where they have not been previously emphasized.

Symptoms

Bone pain is a common presenting feature, but is not necessarily due to Paget's disease. The most difficult problems arise with back and hip pain in the presence of osteoarthrosis (Altman et al, 1987). The distinction may not be possible on clinical grounds. Some investigators have utilized intra-articular local anaesthetic to differentiate joint from bone pain, particularly in the selection of patients for hip surgery (Stevens, 1981), whereas others, including ourselves, assess the response to specific therapy for Paget's disease (Chapter 8).

The converse problem is that signs and symptoms due to Paget's disease may be erroneously considered to be irrelevant. Since the pagetic population is generally elderly, this occurs most frequently with chronic neurological syndromes such as deafness, ataxia, incontinence and impairment of intellectual function with disease of the skull.

Widespread osteosclerosis

Widespread osteosclerosis occurs in many bone diseases which can share some of the features of Paget's disease. These include skeletal fluorosis and rare bone dysplasias such as hyperphosphatasia, Engelmann's disease, pycnodysostosis, osteopetrosis and fibrogenesis imperfecta osseum (Figures 6.1 to 6.3). Widespread osteosclerosis may also arise in metastatic bone disease, myelosclerosis and renal osteodystrophy (Figures 6.4 and 6.5). The distinction is usually straightforward since it is rare for other bone diseases to have more than one of the radiographic features of Paget's disease, and if so the distribution is quite distinct. Deformity, bony enlargement and coarse trabecular markings suggest, but are not specific for, Paget's disease, and occasionally we have resorted to biopsy to exclude coexisting Paget's disease in hyperparathyroidism.

The distinction between widespread sclerosis due to Paget's disease and/or prostatic carcinoma is complicated by the finding of high serum activity of acid phosphatase in patients with extensive Paget's disease, but this is rarely as markedly increased as in extensive prostatic disease. The most common problem is to miss the diagnosis of prostatic cancer in patients with co-existing Paget's disease (Figures 6.6 and 6.7). The presence of atypical lesions in pagetic bone and the abnormal appearance of bone at sites not obviously affected by Paget's disease are helpful in reaching a correct diagnosis (Figure 6.6). So too

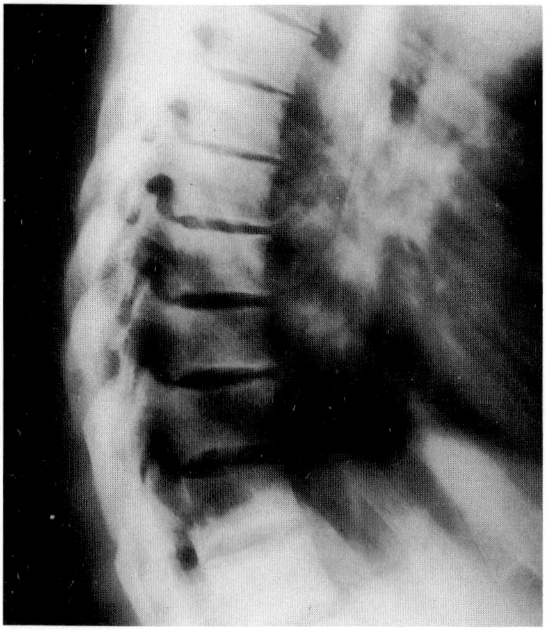

Figure 6.1

Vertebral osteosclerosis due to fluorosis. Sclerosis was evident throughout the vertebral column.

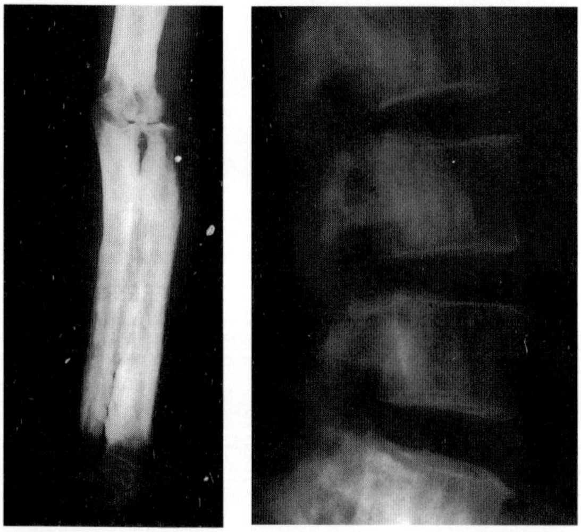

A B

Figure 6.2

Engelmann's disease (progressive diaphyseal dysplasia). The bones are symmetrically enlarged and densely osteosclerotic, but the epiphyses are relatively spared in the forearm (A). At the lumbar spine (B), sclerosis is less marked, there is no bony enlargement and the trabecular markings are accentuated.

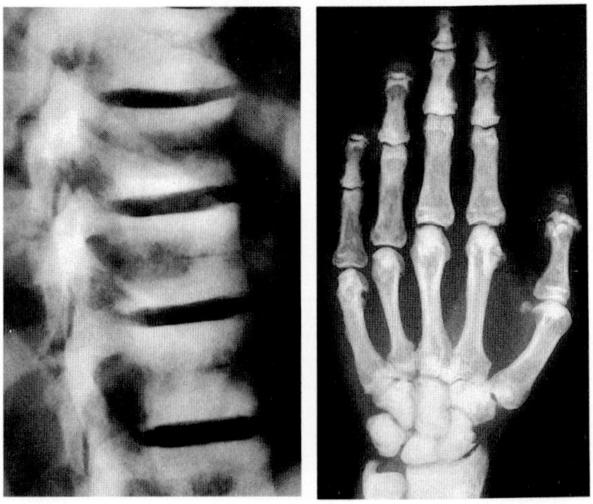

A B

Figure 6.3

Osteosclerosis due to pycnodysostosis. In contrast with Paget's disease sclerosis is predominantly confined to the end-plates and affects all vertebrae (A). Sclerosis at the hand is more patchy (B). The bones are not enlarged and the acro-osteolysis of the terminal phalanges is characteristic of the disorder.

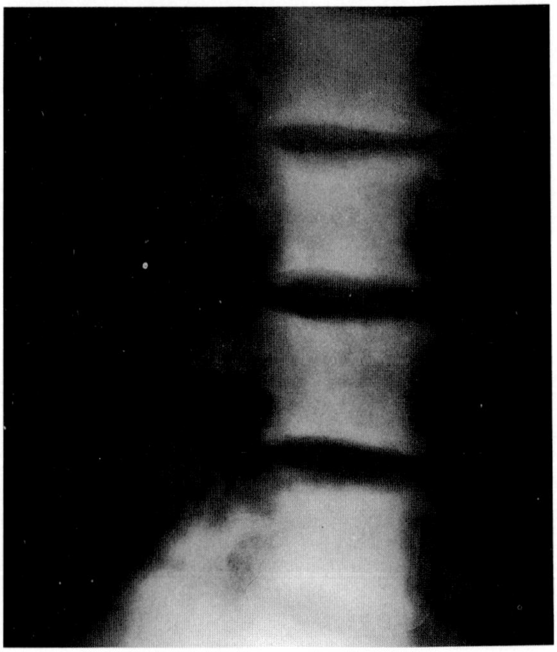

Figure 6.4

Marked vertebral osteosclerosis of the lumbar spine due to extensive secondaries from prostatic cancer. Note the preservation of bone shape and size.

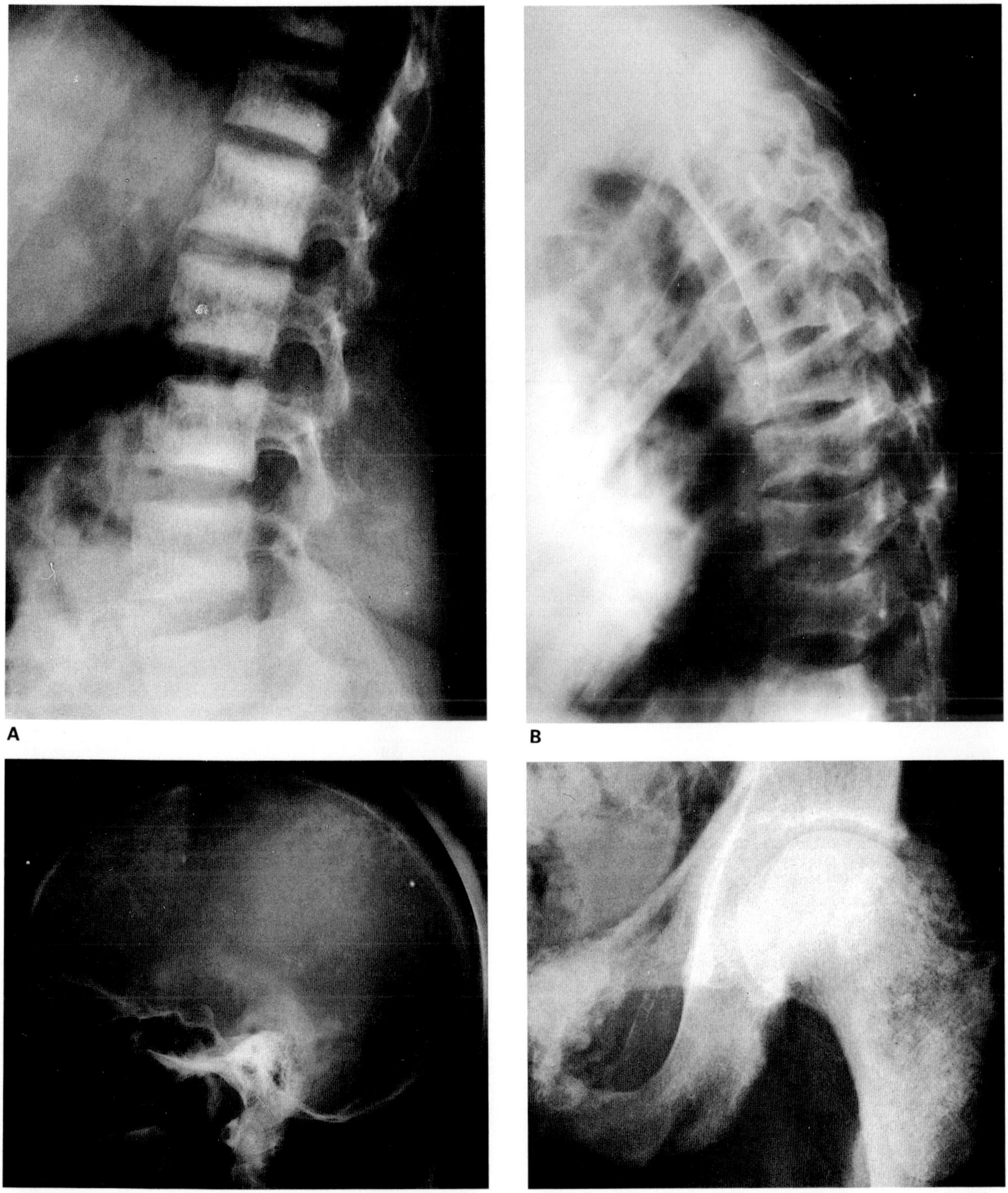

A B C D

Figure 6.5

Osteosclerosis due to hyperparathyroid disease. (A) shows the classic appearance of a 'rugger jersey' spine. More rarely hyperparathyroidism in chronic renal failure may cause enlargement of bones seen here at the vertebral bodies (B). Patchy osteosclerosis and osteolysis may be found in combination (C). More frequently, osteosclerosis alone is found, particularly at epiphyseal sites (D). Note the co-existence of soft tissue and vascular calcification at the hip.

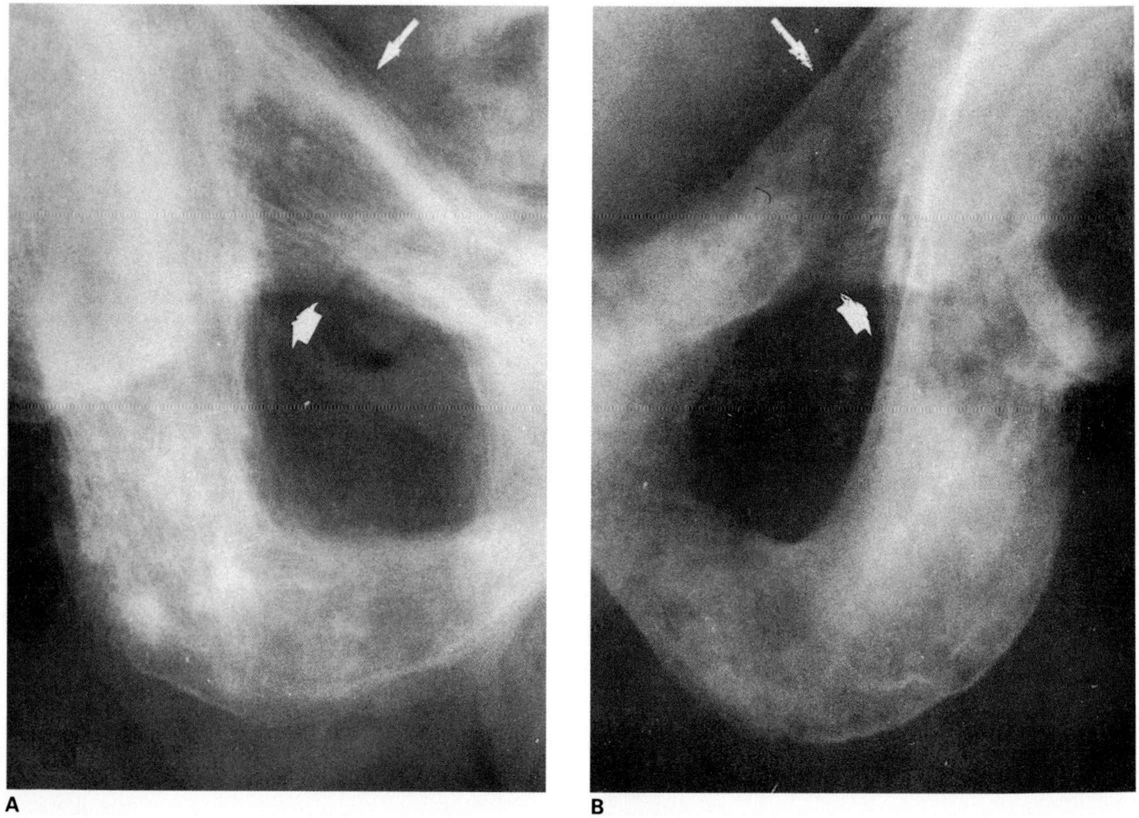

Figure 6.6

Two pelvic views of a patient with coexisting Paget's disease and prostatic carcinoma. (A) (right hemipelvis) shows marked cortical thickening and bony expansion (arrows) due to Paget's disease. The discrete islets of osteosclerosis are atypical. At the left (B) osteosclerosis is not accompanied by cortical thickening or bony enlargement and the features are entirely attributable to prostatic carcinoma. (From Maldague and Malghem, 1989.)

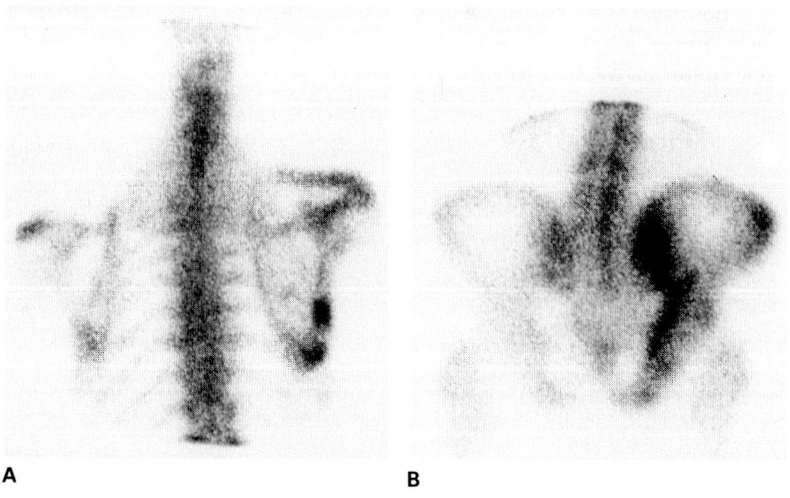

Figure 6.7

Bone scan of a patient with coexisting Paget's disease and prostatic carcinoma. Note the generalized increase in uptake throughout the left scapula (A) but the additional hot spots which were due to prostatic secondaries and were not visible on X-ray examination.

is the distribution of lesions which differs somewhat between the two disorders (Table 6.1), particularly in the predilection of prostatic carcinoma for the ribs, cervical spine and sternum.

The disorder which most resembles Paget's disease is hyperphosphatasia. This is a rare autosomal recessive disorder in which affected infants or children have episodes of fever, bone pain, progressive enlargement and deformity of bones and pathological fractures. The disorder begins in infancy but may not always present then and only be recognized in later life (Kraszeski et al, 1981). Serum activity of alkaline phosphatase and urinary excretion of hydroxyproline are markedly increased and it therefore has some characteristics of Paget's disease. In addition to similar radiographic appearances, bone biopsy may show the mosaic appearance characteristic of Paget's disease (Woodhouse et al, 1972a,b). Unlike Paget's disease it appears to involve the whole skeleton, but is responsive to calcitonin and diphosphonates (Blanco et al, 1977; Doyle et al, 1974b; Kraszeski et al, 1981). Indeed, amongst other names it has been termed 'juvenile Paget's disease', even though it seems to be a quite distinct entity (Thompson et al, 1969). The radiographic appearances are very similar to those of Paget's disease but the early onset, generalized nature, and short stature distinguish the disorder from Paget's disease.

Familial expansile osteolysis (Chapter 1) shares many similarities with Paget's disease, including the presence of viral-like inclusions in giant osteoclasts (Dickson et al, 1990; Figure 6.8) and may in fact be Paget's disease in a highly susceptible family.

Polyostotic fibrous dysplasia may occasionally have a similar appearance, but does not usually have the thickened cortex of Paget's disease (Figures 6.9 to 6.11). It also occurs in younger individuals, and may be unilateral. Affected bone commonly has a knobbly appearance. In the generalized form of polyostotic fibrous dysplasia serum activity of alkaline phosphatase may be increased, but hyperphosphatasia is rarely marked. Unilateral bone lesions, pigmentation and endocrine disturbances when present will distinguish this disorder. Occasionally, bone biopsy may be required and the histological features distinguish the two disorders. Maxillary bone disease resulting in enlargement gives the appearance termed 'leontiasis ossea' and cortical

Table 6.1 Comparative distribution of skeletal foci (percentage of lesions) in prostatic carcinoma and Paget's disease assessed by scintigraphy. Note the predilection of prostatic metastases for the cervical spine, ribs and sternum.

Site	*Prostatic carcinoma (n = 63)*	*Paget's disease (n = 170)*	*Ratio*
Pelvis	82	72	1.1
Thoracic spine	73	45	1.6
Lumbar spine	67	58	1.2
Ribs	65	12	5.4
Shoulder girdle	44	24	1.8
Cervical spine	40	14	2.9
Femora	36	55	0.7
Skull	33	42	0.8
Sternum	32	11	2.9
Humerus	19	31	0.6
Sacrum	19	44	0.4

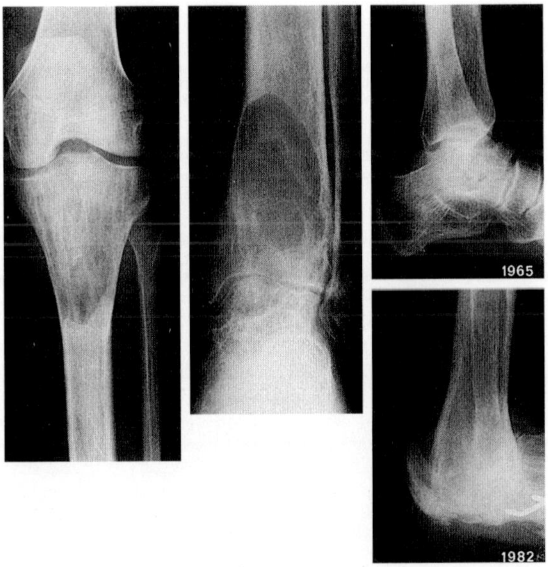

Figure 6.8

Familial expansile osteolysis. Note the marked resorption front and thickened trabecular elements of the proximal tibia.

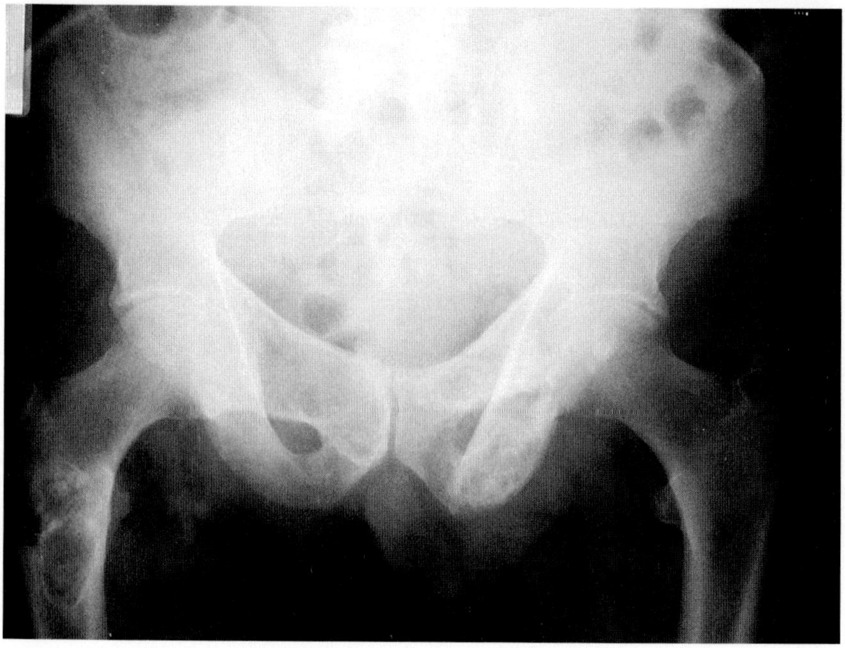

Figure 6.9

Polyostotic fibrous dysplasia. Note the marked bony enlargement but the absence of cortical thickening and destruction rather than enhancement of architectural features.

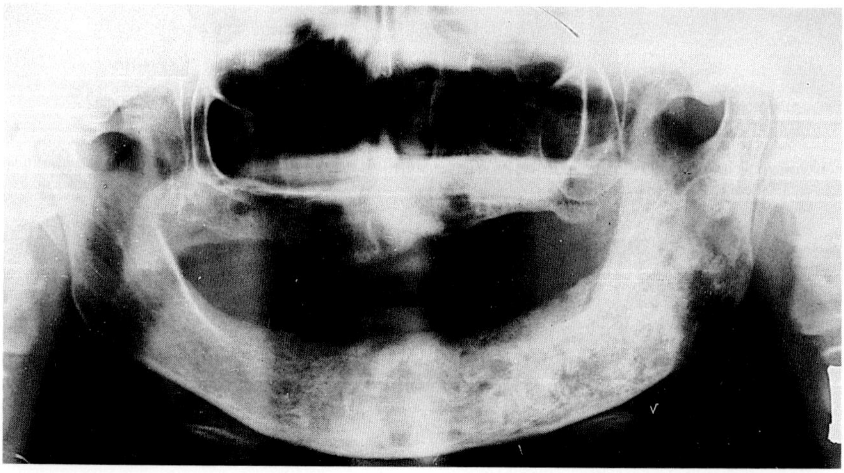

Figure 6.10

Polyostotic fibrous dysplasia of the lower jaw. The left lower jaw is enlarged and has islands of uniform (ground glass) sclerosis. The cortical width is not increased.

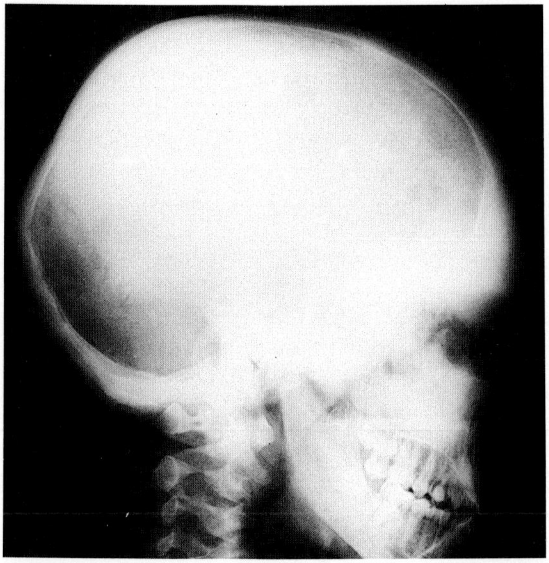

Figure 6.11

Polyostotic fibrous dysplasia of the skull. Note the dense osteosclerosis without skull enlargement. Sclerosis is of the maxilla and frontal sinus has a homogeneous density.

thickening and sclerosis may be marked (Figure 6.11). This abnormality is also seen in Paget's disease, but is rarer and occurs in late life, whereas it usually presents before the age of 30 when due to fibrous dysplasia.

Focal osteosclerosis

There are many causes of focal osteosclerosis (see page 151). Of these, osteosclerotic metastases are the most common. All centres with a large population of Paget's disease have seen patients with a previous history of carcinoma. The occurrence of bone pain and focal osteosclerosis in these patients has on occasion been erroneously attributed to metastatic spread of the disease. We have several patients in whom osteosclerosis was attributed to metastatic disease and in whom iatrogenic opiate addiction has given problems in management.

Focal sclerotic lesions can be confused with chronic osteomyelitis, syphilis, hyperparathyroid bone disease, monostotic fibrous dysplasia, bone infarcts, haemangiomas and neoplasia. Haemangiomas of the vertebral bodies may have a reticulated appearance rather similar to the accentuated vertical trabecular markings of Paget's disease (Figure 6.12). Vertebral collapse may occur and give rise to neurological syndromes. Unlike in Paget's disease, the cortex is not thickened, the vertebral size is normal and involvement of the neural arches is comparatively rare. It commonly involves a single vertebra.

Difficulties may arise in the solitary osteosclerotic lesion of the spine and pelvis (Figures 6.13 and 6.14). In the spine uniformly dense or patchy osteosclerosis may occur without a change in shape (Figure 6.15). There are various causes of the ivory vertebra appearance (see below). Many of these lesions may show a high uptake of isotopes on bone scanning. Moreover, a patient with a single pagetic lesion is not likely to have abnormalities in alkaline phosphatase and other indices of disease activity which further increases the difficulty of accurate diagnosis. Indeed, we have occasionally had to biopsy such lesions.

The most common problem in the diagnosis of isolated sclerotic lesions is to distinguish Paget's disease in the pelvis or more rarely in the spine from changes due to metastatic cancer. A variety of tumours may give rise to osteosclerotic metastases, particularly prostate, breast, lung and

Some causes of a solitary ivory vertebra.

Common
- Metastatic disease
- Compression fracture
- Paget's disease
- Lymphoma

Uncommon
- Osteomyelitis
- Radiation necrosis
- Primary benign tumours
- Primary malignant bone tumours
- Osteoarthrosis
- Monostotic fibrous dysplasia

Rare
- Sarcoidosis
- Myelosclerosis

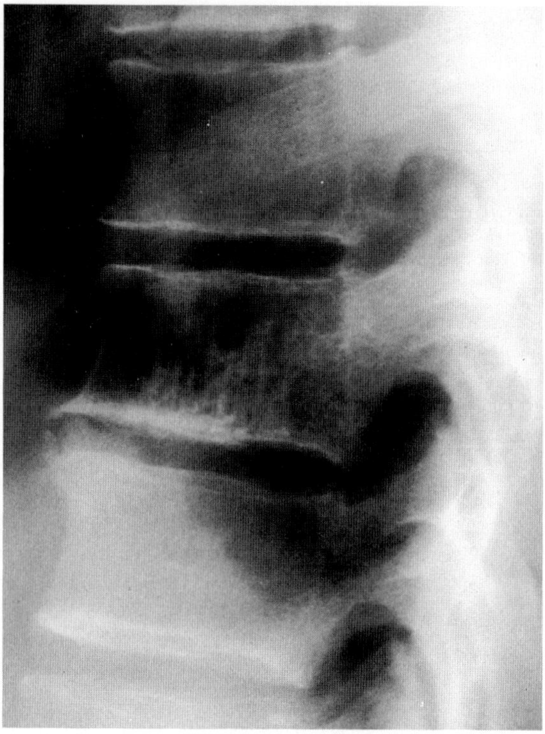

A

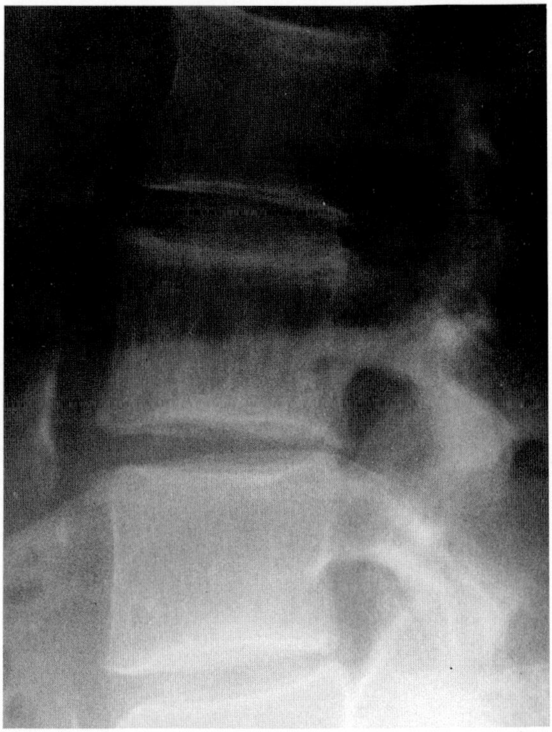

B

Figure 6.12

(A) Lateral radiograph of the lumbar spine showing a haemangioma at T12. Note the accentuated trabecular vertical markings, but the normal shape. (B) Paget's disease of L3. There is an increase in vertical trabecular markings but no increase in bone size. In contrast with haemangioma there is an increase in end-plate sclerosis and pagetic involvement of the neural arch and spinous process.

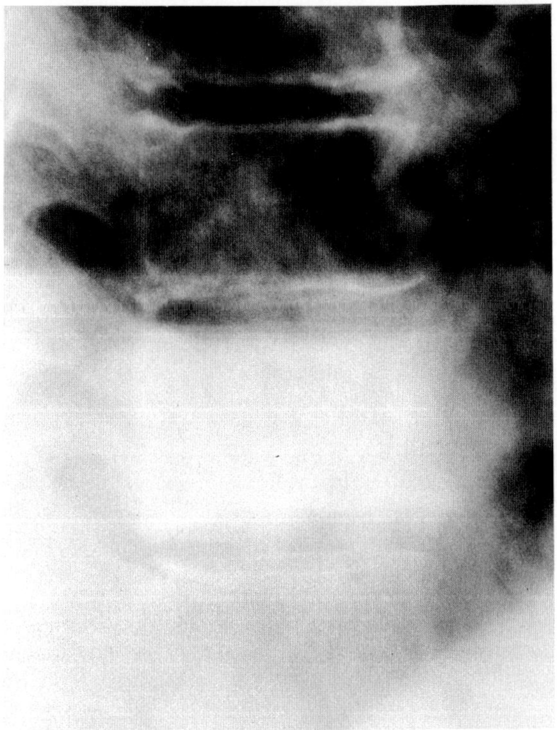

Figure 6.13

Focal osteosclerosis giving the 'ivory vertebra' appearance. The anteroposterior diameter of the vertebral body is increased and was due to Paget's disease.

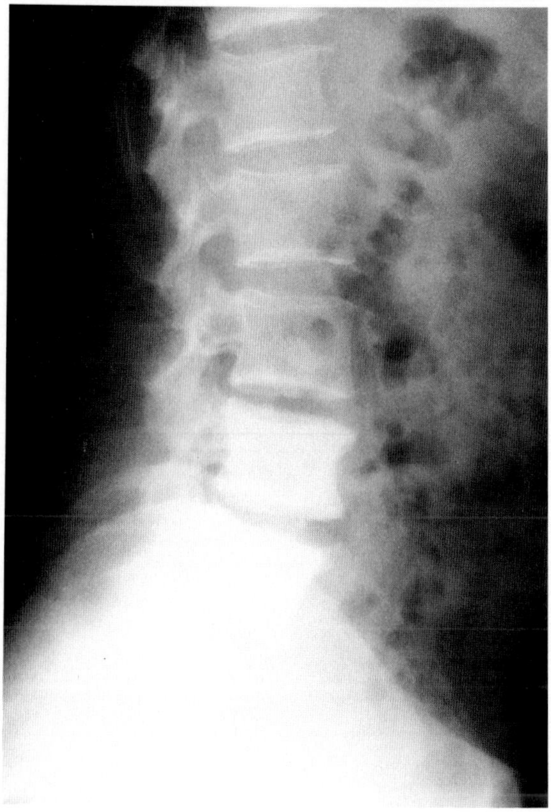

A

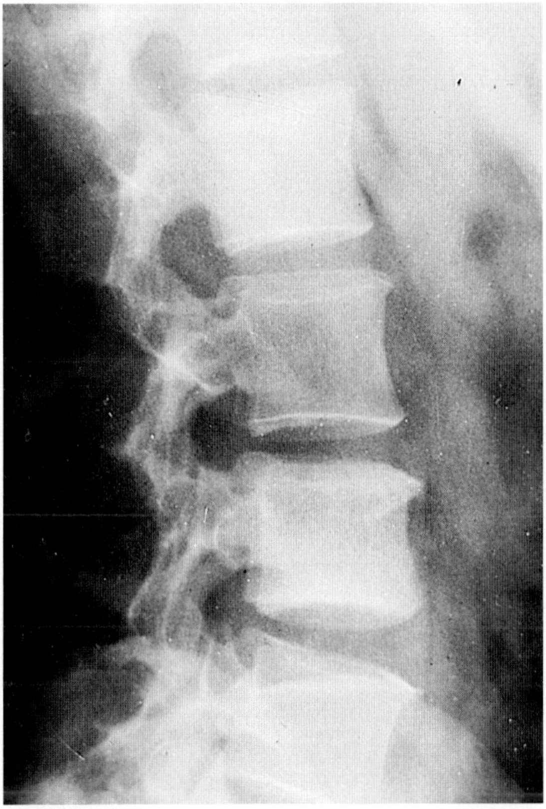

B

Figure 6.14

Dense osteosclerosis at the lumbar spine due to osteoarthrosis (A) and to Hodgkin's disease (B).

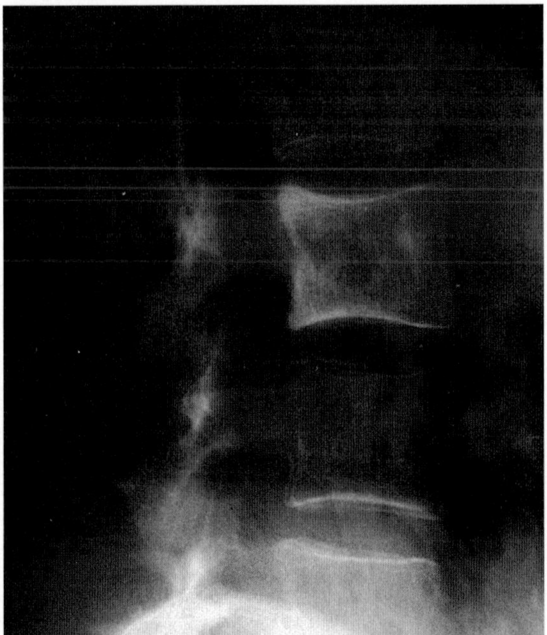

Figure 6.15

Lateral radiograph of lumbar spine showing patchy osteosclerosis of the vertebral body in the absence of bony enlargement. Osteosclerosis of the neural arch was also present and was attributed to Paget's disease because of more characteristic features of Paget's disease elsewhere.

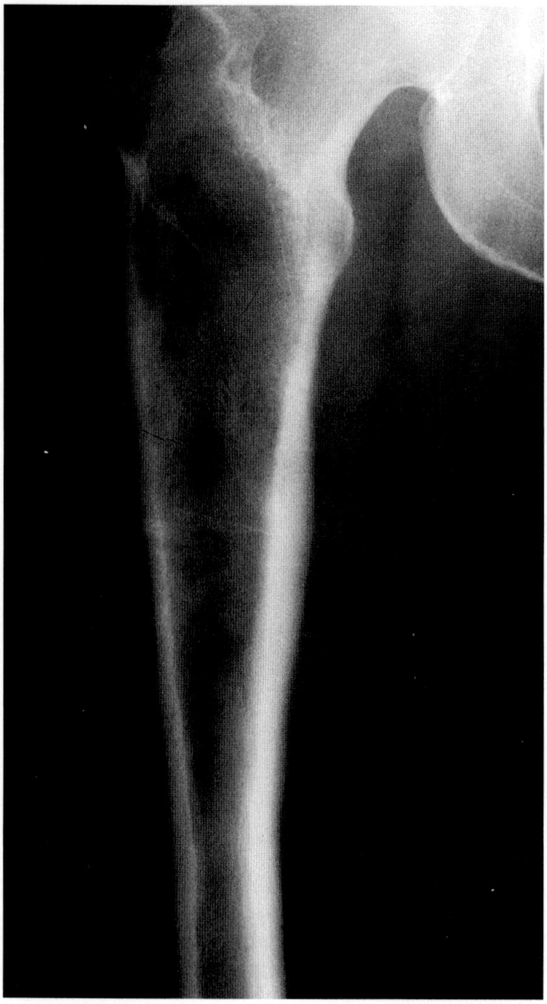

Figure 6.16

Expansile chondrosarcoma of the lower femur causing an increase in cortical diameter. Note the absence of cortical thickening and islands of osteolysis.

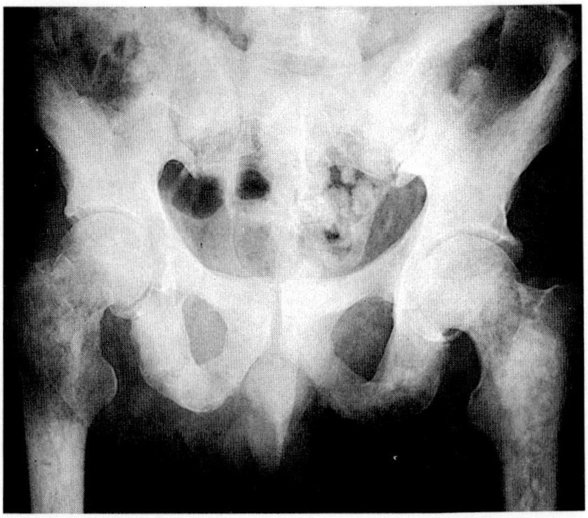

Figure 6.17

Osteosclerosis due to prostatic carcinoma. Note the enlargement of the ischium, more marked on the left. Apart from bony enlargement and patchy osteosclerosis no other features of Paget's disease are evident, but the patient had Paget's disease elsewhere.

pancreas. Secondary deposits can produce radiographic changes somewhat similar to Paget's disease. Osteoblastic metastases may cause periosteal new bone formation both in the vertebrae and pelvis, which increase the size of bone and may be indistinguishable on radiographic criteria from Paget's disease or from carcinoma metastasizing to pagetic bone (Burgener and Perry, 1978; Greenfield, 1980; Edeiken, 1982; Resnik et al, 1984).

Metastatic carcinoma of the prostate is the most common malignancy that causes bony expansion (Jorgens, 1965), but carcinoma of the oesophagus (Greenfield, 1980), melanoma (Fon et al, 1981) and primary bone tumours (Figure 6.16) may also do so. In Paget's disease the enlarged bone usually, but not invariably, retains its shape, but the preservation of the shape of bone may also be found with slow-growing neoplasia. Despite these caveats, bony expansion is rare in the case of osteoblastic metastases, whereas it is very common in Paget's disease.

Although sclerotic metastases may share some similarities with Paget's disease, they rarely have more than one of the radiographic features and careful radiographic examination usually allows a distinction (Figures 6.17 and 6.18).

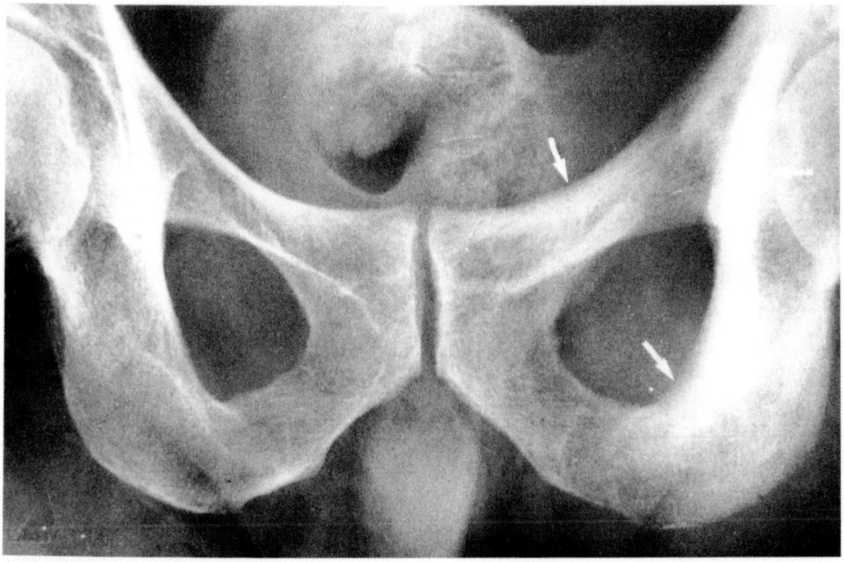

A

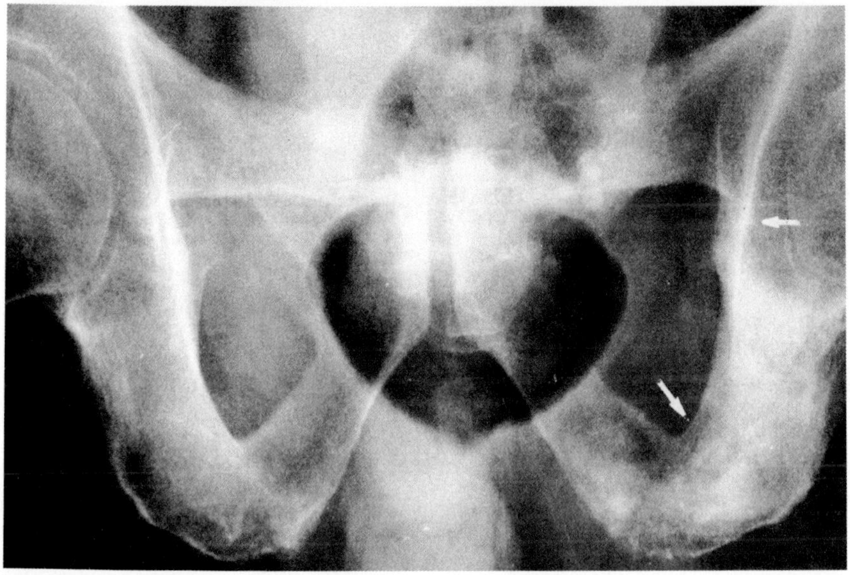

B

Figure 6.18

Comparative radiography of Paget's disease and prostatic carcinoma. (A) shows cortical thickening and enlargement of the descending ramus of the pubis (arrows), characteristic of Paget's disease. (B) shows increased radiodensity, but no cortical thickening nor bone enlargement. (From Maldague and Malghem, 1989.)

Sclerosis near the sacroiliac joints may resemble ankylosing spondylitis and osteitis condensans ilii (Burgener and Perry, 1978). Indeed, a subset of patients with Paget's disease with other features similar to ankylosing spondylitis (B27 negative) have been described (Singer, 1977). The thickening of the iliopectineal line of the pelvic brim is also found in osteopetrosis, but is easily differentiated by other radiographic and clinical features. Rarer causes of focal osteosclerosis which have been confused with Paget's disease include histiocytosis X, osteomyelosclerosis, radiation necrosis, histiocytic lymphoma, sclerosing dystrophies and renal bone disease (Figures

6.19 and 6.20). Other causes are more readily distinguished.

Paget's disease of the spine may sometimes have the appearance of a rugger-jersey spine (see Chapter 3, Figure 3.16). The distinction between this and the florid osteosclerosis of secondary hyperparathyroidism is usually straightforward, but in milder cases the distinction is less obvious. Similar appearances may be seen in pseudohyperparathyroidism (Figure 6.21) and arise during glucocorticoid treatment (Figure 6.22). Trabecular accentuation is not usual – neither is an increase in bone size (but see Figure 6.5). Increased trabecular markings may be seen in a variety of disorders but are not easily confused with Paget's disease (for examples see Figure 6.23).

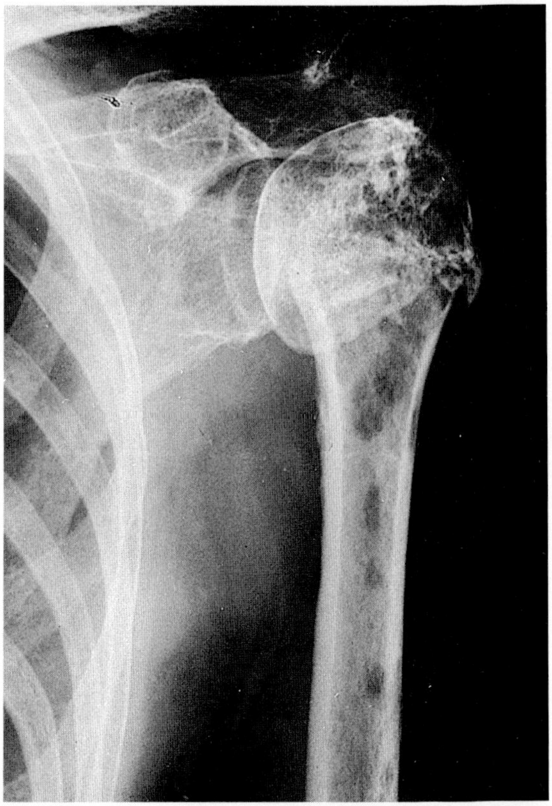

Figure 6.19

Mixed focal osteosclerosis and osteolysis due to radiation and carcinoma. Both sclerosis and lysis are discrete, unlike Paget's disease, and the remaining bone appears normal.

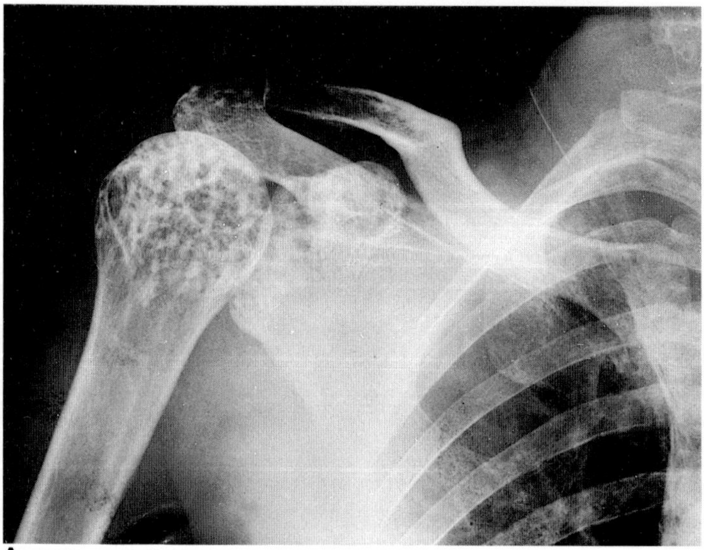

A

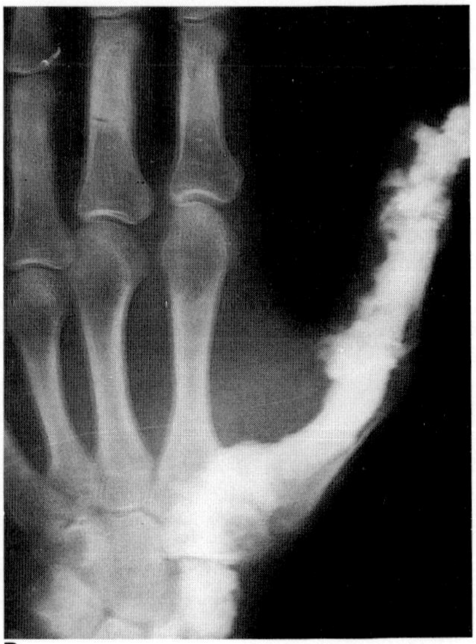

B

Figure 6.20

Focal osteosclerosis due to osteopoikilosis (A) and melorrheostosis (B). Both are distinctive in pattern and distribution from Paget's disease.

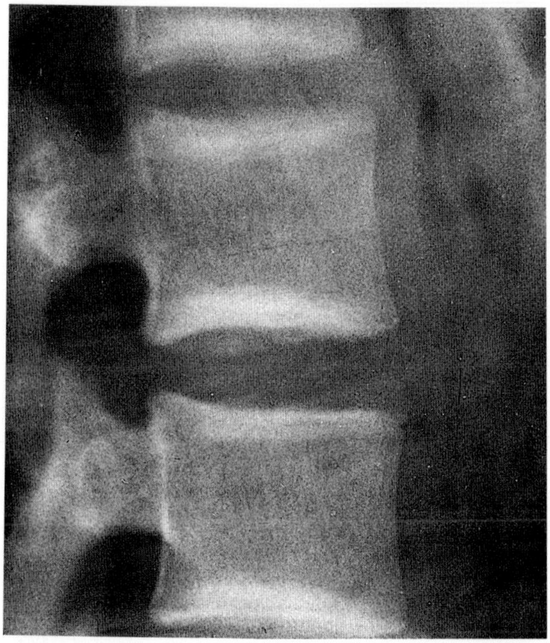

Figure 6.21

Osteosclerosis of the vertebral end-plates due to pseudohyperparathyroidism. In contrast with Paget's disease bony enlargement is not a feature, and the trabecular architecture is blurred rather than accentuated.

Some causes of focal bone sclerosis in adults.

Common
- Paget's disease of bone
- Renal bone disease
- Osteosclerotic metastases

Uncommon
- Haemangioma
- Hodgkin's disease
- Osteomyelosclerosis
- Radiation necrosis
- Histiocytic lymphoma
- Chronic vitamin D poisoning
- Lead poisoning
- Fluorosis
- Hypothyroidism
- Coccidioidmycosis
- Bone islands
- Hyperostosis interna
- Melorheostosis
- Pycnodysostosis
- Osteopoikilosis
- Osteopathia striata

Rare
- Myelomatosis
- Sarcoidosis
- Primary hyperparathyroidism
- Osteopetrosis

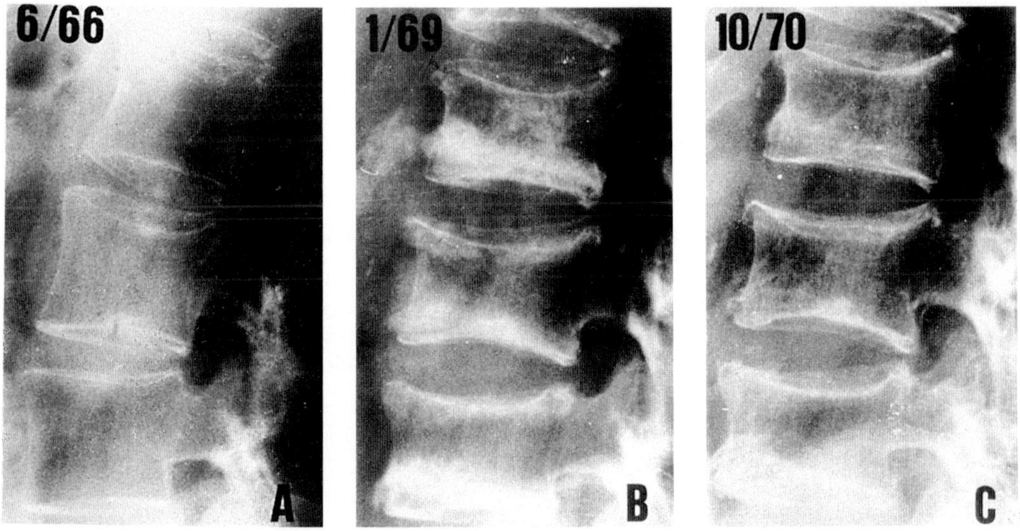

Figure 6.22

Effect of glucocorticoid treatment on trabecular bone architecture at the spine. The increase in radiodensity at the cortical plates is due to the appearance of pseudocallus during treatment (B) which resolved when treatment was stopped (C). Note the lack of accentuation of trabecular markings.

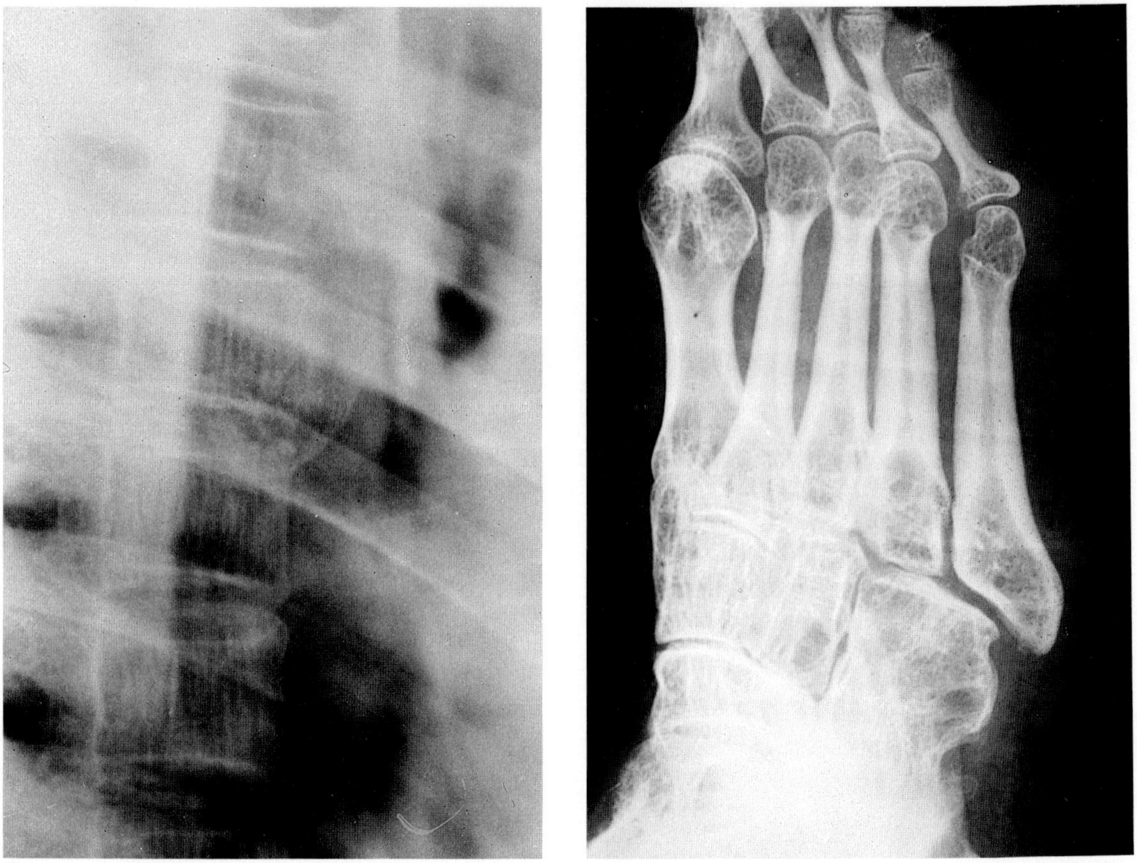

A B

Figure 6.23

Increased trabecular markings due to mechanical stress. The radiograph of the thoracic spine (A) shows increased accentuation of vertical trabeculae due to weight lifting. The radiograph of the foot (B) shows trabecular accentuation following recovery from algodystrophy (Sudek's atrophy). During the algodystrophy trabeculae were lost and the remaining trabeculae have hypertrophied.

Focal osteolysis

Focal areas of osteolysis occurring at pagetic sites may be due to various causes and biopsy may occasionally be necessary to resolve them. Large osteolytic foci should alert one to the possible co-existence of dual pathology (Figure 6.24). It is important to recognize that marked radiotranslucency may arise following treatment with etidronate, particularly in high doses. When this occurs it may be associated with bone pain and should

Some causes of radiotranslucency in areas affected by Paget's disease.

Early Paget's disease – resorption front
Cystic degenerative changes
Following fracture
Treatment with etidronate
Sarcoma
Giant cell tumour
Metastases
Myelomatosis
Brown tumour

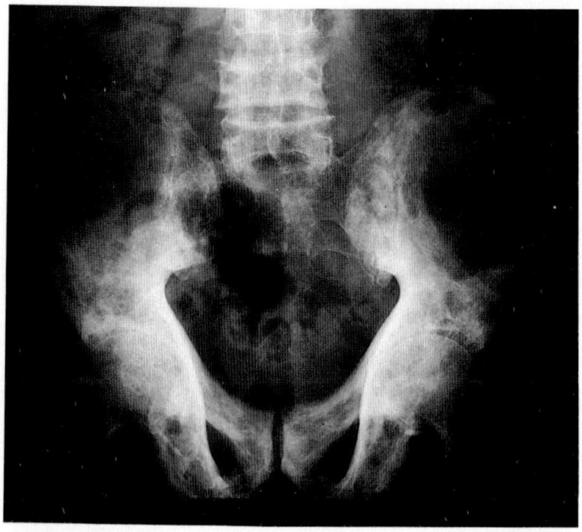

Figure 6.24

Radiograph of pelvis in a patient with extensive Paget's disease. The large osteolytic focus at the left ilium was due to co-existing myelomatosis.

not be mistaken for sarcoma or carcinoma (Rondier et al, 1984; Fedou et al, 1986; Figure 6.25). Similarly marked osteolysis may occur at sites of pathological fracture (see Figure 5.17, Chapter 5) and has been mistaken for sarcoma (Barry, 1969).

Osteolysis in the absence of other pagetic lesions is usually characteristic (Figure 6.26). Occasionally it has been confused with metastatic disease (Kattapuram and Phillips, 1982) and fibrous dysplasia (Figure 6.27) but the distinction is usually obvious. The involvement of bone is irregular rather than diffuse, with disruption rather than enhancement of anatomical features such as trabecular markings. Other helpful distinguishing features are that fibrous dysplasia in long bones is usually diaphyseal whereas this is rare in Paget's disease (Figure 6.27). Recurrence of Paget's disease may, however, show diaphyseal uptake only due to activation at the resorption front (Figure 6.28). Diaphyseal foci do occur in Paget's disease but are rare. Indeed, in a series of five cases of diaphyseal foci of Paget's disease, three required biopsy for diagnosis (Schubert et al, 1984). Similarly, monostotic osteolytic disease of the spine without vertebral enlargement may also require biopsy for confident diagnosis.

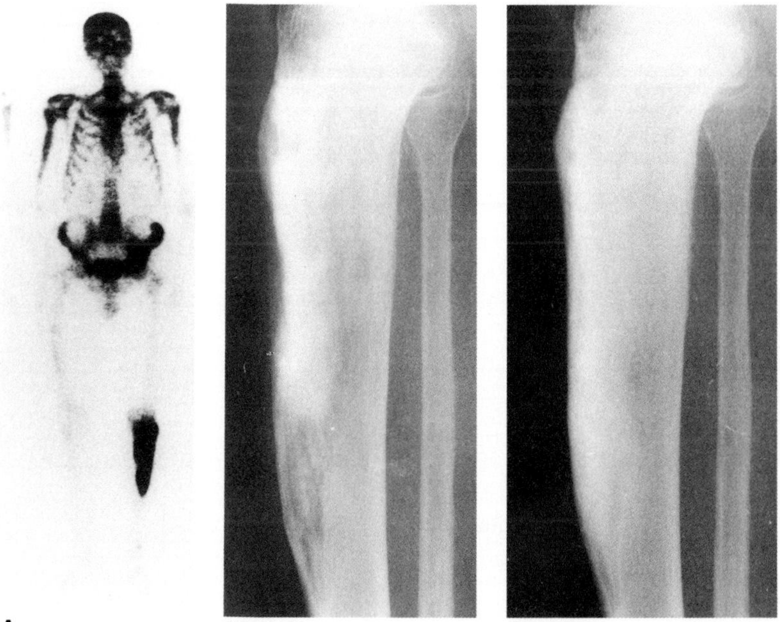

A B C

Figure 6.25

Characteristic bone-scan appearances of Paget's disease affecting the skull, proximal humerus, L4, L5, pelvis and proximal tibia (A). The tibial uptake corresponds to the zone of both sclerosis and rarefaction on the radiographs (B) and (C). The patient was receiving treatment with etidronate. Note the marked rarefaction of the anterior cortex of the tibia which was suspected to be due to sarcoma. The substitution of etidronate with another diphosphonate was associated with remineralization of the cortex and surrounding osteopaenia. (From Maldague and Malghem, 1989.)

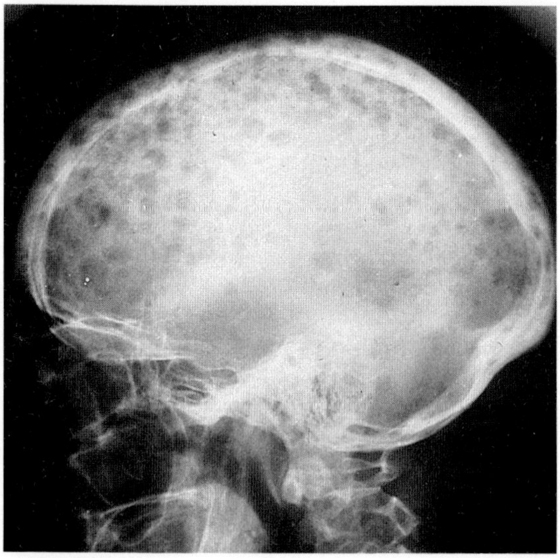

Figure 6.26

Myeloma of the skull showing the characteristic punched-out lesions. Note that the size and shape of the bone is normal.

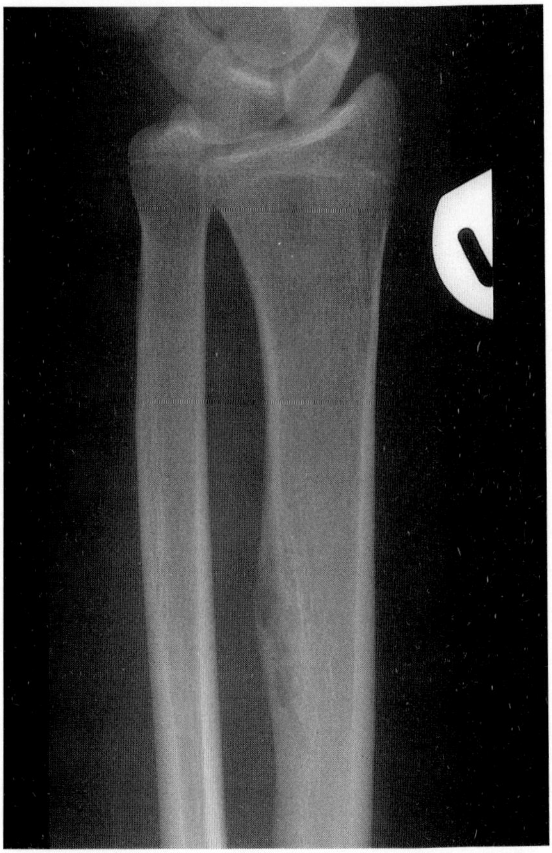

Figure 6.27

Focal osteolytic lesion of the radius due to fibrous dysplasia. Note the mid-diaphyseal location.

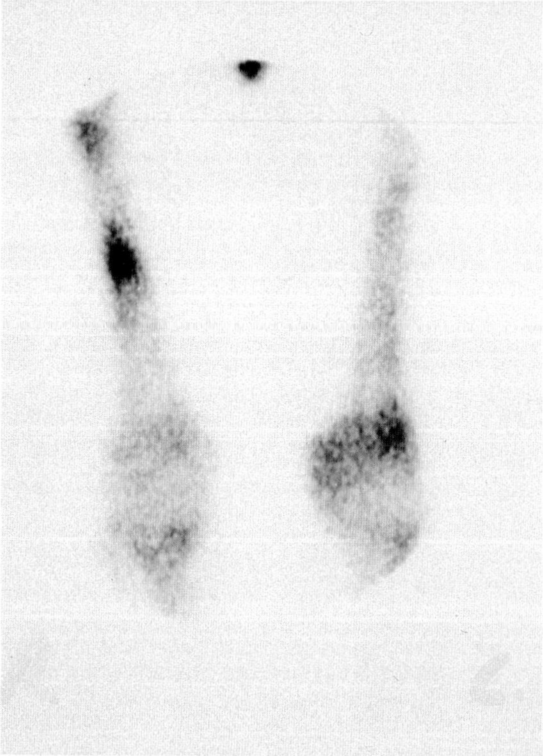

Figure 6.28

Scan appearance in Paget's disease of the femur. The apparent diaphyseal lesion is due to early recurrence of disease activity after a prolonged remission from diphosphonate treatment.

Fissure fractures

Incomplete fissure fractures occur generally on the convexity of long bones in Paget's disease and differ from the distribution pseudo-fractures or Looser's zones seen in osteomalacia. Fissure fractures invariably occur at sites of obvious involvement with Paget's disease, often in association with marked bowing. Looser's zones generally occur on the concave surfaces of long bones, such as the medial shaft of the femur and superior aspect of the neck of the femur. Moreover, they are usually symmetrical. Incomplete fractures on convex surfaces are seen in hypophosphatasia, but the distinction is straightforward (a low activity of alkaline phosphatase).

Cortical thickening

There are many disorders which cause focal or more widespread increases in cortical width. Generalized increases in cortical width occur with the ossification of periosteal new bone formation. They are also a feature of several diaphyseal dysplasias such as Engelmann's disease, Ribbing's disease, hyperphosphatasia and van Buchem's disease. In these disorders, alkaline phosphatase activity may be markedly increased, but their generalized and diaphyseal distribution, and age of onset make the distinction straightforward.

Osteomalacia

It is important to exclude the presence of concurrent osteomalacia where this is suspected, since osteomalacia appears to impair the response to medical treatment of the Paget's disease (Palmieri et al, 1973; Nagant de Deuxchaisnes et al, 1981). Bone pain, when present, commonly responds to vitamin D and the osteomalacia should be treated first for this reason. The diagnosis may be made more difficult by the presence of hyperphosphatasia and secondary hyperparathyroidism commonly seen with extensive disease involvement. Failure to respond to pagetic therapy may bring this to medical attention.

It is important to distinguish the hyperosteoidosis found on bone histology in Paget's disease from osteomalacia resulting in a defect in mineralization. The increase in osteoid volume in Paget's disease is largely attributable to an increase in bone turnover, resulting in an increase in surface coverage with osteoid rather than an increase in its width. The latter is characteristic of osteomalacia (Chapter 2). In addition, mineralization rates are usually high in Paget's disease, as judged by tetracycline labelling in vivo, whereas they are low in osteomalacia. The uptake of tetracycline, however, may be diffuse in both disorders (Plate 24). In Paget's disease diffuse uptake occurs when woven bone formation is marked.

The presence of hypocalcaemia in Paget's disease should suggest osteomalacia since it is rarely a feature of untreated Paget's disease. Note that hypocalcaemia, hypophosphataemia and secondary hyperparathyroidism do occur during the treatment of Paget's disease with mithramycin, the calcitonins and some of the diphosphonates (Chapter 7), but these are expected consequences of the inhibition of bone resorption without clinical significance. Prolonged exposure to the diphosphonate etidronate may, however, induce osteomalacia since high doses impair the mineralization of bone (Chapter 7).

Scintigraphy

Although bone scanning is more sensitive than radiography in the detection of pagetic lesions it is less specific. There are various causes of focal-scan abnormalities (see page 156), but these rarely cause diagnostic problems if the bone scan is interpreted alongside appropriate skeletal radiographs (Figure 6.29). Features which aid in the diagnosis of Paget's disease include its asymmetry (cf hypertrophic pulmonary osteoarthropathy, osteomalacias), homogeneous uptake within foci (cf metastases), confinement of uptake to hard tissue (cf osteomyelitis) and metaphyseal distribution (cf fibrous dysplasia) (Figure 6.30).

As in the case of radiographs, the greatest difficulties are encountered in distinguishing osteoblastic metastases from Paget's disease, particularly at the pelvis and spine and especially

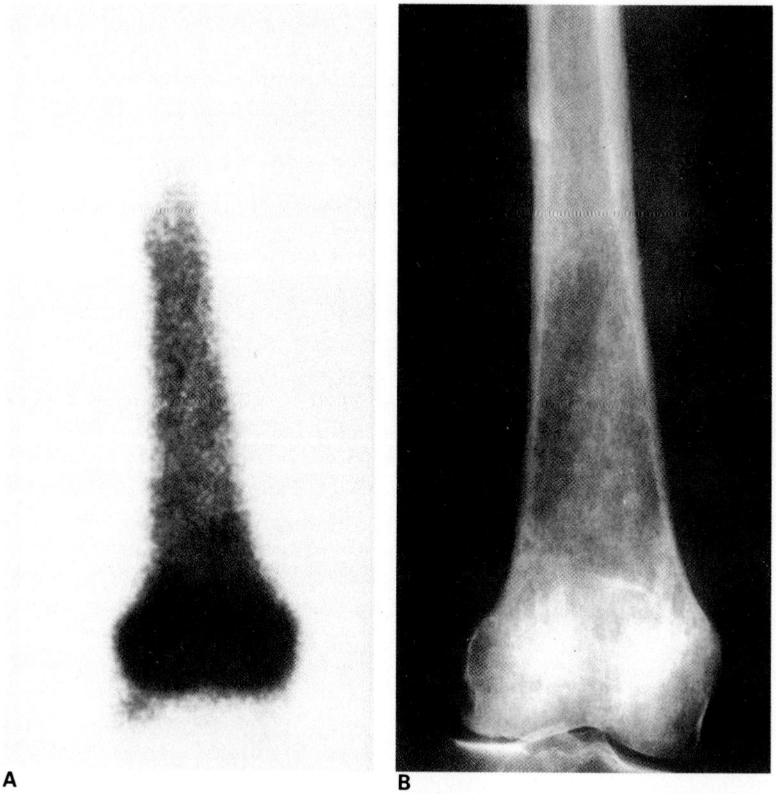

A B

Figure 6.29

Radiograph and bone scan of the distal femur. The bone scan (A) shows intense hyperfixation similar to that observed in Paget's disease. (B) In contrast, the radiograph shows none of the features of Paget's disease, in particular no cortical thickening nor bone enlargement. The discrete zones of osteolysis and sclerosis are also not seen in Paget's disease and were due to carcinoma of the breast. (From Maldague and Malghem, 1989.)

Some causes of focal increases in scintigraphic uptake.

Common
- Recent fracture
- Osteoarthrosis
- Paget's disease
- Skeletal metastases
- Osteomalacia and Looser's zones

Less common
- Fibrous dysplasia
- Osteomyelitis
- Hypertrophic pulmonary osteoarthropathy
- Malignant and benign bone tumours
- Microfractures, eg with fluoride treatment

when the two co-exist. It is important to note that recurrence of Paget's disease, previously treated with diphosphonates, may give rise to a patchy scan appearance more resembling tumour than untreated Paget's disease (Figure 6.28).

Scintigraphic uptake may be markedly increased in fibrous dysplasia, but is more often patchy. Other helpful distinguishing features in more generalized disease have been mentioned previously.

Figure 6.30 (facing page)

Bone scans of the spine. (A) is from a patient with monostotic Paget's disease. Note the intense and homogeneous uptake. The increased scintigraphic uptake of the spine and ribs was due to osteomalacia (B) and gives rise to symmetric uptake. The foci of increased uptake are due to Looser's zones. The increased scintigraphic uptake due to neoplasia (C) (D) shows markedly increased uptake at L2 on the left. In secondary neoplasia, uptake is usually focal, showing multicentric foci within the same bone and variable degrees of asymmetry (bottom right). (From Kanis, 1984b.)

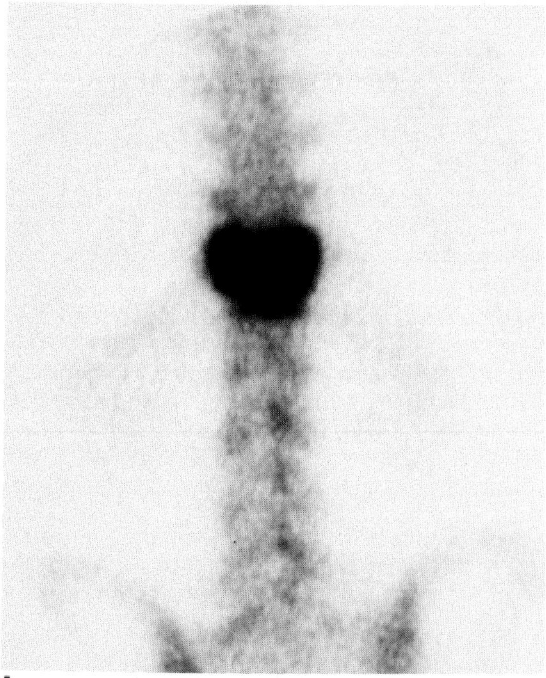

A

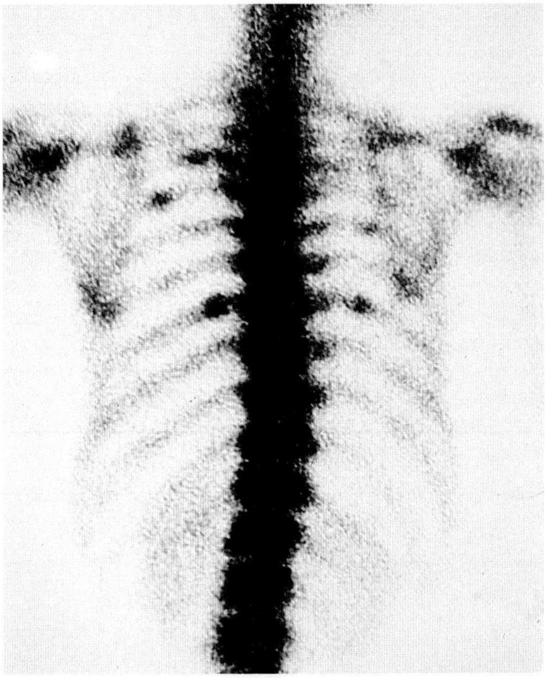

B

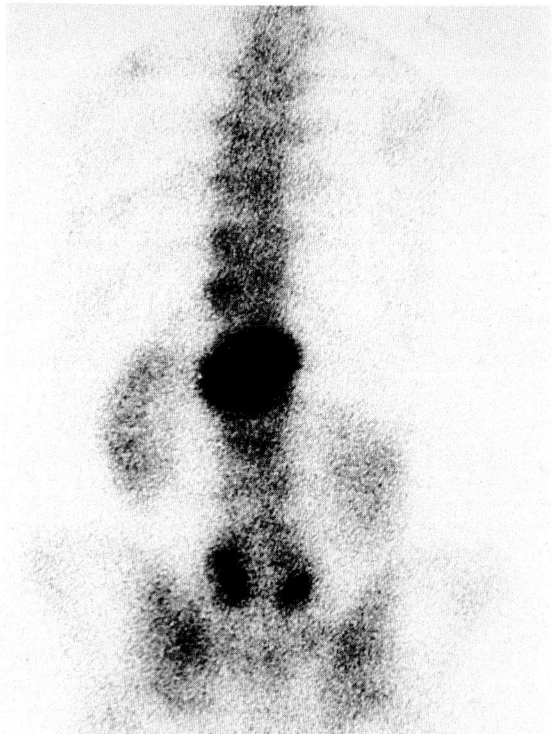

C

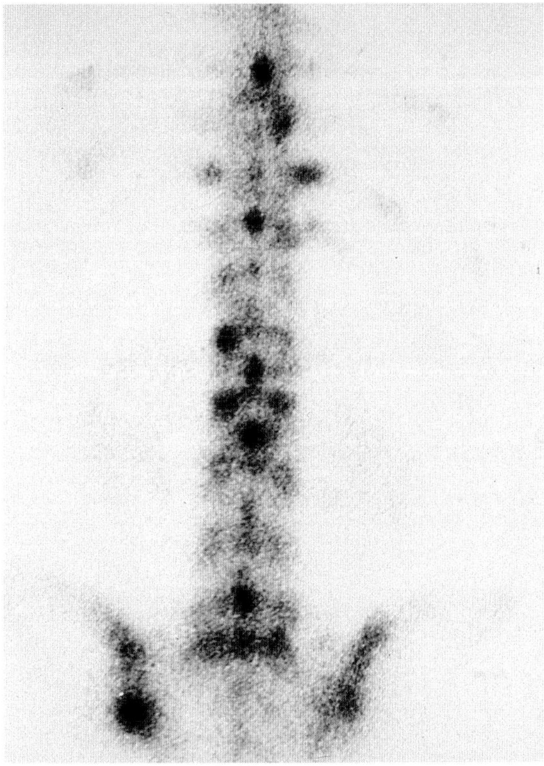

D

Alkaline phosphatase

Not all serum activity of alkaline phosphatase is bone-derived. Significant liver sources can be excluded by appropriate liver-function tests such as gamma glutamyl transferase or 5'-nucleotidase. With co-existing liver disease, measurements of these enzymes or the bone-derived isoenzyme of alkaline phosphatase may be useful in providing a baseline from which to judge the effects of subsequent treatment (Chapter 4). It is important to recognize that a significant minority of patients with Paget's disease have a normal serum activity of alkaline phosphatase, particularly those with monostotic disease. The presence of a normal alkaline phosphatase does not, therefore, exclude the diagnosis of Paget's disease. Problems with the interpretation of urinary hydroxyproline are reviewed in Chapter 4.

Hypercalcaemia

The association of hypercalcaemia with Paget's disease should alert the physician to co-existing pathology. Whereas hypercalcaemia may result solely from immobilization in the presence of extensive disease, it is more commonly due to or is aggravated by other hypercalcaemic pathology such as primary hyperparathyroidism or neoplasia affecting bone. Hypercalcaemia due to primary hyperparathyroidism may be masked in the presence of co-existing vitamin D deficiency.

CHAPTER 7

Drugs used for the treatment of Paget's disease

Twenty years ago Barry (1969) concluded that there were no effective regimens available for the medical treatment of Paget's disease. The introduction of calcitonin for clinical use in the early 1970s and of the diphosphonates some years later has not only revolutionized the medical management of Paget's disease, but has also stimulated renewed interest in its surgical management. Suppression of disease activity is now attainable, and with the realization that disease activity may be controlled for many years, the indications for treatment have expanded and are likely to increase still further in the future.

A wide variety of agents have been proposed for the treatment of Paget's disease, many of which are now obsolete (Albright and Henneman, 1955; McGavack et al, 1961; Maurice et al, 1962; Purves, 1962; Nagant de Deuxchaisnes and Krane, 1964, 1974; Barry, 1969; Levison, 1970; Riggs and Jowsey, 1972; Sekel, 1973; Theodors et al, 1981). Major interest has focused on the use of the calcitonins and the diphosphonates, which have now obtained widespread acceptance. Mithramycin (plicamycin), gallium nitrate and the combination of thiazide diuretics and calcium supplements are also used, but have been less adequately evaluated.

This chapter describes the agents commonly used in the treatment of Paget's disease. It also includes information about their acute and long-term effects on disease activity as judged principally by biochemical, kinetic and histological

Drugs used in the treatment of Paget's disease.

Well established
- Calcitonins: porcine, salmon, human, eel
- Diphosphonates: etidronate, clodronate, pamidronate
- Mithramycin

Less adequately evaluated
- Thiazide and calcium supplements
- Combinations of calcitonin and etidronate
- New diphosphonates, eg tiludronate, aminohexane and aminobutane diphosphonates, risedronate
- Gallium nitrate
- Amylin

Obsolete
- Actinomycin
- Fluoride
- Aspirin (in large doses to inhibit bone turnover)
- Corticosteroids
- Glucagon

Historical interest
- Calcium
- Vitamin D and C
- Colchicine
- Arsenic
- Magnesium carbonate
- Aluminium acetate
- Anabolic steroids
- ACTH
- Phosphate
- Iodides
- Oestrogens
- Folic acid
- Insulin
- Gonadal steroids
- Staphylococcus vaccine

investigation. Their effect on the clinical expression of Paget's disease is considered in Chapter 8.

The calcitonins

Calcitonin is a 32-amino-acid polypeptide considered to be one of the major calcium-regulating hormones (with PTH and the metabolites of vitamin D). It has 32 amino-acid residues with a disulphide bridge between cysteine residues at positions 1 and 7 (Figure 7.1). Its molecular weight is approximately 3.5 kd. It is produced in mammals from the parafollicular cells of the thyroid (Copp et al, 1967), but is found in many vertebrates. The parafollicular or 'C' cells of the thyroid are related embryologically to the ultimobranchial body of lower vertebrate species. Extrathyroidal sites of calcitonin production have been demonstrated in other tissues of neuroectodermal origin such as the thymus and adrenal, and calcitonin-like material is synthesized in the pars intermedia of the pituitary gland (Fischer et al, 1983).

The calcitonin gene encodes other peptides including calcitonin gene related peptide (CGRP) and katacalcin (Jacobs et al, 1981; Amara et al, 1982; Rosenfeld et al, 1983). Katacalcin or carboxyterminal adjacent peptide (PDN-21) is a 21-amino-acid peptide secreted in equimolar concentrations to calcitonin. Calcitonin is genomically translated as a larger peptide (21 kd). The prosequence is a single 57-amino-acid N-terminal peptide. Calcitonin circulates in plasma in heterogeneous form (Singer and Habener, 1974; Deftos et al, 1975; Heynen et al, 1975) and molecular species larger than authentic 1–32 calcitonin may represent calcitonin precursors and glycosylated derivatives. The heterogeneity of circulating calcitonin has presented many problems in the evaluation of its biological function in man since values measured by radioimmunoassay vary widely and some qualitative as well as quantitative differences are found between centres (Heynen et al, 1981; Stevenson et al, 1981). An example is the low values for calcitonin found in postmenopausal osteoporosis found by some (Deftos et al, 1980) whereas others find entirely normal values (Sjoberg et al, 1989).

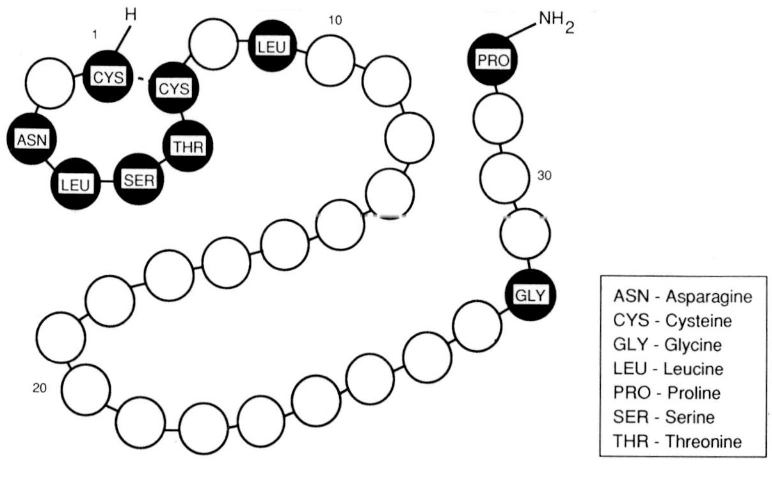

Figure 7.1

Structure of natural calcitonins. The nine invariant amino acids are indicated. In the case of eel calcitonin a synthetic analogue is also used ($Asu^{1,7}$-eel) in which there is an aminosuberic substitution of the two cysteine residues to replace the S–S linkage with an ethylene bridge.

Secretion of calcitonin

The endogenous production rate of calcitonin in man has been assessed by steady-state infusion of human calcitonin. Estimates based on radioimmunoassay suggest that the daily production is approximately 13 IU, but this may be an overestimate due to the uncertain biological activity of large molecular weight fragments (Kanis et al, 1982). A major stimulus to its secretion is an increase in the serum concentration of calcium (Hirsch et al, 1964; Care, 1968; Sjoberg et al, 1989). Since one of its actions is to lower serum calcium it is commonly thought to be a regulator of plasma calcium homeostasis. Many other factors are known to affect the secretion of calcitonin. These include several gastrointestinal hormones such as glucagon and gastrin, beta-adrenergic agents and alcohol (Cooper et al, 1971; Ziegler et al, 1972; Hornum et al, 1975). Calcium, pentagastrin and alcohol have all been used as provocative tests for calcitonin secretion (Cooper et al, 1971; Hillyard et al, 1977; Kanis et al, 1979).

Actions of calcitonin

An obvious action of calcitonin in man and experimental animals is to lower serum calcium levels (Friedman and Raisz, 1965; O'Riordan and Aurbach, 1968). The major reason for the fall in serum calcium is the inhibition of bone resorption (Reynolds and Dingle, 1970). In addition to inhibiting bone resorption it decreases renal tubular resorption of calcium, phosphate, magnesium, potassium, urate and some other ions (Bijvoet et al, 1968, 1971; Singer et al, 1969; Gattereau et al, 1979; Nagant de Deuxchaisnes et al, 1987; Figure 7.2). It also inhibits the secretion of some hormones including gastrin, cholecystokinin, insulin, prolactin, growth hormone, LH, FSH and glucagon (Hesch et al, 1971; Fahrenkrug et al, 1975; Stevenson et al, 1977; Cantalamessa et al, 1978; Petralito et al, 1979; Looij et al, 1988). There is some evidence that calcitonin also stimulates the 1α-hydroxylase enzyme of the kidney to increase the synthesis of calcitriol in vitro and in vivo (Kawashima et al, 1981; Jaeger et al, 1986).

A further action of calcitonin that may have relevance to its use in Paget's disease is its analgesic properties. Experiments and some clinical studies suggest that the administration of calcitonin has analgesic activity (Pecile et al, 1975; Braga et al, 1978; Fiore et al, 1983; Welzel, 1983; Fraioli et al, 1982; Roth and Kolaric, 1986; Pun and Chan, 1989). The mechanism for this effect is controversial, but it could be either a direct central effect of the drug or be mediated by an increase in endogenous opiate secretion (Azria, 1989; Gennari et al, 1989). It is difficult to envisage that parenteral calcitonin has this effect since it is not thought to cross the blood/brain barrier in significant amounts.

Physiological role

Despite or because of the multiplicity of its actions, the physiological role of calcitonin in man

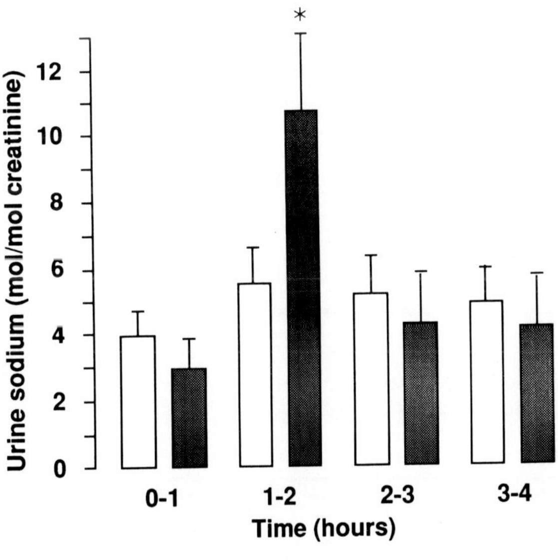

Figure 7.2

Acute effects of human calcitonin on urinary sodium excretion (mean ± SEM) in four healthy subjects. Eight units were given between the first and second hour and compared with a control day. Note the rapid but transient increase in sodium excretion on the day when calcitonin was given (stippled). (Data redrawn from Singer et al, 1969.)

is not clear. It has been suggested that the hormone serves to protect the skeleton against calcium stresses such as dietary loads, pregnancy, lactation and secondary hyperparathyroidism (Heynen et al, 1976; Cooper et al, 1977; Stevenson et al, 1979).

Difficulties in ascribing a physiological role arise for several reasons. The difficulties in the interpretation of radioimmunoassay have been mentioned. In addition, many of the effects of calcitonin have been elicited with large doses (such as 50–100 IU) which are clearly pharmacological. Furthermore, agents which alter calcitonin secretion have generally employed pharmacological quantities, and the effects observed with physiologically appropriate amounts of secretagogues do not always necessarily stimulate calcitonin secretion (Heynen et al, 1981). Further difficulties in ascribing a physiological role to calcitonin are that its deficiency (for example in total thyroidectomy) or excess (medullary carcinoma of the thyroid) are associated with only minor disturbances in skeletal or calcium homeostasis (Woodhouse and Barnes, 1968; Hurley et al, 1987; Figure 7.3). Its physiological role if any is therefore speculative. Nevertheless, there is some evidence that its secretion is regulated in that exogenous infusion of calcitonin appears to inhibit its endogenous secretion (Kanis et al, 1982). Its activity in Paget's disease is nevertheless largely attributable to a pharmacological effect on bone.

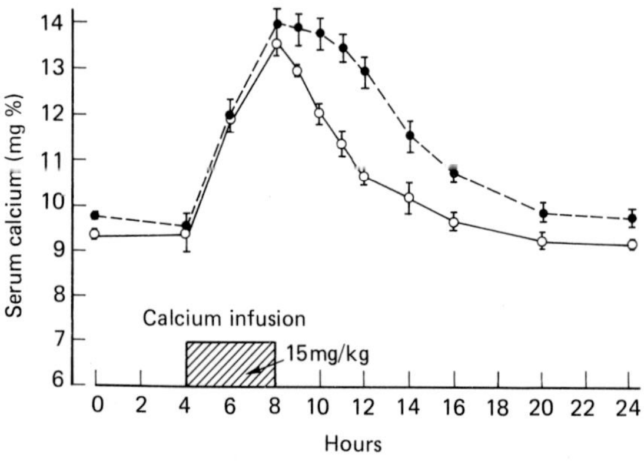

Figure 7.3

The effects of calcium gluconate infusion on serum calcium values (mean ± SEM) in six normal (○) and 6 athyroidal (●) subjected maintained on L-thyroxine. Note the delayed disappearance of the calcium load in the athyroidal subjects. (From Woodhouse and Barnes, 1968.)

Pharmacological preparations

Several different calcitonins are available for the treatment of Paget's disease. The first preparation available for clinical use was porcine calcitonin. Porcine calcitonin (PCT) is extracted from pig thyroid glands, whereas the other calcitonins which are available are synthetic and include synthetic salmon (SCT; salcatonin), human (HCT) and eel calcitonins (ECT; elcatonin). The structure of all the natural calcitonins includes a disulphide bridge, bridging the first amino acid with the seventh. The cysteine residues of the bridge can be replaced by a group giving a carbon rather than disulphide bridge which renders the molecule more resistant to biological degradation (Sakadura et al, 1981). The eel calcitonin analogue ($Asu^{1.7}$) eel CT (carbocalcitonin) is one such analogue available in some countries (Caniggia et al, 1987).

The entire 32-amino-acid sequence is essential for biological activity. There are, however, many differences in amino-acid composition of the calcitonins from different species, and only nine amino acids are invariant (Figure 7.1). These considerations suggest that the tertiary structure of the calcitonins is important in determining biological activity. The marked variation of amino-acid sequence, however, is likely to account for the antigenicity of non-human calcitonins in man.

There are large differences in the potencies of the available forms of calcitonin. For this reason their activity is commonly expressed in international units determined from acute responses in bioassays. Their relative potencies in various bioassay systems vary (Maier et al, 1970) and do not always accord with the doses that have been effectively used in clinical practice. Very few long-term comparisons have been made between the activity of the various forms of calcitonin in

Paget's disease, but differences of possible therapeutic significance are reviewed later.

Surprisingly, the salmon hormone (salcatonin) resembles the human hormone more than do other mammalian calcitonins, and it is interesting to note that both salmon and eel calcitonin are more potent in man than the porcine or human hormone (Galante et al, 1973; Azria, 1989; Figure 7.4). In addition, the salmon and eel hormones have a longer duration of hypocalcaemic activity. The reasons for these differences in potency are not known, but may be due to differences in receptor-binding affinity or metabolic clearance (Marx et al, 1972; Singer et al, 1977; Huwyler et al, 1979; Azria, 1989). Lower estimates of potency in the clinical literature than those shown in Figure 7.4 are due to variable degrees of purity of the hormone (for example Doyle et al, 1974a; Kanis et al, 1974; Evans, 1977).

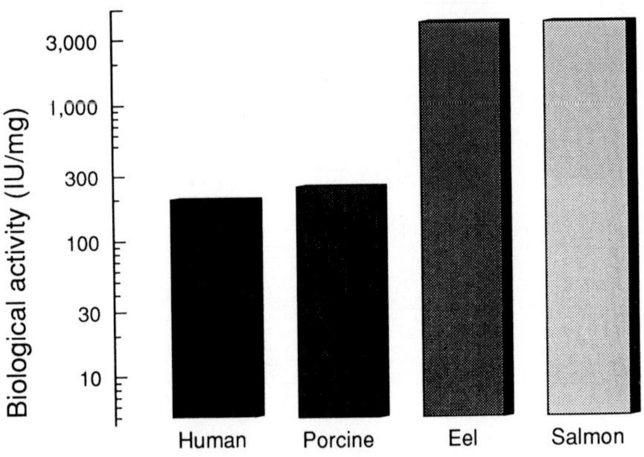

Figure 7.4

Comparative activity of the calcitonins.

Acute effect of calcitonin on bone and serum calcium

The major action of calcitonin is to inhibit bone resorption and thereby to decrease plasma calcium and the urinary excretion of hydroxyproline (Bijvoet et al, 1968; Haddad et al, 1970a; Nagant de Deuxchaisnes, 1989). It may also decrease calcium efflux from bone across quiescent skeletal surfaces (Talmage et al, 1983). In addition, calcitonin decreases renal tubular reabsorption of calcium, but this probably contributes little to its acute hypocalcaemic effect in Paget's disease.

Calcitonin acts directly on osteoclasts (Chambers and Magnus, 1982) and receptors have been identified in the isolated rat osteoclast (Nicholson et al, 1986). Exposure of rat osteoclasts to calcitonin causes invagination of the brush border, retraction from the bone surface (Kallio et al, 1972; Holtrop et al, 1974) and a decrease in their motility (Chambers and Magnus, 1982; Kanehisa, 1989). The number of osteoclasts visible and applied to bone decreases in vivo within half an hour but returns to normal after a few hours (Baron and Vignery, 1981; Hedlund et al, 1983). As in the case of other target tissues it is possible that these actions are mediated by the activation of adenylate cyclase (Chierichetti et al, 1985; Nicholson et al, 1986).

Since the pharmacological effect of calcitonin on bone is largely attributable to the number of functional osteoclasts, the degree of hypocalcaemia attained acutely after the injection of a fixed dose of calcitonin is proportional to the prevailing rate of bone resorption. Thus, in patients with Paget's disease, the hypocalcaemic response is greater than in normal subjects and is most marked in those patients with the more extensive disease activity, whether judged by scintigraphy or by biochemical markers of disease activity (Bordier et al, 1970; Gershberg et al, 1973; Fournie et al, 1977; Hosking et al, 1979; Meunier et al, 1987; Figure 7.5). Similarly, when Paget's disease is treated with any agent (including calcitonin), the acute hypocalcaemic response decreases with the decrease in disease activity (Figure 7.6). Indeed, the 'calcitonin test' has been used to assess prevailing rates of bone resorption in many disorders, and in Paget's disease as a (rather unreliable) test of responsivity to calcitonin in drug-induced resistance (Salson, 1981; Hosking, 1983). A corollary is that when the activity of calcitonin is tested in man, account needs to be taken of the prevailing rate of bone resorption. When patients with Paget's disease

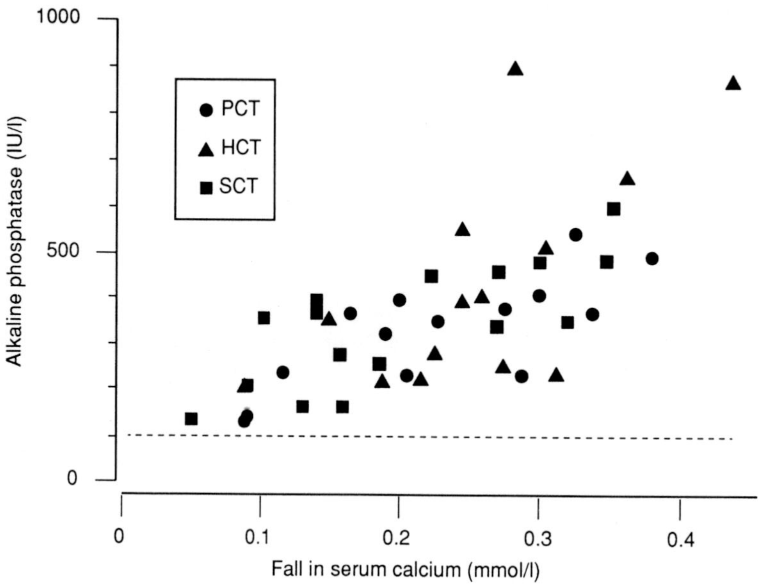

Figure 7.5

Acute hypocalcaemic effect of the calcitonins given subcutaneously. The fall in serum calcium at 6 hours correlated with disease activity as judged by alkaline phosphatase. There was no marked difference in responses between salmon (SCT; 100 IU), porcine (PCT; 160 IU) or human calcitonin (HCT; 100 IU).

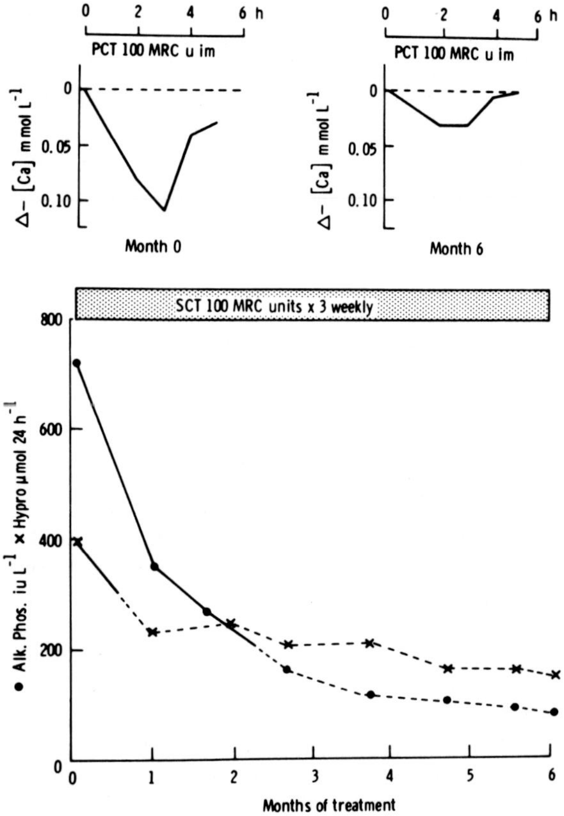

Figure 7.6

Changes in the acute hypocalcaemic response to porcine calcitonin (PCT) in a patient before and during treatment of Paget's disease with salmon calcitonin (SCT). Note that the hypocalcaemic response diminished as bone turnover decreased. (From Hosking, 1983.)

are matched for disease activity a dose dependent effect of calcitonins on serum calcium is observed (Galante et al, 1973; Gennari et al, 1981, 1985; O'Doherty et al, 1990a), and doses approaching physiological have the less marked hypocalcaemic effects (Figure 7.7).

It is to be expected that the decrease in serum calcium would provoke a homeostatic response. Secondary hyperparathyroidism occurs as expected (Burckhardt et al, 1973; DeRose et al, 1974), but this is transient and matches the acute fall in serum calcium. Thus, repeated daily injections are associated with repeated but transient increases in PTH secretion. The sustained effect of calcitonin on bone resorption, but transient

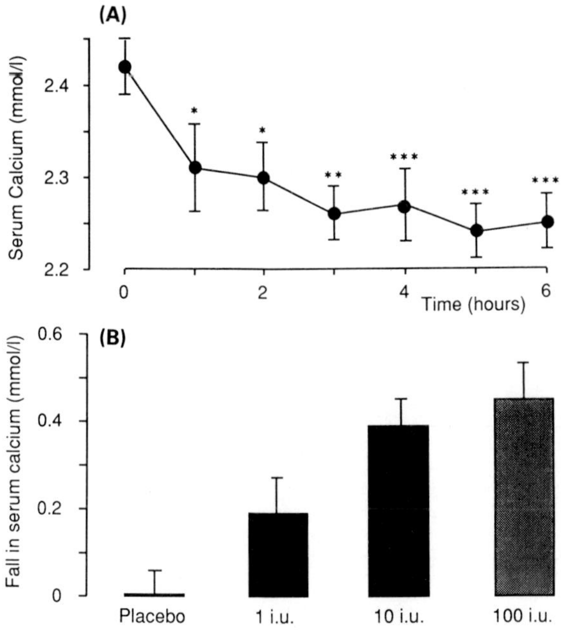

Figure 7.7

Acute effect of synthetic salmon calcitonin in Paget's disease. (A) shows the sequential changes in serum calcium (mean ± SEM) after 100 IU were given subcutaneously to nine patients. (B) shows the hypocalcaemic response (cumulative change in serum calcium between the fourth and sixth hour) with this and lower doses in the same patients.

effects on serum calcium, suggests that the hypocalcaemic response is due in part to changes in calcium fluxes across quiescent surfaces of bone.

Long-term effects on bone remodelling

The effects of calcitonin in Paget's disease were first demonstrated by Bijvoet and his colleagues (Bijvoet and Jansen, 1967; Bijvoet et al, 1968). They demonstrated the ability of calcitonin to decrease bone resorption, as judged by a decrease in the urinary excretion of hydroxyproline. Its repeated administration maintains this effect and is followed by a subsequent decrease in serum activity of alkaline phosphatase (Figure 7.8; Haddad et al, 1970b; Shai et al, 1971; Krane et al, 1973; DeRose et al, 1974; Avramides, 1977; Singer, 1977). The most conspicuous action of calcitonin is to inhibit the activity and numbers of osteoclasts, effects which are amply demonstrated in experimental studies but which have also been demonstrated in patients with Paget's disease (Bordier et al, 1970; Singer et al, 1976). Early effects shown in man include the detachment of osteoclasts from the erosion surfaces and a decrease in osteoclast nuclearity (Table 7.1). These effects are sustained by continued treatment (Bordier et al, 1970; Woodhouse et al, 1971; Rasmussen and Bordier, 1974; Eisinger and Laponche, 1976; Martin et al, 1977; Delling et al, 1977; Singer et al, 1977; Fornassier et al, 1978; Williams et al, 1978). Osteoclast numbers and nuclearity decrease, as does the resorbing surface. Viral inclusions persist, however, despite the decrease in osteoclast numbers (Rebel et al, 1977; Harvey et al, 1982).

The question arises why an inhibitor of bone resorption without conspicuous effects on bone formation should lead to a decrease in bone formation. The reasons for this almost certainly relate to the coupled nature of bone remodelling present in Paget's disease (Chapter 2). A substantial decrease in numbers of osteoclasts and their formation would not only decrease the prevailing rate of bone resorption, but also the recruitment of osteoclasts to future remodelling sites. At those remodelling sites which were in the process of formation, bone formation would continue after the administration of calcitonin. At those sites where resorption had been occurring at the time of administration, formation would also be likely to occur as a later event (Figure 7.9). This explains why the administration of calcitonin has no acute action on the activity of alkaline phosphatase. As treatment continues, however, fewer new osteoclasts and resorption cavities are formed and the eroded or resorption surfaces on bone are decreased. Since progressively less and less of the surface of bone undergoes bone resorption, less surface is available for the subsequent attraction of osteoblasts. It would be expected then that calcitonin should decrease the

Table 7.1 Acute effects of calcitonin on osteoclasts in Paget's disease (number/mm^2). Biopsies were taken before and 30 minutes after the injection of calcitonin. Treatment was associated with a decrease in the number of osteoclasts and a decrease in the proportion of remaining osteoclasts attached to bone. (From Singer et al, 1976.)

	Total		*Free*		*Attached*		*Free/attached*	
	Before	*After*	*Before*	*After*	*Before*	*After*	*Before*	*After*
SCT 20 μg	4.8	2.0	3.2	1.7	1.6	0.3	2.0	5.9
SCT 20 μg	9.5	4.0	6.5	3.2	3.0	0.8	2.2	4.0
SCT 20 μg	1.3	2.8	0.4	1.6	0.9	1.2	0.4	1.3
HCT 500 μg	2.6	1.1	1.0	0.3	1.6	0.8	0.6	0.4
HCT 500 μg	2.5	1.4	1.4	1.1	1.1	0.3	1.3	3.7

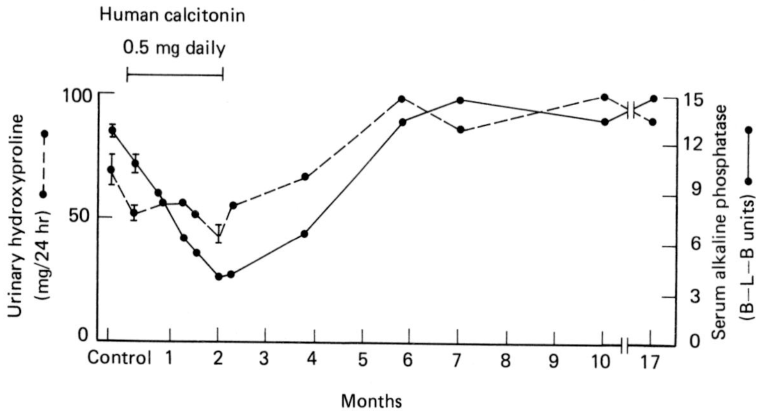

Figure 7.8

Pattern of response to calcitonin and relapse in a patient treated for 2 months with human calcitonin, 0.5 mg daily. Note the early fall in hydroxyproline and later fall in alkaline phosphatase. Similarly, during relapse, hydroxyproline rose earlier than did values for phosphatase. (From Singer et al, 1977.)

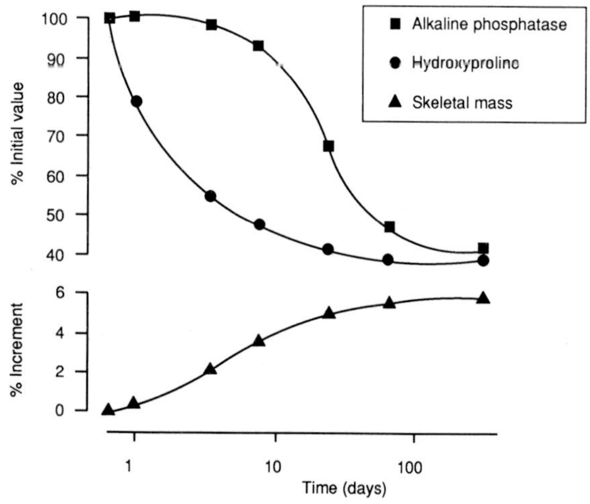

Figure 7.9

Expected consequences of the inhibition of bone resorption on bone formation and skeletal mass. During the early phase of treatment, bone formation continues despite the inhibition of bone resorption, and skeletal mass increases due to a decrease in remodelling space. Later, as bone formation matches bone resorption, skeletal mass remains constant, albeit at a higher value than before treatment. Data on the change of phosphatase and hydroxyproline were taken from responses observed with clodronate.

rate of bone resorption and be followed some time later by a decrease in bone formation.

This sequence of events – the inhibition of resorption and later decrease in formation – predicted from knowledge of bone remodelling and the coupling of bone formation to prior resorption appears to occur in practice. It can be monitored indirectly in Paget's disease after the start of treatment with calcitonin by an early decrease in urinary excretion of hydroxyproline followed later by a decrease in serum activity of alkaline phosphatase (Figure 7.8). This dissociation between the various aspects of bone remodelling is similar to that observed with the diphosphonates (see later), but the fall in alkaline phosphatase occurs more rapidly with the use of calcitonin than with some of the diphosphonates. There is some evidence that calcitonin decreases the reversal surface in normal mammals (DeVernejoul et al, 1989), implying that the time interval between the completion of resorption and the onset of bone formation is decreased. This would provide a reasonable explanation for the more rapid suppression of phosphatase with calcitonin than with etidronate or clodronate.

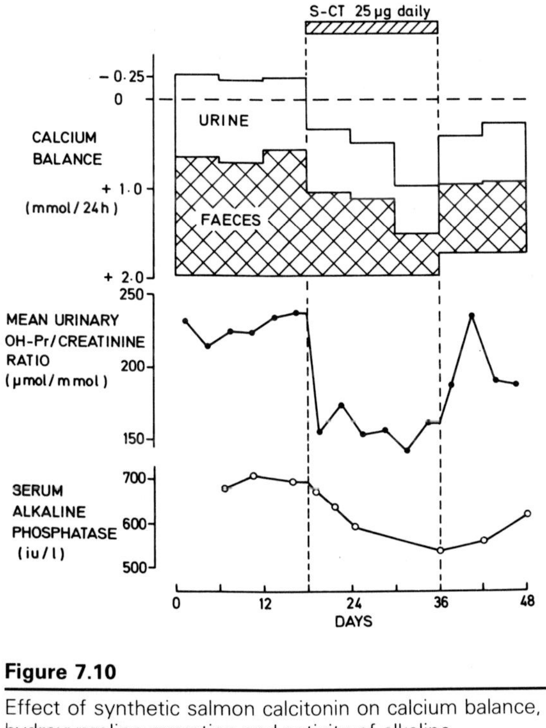

Figure 7.10

Effect of synthetic salmon calcitonin on calcium balance, hydroxyproline excretion and activity of alkaline phosphatase. Before treatment, the patient was in moderate negative balance for calcium. Treatment was associated with a marked decrease in hydroxyproline and slower fall in alkaline phosphatase. Calcium balance increased, reflecting continued bone formation at a time when resorption was inhibited. These effects reversed when treatment was stopped.

Calcitonin receptors have not been found in mammalian osteoblasts (Warshowsky et al, 1980; Nicholson et al, 1986) and on that basis it is assumed that any changes in bone remodelling are secondary to a decrease in endosteal resorption surfaces. This seems to provide a satisfactory explanation for the decrease in bone formation, but it does not exclude other indirect effects of calcitonin on osteoblasts (for example by increased secretion of PTH and synthesis of $1,25(OH)_2D_3$). Indeed, when calcitonin is given to patients with Paget's disease, decreases are seen in the urinary excretion of non-dialysable hydroxyproline peptides within a few hours of administration (Krane et al, 1973). Since these peptides are thought to be derived from collagen during its synthesis this might suggest acute inhibitory effects of calcitonin on collagen formation. We have recently shown an increase in the urinary excretion of hydroxyproline within the first hour of the administration of calcitonin (O'Doherty et al, 1990a). The mechanism is not known, but it is apparently not due to an effect of calcitonin on the renal clearance of hydroxyproline (Bijvoet et al, 1968). These observations suggest that calcitonin, in addition to its effect on bone resorption, has a wide range of effects on bone metabolism.

During the early phase of treatment when bone resorption is inhibited but formation is still occurring at sites of previous bone resorption, it is to be expected that skeletal mass will increase (Figure 7.9). Traditional metabolic balance studies have shown an early increase in calcium balance (Shai et al, 1971; Kanis et al, 1975; Figure 7.10). More modern techniques have shown an increase in regional bone density as judged by photon absorptiometry (Chandler and Chandler, 1982). The increase in skeletal mass does not continue indefinitely, but a new steady state is achieved when bone formation has been suppressed, and bone formation once more matches bone resorption, albeit at a lower rate than before treatment. Thus, increments in calcium balance become less marked with continued treatment (Kanis et al, 1975; Oreopoulos et al, 1977; Sturtridge et al, 1977). This new steady state of bone turnover may take several months to be achieved.

The decrease in bone turnover induced by long-term treatment with calcitonin has several important other effects. As reviewed in Chapter 2, the increased bone remodelling that occurs in Paget's disease causes a decrease in skeletal mass by increasing the number of sites on bone surfaces occupied by resorption. Conversely, when bone remodelling is decreased with calcitonin (or with other agents) an increase in skeletal mass and in radiographic density may be apparent. This has been well described with calcitonin (Chapter 8). A second and important effect of calcitonin in Paget's disease is to halt the advance of the resorption front and therefore the progressive involvement of normal bone by the pagetic process. Third, the new bone formed under the influence of calcitonin appears to be lamellar rather than woven in structure (Woodhouse et al, 1971). Thus, treatment appears to be associated, not only with a halt in its extension, but also with the production of more normal bone. This has obvious implications for long-term management which are reviewed in the next chapter.

A number of other changes are described with the use of calcitonin. As expected, scintigraphic abnormalities become less prominent (Lavender et al, 1977; Waxman et al, 1980), as do kinetic indices of bone turnover (Hosking et al, 1981). Treatment is also associated with a decrease in vascularity as judged by changes in skin temperature (Bouvet, 1977; Ring et al, 1977), bone blood flow (Wooton et al, 1978) and cardiac output (Chapter 8). These effects occur within days of administration, before the suppression of bone formation, suggesting that calcitonin may have direct effects on blood flow. The effects of calcitonin on bone pain are also rapid (Chapter 8), and this is one of the reasons for thinking that increased bone blood flow might contribute to pagetic pain.

Parenteral therapeutic regimens

Calcitonin is generally given by subcutaneous or intramuscular injection. The responses described above do not depend on the type of calcitonin used. A number of studies have examined the acute hypocalcaemic activity of various calcitonins in patients with Paget's disease. In general, the response conforms to the known differences in potency between the various calcitonins when given by subcutaneous or intramuscular injection (Figure 7.4). For example, similar responses are evoked with equimolar doses of salmon and eel calcitonins (Chapuy and Meunier, 1982; Chierichetti et al, 1985), whereas the salmon hormone is 10 times more potent than human calcitonin which in turn is more potent than porcine (Galante et al, 1973; Chapuy et al, 1980; Gennari et al, 1981, 1985).

Very little detailed dose-response work has been undertaken with the long-term use of calcitonin in Paget's disease, principally because of its safety, irrespective of the dose used. There are, however, sufficient data to enable some generalizations to be made concerning the effects of different calcitonins, different doses and different frequencies of administration.

All the commercially available forms of calcitonin are effective in relieving bone pain and in reducing plasma alkaline phosphatase and urinary hydroxyproline if given in sufficient dose. As for the acute response, there are more similarities than differences in the long-term responses of bone to different calcitonins. Dosage regimens which induce significant effects vary from 50 IU on alternate days (or thrice weekly) to 100 or 200 units daily. Weekly injections, of 50 IU SCT or HCT for example, appear to give submaximal responses (Figure 7.11; Avramides et al, 1975; Evans et al, 1977) but may be sufficient to maintain a response once a decrease in bone turnover has been induced (Kanis et al, 1974; Figure 7.12).

In the case of salmon calcitonin, 50 IU thrice weekly is probably the minimum effective dose (DeRose et al, 1974; Kanis et al, 1974) and others prefer to give 100 IU thrice weekly (Woodhouse et al, 1977; Martin, 1979; O'Donoghue and Hosking, 1987) or daily administration of 50–100 IU (Hamilton, 1974; Bastian et al, 1977; Grunstein et al, 1981). A daily regimen appears to induce a more rapid suppression of bone turnover than

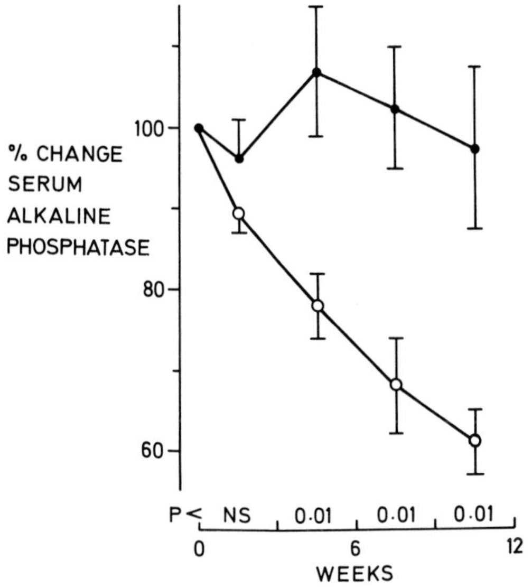

Figure 7.11

Responses of alkaline phosphatase (mean ± SEM) to two treatment regimens of synthetic salmon calcitonin: 50 μg given either thrice weekly (16 patients; ○) or weekly (5 patients; ●). The weekly dose was without effect (Kanis and Strong, unpublished).

thrice-weekly injections (Chapuy et al, 1975), but the ultimate response is probably similar. These thrice weekly or daily regimes induce about a 50 per cent reduction in disease activity (Figure 7.13).

Similar conclusions have been derived with the use of HCT (Evans, 1977a; Singer, 1977; Lang et al, 1981; MacIntyre et al, 1980). Radiographic studies following the long-term use of human calcitonin have suggested that 50 IU daily is the minimum dose necessary to maintain radiographic improvement (Doyle et al, 1974a). The optimal dose regimen of porcine calcitonin has not been as extensively studied as for the salmon or human hormone, but effective regimens are 50–200 IU daily or on alternate days (Bastian et al, 1977). These treatment schedules are similar to those described for salmon and human calcitonin (Figure 7.14). There are as yet few data concerning the long-term use of eel calcitonin or carbocalcitonin (Nuti, 1986). Reports of suboptimal effects of 40 IU carbocalcitonin given every other day may be due to problems present at that time with its formulation (Caniggia et al, 1987) which have now been resolved.

Apart from the differences in relative potency between the calcitonins, the question arises whether the different calcitonins evoke different clinical responses. The analgesic effects of salmon and eel calcitonin appear to be greater than

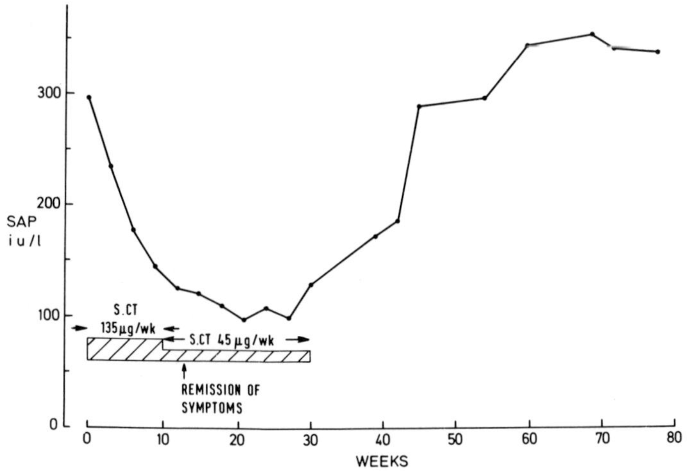

Figure 7.12

Serum activity of alkaline phosphatase following the administration of synthetic salmon calcitonin in a patient with Paget's disease. Note the suppression of disease activity with 45 μg (136 IU) thrice weekly. Disease activity remained suppressed with weekly injections, but relapse occurred immediately after treatment was stopped. (From Kanis et al, 1974.)

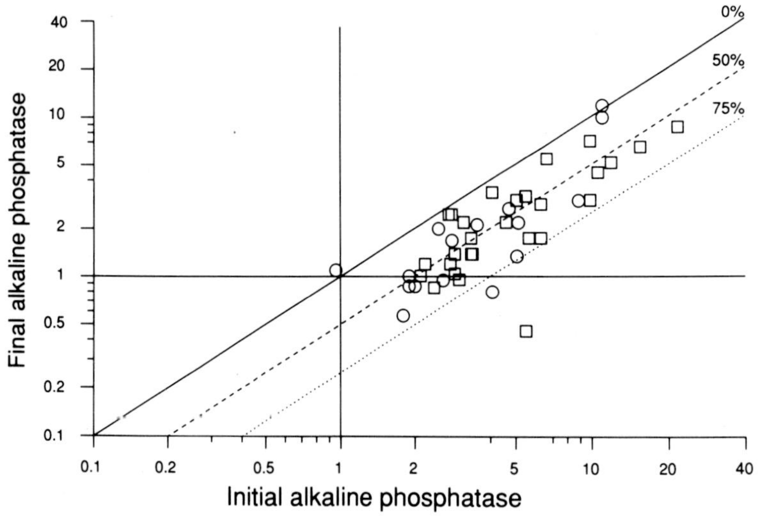

Figure 7.13

Serum activity of alkaline phosphatase (expressed as a ratio of the upper limit of the reference range) before and during treatment with synthetic salmon calcitonin. Values during treatment are nadir values observed after treatment for 3 months or longer. Round symbols denote responses to 50–100 IU daily and square symbols responses to thrice weekly injections of 100 IU. The solid lines denote the normal range and the line of identity. Dotted lines denote the expected relationship assuming a reduction of 50 or 75 per cent of disease activity. Note the logarithmic coordinates. (Data from Hamilton, 1974, and O'Donoghue and Hosking, 1987.)

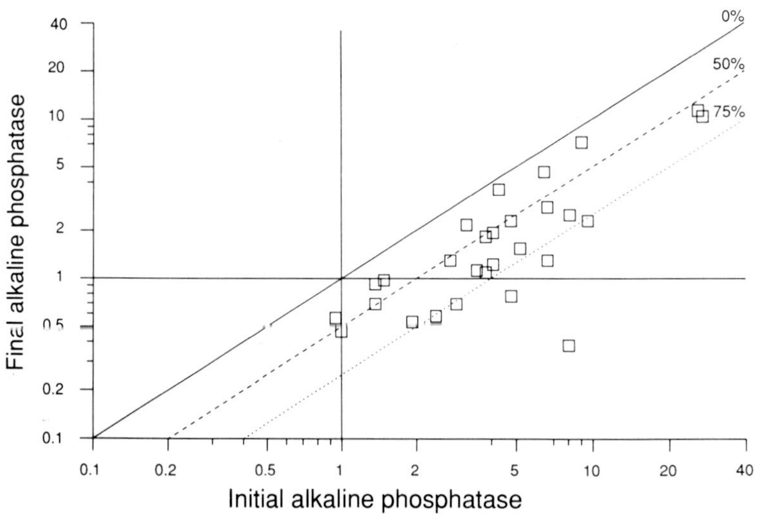

Figure 7.14

Serum activity of alkaline phosphatase (expressed as a ratio of the upper reference range) before and during treatment with human calcitonin, 100 IU daily. Values during treatment are nadir values after 3–34 months of continuous treatment. The solid lines denote the normal range and the line of identity. Dotted lines denote the expected relationship assuming a reduction of 50 or 75 per cent of disease activity. Note the similarity of response with salmon calcitonin, Figure 7.13. (Data from MacIntyre et al, 1980.)

equivalent doses of HCT (Gennari et al, 1983, 1985). There is some evidence for calcitonin-like peptides in the brain which are more closely related to SCT than HCT (Fischer et al, 1983). Their role is not known, but they might conceivably be important in the regulation of the perception of pain. No other differences in therapeutic effect have been reported.

Despite general agreement about the optimal doses of calcitonin for populations, the question arises whether dose requirements vary significantly between individuals. There is some evidence that patients with more extensive disease require larger doses of calcitonin, based on both the acute and longer-term effects of calcitonin (O'Doherty et al, 1990a).

The acute effects of calcitonin can be readily assessed by the hypocalcaemic response to a single injection which, for any given dose of calcitonin, is proportional to the prevailing rate of bone turnover. When relatively low doses of calcitonin are utilized (such as 10 IU) then the hypocalcaemic effect is attenuated in patients with extensive Paget's disease as might be expected (Figure 7.7). However, the response in patients with less extensive disease is similar to that expected with much larger doses: it is those patients with extensive disease in whom responses are attenuated. It appears therefore that patients with minimal disease require less calcitonin to have complete effects than do patients with extensive disease (O'Doherty et al, 1990a). The reasons for this are not known, but do not relate to any known differences in metabolic clearance of calcitonin between patients (Kanis et al, 1982).

The differing sensitivity of patients to the calcium-lowering effects of calcitonin thus appears to depend in part upon the extent of the disease. The evidence that patients with a range of disease activity require different doses of calcitonin is less complete. It has been noted that patients with skull involvement may require larger doses of calcitonin (Hamdy, 1981) and patients with disease of the skull generally have more extensive disease (Chapter 3). Against this view, the degree of suppression of disease activity (approximately 50 per cent of initial alkaline phosphatase) is similar over a wide range of disease activity (Figures 7.13 and 7.14). This suggests no simple relationship between dose, response and extent of disease, and that higher doses than generally recommended are unlikely to be of greater value in those patients with extensive disease. On the other hand, lower doses of calcitonin than currently used are likely to evoke worthwhile clinical responses in patients with very mild disease, but be suboptimal in those patients with more extensive disease.

Therapeutic responses to calcitonins

Primary resistance to calcitonin is rarely if ever observed provided that the dose given is adequate (Hamilton, 1974; Evans, 1977). When doses of at least 50 IU (daily or thrice weekly) are given, responses are observed in nearly all patients, irrespective of the type of calcitonin. Indeed, no distinction is made between porcine, human or salmon calcitonins in the degree of response (DeRose et al, 1974; Greenberg et al, 1974; Wallach, 1983; see Figures 7.13 and 7.14).

The effects of calcitonins on disease activity are, however, not always complete. On average, serum activities of alkaline phosphatase and urinary excretion of hydroxyproline fall to between 40 and 50 per cent of pretreatment values (Bastian et al, 1977; Hosking, 1981a, 1982; Wallach, 1983). When combined series are examined the average suppression of disease activity is up to 55 per cent of initial activity as judged by both urinary hydroxyproline and serum activity of alkaline phosphatase (Wallach, 1983). There is no apparent difference between the porcine, human or salmon hormone. A similar degree of suppression occurs in the majority of patients irrespective of the extent of disease activity (Figures 7.13 and 7.14). For this reason serum alkaline phosphatase is likely to fall to normal in patients with modest disease activity (for example those with initial values up to twice the upper limit of normal). In patients with more extensive disease activity values do not usually return to the normal range (DeRose et al, 1974).

The rate at which alkaline phosphatase falls may be dose-dependent (Chapuy et al, 1975), but this has not been well studied. With the use of high doses (100 IU or more) the rate of fall of alkaline phosphatase is mono-exponential after the initial lag period. This means that those patients with higher degrees of hyperphosphatasia take longer to attain their new steady state. In some patients the rate of fall is close to the half-life of the skeletal enzyme (1.7 days) (Figure 7.15).

The new steady state of serum activity of alkaline phosphatase has been termed the 'plateau response' when values of alkaline phosphatase remain above the upper end of the reference range. Increasing the dose of calcitonin generally has little effect on this plateau (DeRose et al, 1974; Singer et al, 1974), but the addition of another agent such as the diphosphonates or mithramycin can result in further suppression (Hosking et al, 1976; Bijvoet et al, 1978; Hosking, 1981a; Adami et al, 1984; Figure 7.16). The plateau effect is not due to an acquired lack of sensitivity to calcitonin, at least as judged by the acute hypocalcaemic response which remains appropriate for the prevailing rate of bone turnover (Hosking et al, 1979).

The plateau phenomenon described above suggests that some patients, for example those patients with serum activity of alkaline phosphatase greater than twice normal, fail to respond completely. A corollary is that in patients with the

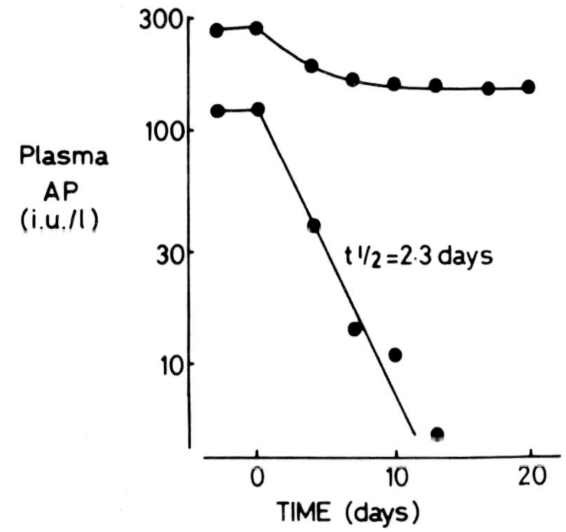

Figure 7.15

Rates of fall of alkaline phosphatase (AP) in a patient given porcine calcitonin, 160 MRCu daily. Note the mono-exponential fall in phosphatase with a half-life of 2.3 days. This compares with a half-life of the skeletal enzyme of 1.7 days.

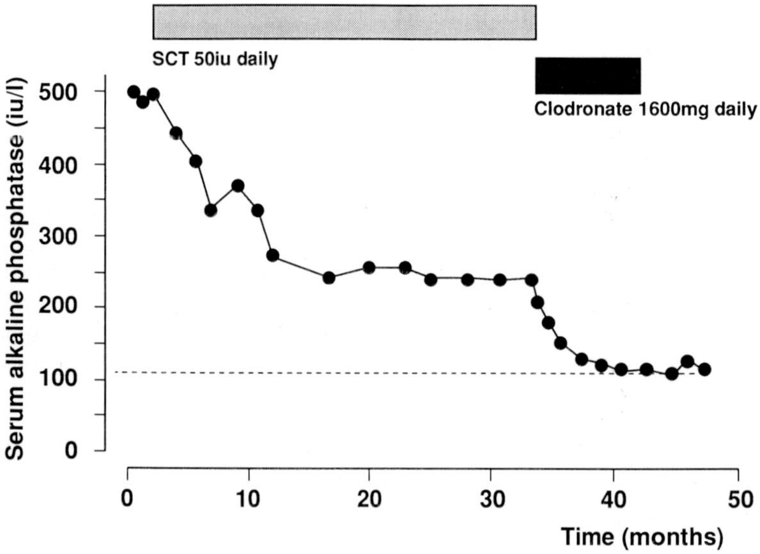

Figure 7.16

Long-term treatment of Paget's disease with calcitonin. Treatment was associated with sustained suppression of disease activity. When clodronate was given, further suppression occurred with the attainment of a new plateau.

less extensive disease, a complete suppression of disease activity is observed. This is likely to be an oversimplification. Just as some untreated patients have activities of alkaline phosphatase within the laboratory reference range, so too may treated patients with normal values for phosphatase have residual disease activity. It is possible, therefore, that the plateau is observed in all patients and that the suppression of phosphatase to 'normal' is misleading in a therapeutic sense. Incomplete response implies incomplete effects on osteoclasts. Incomplete suppression may be one of the reasons why relapse occurs rapidly when treatment is stopped–because of the continued existence of a population of abnormal osteoclasts.

In distinction to the plateau phenomenon, the rebound phenomenon (also termed 'escape') describes the failure to maintain a biochemical response despite continuing treatment or even increasing the dose (Haddad and Caldwell, 1972; Singer et al, 1972, 1980; DeRose et al, 1974; Martin and Woodhouse, 1977; Woodhouse et al, 1977a; Figure 7.17). Resistance to calcitonin is not a predictable event and may occur after several months or after several years of continuous treatment (Kanis et al, 1981). It has been reported in 5–40 per cent of patients receiving long-term treatment (Haddad and Caldwell, 1972) but its frequency may have been overemphasized. Patients in whom medical control has been attained for many years are well documented (DeRose et al, 1974; MacIntyre, 1977; Singer, 1977), though possibly less frequently reported than those developing resistance. A reasonable estimate for the frequency of resistance is 20 per cent.

In some cases acquired resistance appears to be associated with the development of IgG antibodies to either porcine or salmon calcitonin (Haddad and Caldwell, 1972; Singer et al, 1972), but more usually patients develop high antibody titres without becoming resistant to treatment (DeRose et al, 1974; Martin and Woodhouse, 1977; Woodhouse et al, 1977b; Hosking et al, 1979). In addition, resistance has been observed

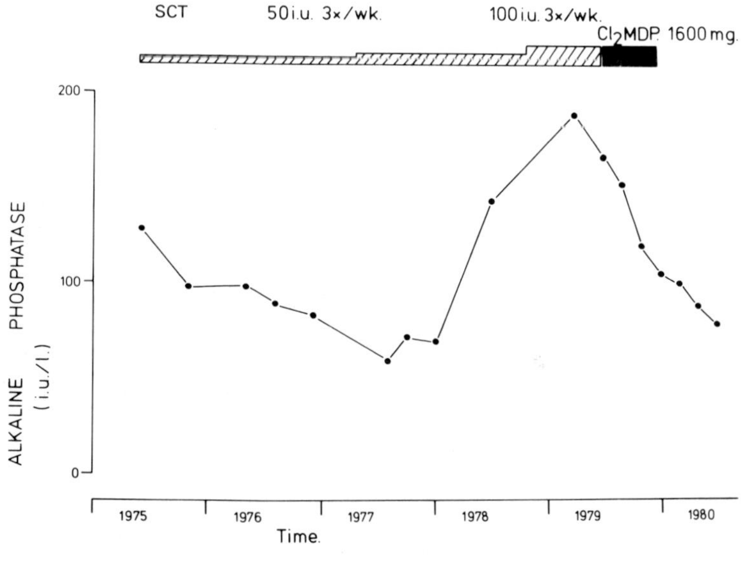

Figure 7.17

The effects of long-term treatment with synthetic salmon calcitonin on alkaline phosphatase in Paget's disease. Treatment was associated with the suppression of alkaline phosphatase to normal values (reference range <100 IU/l), an effect that persisted for more than 2 years. Note the increase in alkaline phosphatase despite continuing the treatment and increasing the dose. Treatment with clodronate, 1600 mg daily, resulted in a further suppression of disease activity. (From Kanis and Gray, 1987.)

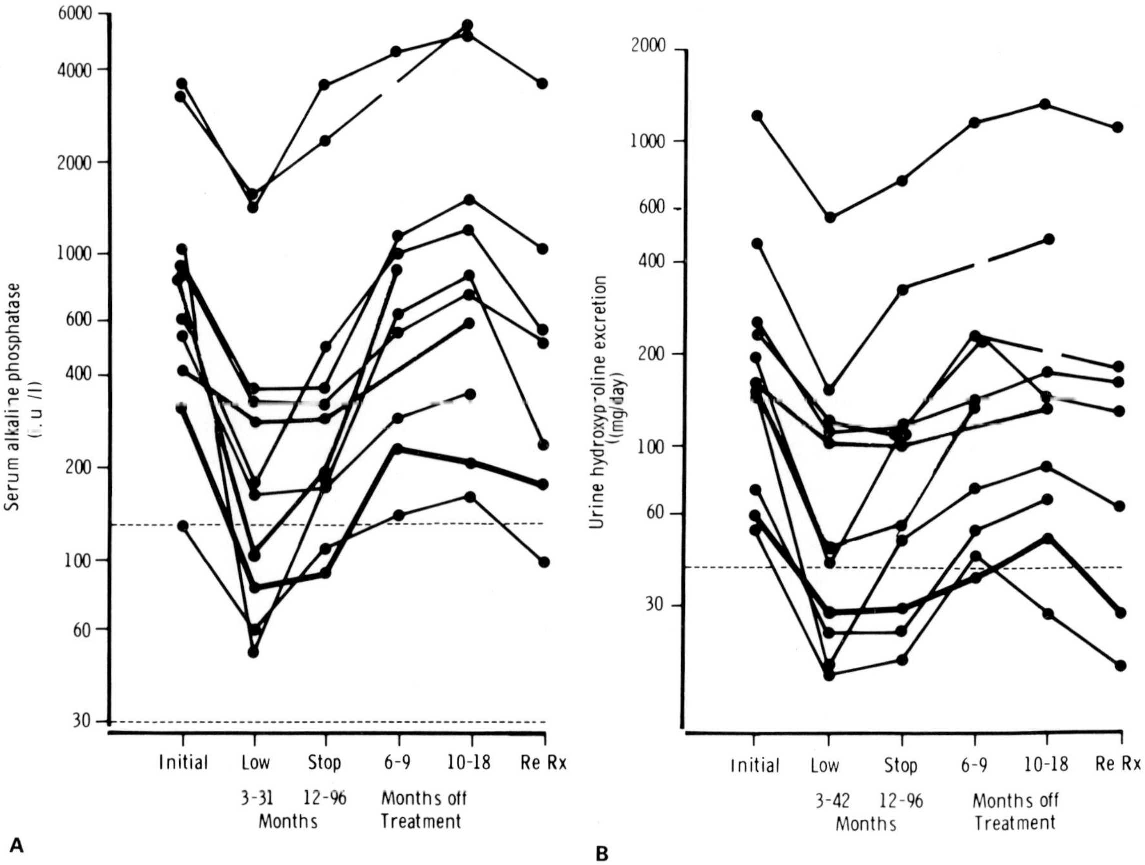

Figure 7.18

Serum activity of (A) alkaline phosphatase and (B) urinary hydroxyproline in patients treated with human calcitonin, 100 IU daily for 12–96 months. Note the rebound phenomenon and the further rise in values when treatment is stopped. (From MacIntyre et al, 1980.)

in patients without demonstrable antibodies, after porcine, salmon or human calcitonin (DeRose et al, 1974; Evans et al, 1980; MacIntyre et al, 1980; Singer et al, 1983; Figure 7.18). Thus, the relationship between antibody formation and resistance is not always causal, perhaps even rarely so. If true, the potential advantage of human calcitonin in being non-immunogenic (or less immunogenic) may not, therefore, offer major practical benefits.

The diagnosis of antibody-based resistance is made on the presence of high titres (greater than 1 in 1500) and a biochemical response to an alternative calcitonin (Singer et al, 1980). Patients fulfilling these requirements have been well described (Singer et al, 1972; Rojanasathit et al, 1974; Altman, 1987). As might be expected, patients with rebound also respond to diphosphonates (Figure 7.19). The effects of salmon, porcine or eel calcitonin on patients with acquired

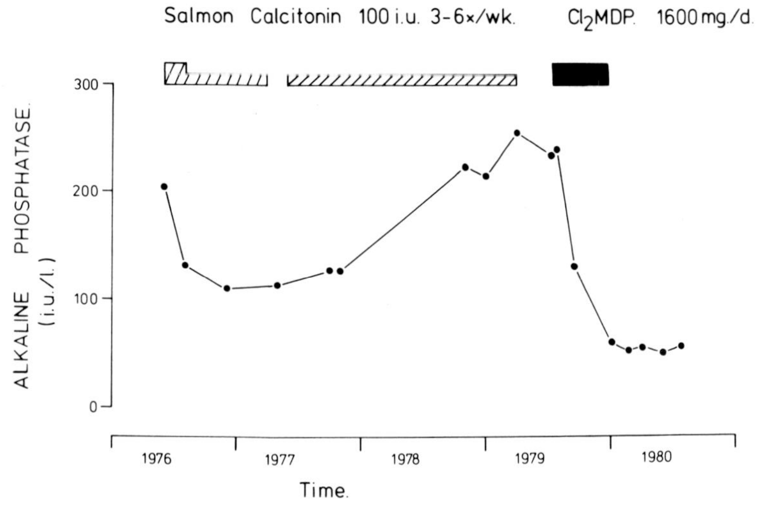

Figure 7.19

Sequential measurements of alkaline phosphatase over 4 years of treatment. Treatment with salmon calcitonin, 100 IU daily, induced a decrease in disease activity which was maintained when the dose was decreased to 100 IU thrice weekly. Rebound and acquired resistance occurred during the 3 years of treatment. Suppression of disease activity occurred when diphosphonate treatment was given.

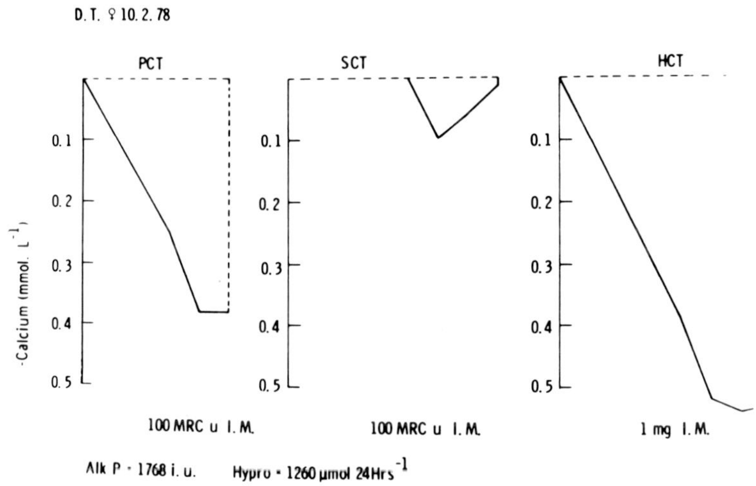

Figure 7.20

The loss of hypocalcaemic response to salmon calcitonin (SCT) in a patient with high titres of SCT antibodies. The hypocalcaemic response to human and porcine calcitonin was appropriate for the prevailing bone turnover. (From Hosking, 1983.)

resistance to human calcitonin has not been examined.

Resistance may be associated with a blunted acute response to calcitonin (Figure 7.20), but a blunted acute response is not always associated with high antibody titres (Singer et al, 1972). Thus, the acute hypocalcaemic response to calcitonin is not a reliable criterion for the presence of antibody-based resistance. Moreover, patients with modest antibody titres to calcitonin (for example 1 : 200) may also lose the acute hypocalcaemic response even when in the plateau, suggesting that the lack of a hypocalcaemic response is not invariably associated with rebound. Apart from the question of resistance, no adverse effects of antibody formation have been reported.

Down regulation of calcitonin receptors has been suggested as a mechanism for rebound (Singer et al, 1980), mainly on the basis of short-term experimental observations (Wener et al,

1972). The down regulation of calcitonin receptors in vitro is rapid (hours) (Chao and Forte, 1982, 1983; Kanehisa, 1989) and there is no direct evidence to indicate that down regulation accounts for the rebound phenomenon in calcitonin-treated patients which occurs over months or years. Stopping treatment temporarily does not restore sensitivity, whereas the reversal of desensitization in vitro is rapid. It is possible but speculative that prolonged exposure results in the preferential survival of calcitonin-resistant osteoclasts.

Some have argued that the plateau and rebound do not represent an incomplete action of calcitonin or a loss of its activity, since symptomatic relief may continue and healing of radiographic lesions may occur during the rebound phase (Greenberg et al, 1974; Nagant de Deuxchaisnes, 1989). It has even been suggested that the rise in phosphatase represents healing. This seems unlikely, and there is now good evidence that clinical control of Paget's disease with calcitonin depends upon effective and sustained suppression of both alkaline phosphatase and hydroxyproline (Chapter 8).

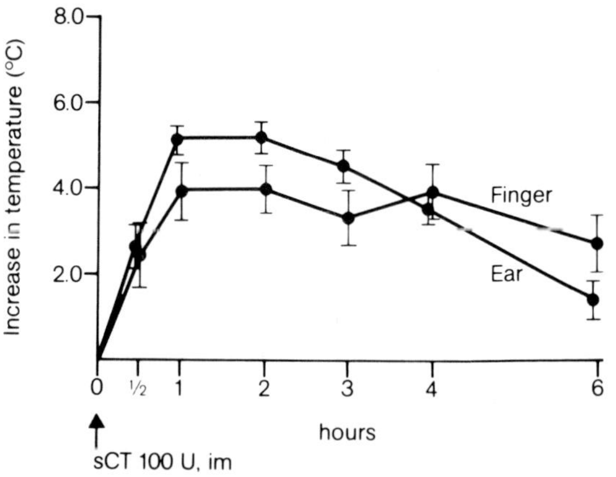

Figure 7.21

The effect of salmon calcitonin (SCT; 100 IU) on skin temperature in normal volunteers. (From Nagant de Deuxchaisnes, 1983.)

Side effects

All the calcitonins induce side effects which are inconvenient rather than serious. Their frequency and severity are dose-dependent (Grunstein et al, 1981). The most frequent effect is nausea which occurs shortly after injection in up to 30 per cent of patients (Bastian et al, 1977). Nausea may be transient or may persist for several hours. Occasionally, it may persist until the next injection and 5–10 per cent of patients cannot tolerate long-term treatment (Grunstein et al, 1981; Nagant de Deuxchaisnes, 1989). Nausea can be managed to some degree by the concurrent administration of anti-emetics.

Other symptoms include flushing, vomiting, diarrhoea and local pain at the site of injection. The vascular side effects are more marked in the young. It is of interest that skin temperature rises over the extremities such as the ear lobe and fingers within minutes (Figure 7.21), but decreases over bony pagetic sites such as the tibia (Nagant de Deuxchaisnes, 1983). Less frequent side effects include a metallic taste in the mouth, urticaria at the site of injection and polyuria. Generalized urticaria has been reported but is exceptionally rare (DeRose et al, 1974; Lang et al, 1981). Apart from these side effects, calcitonin appears to be remarkably safe and there are no known interactions of calcitonin with other drugs and no evidence of systemic toxicity to any organ.

Side effects often, but not invariably, decrease in severity or disappear altogether with continued treatment (DeRose et al, 1974; Kanis et al, 1974). They are less frequent with subcutaneous than with intramuscular or intravenous injection. Side effects can also be minimized by giving injections at night before the patient sleeps if the patient or a relative is taught to administer the drug. Nausea can also be minimized with the use of anti-emetics given an hour before injection.

It is our impression that the frequency of side effects is inversely proportional to age, and there is some evidence that women are more susceptible than men (Bouvet, 1977; Grunstein et al, 1981). The cause of many of these side effects is not known. It has been suggested that the vascular and intestinal effects may be due to the release of vasoactive substances such as serotonin (Crisp, 1981). The side effects are somewhat similar to the effects of calcitonin gene related peptide (CGRP) (MacIntyre et al, 1987), and it is possible that these effects of calcitonin could be due to the activation of CGRP receptors by high concentrations of calcitonin.

There are few comparative data concerning the frequency and severity of side effects with different calcitonins. There seems to be no difference in the range of side effects observed. There is some evidence to indicate, however, that the side effects of HCT (100 IU) occur more frequently and are of greater severity than those of SCT (Gennari et al, 1983, 1985). Side effects are also more frequent with porcine than with equipotent doses of salmon calcitonin (Bastian et al, 1977). Less frequent side effects have been reported with ECT than with SCT (Chapuy and Meunier, 1982), but the formulation of ECT may not have been adequate at that time, and more recent studies have not confirmed this (Gennari et al, 1985). Nevertheless, patients with unacceptable side effects from salmon calcitonin may tolerate other calcitonins and vice versa. The small differences in the frequency and severity of side effects of different calcitonins probably have relatively little impact on the proportion of patients who do not tolerate long-term treatment (Lesh et al, 1974).

Stopping treatment

The action of calcitonin on Paget's disease is relatively short lived and, when treatment is stopped, disease activity increases more or less immediately and complete relapse occurs within months (Woodhouse et al, 1971; Greenberg et al, 1974; Kanis et al, 1974; Avramides et al, 1976; MacIntyre et al, 1980; see Figures 7.10, 7.12 and 7.18). It has been suggested that treatment for a year or more may be associated with longer remissions (Avramides et al, 1976), but this has been rarely observed by others (MacIntyre et al, 1980; Hosking, 1982).

From a consideration of the actions of calcitonin and the nature of bone remodelling, it would be expected that relapse after stopping treatment would be indicated first by an increase in the urinary excretion of hydroxyproline, reflecting increased bone resorption, and later as an increase in the rate of bone formation, as judged by the activity of alkaline phosphatase. The pattern of relapse has not been well studied. One report suggests that alkaline phosphatase increases many months before a rise in hydroxyproline excretion (Avramides et al, 1976), but this has not been the pattern observed by others where rises in hydroxyproline excretion have preceded changes in phosphatase (Figure 7.8). This pattern of relapse is similar during the course of the rebound phenomenon (Figure 7.22).

It is of interest to observe that early signs of relapse may be visible radiographically as a radiotranslucency at the site of the old resorption front. This suggests that osteoclasts at the junction of normal and pagetic bone undergo the earliest reactivation, a phenomenon which has also been observed with the use of the diphosphonates.

The relapse of Paget's disease after stopping treatment with calcitonins is a major disadvantage of these agents for the long-term control of disease activity. Thus in patients in whom long-term control of disease is desirable, treatment must be continued indefinitely, a particular problem since its normal route of administration is parenteral. Novel routes of administration of calcitonin are, however, being developed, and non-injectable formulations with sufficient bioavailability will overcome some of these difficulties.

Novel formulations of calcitonin

The calcitonins are generally given parenterally. A considerable research effort is currently underway to develop novel methods of delivery such as by suppository, nasal insufflation and by mouth. Calcitonin is absorbed from the nasal mucosa and a nasal spray has been used in the treatment of Paget's disease. Significant suppression of disease activity has been reported with doses of up to 400 units daily (Reginster et al, 1985, 1988b; Nagant de Deuxchaisnes et al, 1987) but is not nearly as marked as with parenteral calcitonin (Figure 7.23) suggesting decreased activity of the

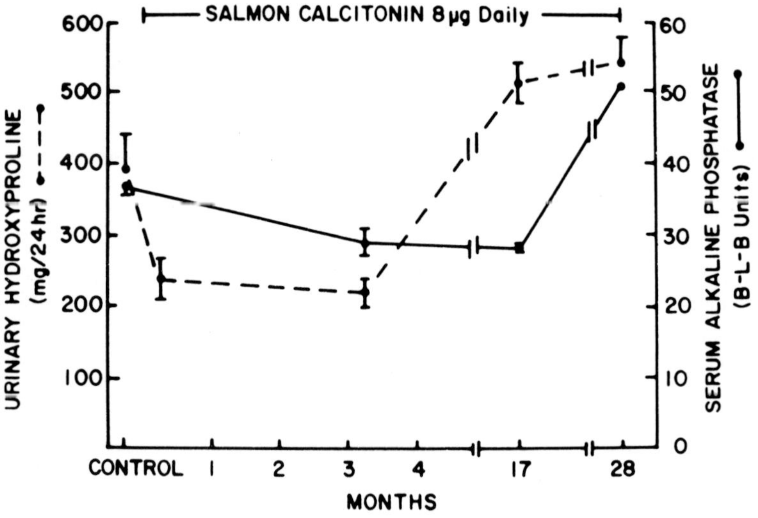

Figure 7.22

Response and rebound to salmon calcitonin in a patient who developed high antibody titres. Note that hydroxyproline excretion increased during the rebound at a time when alkaline phosphatase values were still suppressed. (From Singer et al, 1980.)

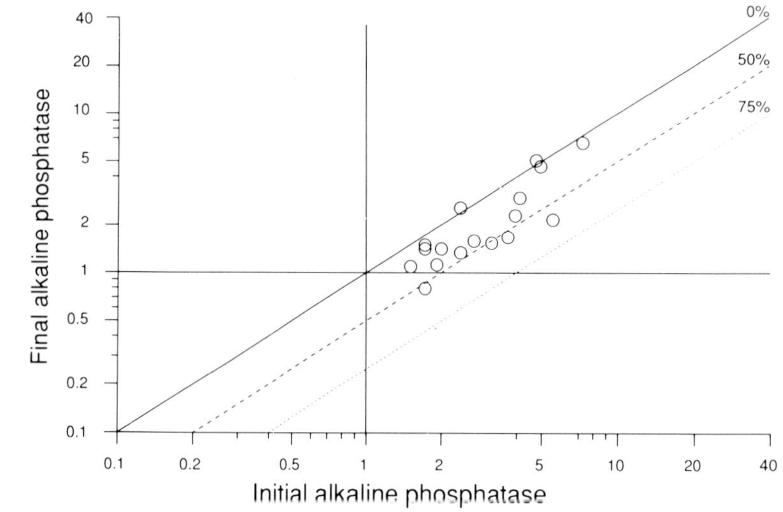

Figure 7.23

Serum activity of alkaline phosphatase (expressed as a ratio of the upper limit of the reference range) before and after one year of treatment with salmon calcitonin (200–400 IU daily) administered by nasal spray. The solid lines denote the normal range and the line of identity. Dotted lines denote the expected relationship assuming a reduction of 50 or 75 per cent of disease activity. Note the logarithmic scales. (Data from Reginster et al, 1988b.)

nasal spray. Indeed, the acute hypocalcaemic response to 400 units is similar to that observed with 30 units by injection (O'Doherty et al, 1990a), suggesting a relatively low bioavailability for the spray.

Studies with the use of nasal or rectal calcitonin suggest that side effects are rarely, if ever, encountered (Reginster et al, 1985; Nagant de Deuxchaisnes et al, 1987). It is likely, however, that this is also related to the relatively low bioavailability of those formulations which are currently available (Gonzalez et al, 1987), and thus the low dose of calcitonin delivered. Nevertheless, these small doses are effective in the control of increased bone losses due to other disorders such as osteoporosis (Reginster et al, 1987;

Overgaard et al, 1989) where resorption rates are less markedly increased, and it is probable that nasal calcitonin as currently formulated might provide a satisfactory treatment for patients without extensive disease. The development of sprays with non-irritant enhancers and other formulations are likely to extend its use in Paget's disease.

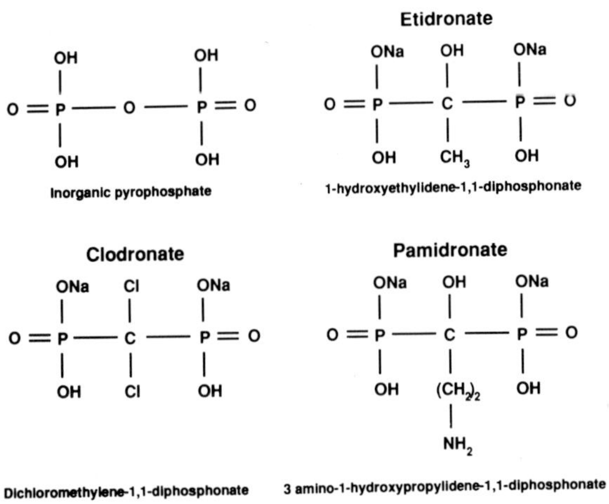

Figure 7.24

Structural formula of pyrophosphate and the geminal diphosphonates used in Paget's disease.

Diphosphonates

The geminal diphosphonates (also known as bisphosphonates) are compounds characterized by two P–C bonds. The geminal diphosphonates share the same carbon atom (P–C–P). They are analogues of pyrophosphate (P–O–P) (Figure 7.24; Fleisch, 1981, 1987). The carbon backbone renders these compounds resistant to chemical and enzymic hydrolysis, but like pyrophosphate they inhibit the growth and dissolution of hydroxyapatite crystals in vitro (Russell and Fleisch, 1970). In tissue culture the diphosphonates also inhibit normal and stimulated bone resorption, and prevent osteolysis due to parathyroid hormone, calcitriol, prostaglandins and lymphokines (Fleisch, 1981, 1983). The wide spectrum of inhibitory actions suggests that the diphosphonates interfere at a distal step in the biochemical and physicochemical events leading to bone resorption. It was once thought that this action of diphosphonates was due to inhibition of bone crystal dissolution, but more recent evidence suggests that the diphosphonates also directly affect the activity of osteoclasts and the interaction between mononuclear cells and their recruitment to the osteoclast pool (Boonekamp et al, 1986).

The activity of various diphosphonates on skeletal metabolism is markedly different with up to 1000-fold range in potency (Shinoda et al, 1983), and few convincing relationships have been observed between their structure and metabolic activity. Many metabolic effects of diphosphonates have been described. These include variable effects on glycolysis (Fast et al, 1978; Felix and Fleisch, 1983), oxidation of fatty acids (Felix and Fleisch, 1981), the Kreb's cycle (Ende and van Rooijen, 1979), acidification (Carano et al, 1990) and on prostaglandin synthesis (Ohya et al, 1985), presumed to be related to cellular uptake of the diphosphonates (Felix et al, 1984). Their pharmacological relevance is uncertain since these effects vary between diphosphonates and bear little relationship to their relative potencies (Fleisch, 1989).

Diphosphonates may inhibit the proliferation of human bone-derived cells in vitro (Khokher and Dandona, 1989), but such effects are described in osteoblasts and do not explain their major activity in vivo. Diphosphonates also inhibit the growth of cultured macrophages, an effect more marked when the diphosphonates are bound to bone (Chambers, 1980). Pamidronate is also a potent inhibitor of mitogen-stimulated cell proliferation (deVries et al, 1982), suggesting effects on osteoclast precursors or cells which modulate their behaviour. More recently the diphosphonates have been shown to inhibit the recruitment of mononuclear cells to the osteoclast pool in vitro, an effect consistent with their effects in vivo (Boonekamp et al, 1986).

The diphosphonates are currently being used or evaluated for the treatment of several disorders of calcium and skeletal metabolism, including Paget's disease, increased bone resorption due to malignancy, osteoporosis, immobilization bone loss, renal nephrolithiasis and heterotopic ossification (Bijvoet et al, 1974; Lockwood et al, 1975; Stover et al, 1976a,b; Finerman and Stover, 1981). They are also used in medicine as bone-scanning agents.

Three diphosphonates have been used extensively in Paget's disease and are commercially available in various countries. They are etidronate, clodronate and pamidronate (Figure 7.24). Four further diphosphonates, aminohexane diphosphonate, aminobutane diphosphonate, dimethyl APD and tiludronate, are undergoing clinical trials, and many more have been synthesized and will be tested in the near future. The disodium salt of etidronate is widely available for the management of Paget's disease, but clodronate and pamidronate (APD) are available in Europe, although not yet licensed for use in Paget's disease.

The effects of the diphosphonates in Paget's disease of bone share many similarities in terms of their effects on bone remodelling, even though there are marked differences in potency, and some more subtle differences which in some instances have clinical significance. As in the case of calcitonin, their common features are reviewed before considering their unique features.

Pharmacokinetics

Studies of the pharmacokinetics of diphosphonates have several difficulties, not least of which is the lack, until recently, of suitable and sensitive assays. Much of the information available has been collected from studies using carbon-labelled diphosphonates. In addition, the kinetics of diphosphonates are complex.

The absorption of diphosphonates from the gastrointestinal tract is low (Recker and Saville, 1973b; Yakatan et al, 1982; Fogelman et al, 1986). The bioavailability ranges from 1 to 10 per cent but also varies markedly in individuals. The bioavailability of pamidronate has not been tested, but indirect evidence suggests that this too is low – perhaps 1 per cent of an oral dose (Harinck et al, 1987a). In addition, the diphosphonates have a strong affinity for calcium and therefore their administration must not be combined with food, particularly foods rich in calcium. Combinations of the diphosphonates with antacids and iron preparations must be avoided for the same reasons. The low and variable absorption poses problems, particularly with the use of etidronate where the windows between ineffective, therapeutic and toxic dose are relatively narrow.

After intestinal absorption or intravenous administration, the disappearance of the diphosphonates from the circulation is extremely rapid (Yakatan et al, 1982). They are thought not to be metabolized (Steber and Wierich, 1986), and in health, approximately 75 per cent is excreted by the kidney unchanged and the remainder is taken up by the skeleton (Michael et al, 1972). There is some experimental evidence for the renal tubular secretion of diphosphonates (Troehler et al, 1975).

There are some differences in skeletal uptake between the different diphosphonates (Fogelman et al, 1981b), but this is of little significance in Paget's disease. In health the uptake of diphosphonates by the skeleton is not uniform and in Paget's disease this heterogeneity is increased and forms the basis for bone scanning. Uptake appears to be dependent in part on bone blood flow, but is particularly dependent on skeletal activity and uptake occurs at sites of active bone formation and mineralization. Markedly increased uptake is also seen in osteomalacia and in metastatic bone disease, also a feature exploited for bone scanning. The new aminophosphonates appear to localize preferentially at sites of resorption (G. Rodan, personal communication) and their skeletal uptake is greater (50 per cent of a daily dose).

The patchy distribution of diphosphonates within the skeleton may have important therapeutic implications for Paget's disease since a proportionately greater dose is delivered to the site of the disorder than elsewhere. This targeting effect may have obvious pharmacological advantages in sparing non-affected sites, but it may also cause problems when a fixed dose is given to patients with widely differing extents of disease activity. Thus, in very extensive Paget's disease a given dose of diphosphonate will deliver less compound to any one site of disease activity than the same dose delivered to a patient with limited skeletal involvement. Indeed, this may account to some extent for the heterogeneity of responses observed in some clinical studies. Several investigators have commented that patients with limited disease activity respond more completely with a given dose of diphosphonate (Fromm et al, 1979; Vega et al, 1987) which may be attributable in part to such an effect.

The diphosphonates are commonly prescribed on the basis of body weight (for example 5–10 mg/kg per day for etidronate). Since their distribution and activity are dependent upon disease activity, which varies markedly from patient to patient, it would seem more logical to calculate the dose of diphosphonates on the basis of disease activity, but this is rarely done. The lack of precision of a dose based on body weight is increased in the case of oral formulations with the provision of relatively large tablet or capsule size and the variable degree of drug absorption.

As reviewed in Chapter 3, technetium-labelled diphosphonates (such as ^{99m}Tc-Sn-EHDP) have been extensively used to study distribution of disease and the estimation of whole-body retention of diphosphonates can be used as an integrated index of disease extent (Fogelman et al, 1981b). Retention techniques have been used to determine whether treatment with diphosphonates might influence the disposition of further diphosphonate by the saturation of skeletal sites. This is important in the assessment of scintigraphic responses to treatment, since a decrease in scan uptake might variously indicate suppressed disease activity or the saturation of skeletal sites with diphosphonates. In the case of Paget's disease the decrease in whole body retention of diphosphonate after treatment with diphosphonates appears to be due to the decrease in bone turnover rather than to any saturation of skeletal sites (see Chapter 3, Figure 3.72).

The diphosphonates are retained in the skeleton by their adsorption onto hydroxyapatite, and their half-life is probably proportional to the local rates of bone turnover at sites of uptake. Since turnover rates vary markedly from site to site, particularly in Paget's disease, the skeletal half-life will also vary markedly. In addition, the diphosphonates themselves affect bone turnover which increases the complexity of kinetic studies.

It is notable that, unlike calcitonin, the effects of diphosphonates on bone resorption in Paget's disease persist, even when treatment is stopped. This property is of great importance for the long-term control of disease activity. It has been suggested that the prolonged duration of their effect is due to their skeletal localization, but this is by no means certain and the prolonged effect may be due to other causes. The skeletal sequestration of diphosphonate may be therefore irrelevant.

Activity of diphosphonates on bone

Because the diphosphonates are inhibitors of bone resorption, there are several similarities between responses to these agents and responses to calcitonin. In general, the diphosphonates induce a dose-dependent suppression of bone resorption, as judged by histological, kinetic and indirect biochemical measurements. A decrease in bone resorption is seen within days of administration of the diphosphonate, particularly when it is given intravenously, which can be monitored by following the urinary excretion of hydroxyproline (Figure 7.25). The decrease in hydroxyproline excretion is exponential with a half-life of several days compared to the more rapid effects of calcitonin (Figure 7.26). The half-life appears to be dose-dependent with any one diphosphonate regimen and can be used to calculate the relative potencies of different diphosphonates in vivo (Harink et al, 1987a).

Because of the coupling mechanism, a decrease in bone resorption is followed by a later decrease in bone formation. For this reason, as for calcitonin, there is a transient state where bone formation rates exceed those of bone resorption, and a later steady state where bone formation once more approximates the rate of bone resorption at rates lower than pretreatment values. At this time the relationship between serum alkaline phosphatase and urinary hydroxyproline is unchanged, suggesting that bone formation and resorption rates are once more matched (Figure 7.27). This pattern of response is characteristic of all the diphosphonates tested in Paget's disease.

Histological studies have confirmed that the surface of bone undergoing resorption decreases

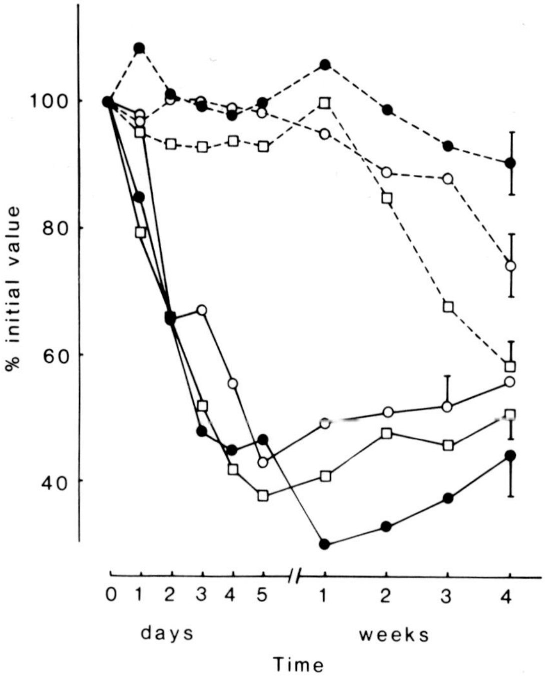

Figure 7.25

Effect of three diphosphonates in Paget's disease. The diphosphonates clodronate (Cl_2MDP; squares), etidronate (EHDP; closed circles) and aminohexane diphosphonate (AHDP; open circles) were given intravenously for five consecutive days. Note the early fall in hydroxyproline (solid lines). Serum alkaline phosphatase values (dotted lines) began to fall 3–4 weeks after treatment.

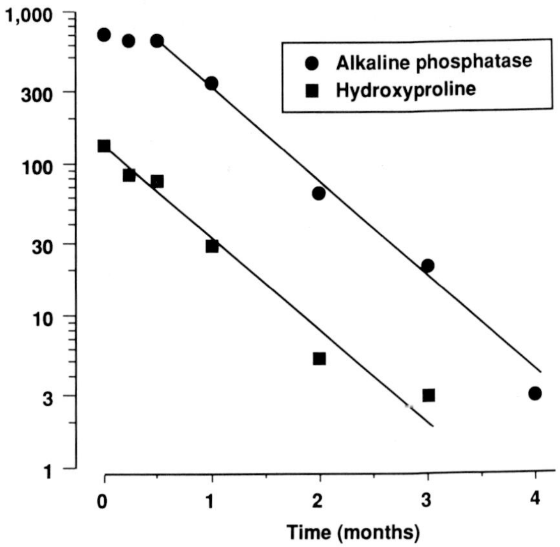

Figure 7.26

Responses of alkaline phosphatase (IU/l) and urinary hydroxyproline (mmol/mol creatinine) to treatment with clodronate, 800 mg daily by mouth for 6 months. Values shown are observed values minus asymptotic values and are plotted on a logarithmic scale. Both hydroxyproline and alkaline phosphatase values fell in a mono-exponential manner with a similar half-time of 13 days, but the response of alkaline phosphatase lagged behind that of hydroxyproline.

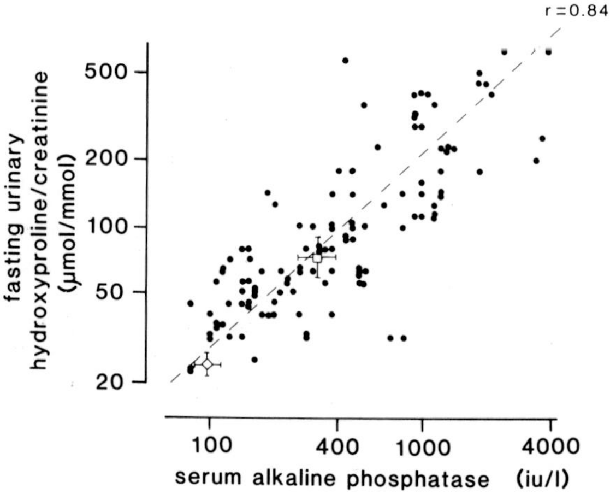

Figure 7.27

Relationship between serum activity of alkaline phosphatase and urinary excretion of hydroxyproline in patients with Paget's disease. Solid symbols refer to untreated patients and the dotted line to the slope of the bivariate regression. Open symbols refer to mean values (± SEM) observed before (□) and following the completion of a biochemical response to treatment (◇) with etidronate (20 mg/kg per day by mouth for one month) in 19 patients. (From Kanis and Gray, 1987.)

Table 7.2 Effects of clodronate on histomorphometric measurements in iliac trabecular bone. Ten patients were given 0.8 to 3.2 g clodronate for 3 to 6 months and biopsied 0 to 6 months after the end of treatment.

	Before treatment	*After treatment*	*p<*
Bone volume (% tissue volume)	37.4 ± 6.2	46.5 ± 8.5	0.01
Osteoid volume (% bone volume)	6.0 ± 1.3	2.4 ± 0.3	0.05
Osteoid thickness (μ)	11.0 ± 1.0	10.0 ± 1.0	NS
Maximum number of osteoid lamellae	3.2 ± 0.3	3.0 ± 0.6	NS
Osteoblast density (/mm bone surface)	2.4 ± 1.2	0.7 ± 0.4	0.05
Osteoclast density (/mm bone surface)	1.14 ± 0.44	0.36 ± 0.18	0.05

NS: not significant.

as expected. An early effect appears to be the withdrawal of osteoclasts from the bone surface (Plate 25) in much the same way as is seen with calcitonin. Later, giant osteoclasts disappear and secondary decreases in bone formation also occur (Khairi et al, 1977; Frijlink et al, 1979; Harink et al, 1987; Table 7.2). The decrease in bone formation is associated with a decrease in bone blood flow (Walton et al, 1985) and a decrease in marrow fibrosis. When osteoclasts persist after treatment viral like inclusions are found to persist (Harvey et al, 1982), but may be difficult to identify when resorption is markedly inhibited (Alexandre et al, 1981b). New bone formed is characteristically lamellar in structure (Yates et al, 1985; Atkins et al, 1987). As might be expected, suppression of disease activity is associated with scintigraphic and in some cases with radiographic improvements (Chapter 8). Other changes include reduction in skin temperature over affected sites.

There may well be differences between diphosphonates in the manner in which they affect osteoclasts, in accordance with their different effects in vitro. In our own studies, treatment with clodronate is associated with early detachment of osteoclasts from bone surfaces but later with a decrease in osteoclast numbers, both on the bone surface and in the marrow cavity. Pamidronate is associated with the persistence of giant osteoclasts, albeit in fewer numbers, within the marrow cavity even after several months. In the case of aminobutane diphosphonate, osteoclasts appear to perish in situ within resorption cavities (unpublished observations) and are not seen in the marrow cavity at all. There is currently no evidence that these interesting differences are of therapeutic significance in Paget's disease.

During the early phase of diphosphonate treatment it would be expected that the inhibition of bone resorption, but continued bone formation, would decrease the net efflux of calcium from the skeleton to the extracellular pool. For this reason the early effects of treatment include a decrease in serum calcium and the fasting urinary excretion of hydroxyproline as seen with the calcitonins, but more slowly. The fall in serum calcium increases the secretion of PTH and secondary hyperparathyroidism has been well documented in the case of clodronate (Delmas et al, 1982), pamidronate (Heynen et al, 1982; Papapoulos et al, 1986), aminobutane (O'Doherty et al, 1990b) and aminohexane diphosphonates (Atkins et al, 1987; Figure 7.28). Although these effects can be observed acutely after the administration of calcitonin, the fall in serum calcium is short-lived and usually persists for less than 24 hours. In contrast, the effect with these diphosphonates is much longer lived, and a sustained increase in the secretion of PTH is observed during this early phase of treatment. The increase in PTH serves to minimize the hypocalcaemic challenge by increasing the synthesis of calcitriol and stimulates intestinal absorption of calcium (Heynen et al, 1982; Papapoulos et al, 1986; McCloskey et al, 1987; Lawson-Matthew et al, 1988). In addition, increased secretion of PTH decreases renal tubular resorption of phosphate and thereby lowers serum phosphate concentrations.

It would be expected that the fall in serum calcium and phosphate and rise in PTH and calcitriol would reverse when maximum suppression of disease activity had occurred, where bone formation more closely matched bone resorption. At this time, there would no longer be a net decrease in the efflux of calcium from bone to the extracellular fluid. This transient sequence of events has been observed with the several

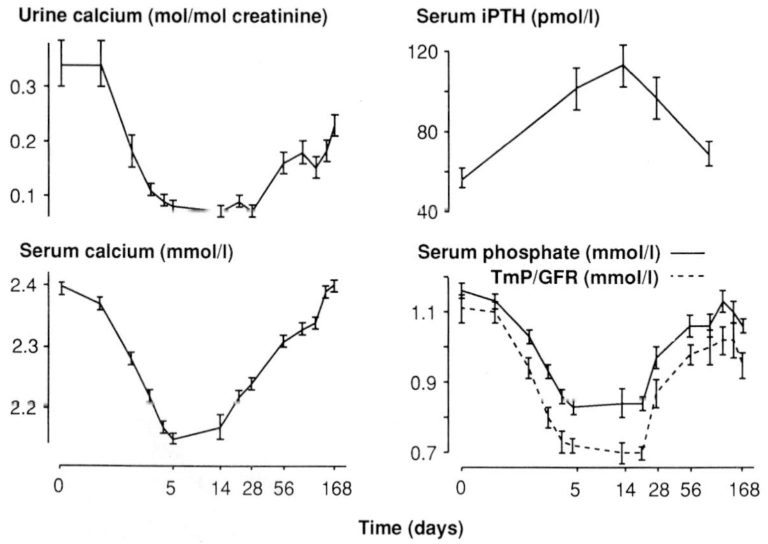

Figure 7.28

Effect of the aminobutane diphosphonate on calcium and phosphate homeostasis. Intravenous treatment for 5 days resulted in a decrease in net efflux of calcium from bone and hence a decrease in mean (± SEM) serum calcium and fasting calcium excretion. Note the fall in serum phosphate and Tmp/GFR attributable to the secondary hyperparathyroidism. These effects persisted when treatment was stopped, but reversed when bone formation and resorption became matched 6 months after the onset of treatment.

diphosphonates mentioned and has also been noted with mithramycin (Bilezikian et al, 1978; Meunier et al, 1979; Bijvoet et al, 1980b; Douglas et al, 1980a,b; Adami et al, 1982; Delmas et al, 1982; Heynen et al, 1982; Yates et al, 1985; Atkins et al, 1987; Thiebaud et al, 1987). Whereas similar effects have been reported with low oral doses of etidronate these effects have not been consistently shown after higher doses due to additional effects of etidronate on the mineralization of bone (see below).

It has been suggested that the secondary hyperparathyroidism induced by diphosphonates might limit their effectiveness (Delmas et al, 1982). Whereas secondary hyperparathyroidism can be attenuated by the concurrent use of vitamin D and calcium, it does not appear to influence markedly the ultimate response. Small differences in response between diphosphonate-treated patients with and without vitamin D (Delmas et al, 1982) are probably attributable to differences between patient groups in their disease activity. Whether or not the clinical response to diphosphonates in patients is more or less adequate than the clinical response to calcitonin has not been formally tested, but the biochemical responses to the diphosphonates are certainly more complete. It is important to recognize, however, that incomplete biochemical effects are also observed with the diphosphonates (Altman et al, 1973; Russell et al, 1974; Canfield et al, 1977; Khairi et al, 1977; Douglas et al, 1980a,b; Delmas et al, 1982; Dewis et al, 1985; Mautalen et al, 1985) but the plateau phenomenon is more marked with calcitonin than with the diphosphonates. Where information is available, some comparisons of different diphosphonates and calcitonins are reviewed under the appropriate diphosphonate.

Etidronate

Etidronate is normally given by mouth. The dose regimen recommended by the manufacturers for Paget's disease is 5–10 mg/kg per day for 3–6 months. The doses which have been studied in Paget's disease range from 1–20 mg/kg body weight per day. Between 5 and 20 mg/kg per day there is a dose-dependent decrease in bone turnover (Altman et al, 1973; Russell et al, 1974;

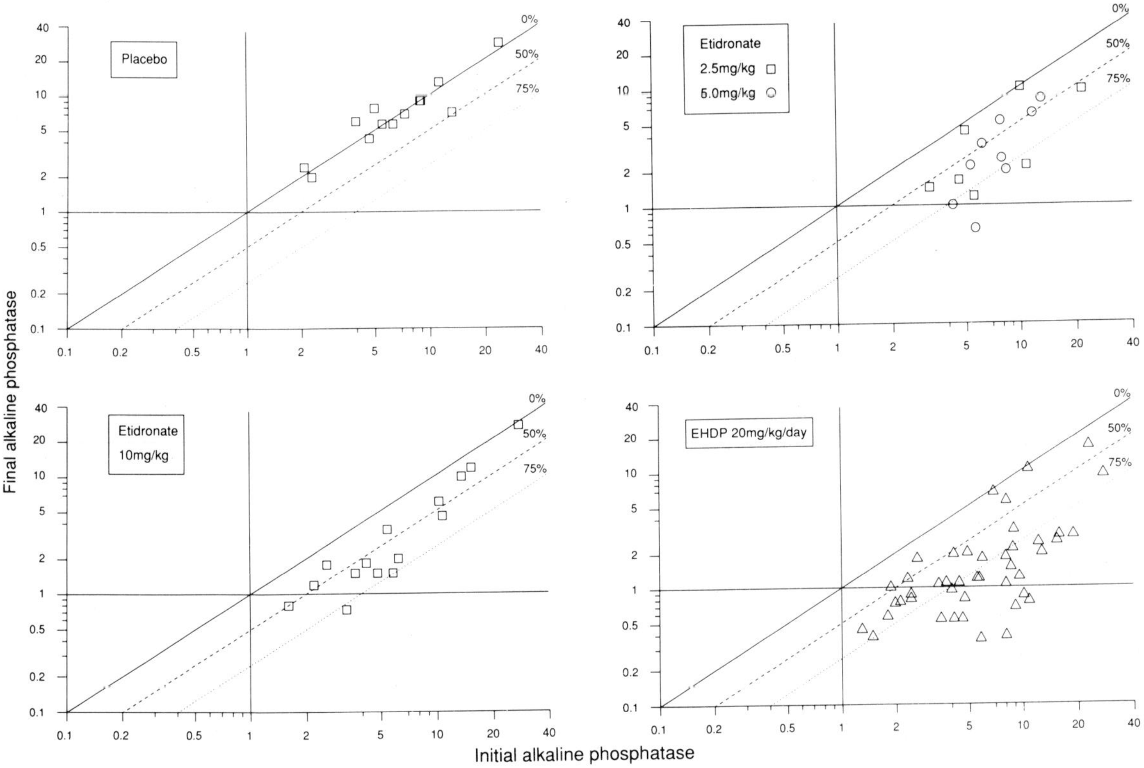

Figure 7.29

Serum activity of alkaline phosphatase (expressed as a ratio of the upper limit of the reference range) before and after 6 months' treatment with etidronate at the doses shown. The solid lines denote the normal range and the line of identity. Dotted lines denote the expected relationship assuming a reduction of 50 or 75 per cent of disease activity. Note the logarithmic scales. (Data from Canfield et al, 1977.)

Canfield et al, 1977; Figure 7.29). The early fall in hydroxyproline is followed by a later decrease in serum activity of alkaline phosphatase. These effects have been confirmed by histological and scintigraphic studies (Russell et al, 1974; Goldman et al, 1975; Meunier et al, 1975; Alexandre et al, 1981a, 1983; Baslé et al, 1984; Figure 7.30). In this regard the responses to etidronate resemble those of all the other diphosphonates tested in man.

In contrast, the secondary endocrine effects of etidronate administration differ from those observed with the other diphosphonates used in clinical practice. When high oral or intravenous doses of etidronate are given, no fall in serum calcium is observed, and subsequently no increase in PTH secretion, calcitriol production or calcium balance is observed (Altman et al, 1973; Smith et al, 1973; Figure 7.31). Indeed, high doses may suppress the production of calcitriol (Lawson-Matthew et al, 1988; Figure 7.32).

These differences almost certainly relate to the fact that high doses of etidronate delay the mineralization of bone. This delay might be expected to attenuate any hypocalcaemic effect resulting from the inhibition of bone resorption,

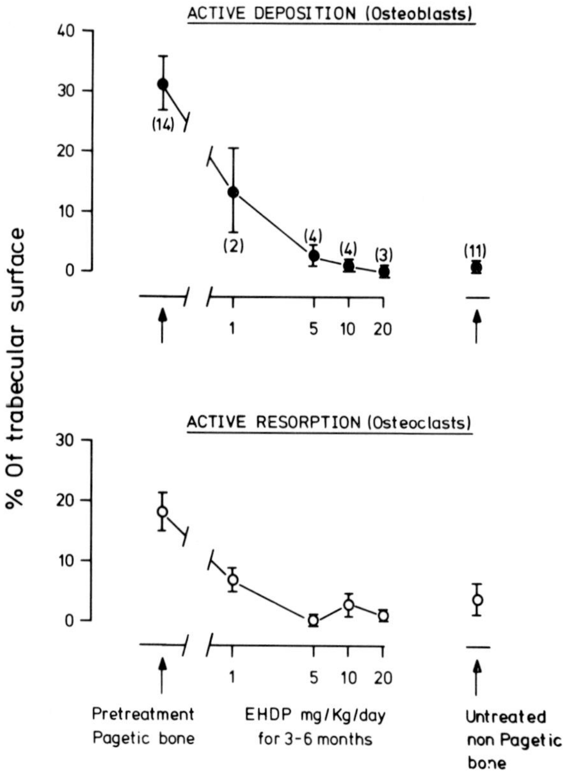

Figure 7.30

Effect of various doses of etidronate (EHDP) on surface coverage of trabecular bone by active bone cells. After 3–6 months of treatment the osteoclast and osteoblast surface decreased to normal values. The effect was suboptimal with a daily dose of 1 mg/kg per day, but was nearly complete with the 5 mg dose. (Walton, 1978.)

an effect which would be greater the higher the rate of bone formation. Thus, in Paget's disease where bone resorption and bone formation rates are increased, high doses of etidronate (for example 20 mg/kg per day) effectively inhibit bone resorption, as judged by urinary excretion of hydroxyproline, but do not induce a fall in serum and urinary calcium (Kanis et al, 1987; Figure 7.32). This action of etidronate on mineral influx into bone probably explains why etidronate by mouth is less effective in lowering serum calcium than other diphosphonates in other disorders associated with increased bone turnover (Kaplan et al, 1977; Kanis et al, 1987).

This pattern of response contrasts with high doses of intravenous clodronate, pamidronate or other diphosphonate which cause significant falls in serum and urinary calcium for a similar degree of inhibition of bone resorption. These differences in early effects of etidronate from other diphosphonates are associated with different effects on the mineralization of bone. Histological studies examining the rate of mineralized bone formation have shown that mineralization ceases abruptly but transiently following the intravenous use of etidronate. In contrast, clodronate, aminohexane and aminobutane diphosphonates do not decrease mineralization below normal values (Kanis et al, 1985a; McCloskey et al, 1987; Figure 7.33).

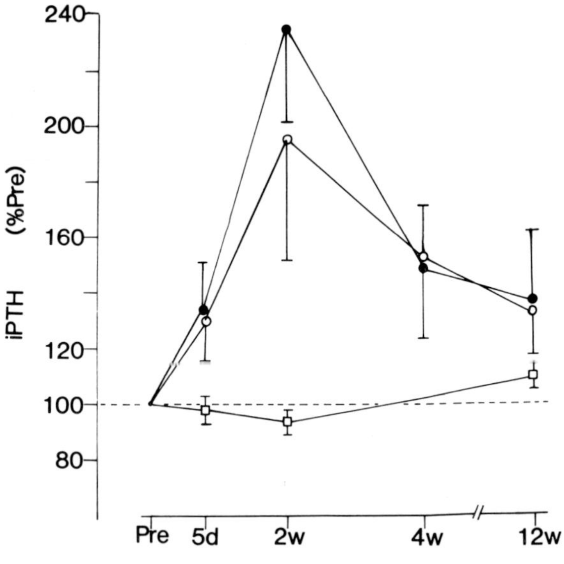

Figure 7.31

Effects of three diphosphonates on serum immunoreactive parathyroid hormone values (percentage of pretreatment values). The patients were given intravenous etidronate (□), clodronate (●) or aminohexane diphosphonate (○) for 5 days. Note that transient secondary hyperparathyroidism was not induced with etidronate. (From McCloskey et al, 1987.)

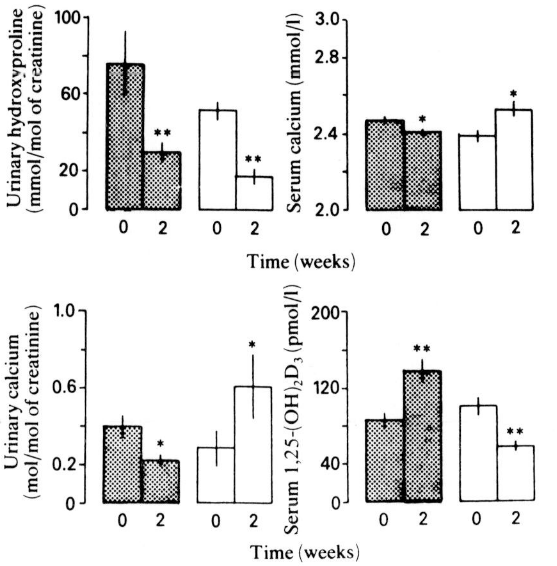

Figure 7.32

Mean biochemical values (± SEM) before and two weeks after starting treatment with oral (stippled) and high intravenous (open) doses of etidronate. Note that both regimens decrease bone resorption but that with the intravenous etidronate this is associated with a rise in fasting serum and urinary calcium and suppression of calcitriol synthesis (** $p < 0.01$; * $p < 0.05$, compared with pretreatment values). (From Lawson-Matthew et al, 1988.)

The impairment of mineralization is an effect of etidronate which is exploited in the management of heterotopic ossification (Bijvoet et al, 1974; Stover et al, 1976a,b; Finerman and Stover, 1981), but is an unwanted effect in the treatment of Paget's disease, particularly if treatment is given for long periods. Indeed, studies with the use of 20 mg/kg per day given for 6 months or longer indicate that the osteomalacia induced by etidronate increases the risk of pathological fracture (Kantrowitz et al, 1975; Canfield et al, 1977; Khairi et al, 1977; Mautalen et al, 1986). An increased frequency of fracture can also be reproduced experimentally (Flora et al, 1981).

The effects of etidronate on calcium and skeletal metabolism are less marked when lower doses are used. With a daily dose of 5 mg/kg, skeletal calcium retention has been demonstrated (DeVries and Bijvoet, 1974; Bijvoet et al, 1978) as would be expected from the inhibition of bone resorption and continued bone formation which underwent mineralization. Histological indices of turnover also decrease (Alexandre et al, 1981a) but are less marked than the effects of higher doses (Figure 7.30; Johnston et al, 1980). This dose (5–10 mg/kg per day by mouth) does, however, appear to be a reasonable compromise between wanted and unwanted effects (Canfield

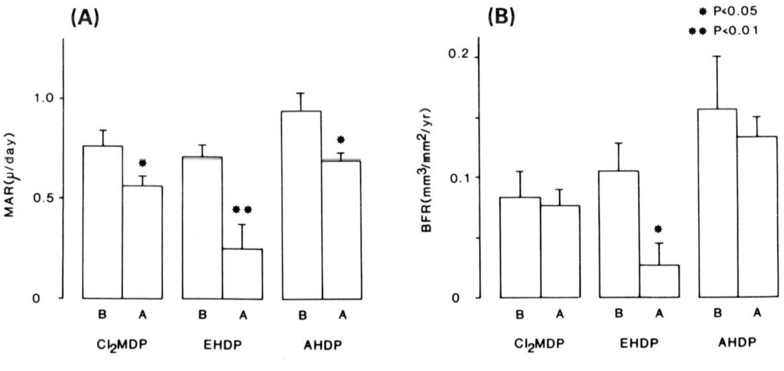

Figure 7.33

Effect of three diphosphonates, clodronate (Cl_2MDP), etidronate (EHDP) and aminohexane diphosphonate (AHDP) on (A) mean mineral apposition rate (MAR) and (B) bone formation rate (BFR). Rates were calculated by triple labelling with tetracycline. The first two courses were given before treatment and the third 10 days after the start of treatment. Note the inhibitory effect of intravenous etidronate on mineralization, an effect much less marked when lower doses were given by mouth. (From McCloskey et al, 1987.)

Table 7.3 Comparison of five treatment regimens with two diphosphonates. There were no significant differences in disease activity between patients before treatment. Note that fewer patients responded to etidronate 5–10 mg/kg per day for 6 months than to other regimens as judged by a 25 per cent or greater decrease in disease activity. The most durable responses were observed with clodronate 1600 mg daily for 6 months. (From Gray et al, 1987.)

Agent	*Daily dose*	*Duration (months)*	*No of patients*	*Percentage responding*	*Percentage normalizing**	*Percentage relapse-free**	
						1 year	*2 years*
Etidronate	5–10 mg/kg	6	24	71†	65	61	15
	20 mg/kg	1	19	95	57	62	29
	20 mg/kg	6	41	95	59	51	20
Clodronate	800 mg	6	18	89	69	66	37
	1600 mg	6	45	100	60	90†	60†
	1600 mg	1	20	90	44	64	27

*Proportion of patients who responded to treatment, ie excluding non-responders.
†Significantly different from other treatments.

et al, 1977) and is the dose most frequently recommended.

The experience with the use of the above dose for 3 or 6 months has been varied. In our own hands and in many other centres this dose has provided effective suppression of bone turnover without unwanted effects, either clinically or by bone histology (Canfield et al, 1977; Khairi and Johnston, 1977; Khairi et al, 1977; Johnston et al, 1980; Alexandre et al, 1981a; Figure 7.34). About 30 per cent of patients do not apparently respond to treatment, as judged by a decrease of 25 per cent or more in serum activity of alkaline phosphatase.

In the case of high doses (20 mg/kg per day) virtually all patients appear to respond when a change in alkaline phosphatase of more than 25 per cent is used as a criterion of response (Smith et al, 1971; Altman et al, 1973; Guncaga et al, 1974; Russell et al, 1974; Meunier et al, 1975; Canfield et al, 1977; Gray et al, 1987; Table 7.3). In contrast, the response rate in patients given the lower doses (such as 5 mg/kg) is significantly less; but in those who respond the degree of disease suppression is similar to patients given higher doses.

In contrast to this general experience, at other centres this dose appears to be without pharmacological effect, perhaps due to its inappropriate administration with food (Peacock M, personal communication), whereas in others this dose is associated with a high incidence of focal osteomalacia, bone pain and in some cases fracture (Nagant de Deuxchaisnes et al, 1979; Boyce et al, 1984). The reasons for this are discussed later, but have led to the development of alternative regimens for the administration of etidronate.

Alternative drug regimens

Because of the variable experience with the use of recommended doses there has been a great deal of interest in developing new treatment regimens (Siris et al, 1980, 1981; Preston et al, 1986; Kanis et al, 1987). Our own observations suggested that high doses of etidronate by mouth (20 mg/kg per day) given for only one month suppressed biochemical indices of disease activity in Paget's disease as completely as a 6-month

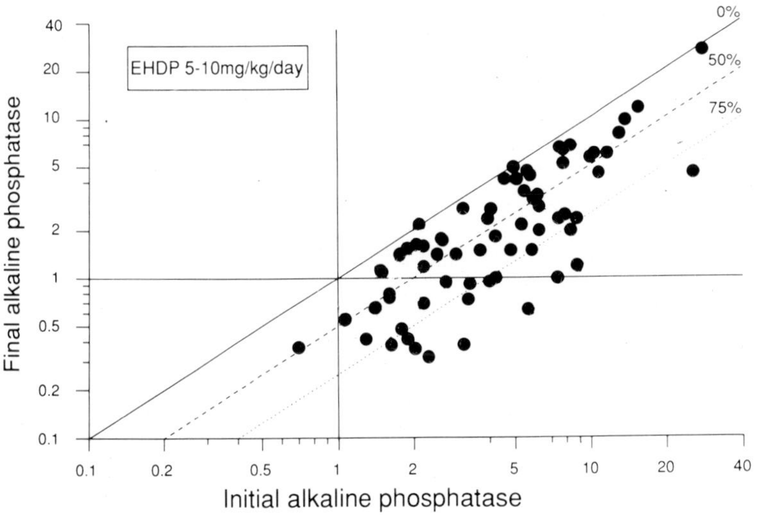

Figure 7.34

Serum activity of alkaline phosphatase (expressed as a ratio of the upper limit of the reference range) before and after 6 months' treatment with oral etidronate (5–10 mg/kg per day). Dotted lines denote the expected relationship assuming a reduction of 50 or 75 per cent of disease activity. Note the logarithmic coordinates. (Data plotted from Canfield et al, 1977; O'Donoghue and Hosking, 1987 and a personal series.)

treatment with this dose (Figure 7.35; Preston et al, 1986). In contrast to the 5 mg dose, responses were observed in nearly all patients, and remission from disease activity continued for at least one year (Table 7.3). Moreover, the effect on biochemical indices of disease activity was more complete than the lower dose given for 6 months. This suggested that there was little benefit in giving high doses for longer than one month.

The one-month high-dose regime is associated with an abrupt decrease in the rate of mineralization (Gibbs et al, 1986; Preston et al, 1986), but this is reversed when treatment is stopped (Table 7.4), whereas the effects on disease activity persist for many months and in some cases for years after stopping treatment. Indeed, the duration of response after high doses of etidronate given for one month is comparable to that observed after longer courses of treatment (Figure 7.36). The regimen also gives more consistent effects than lower doses. Although treatment impairs the mineralization of bone, the impairment is transient.

Others have devised similar regimens for similar reasons. For example, etidronate has been given intermittently for one month out of four in high doses, or in 6-monthly alternating cycles of etidronate and drug-free interval (Siris et al, 1981). The prolonged duration of a single short course of treatment suggests, however, that repetitive cycles may not be necessary.

Table 7.4 Effect of high oral doses (20 mg/kg per day) of etidronate on histological measurements (mean ± SEM) in trabecular bone. Note the significant delay (*$p<0.05$) in mineralization during treatment and its reversal 4 to 12 months after treatment, but the persistent effect on osteoclast surfaces. (From Preston et al, 1986.)

	Before treatment	*During treatment*	*After treatment*
Osteoid area (% matrix area)	5.8	14.6*	7.3
Osteoid surface (% trabecular surface)	46	60	47
Osteoid seam width (μ)	13	21*	13
Calcification front (% osteoid surface)	57	28*	49
Osteoclast surface (% trabecular surface)	4.6	Not measured	1.3*

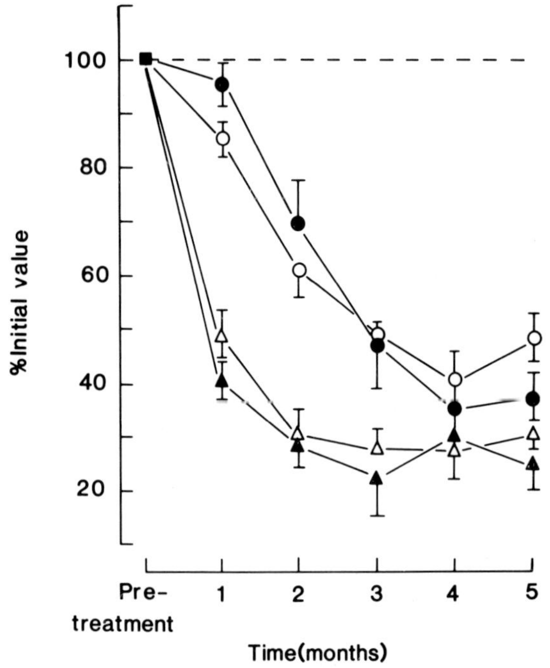

Figure 7.35

Effects of etidronate (20 mg/kg per day) on disease activity as judged by serum alkaline phosphatase (circles) and urine hydroxyproline (triangles). One group of patients received the daily dose for 6 months (open symbols) and the other for 1 month (solid symbols). Note the similarity of response. (Data from Preston et al, 1986.)

An extension of this kind of treatment strategy has been to give the drug intravenously in high doses. Intravenous etidronate is available for the management of malignant hypercalcaemia, and its use in Paget's disease is still experimental. Nevertheless, clinical experience in limited numbers of patients suggests that intravenous etidronate (300–600 mg) given for 5 days can effectively suppress disease activity (Kanis et al, 1987). The doses used are comparatively large and from the known bioavailability of etidronate are equivalent to 6–10 g daily by mouth. Thus, the total dose delivered over the 5-day treatment is equivalent to a 20 mg/kg dose given for one month. Since the effects of the two regimens are similar in terms of disease suppression (Figure 7.37) this might suggest that, to attain a given degree of disease suppression, the total dose given is more important than the duration of its administration.

Duration of effect

All the oral and intravenous regimens are capable of inducing biochemical and histological suppression of disease activity, which may persist for a long time, even for several years after treatment has stopped. This contrasts markedly with the use

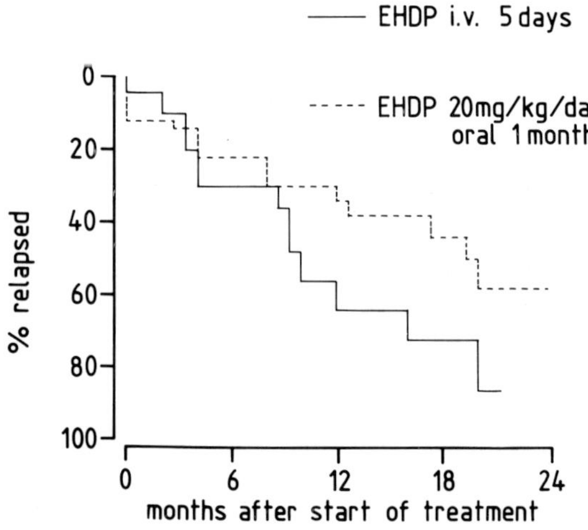

Figure 7.36

Kaplan–Meier analysis of relapse of hyperphosphatasaemia after treatment with etidronate (20 mg/kg per day) for 6 months (solid line) and for 1 month (broken line). In 19 patients given the one-month treatment 62 per cent remained in remission at one year compared with 51 per cent of 41 patients given the longer treatment (NS). A similar proportion of patients given each treatment were in remission at 2 years (29 vs 20 per cent respectively). Relapse was defined as a consistent increase in serum alkaline phosphatase of >25 per cent of the minimum values. (From Kanis et al, 1986.)

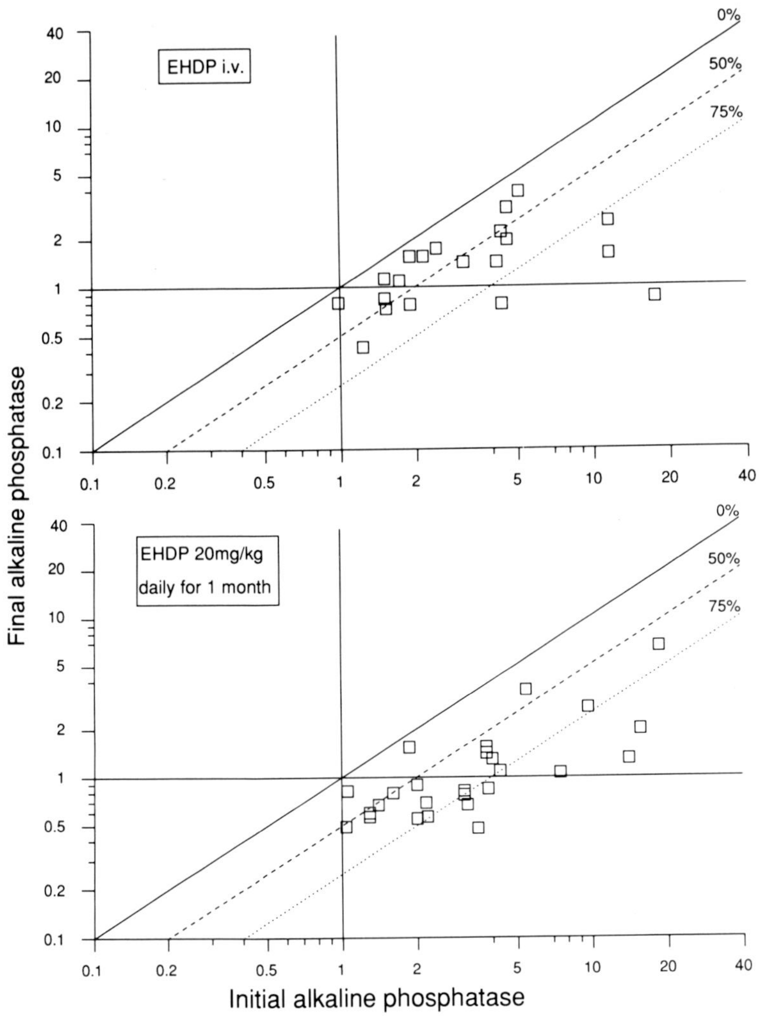

Figure 7.37

Serum activity of alkaline phosphatase (expressed as a ratio of the upper limit of the reference range) before and after treatment with etidronate, 300–500 mg iv daily for 5 days (top panel) or 20 mg/kg per day for 1 month by mouth (lower panel). Dotted lines denote the expected relationship assuming a reduction of 50 or 75 per cent of disease activity. Note the logarithmic coordinates.

of calcitonin where stopping treatment results in an early relapse. Suppression of disease activity characteristically continues for many months after stopping treatment (Khairi et al, 1977a; Johnston et al, 1980). Using drug-free interval as an index, this is significantly longer with a daily dose of 20 mg/kg than with 5 mg/kg per day (Table 7.5). In another study the drug-free interval was 3 years for the 5 mg dose but only 18 months for the higher dose (Altman, 1985). This accords more closely with our own data where response and relapse are defined as a given (25 per cent) change in serum alkaline phosphatase. We found that a smaller proportion of patients responded to the lower dose, but when responses were evoked the duration of response was significantly greater than that achieved with the 20 mg dose (Gray et al, 1987; Table 7.3).

Table 7.5 Patients (per cent ± SEM) remaining drug-free, having been given etidronate at the doses shown for 6 months (from Johnston et al, 1980).

Time (months)	*5 mg/kg*	*20 mg/kg*
12	71 ± 9	89 ± 7
24	49 ± 10	72 ± 11
36	41 ± 10	61 ± 12
48	–	56 ± 12
Median drug-free time (months)	19.5	54.0

Retreatment with etidronate

The question has arisen whether patients might develop resistance to repeated treatment with etidronate or with other diphosphonates. The general experience has been that a repeat treatment is equally effective in that the same mean nadir value for alkaline phosphatase is induced (Johnston et al, 1980; Table 7.6). Similar observations have been made for clodronate (Yates et al, 1985) and pamidronate (Harinck et al, 1987a,b) where populations have been studied. It has been suggested that resistance to etidronate might occur in a few individuals (Delmas et al, 1987), but the failure to respond to the small dose used (5 mg/kg per day) might have been due to inadequate absorption of the drug since, as described above, the responses to this dose can be variable. On the other hand, Altman (1985) also describes resistance, and although details are not provided, some patients previously sensitive to a 5 mg/kg daily dose proved resistant to much higher doses (20 mg/kg per day). Drug-induced bone pain was a common feature in these cases. If true drug resistance does occur, such patients appear to respond to an alternative diphosphonate (Delmas et al, 1987).

Side effects

Etidronate is remarkably free from toxicity in animal studies apart from its skeletal effects. Side effects reported with oral treatment include intestinal upset, changes in serum phosphate, bone pain and fracture. A skin rash has been rarely reported and other effects are probably fortuitous (Reginster et al, 1985).

The most frequent unwanted effect is diarrhoea or mild intestinal upset which occurs in 15 per cent or so of patients (Russell et al, 1974; Canfield et al, 1977; Khairi et al, 1977; Ibbertson et al, 1979; Siris et al, 1980). The effect is dose-dependent and is usually managed by dividing the daily dose into a twice-daily regimen. Intestinal effects are not observed with intravenous administration, indicating a local effect of the drug on the intestine.

Intravenous infusions of etidronate induce an abnormality of taste in approximately one-third of patients (Jones et al, 1987). This is variously described as a loss of taste or a metallic taste and is short-lived. It usually resolves within an hour of stopping the infusion, but may persist for up to 24 hours.

Etidronate induces a dose-dependent rise in plasma phosphate due to enhanced renal tubular resorption of phosphate (Recker et al, 1973; Walton et al, 1975; Figure 7.30). This commonly occurs with the higher doses, above 10 mg/kg per

Table 7.6 Effect of retreatment of 12 patients with Paget's disease with etidronate. All values expressed as a percentage of mean values (± SEM) observed before the first treatment. (From Johnston et al, 1980.)

	Initial value	*After first treatment*	*Before second treatment*	*After second treatment*
Alkaline phosphatase	100	40 ± 6	52 ± 6	37 ± 5
Hydroxyproline	100	45 ± 8	61 ± 10	56 ± 10

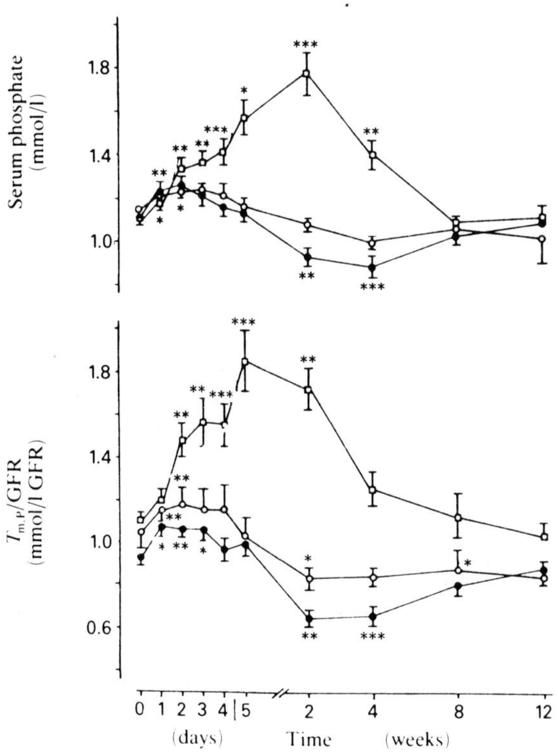

Figure 7.38

Mean serum phosphate and TmP/GFR (± SEM) before and following treatment with intravenous etidronate (□), clodronate (●), and aminohexane diphosphonate (○). Note the significant rise in serum phosphate and TmP/GFR with etidronate and the fall with the other diphosphonates. Asterisks denote the significance of mean values compared with pretreatment values (*$p < 0.05$; **$p < 0.01$; ***$p < 0.001$). (From McCloskey et al, 1988.)

day, and has no known clinical consequences. It may be useful, however, to monitor serum phosphate during treatment (Nagant de Deuxchaisnes et al, 1977, 1982a; Kanis, 1984). In patients given high doses for short periods it provides a useful index of compliance or absorption. With the use of lower doses, such as 5 mg/kg per day, the occurrence of hyperphosphataemia should alert the physician that the patient is taking (or absorbing) too much of the diphosphonate.

Like all diphosphonates, etidronate is excreted unchanged in the urine and consideration should be given to decreasing the duration of treatment in patients with markedly impaired renal function. High doses of intravenous diphosphonates (etidronate and clodronate) have been reported to decrease glomerular function in three patients with hypercalcaemia due to malignancy (Bounameaux et al, 1983). Although there may be no causal relationship (Kanis et al, 1983) it is possible that renal failure was due to the bolus injection of diphosphonates. Effects on renal function have not been shown following its slow intravenous infusion, even in patients with mild renal failure (Urwin et al, 1987).

New bone pain or an exacerbation of pain at pre-existing sites of pain occurs in approximately 5–10 per cent of patients treated with etidronate (Altman et al, 1973; Canfield et al, 1977; Khairi et al, 1978; Fromm et al, 1979; Ibbertson et al, 1979; Johnston et al, 1980; Altman, 1985) and may resolve with continued treatment. The mechanism is not known but may be associated with increases in radiographic lucency (Figure 7.39) suggesting that radiotranslucency is caused by continued bone formation without subsequent mineralization. The incidence of bone pain is dose-related and rises to 20 per cent or so when a dose of 20 mg/kg is used for more than a few months (Kantrowitz et al, 1975; Canfield et al, 1977; Khairi et al, 1977; Evans, 1983). It seems to be a feature of long-term treatment and studies giving short courses of high doses for 1–3 months have not shown a high frequency of bone pain (Dewis et al, 1985; Gray et al, 1987).

Increased or new bone pain from pagetic sites has been reported with increased frequency from two centres using recommended doses (Nagant de Deuxchaisnes et al, 1979; Boyce et al, 1984). In both these series, hyperphosphataemia was a common observation, suggesting that these patients were given or absorbed higher doses of diphosphonate than expected. The patients from Leuven generally had marked osteolytic disease and bone pain may be more common in these patients. An increased frequency (15 per cent) has also been reported in patients who have taken multiple courses of etidronate (Altman, 1985) and in patients with monostotic disease (Fromm et al,

1979). These latter observations suggest that high focal concentrations of etidronate are the cause for pain, but the mechanism is unknown.

Etidronate induces a dose-dependent delay in the mineralization of bone which is most marked when doses of 20 mg/kg per day are used. Etidronate-induced osteomalacia is not reversed by alfacalcidol (Ralston et al, 1987). Since remineralization of bone occurs rapidly after short courses of treatment (one month, for example) but bone turnover is suppressed for many months thereafter, the use of a short high-dose treatment exposes patients to osteomalacia for a short period of time.

A major concern with the osteomalacia induced by high doses for long periods relates to the possibility that the risk of fracture is increased. Studies using 20 mg/kg per day for 6 months or longer indicated marked osteomalacia (Plates 26 and 27; Smith et al, 1971) and an increased incidence of fracture (Kantrowitz et al, 1975; Canfield et al, 1977).

The relationship between osteomalacia and fracture is not, however, straightforward. Spontaneous fractures do occur in experimental animals given high doses of etidronate for prolonged periods. However, prolonged administration of clodronate to experimental animals also induces fractures but does not induce osteomalacia (Flora et al, 1980). This suggests that fractures are due to greatly decreased bone turnover, which inhibits the repair of fatigue damage in the skeleton, rather than due to a defect in mineralization.

The incidence of osteomalacia is much lower when doses between 5 and 10 mg/kg daily are used (Russell et al, 1974; Meunier et al, 1975; Alexandre et al, 1981, 1983). However, focal osteomalacia may be overlooked on quantitative bone histology where conventionally average rates of mineralization or osteoid seam width are calculated. Mild degrees of osteomalacia probably occur in a substantial minority of patients. The duration of exposure to etidronate (generally 3–6 months) and the relatively modest suppression of bone turnover (generally to within the normal range) suggests that any osteomalacia may not have adverse clinical consequences. One centre has reported a high frequency of focal osteomalacia associated with bone pain (Boyce et al, 1984) with moderate doses of etidronate. These patients were generally hyperphosphataemic and may have been exposed therefore to higher doses than appreciated by the investigators at the time.

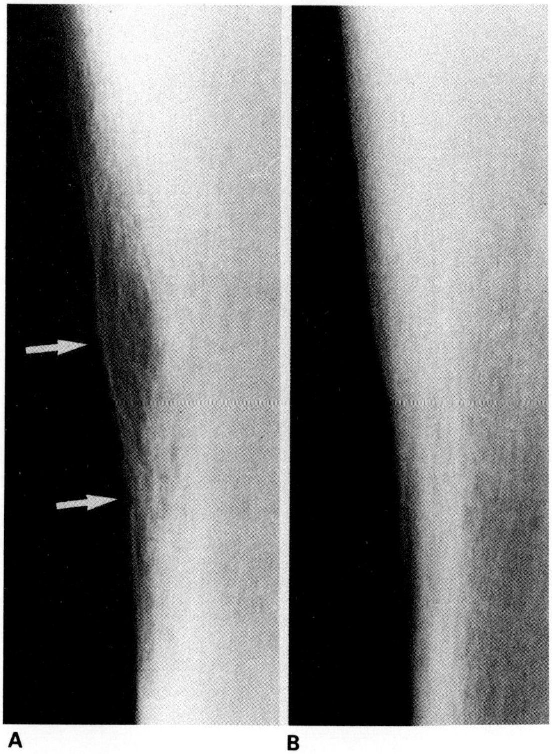

Figure 7.39

Radiographic appearances in a patient who developed bone pain after 5 months' treatment with etidronate. X-ray examination at that time (A) showed two intracortical resorption clefts (arrows) at the site of pain which resolved with subsequent treatment (for 3 months) with calcitonin (B). (From Maldague and Malghem, 1989.)

Increased radiotranslucency has also been reported in patients with predominantly extensive osteolytic disease in long bones (see Figure 7.39), particularly with the higher doses (Kantrowitz et al, 1975; Nagant de Deuxchaisnes et al, 1979). This presumably is related to rapid rates of new bone formation which fail to mineralize under the influence of etidronate, but which mineralize when treatment is stopped (Figure 7.40). For this

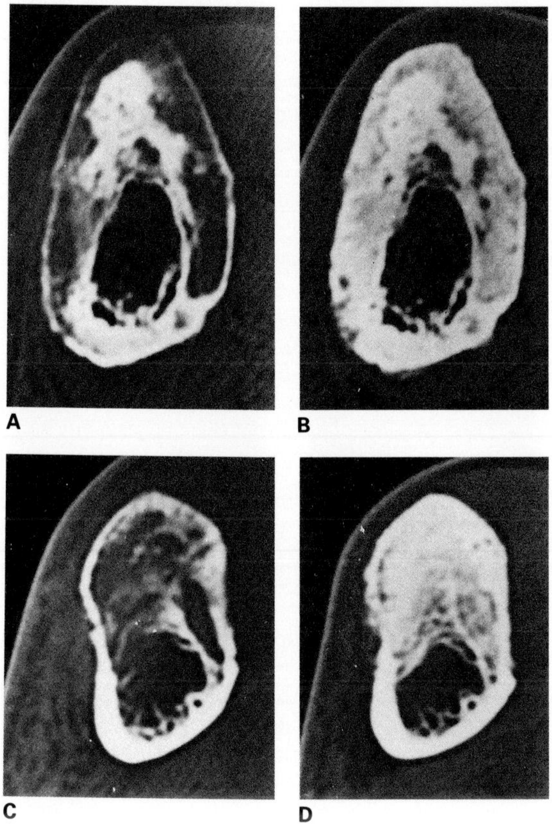

Figure 7.40

Computerized axial tomography of the proximal (A) (B) and mid-diaphyseal (C) (D) region of the tibia in a patient during (left) and after (right) treatment with etidronate. Bone remodelling was associated with impaired mineralization of bone but rapidly remineralized when another diphosphonate was substituted. (From Maldague and Malghem, 1989.)

reason we and others consider extensive osteolytic disease of long bones, particularly the weight-bearing long bones, as a contraindication to the use of high doses of etidronate (Nagant de Deuxchaisnes et al, 1977; Krane, 1982). There is no firm evidence that this is a concern with the use of low doses, and arrest of advancing osteolytic lesions has been observed with the use of etidronate in the same way as with calcitonin and other diphosphonates. The available evidence would suggest that etidronate in the doses recommended by the suppliers (5–10 mg/kg for 3–6 months) is unlikely to increase the risk of fracture. The evidence for and against this view is discussed in the following chapter.

Clodronate

Dichloromethylene diphosphonate (clodronate; Cl_2MDP) is a potent inhibitor of bone resorption. Experimental studies suggest that clodronate inhibits bone resorption with much less marked effects than etidronate on the mineralization of bone (Francis et al, 1969). In man its potency on bone resorption is similar to that of etidronate.

Published studies in Paget's disease have used oral doses between 400 and 3200 mg per day. These indicate that there is a rapid decrease in urinary excretion of hydroxyproline and a later decrease in activity of plasma alkaline phosphatase (Meunier et al, 1979; Douglas et al, 1980a; see Figure 7.26). Histological improvement is also observed to the same extent as with adequate treatment with etidronate (Table 7.2; Delmas et al, 1982). Suppression of disease activity is associated with the resumption of lamellar bone formation (Meunier et al, 1979; Yates et al, 1985) and a decrease in scintigraphic uptake (Figure 7.41). Unlike etidronate, it does not impair the mineralization of bone with the doses used in clinical practice (Meunier et al, 1979; Douglas et al, 1980a,b; Delmas et al, 1982; Yates et al, 1985; Figure 7.33 and Plate 27).

There is little difference in the degree of suppression achieved with doses between 800 and 1600 mg daily given for 3–6 months (Douglas et al, 1980; Figure 7.42), but the duration of remission appears to be longer with the higher doses (Gray et al, 1987; Table 7.3). The response to 400 mg daily or less may be less complete and relapse occurs more rapidly (Meunier et al, 1979). Suppression of disease activity is associated with scintigraphic changes (Espinasse et al, 1981; Delmas et al, 1982) and clinical benefits are reviewed in Chapter 8. As with other diphosphonates, disease activity remains suppressed for many months after stopping treatment. The most long-lasting remissions have been observed with a 6-month treatment of 1600 mg daily (Table 7.3;

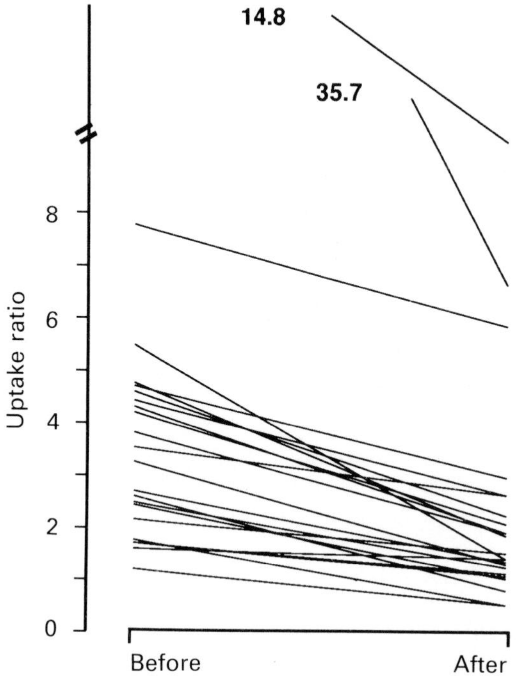

Figure 7.41

Effect of clodronate on scintigraphic uptake. Uptake was assessed as the ratio of uptake at an affected site to that of a corresponding unaffected contralateral site utilizing the same area of interest. Treatment (800–1600 mg daily) was associated with a significant decrease in uptake ratio (5.32 ± SEM 1.5 to 2.39 ± 0.45; $p<0.05$) 2 to 4 months after the start of treatment.

Figure 7.43) and in a few individuals remission has been observed for more than 9 years.

As in the case of etidronate, it is now evident that treatment for one month is capable of suppressing disease activity to an extent similar to that observed with a 3- or 6-month treatment (Chapuy et al, 1983; Gray et al, 1987; Figure 7.44). Similarly, the use of intravenous clodronate (300 mg daily for 5 days) will also induce suppression of disease activity (Yates et al, 1985), an effect which lasts for many months after treatment has stopped. There is no marked difference in the degree of disease suppression comparing these short treatments to longer regimens, but the duration of response may be shorter with the intravenous regimen (Figure 7.43). Acquired resistance to clodronate has not been described and the response to retreatment is similar (Yates et al, 1985).

As in the case with etidronate, the effects of clodronate on disease activity are greater than those with calcitonin. When patients attain the plateau response with calcitonin, the addition of clodronate induces a substantial further decrement in disease activity (Figure 7.16; Adami et al, 1984).

Side effects

There are few reported side effects. These include mild intestinal intolerance with oral treatment and transient proteinuria during intravenous infusions (Yates et al, 1985). In addition, there have been concerns about suspected drug-induced leukaemia, discussed later. Mild intestinal intolerance is dose-dependent and occurs in 5–20 per cent of patients. It is usually resolved by giving the daily dose in two aliquots (Douglas et al, 1981b).

Unlike the continued administration of etidronate, clodronate does not impair the mineralization of bone and histological studies undertaken after 6 months of continuous treatment have shown no abnormal suppression of mineralization or bone formation at pagetic or non-involved sites (Meunier et al, 1979; Table 7.2). Mineralization also proceeds normally after intravenous infusions of large doses (Yates et al, 1985; McCloskey et al, 1987; Figure 7.33). Fractures appear to heal normally during treatment (Douglas et al, 1980). These observations suggest that there are no skeletal risks even with prolonged treatment.

Adverse effects of clodronate on renal glomerular function have not been reported, with the possible exception of rapid intravenous bolus injection (see etidronate). Liver-function tests do not change, although small but not significant increases in lactate dehydrogenase have been reported (Douglas et al, 1980).

High doses of clodronate may induce an osteopetrotic-like lesion in experimental animals (Labat et al, 1984). This effect is what might be

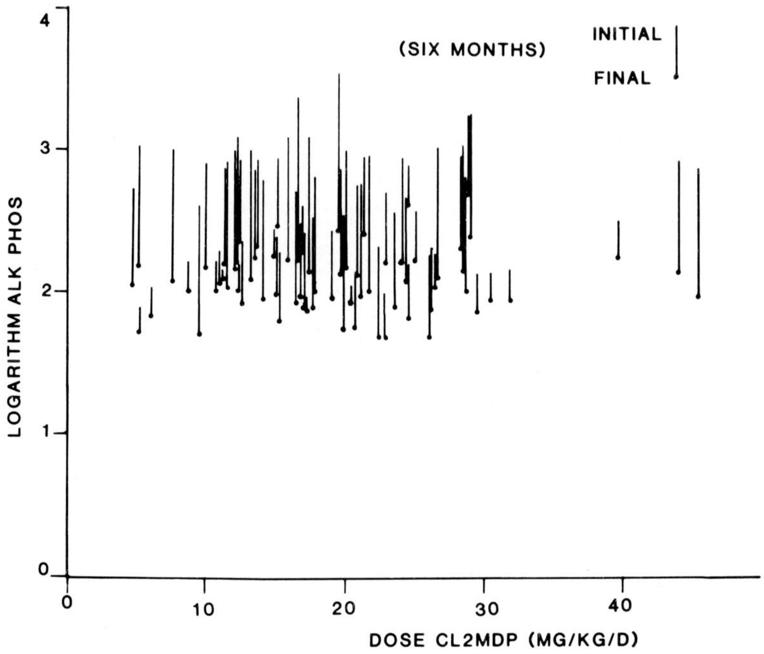

Figure 7.42

Effect of different doses of clodronate given by mouth for 6 months on suppression of disease activity in Paget's disease. The lines connect values before and after 6 months' treatment.

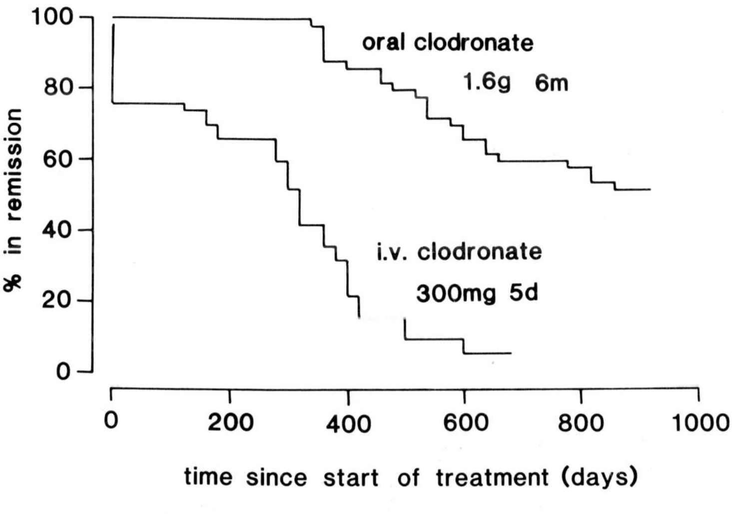

Figure 7.43

Actuarial analysis of the duration of biochemical responses after treatment with clodronate given either by mouth (1.6 g daily for 6 months) or intravenously (300 mg daily for 5 days). At 3 years, more than 50 per cent of patients given the oral regimen continued to show suppressed disease activity. (Gray and Kanis, unpublished.)

expected of an inhibitor of bone resorption in a growing animal. They also deplete the natural killer lymphocytes and on this basis it has been suggested that this effect might compromise neoplastic surveillance of the immune system. Similar effects on NK cells are observed, however, with many drugs and the immunological changes and osteopetrosis are probably coincidental. There have been concerns, however, that the use of clodronate may induce leukaemia, and the occurrence of three cases (excluding a diagnostic error) led to a suspension of clinical

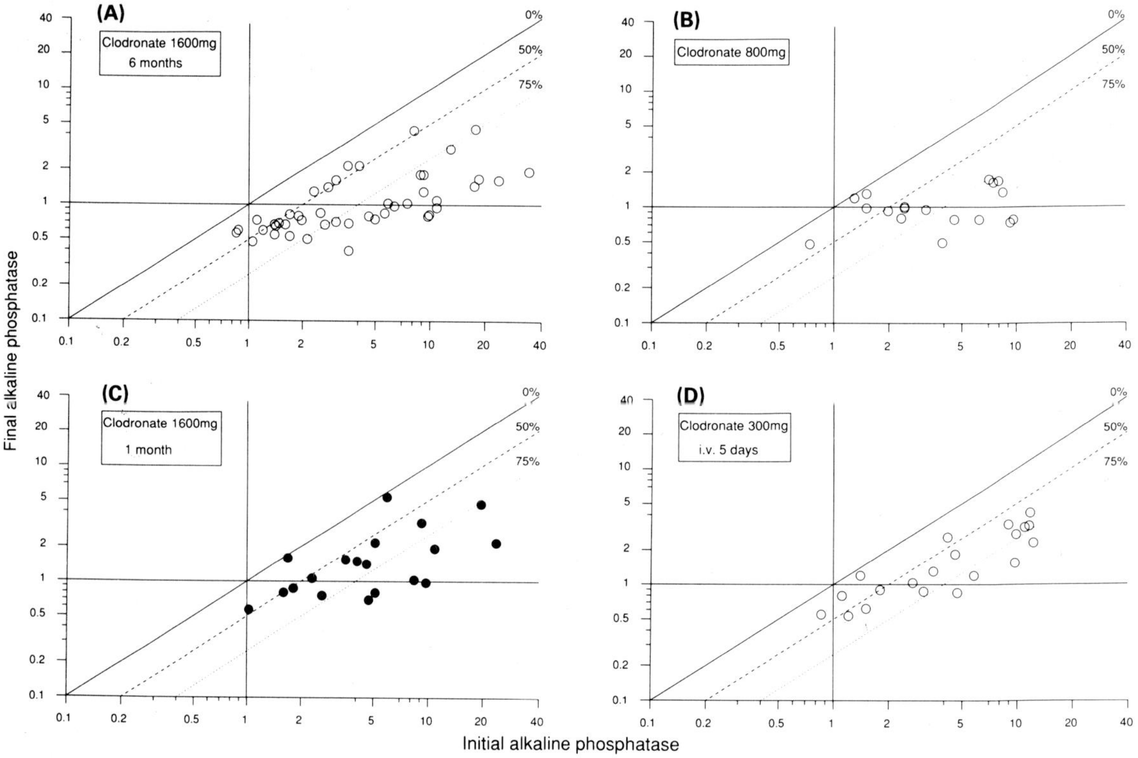

Figure 7.44

Serum activity of alkaline phosphatase (expressed as a ratio of the upper limit of the reference range) before and after treatment with clodronate utilizing four different regimens. (A) 1600 mg daily by mouth for 6 months; (B) 800 mg daily for 6 months; (C) 1600 mg daily for 1 month; (D) an intravenous regimen of 300 mg daily for 5 days. Values after treatment are nadir values. Dotted lines denote the expected relationship assuming a reduction of 50 or 75 per cent of disease activity. Note the logarithmic coordinates.

trials in the USA in 1981. Since the suspension of these studies no new cases of leukaemia have been reported, and many additional hundreds of patients have received clodronate. These observations together with the predisposing factors identified in two of the three patients reported – that is, prolonged exposure to benzene (Delmas et al, 1982) and myelomatosis – indicate that the association is coincidental. In addition, studies of the long-term effects of clodronate on chromosomal damage have shown no increased incidence of chromosome/chromatid breaks (Borgstrom et al, 1987).

The effect of etidronate to raise serum phosphate concentrations by increasing its renal tubular resorption (TmP/GFR) has not been observed with clodronate when given orally to patients with Paget's disease. However, a small and transient increase in TmP/GFR has been observed one or two days after its intravenous administration (McCloskey et al, 1988; Figure 7.38). It is notable that etidronate-induced hyperphosphataemia can be reversed by the administration of parathyroid hormone (Recker et al, 1973). The administration of clodronate increases the secretion of parathyroid hormone (due to its hypocalcaemic activity)

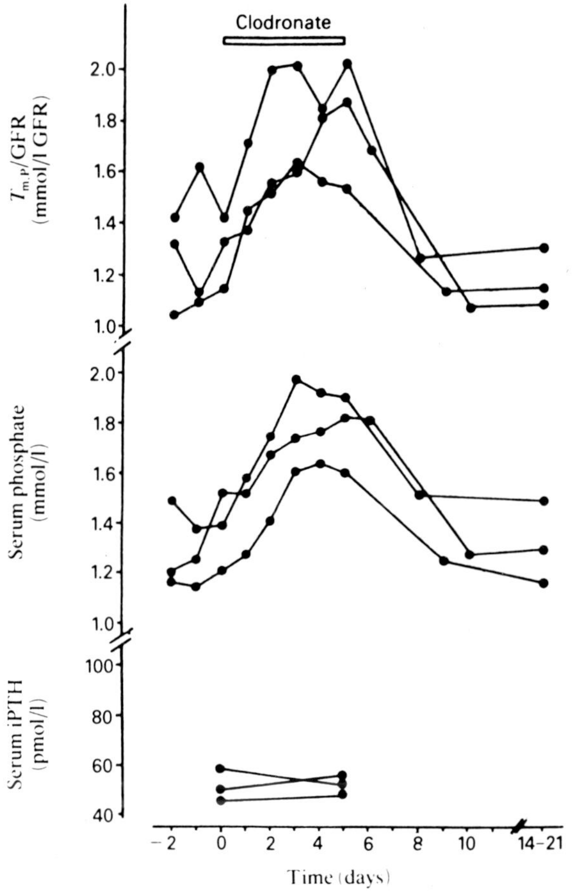

Figure 7.45

Effect of clodronate to increase serum phosphate and estimated TmP/GFR following a 5-day treatment with intravenous diphosphonate. These patients were hypoparathyroid and, unlike patients with Paget's disease, the diphosphonate-induced hypocalcaemia did not stimulate the secretion of PTH. (McCloskey et al, 1988.)

which may mask any intrinsic hyperphosphataemic effect. Indeed, when clodronate (or aminohexane diphosphonate) is administered to hypoparathyroid patients who are unable to mount an effective PTH response, these diphosphonates induce marked hyperphosphataemia (Figure 7.45). This suggests that many diphosphonates increase renal tubular resorption of phosphate, but that this is masked by secondary hyperparathyroidism with those that do not impair the mineralization of bone.

Pamidronate (APD)

Pamidronate or 3-amino-hydroxypropylidene-1,1-diphosphonate (APD) is a potent inhibitor of bone resorption. Observations in experimental animals indicate that pamidronate is more potent than clodronate or etidronate (Shinoda et al, 1983), but estimates of relative potency in animal studies or in vitro do not generally match clinical experience. Clinical studies suggest that pamidronate is 4–20 times more potent than etidronate (Dewis et al, 1985; Harinck et al, 1987). The only direct comparison in patients indicated that the response to pamidronate (4.5 mg/kg per day) for 3 months was similar to that induced by 20 mg/kg per day of etidronate for a similar period (Dewis et al, 1985).

Pamidronate has been extensively investigated in Paget's disease, particularly in Holland, Belgium, the UK and Argentina (Frijlink et al, 1979; Bijvoet et al, 1980a, 1982; Heynen et al, 1982; Nagant de Deuxchaisnes et al, 1982; Mautalen, 1983; Dewis et al, 1985; Mautalen et al, 1985; Harinck et al, 1987). These studies indicate that it is rapidly effective in suppressing bone turnover. Like clodronate and etidronate it has also been used to treat hypercalcaemia associated with myeloma and malignant disease (Van Breukelen et al, 1979; Sleeboom et al, 1983).

A bewildering array of doses and regimens have been used, either by mouth or by intravenous infusion. The oral doses used have ranged from 50 to 1600 mg daily for 1 week to more than 6 months (Harinck et al, 1987b; Heynen et al, 1982; Mautalen, 1983, 1985; Dodds et al, 1987; Thiebaud et al, 1987). Few dose-ranging studies have been made but a daily dose of 50 mg for 6 months is suboptimal (Heynen et al, 1982). More complete responses are observed with doses greater than 250 mg daily (Heynen et al, 1982; Nagant de Deuxchaisnes et al, 1982b; Fraser et al, 1984; Dewis et al, 1985; Dodd et al, 1987). Early suppression of bone resorption is later followed by a fall in alkaline phosphatase (Cantrill et al, 1986).

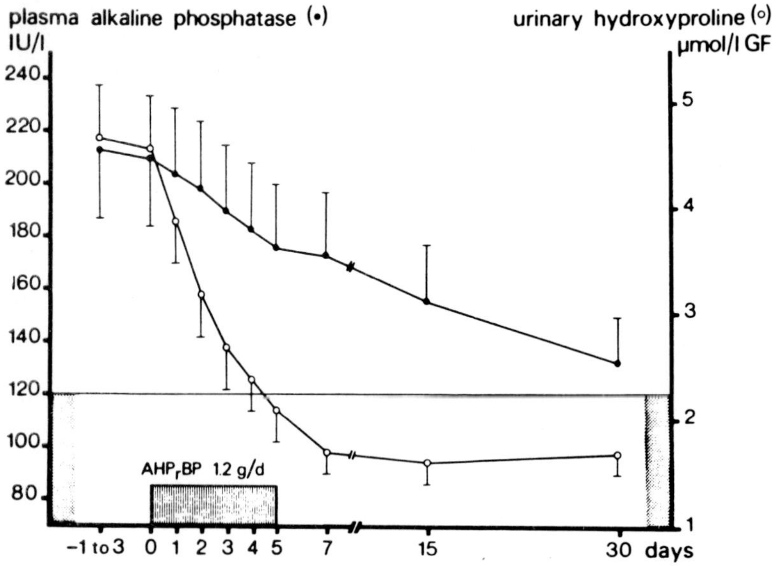

Figure 7.46

Biochemical indices of disease activity (mean ± SEM) before, during and after pamidronate, 1200 mg daily for 5 days by mouth. The pattern of response in the 11 patients is similar to that observed with intravenous clodronate in that inhibition of bone resorption is maximal 5–10 days after the start of treatment. The fall in activity of phosphatase in contrast occurs more rapidly. (From Thiebaud et al, 1987.)

Apart from the question of effective dose and side effects, there are more similarities than differences between pamidronate and clodronate. A notable difference is the rate of fall of alkaline phosphatase which is more rapid in the case of pamidronate (and aminobutane diphosphonate) than with the other diphosphonates thus far studied (Figure 7.46). It is not known whether this represents an adverse or advantageous effect. In addition, urinary excretion of hydroxyproline may rise transiently during the first day of treatment (Harinck et al, 1987).

As expected, suppression of disease activity is associated with decreased scintigraphic uptake (Vellenga et al, 1984a, 1985b) and decreased radiotranslucency of radiographs (Vellenga et al, 1985c; Anderson et al, 1988), consistent with a decrease in bone remodelling. Adverse effects on mineralization have not been observed (Frijlink et al, 1979). Unlike treatment with clodronate or etidronate, osteoclast numbers may not decrease to normal, but abundant abnormal osteoclasts may persist in the marrow cavity detached from bone surfaces. This suggests that pamidronate prevents the accession of new osteoclasts to the bone surface but does not invariably block their formation. The implications of this for long-term control of disease activity are not known. Durable suppression of disease activity does occur with pamidronate in many patients (Harinck et al, 1987a), but it is possible that relapse might occur earlier in those patients with the more incomplete suppression of abnormal osteoclast formation.

Intravenous pamidronate has also been used and the regimens given have varied widely. Some have given 2–30 mg daily for up to 10 days (Cantrill et al, 1986; Harinck et al, 1987a,b) or weekly or twice weekly infusions (Anderson and Cantrill, 1988). The total dose infused has ranged from 10 to 400 mg. As in the case of oral treatment, intravenous regimens may induce sustained remissions (Buckler et al, 1986; Cantrill et al, 1986; Dodds et al, 1987; Harinck et al, 1987a; Vega et al, 1987; Thiebaud et al, 1988; Cantrill, 1989; Figure 7.47). The effects are comparable in degree to clodronate and etidronate. It is of great interest that its continuous intravenous infusion for a single day (60 mg) can also result in

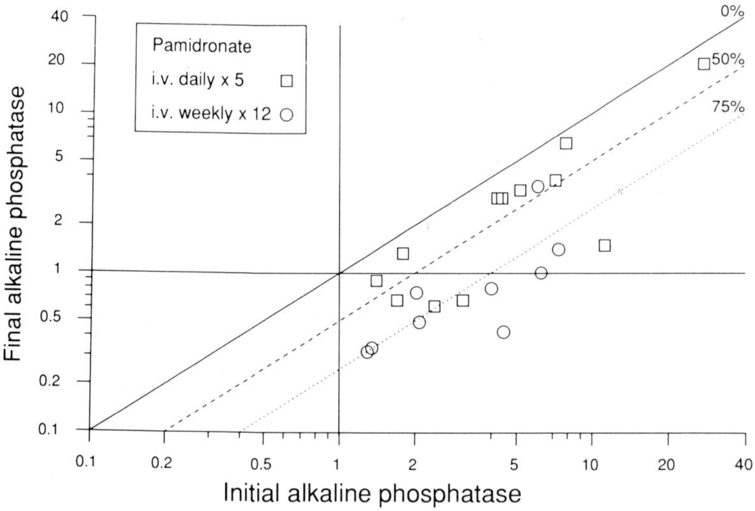

Figure 7.47

Serum activity of alkaline phosphatase (expressed as a ratio of the upper limit of the reference range) before and after treatment with intravenous pamidronate, 15 mg given either on 5 consecutive days or weekly for 12 weeks. Dotted lines denote the expected relationship assuming a reduction of 50 or 75 per cent of disease activity. Note the logarithmic coordinates. (From Cantrill et al, 1986.)

sustained remissions for up to one year (Thiebaud et al, 1988). In one large series, 80 per cent of treated patients showed suppression of disease activity to within the laboratory reference range (Richardson et al, 1990).

Few comparisons between treatment regimens have been made, but as for etidronate, the responses to oral treatment appear to be more heterogeneous than after intravenous treatment (Dewis et al, 1985) perhaps due to variations in absorption. The optimal dose, route of administration and duration of treatment to obtain the maximum duration of biochemical control is not yet known. The degree of disease suppression with pamidronate is similar to that with etidronate and clodronate and, as with these agents, prolonged remissions have been observed. In one series 50 per cent of patients remained in remission 2 years after the normalization of disease activity and 25 per cent remained relapse-free at 4–5 years (Harinck et al, 1987a). The reported effects have not always been so marked even after 6 months treatment (Mautalen, 1983).

As with the other diphosphonates, acquired resistance has not been described and the responses to retreatment are similar to the initial treatment (Harinck et al, 1987b).

Side effects

A major problem with the use of oral pamidronate has been gastrointestinal intolerance. This is dose-dependent and is found in 30 per cent of patients given 600 mg daily, but occurs less frequently with lower doses (Heynen et al, 1982; Mautalen et al, 1984; Harinck et al, 1987b). Improvements in oral formulation appear to have decreased the frequency of this unwanted effect.

The use of pamidronate and some other amino diphosphonates is associated with a transient leucopaenia and rise in body temperature during the early phase of treatment (Figures 7.48 and 7.49; Bijvoet et al, 1980, 1982; Heynen et al, 1982; Nagant de Deuxchaisnes et al, 1982; Mautalen et al, 1984; Vega et al, 1987). The effect appears to

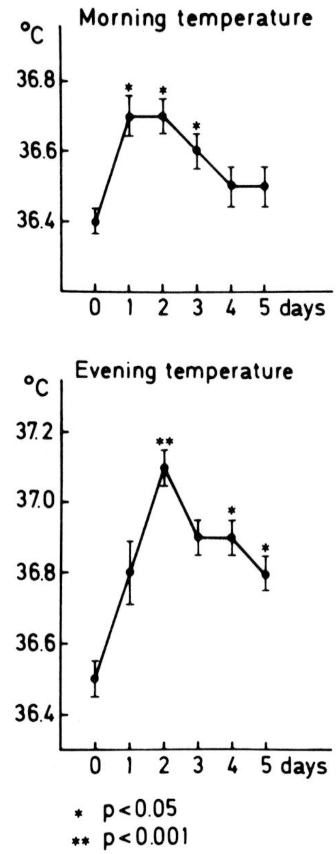

Figure 7.48

Effects of oral pamidronate (600 mg daily) on body temperature (from Nagant de Deuxchaisnes et al, 1982).

be dose-dependent. It generally occurs 24 hours after the start of treatment and is maximal at 48 hours. Lymphopaenia occurs more consistently than fever and is evident by 24 hours and followed by a fall in neutrophils. The effect seems to be transient, but few long-term data are reported. It is of interest that even large doses, such as 60 mg intravenously, do not consistently induce fever (Thiebaud et al, 1988). It has been suggested that re-exposure of patients to pamidronate does not induce a second reaction (Harinck et al, 1987b). This is partially true in that fever following a single infusion does not recur when weekly infusions are given thereafter. Such desensitization does not appear to be permanent, however, and re-exposure may result in a further reaction after a prolonged period (unpublished observations). It is of particular interest that desensitization appears to occur following infusions of clodronate, even though no acute phase response occurs with this agent (Adami et al, 1987).

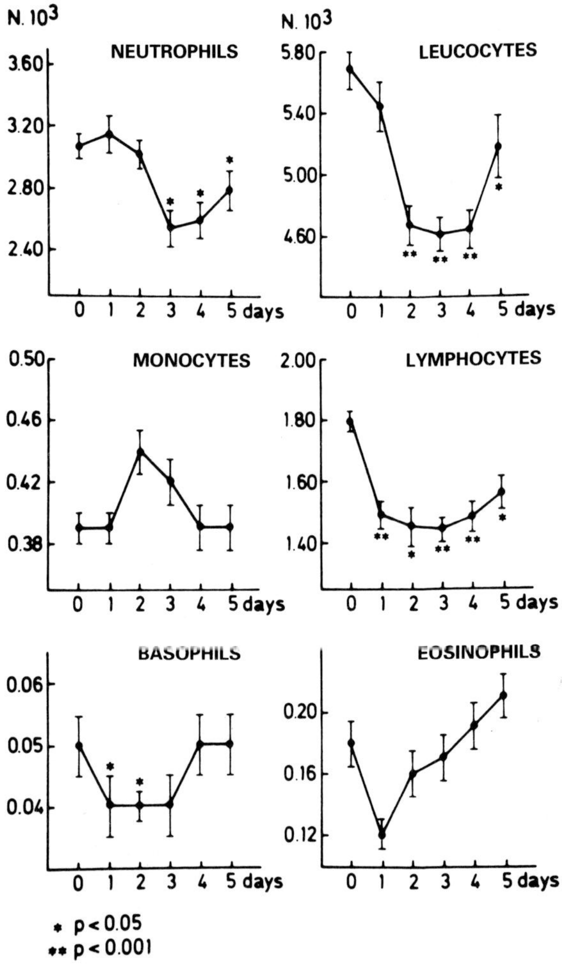

Figure 7.49

Effect of oral pamidronate (600 mg daily) on white blood cells counts (from Nagant de Deuxchaisnes et al, 1982).

The mechanism responsible for fever and leucopaenia is unknown, but it is thought that this represents an acute phase reaction, and is associated with the expected changes in serum zinc and in acute-phase proteins (Bijvoet et al, 1980; Adami et al, 1987). The acute-phase reaction is in part dependent upon the production of interleukin-1 and 6 (Dinarello, 1984), both potent bone-resorbing cytokines, suggesting that the reaction itself is not responsible for the suppression of osteoclast activity. A transient rise in hydroxyproline may be observed early after the start of treatment and may be due to the release of these cytokines. The acute-phase response occurs in bone disorders other than Paget's disease and is dose-dependent. Intravenous doses of 10 mg have modest if any effect on white-cell counts, whereas infusions of 30 mg or more have marked effects. The clinical significance of these effects is not known.

Transient proteinuria has been observed after intravenous infusion in 30 per cent of patients (Vega et al, 1987). Other side effects include increases in bone pain (Thiebaud et al, 1988) and thrombophlebitis at the site of infusion which is reported in 20 per cent of patients (Harinck et al, 1987b). Other infrequently reported side effects include rash, thrombocytopaenic purpura (Mautalen et al, 1984) and an increase in bone pain (Cantrill et al, 1986).

AHDP

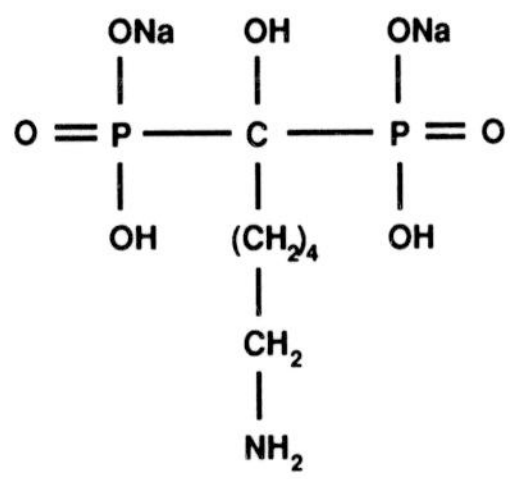

6 amino-1-hydroxyhexylidene-1,1-diphosphonate

ABuPD

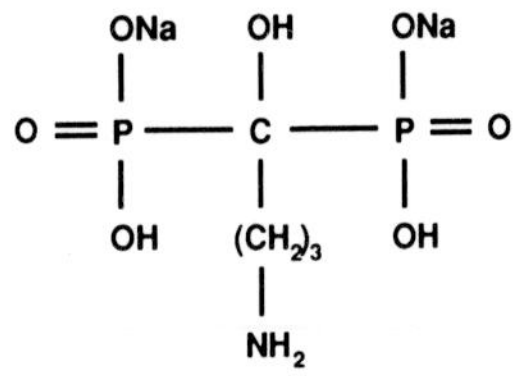

4 amino-1-hydroxybutylidene-1,1-diphosphonate

Figure 7.50

Structural formula of two amino diphosphonates being tested for the treatment of Paget's disease.

Other diphosphonates

Recently, four new diphosphonates have been used experimentally in the treatment of Paget's disease; these are tiludronic acid ((4-chlorophenyl) thiomethylene diphosphonate or SR 41319B) (Audran et al, 1985; Reginster et al, 1988), dimethyl APD (Papapoulos et al, 1989), aminohexane diphosphonate (AHDP) (Atkins et al, 1987) and aminobutane diphosphonate (alendronic acid, ABDP) (O'Doherty et al, 1990b; Figures 7.50 and 7.51). Preliminary results with tiludronate (200–400 mg daily) have suggested less complete suppression of Paget's disease than is commonly observed with the diphosphonates (Figure 7.52), but similar to the effects of calcitonin (Figure 7.13; Reginster et al, 1988; Amor et al, 1989; DeVogelaer et al, 1989).

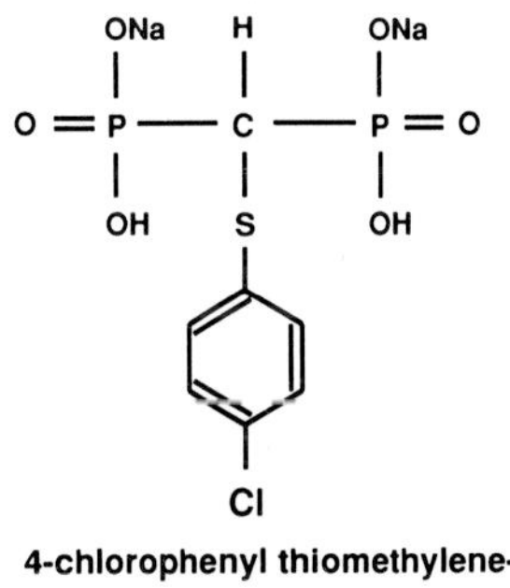

Tiludronate

4-chlorophenyl thiomethylene-1,1-diphosphonate

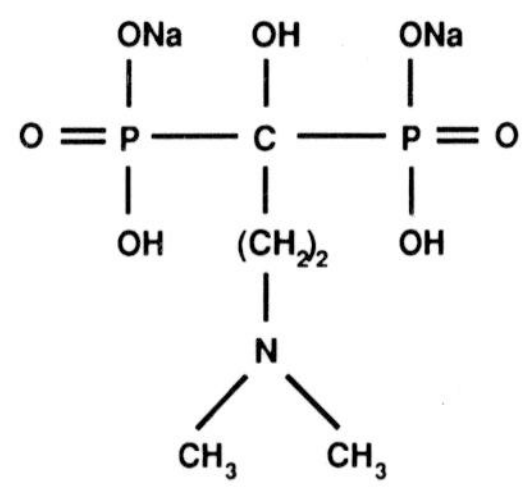

Dimethyl APD

N,N,dimethyl-3-amino-1-hydroxypropylidene-1,1-diphosphonate

Figure 7.51

Structure of tiludronate (top) and dimethyl APD (bottom).

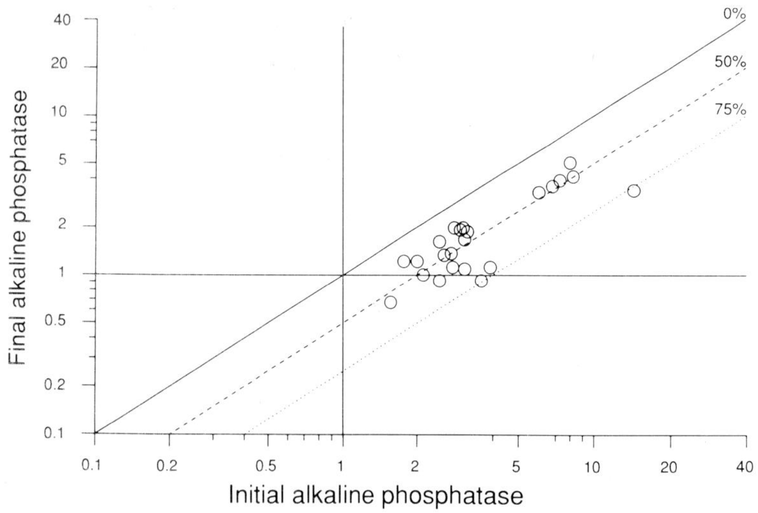

Figure 7.52

Serum activity of alkaline phosphatase (expressed as a ratio of the upper limit of the reference range) before and after treatment with tiludronate, 200–400 mg daily by mouth for 6 months. Dotted lines denote the expected relationship assuming a reduction of 50 or 75 per cent of disease activity. Note the logarithmic coordinates. (After Reginster et al, 1988a.)

The new aminoderivatives appear to be highly potent agents. Daily intravenous infusions of ABDP for 5 days induce a dose-dependent suppression of disease activity over the range of 2.5 to 10 mg daily (Figure 7.53). A febrile reaction is observed in a minority of patients together with the other changes expected of an acute-phase response in much the same way as observed with pamidronate (Figure 7.54; Adami et al, 1986; O'Doherty et al, 1990b). Similarly, the fall in alkaline phosphatase is more rapid than with other diphosphonates (compare Figures 7.55 and 7.46)

AHDP is 10 times less potent than ABDP. A daily dose of 400 mg by mouth for 1–3 months induces marked biochemical suppression, healing of osteolysis and does not impair the mineralization of bone (Figure 7.33). Similar effects are reported with five daily infusions of 20–50 mg (Atkins et al, 1987; Delmas et al, 1987). These regimens do not induce fever, lymphopaenia or rapid suppression of alkaline phosphatase (Atkins et al, 1987; Delmas et al, 1987), but higher doses (such as 75 mg iv) have been reported to induce fever in some patients (Adami et al, 1987). Neither ABDP nor AHDP impair the mineralization of bone (Atkins et al, 1987; O'Doherty et al, 1990).

Many other diphosphonates are likely to become available shortly (Abe et al, 1989; Muhlbauer et al, 1989; Pluijm et al, 1989; Stutzer et al, 1989; Valentin-Opran et al, 1990). Pilot work has begun with risedronate, but much more work will be required to determine whether this and other compounds offer advantages over the other diphosphonates used in Paget's disease.

Combined use of diphosphonates and calcitonins

There are now several reports of treatment of Paget's disease using low doses of etidronate (7.5–10 mg/kg per day for 6 months) combined with human or salmon calcitonin (Hosking et al, 1976; Bijvoet et al, 1977, 1978a; Fraser et al, 1984; O'Donoghue and Hosking, 1987). The rationale has been to try to combine the potential advantages of each regimen without the disadvantages: namely to use low doses of etidronate and thereby avoid impairment of bone mineralization while still inducing the marked suppressive effects normally seen with higher doses of etidronate.

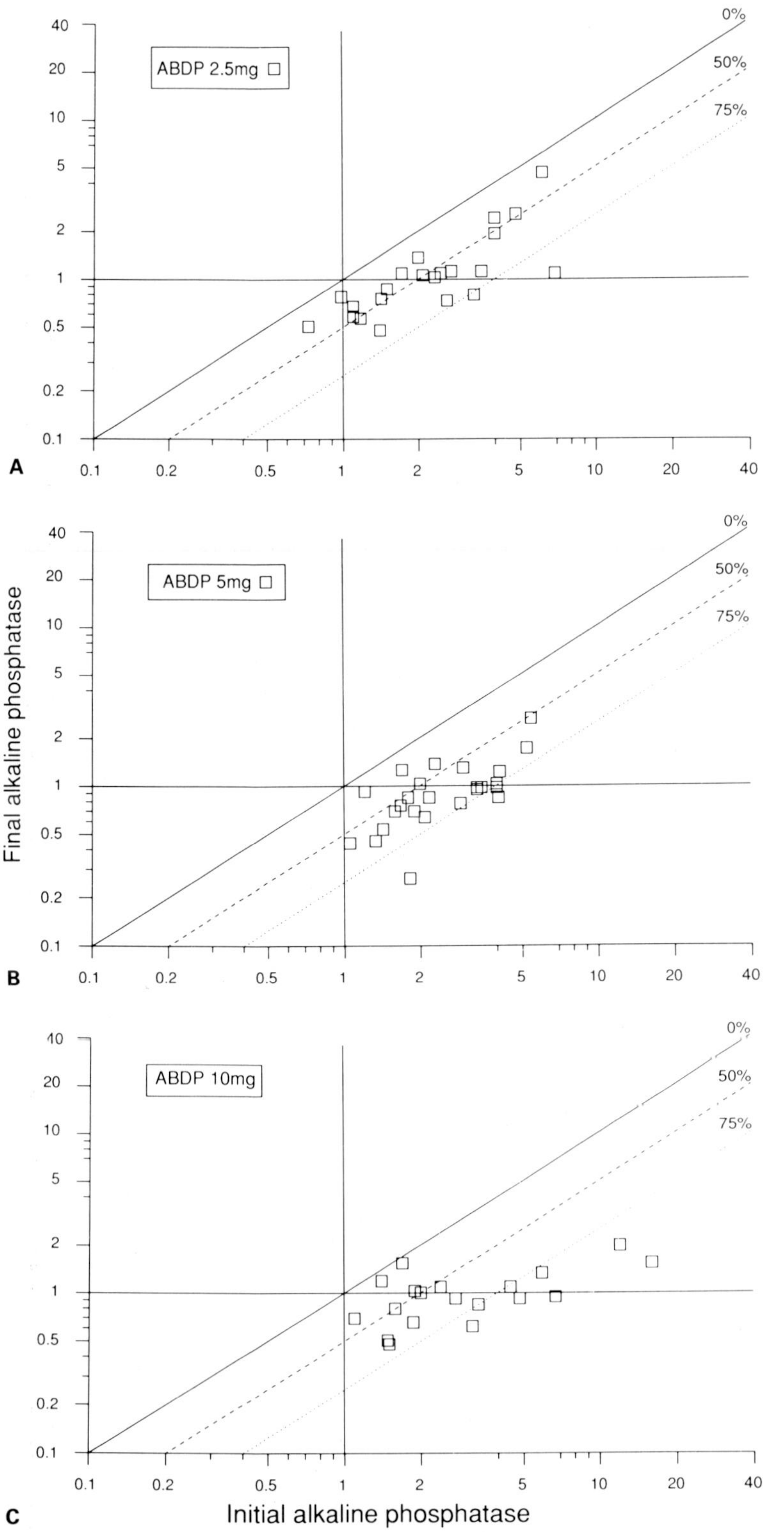

Figure 7.53

Serum activity of alkaline phosphatase (expressed as a ratio of the upper limit of the reference range) before and after intravenous aminobutane diphosphonate given daily for 5 days using a daily dose of 2.5 (A), 5.0 (B) or 10 mg (C). Dotted lines denote the expected relationship assuming a reduction of 50 or 75 per cent of disease activity. Note the logarithmic coordinates.

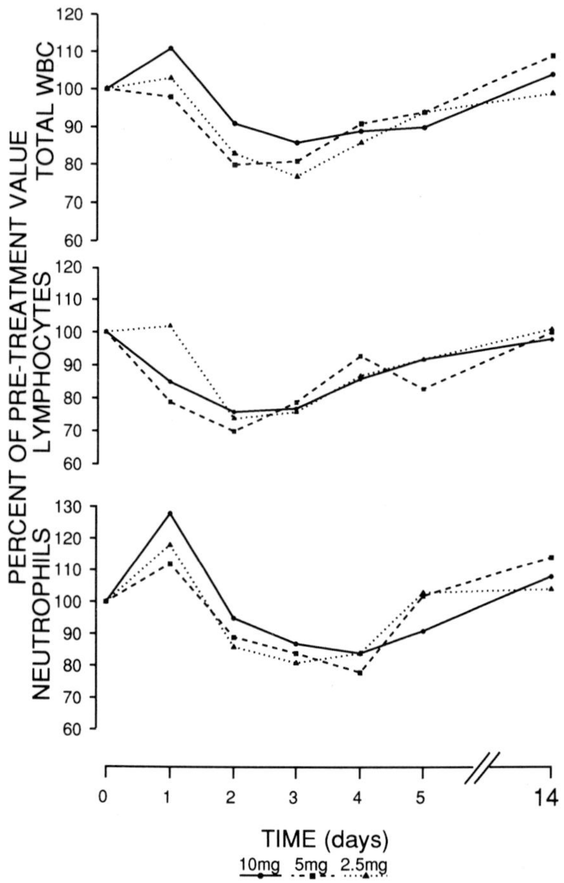

Figure 7.54

Mean haematological measurements in 30 patients treated with one of three doses of aminobutane diphosphonate by iv infusion for Paget's disease of bone. Each dose regimen (2.5, 5 and 10 mg iv daily for 5 days) induced changes in white cell counts which had reversed 2 weeks after the start of treatment.

When account is taken of disease activity, then the effects of the combined regimen seem to be more marked than either agent alone (O'Donoghue and Hosking, 1987; Figure 7.57). However, the effects of etidronate alone in this series were not as impressive as in some other series. The combined regimen does not prevent the increased bone pain sometimes seen with etidronate, and osteomalacia has also been observed with the combination (O'Donoghue and Hosking, 1987). As expected, bone scans show suppression of uptake.

Some experimental studies suggest that calcitonin might have effects on the mineralization of bone. In the rat, calcitonin appears to affect favourably etidronate-induced osteomalacia (Boris et al, 1979). Calcitonin in man has also been reported to improve radiographic osteolysis induced with etidronate (Nagant de Deuxchaisnes et al, 1979, 1980; Maldague and Malghem, 1989; see Figure 7.39). Conversely, when combined treatment is stopped etidronate-like radiographic abnormalities may appear de novo (Maldague and Malghem, 1989). These observations suggest a role for calcitonin in the treatment of etidronate-induced abnormalities in mineralization, but not necessarily for its concurrent use. For reasons which are not known the injection of calcitonin may increase serum calcium in etidronate-treated patients (Alexandre et al, 1979a). These observations suggest fascinating but unexplained interactions between the two agents.

Whereas any advantages of the combined regimen seem modest, it is clear that the addition of calcitonin in patients who have failed to respond adequately to a disphosphonate, or conversely the addition of diphosphonate in patients with incomplete responses to calcitonin, may confer advantages in particular individuals (Figures 7.16, 7.17, 7.19 and 7.58; Adami et al, 1984; Altman et al, 1987).

Mithramycin

Mithramycin or aurelcolic acid (known as plicamycin in the USA) is a cytotoxic antibiotic (Figure 7.59) which operates by inhibiting RNA synthesis (Yarbro et al, 1966). It has been used as an anti-tumour agent, but is also effective in relatively small doses in reducing osteoclast-mediated bone resorption. Indeed, it is used in the management of hypercalcaemia and has also been shown to be effective in patients with Paget's disease of bone.

Effective regimens have been 15–25 μg/kg per day, given by intravenous infusion over a 10-day

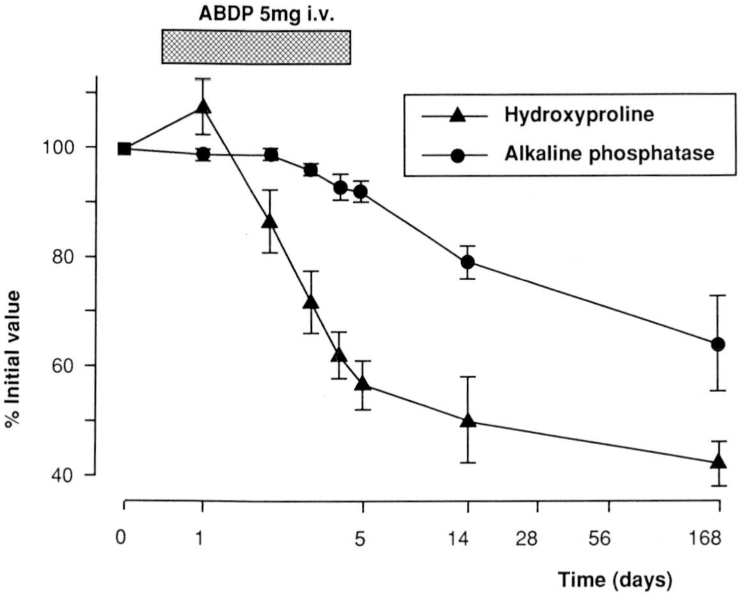

Figure 7.55

Effects of intravenous alendronate biochemical indices of disease activity (mean ± SEM). Note the dissociation in time of the response of alkaline phosphatase from that of hydroxyproline. Nevertheless, the fall in alkaline phosphatase occurred earlier than with etidronate or clodronate (see Figures 7.25 and 7.36).

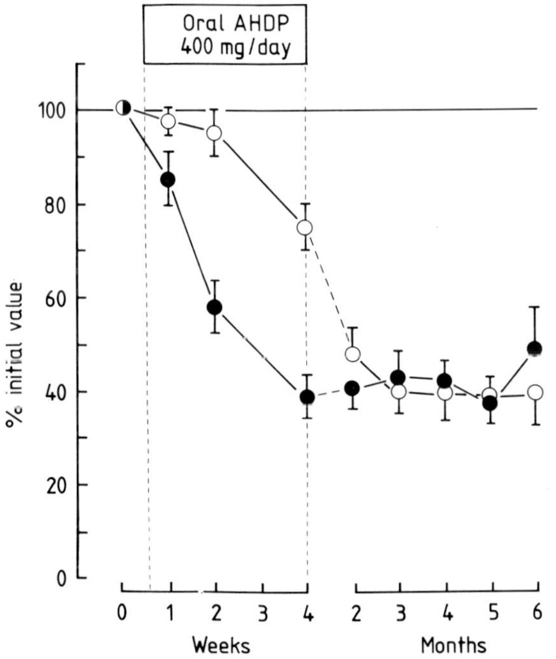

Figure 7.56

Mean values (± SEM) for alkaline phosphatase (○) and urinary hydroxyproline (●) before, during and after treatment with aminohexane diphosphonate by mouth (from Atkins et al, 1987).

period. Alternatively, the same dose has been used weekly rather than daily (Lebbin et al, 1974; Ryan, 1977). There is little doubt that this is an effective drug for reducing symptoms and biochemical indices of disease activity (Condon et al, 1972; Lebbin et al, 1974; Hadjipavlou et al, 1977; Ryan and Schwartz, 1980). Early responses are a decrease in urinary hydroxyproline together with a fall in serum calcium (Condon et al, 1972). Secondary hyperparathyroidism and an increase in $1,25(OH)_2D_3$ have been described, as with the diphosphonates (Bilezekian et al, 1978). The fall in alkaline phosphatase occurs later (Condon et al, 1971) consistent with a primary effect on bone resorption. The degree of suppression of disease activity is less marked than with the diphosphonates (Figure 7.60). A single course of treatment may produce a remission lasting for many months. Remissions have been noted for up to 2 years – and in one patient for 17 years (Ryan, 1989) – but most patients relapse shortly after stopping treatment.

As in the case of calcitonin, pain relief may persist despite biochemical relapse (Hadjipavlou et al, 1977; Ryan, 1977; Russell et al, 1979) and scintigraphic, radiographic and histological improvements have also been observed (Shirazi et al, 1974; Ryan, 1977). The disadvantages with

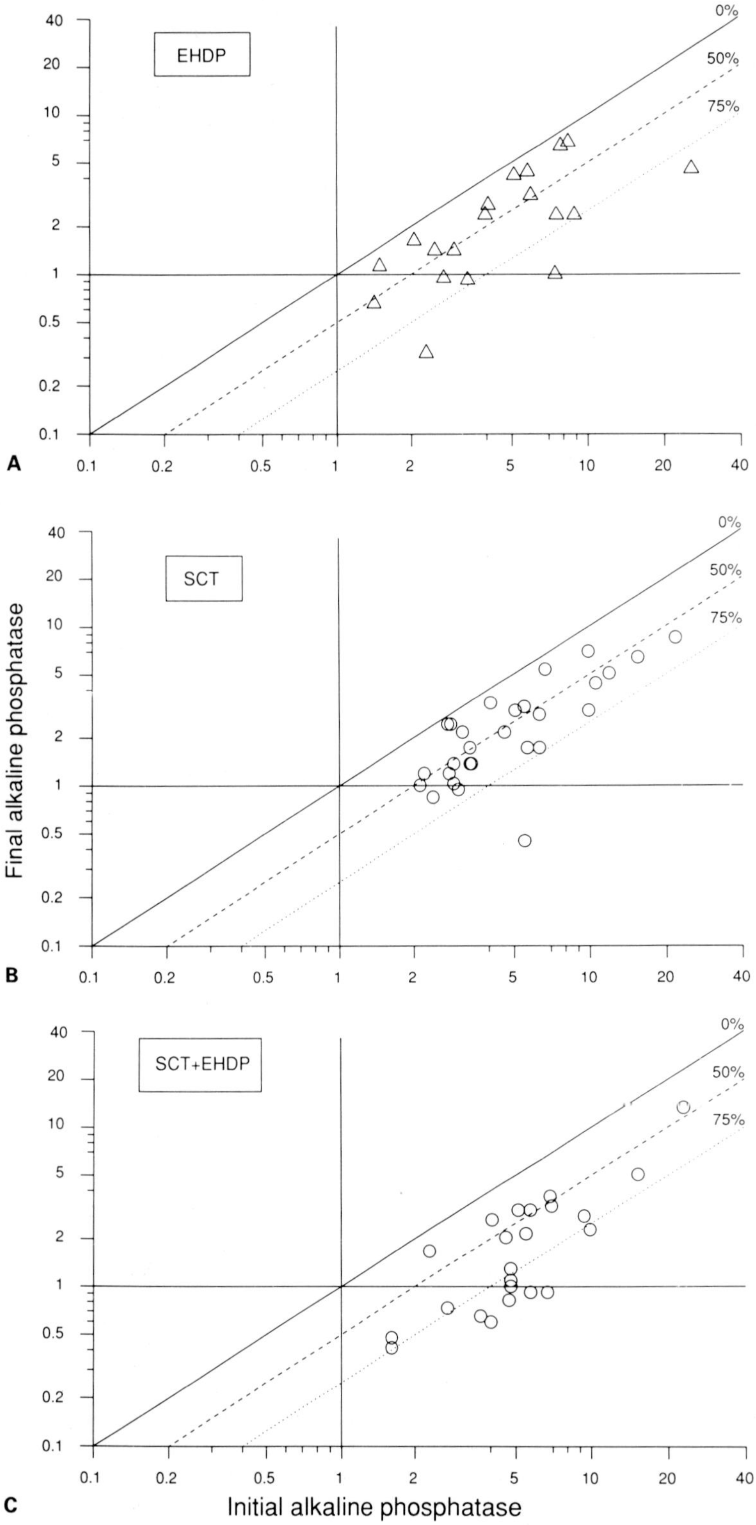

Figure 7.57

Serum activity of alkaline phosphatase (expressed as a ratio of the upper limit of the reference range) before and after etidronate 400 mg daily by mouth for 6 months (A), calcitonin 100 IU thrice weekly for 6 months (B) and the combination (C) (from O'Donoghue and Hosking, 1987).

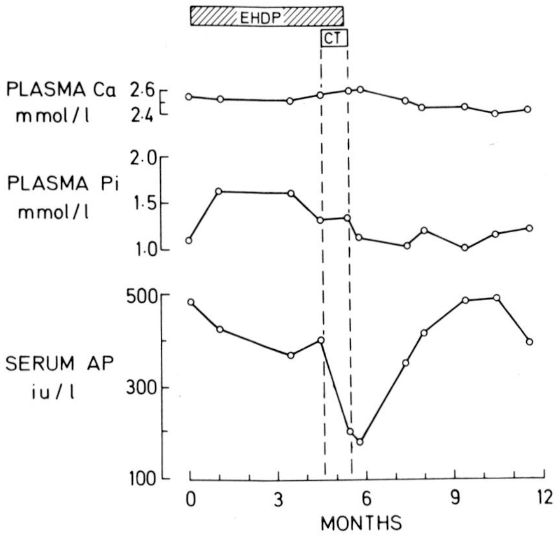

Figure 7.58

Effect of etidronate (EHDP 20 mg/kg per day) and porcine calcitonin (CT 160 MRC units daily) in a patient previously given several courses of diphosphonates. Note the incomplete response to the diphosphonate and the efficacy of additional treatment with calcitonin. (From Kanis et al, 1981.)

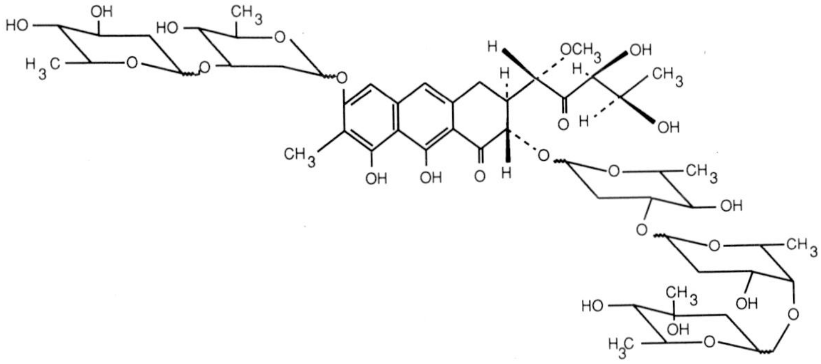

Figure 7.59

Structure of mithramycin.

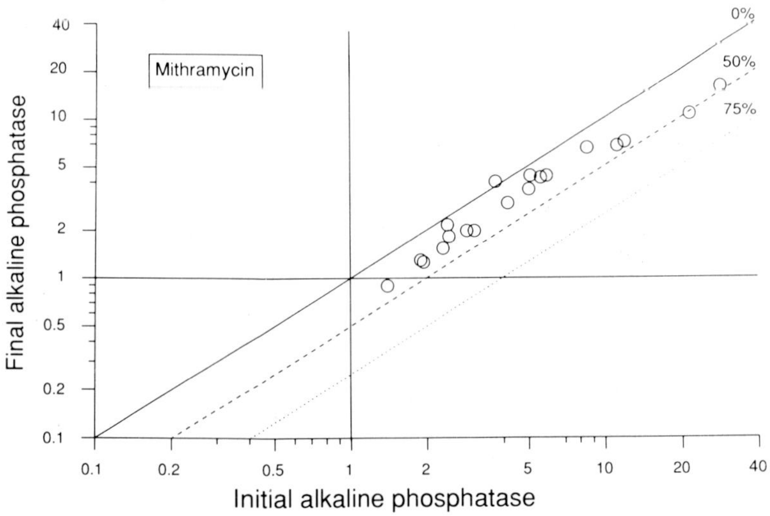

Figure 7.60

Relationship between serum activity of alkaline phosphatase (expressed as a ratio of the upper limit of normal) before and after treatment with mithramycin (11.5 μg/kg daily) for 10 days. The solid lines denote the normal range and the line of identity. The dotted lines denote the relationships assuming a reduction of 50 or 75 per cent of disease activity. Note the logarithmic scales. (Data from Russell et al, 1979.)

its use are that it must be given by intravenous infusion and it has some potentially serious toxic effects, particularly on the liver (Condon et al, 1971; Aitken and Lindsay, 1973; Ryan et al, 1980). The most obvious hepatotoxic effect is a rise in LDH. Indeed, it has been noted that a 10-fold or greater rise in LDH is associated with a more favourable effect on bone turnover, indicating the close relationship between systemic toxicity and effective dose. Permanent liver damage has not been reported in Paget's disease. Transient increases in plasma creatinine (Ryan, 1977; Ryan and Schwartz, 1980) and thrombocytopaenia are also reported (Kennedy, 1970; Ryan, 1977). Subjective side effects include nausea, vomiting and diarrhoea, which are more marked in the elderly. Their severity is decreased by lengthening the period of infusion and by administration of antihistamines.

In an attempt to minimize the serious side effects a dose of 10 μg/kg per day has been successfully used (Heath, 1981). However, a 10-day treatment evokes poor biochemical responses (Figure 7.60), and does not attain good long-term results since relapse occurs after 2–4 months.

In view of the side effects and the existence of safer drugs, mithramycin is not commonly given. Nevertheless, it may be useful in selected patients with severe disease or concurrently with other treatments in those patients in whom rapid responses are desired – for example, in progressive paraplegia (Douglas et al, 1981). It may be given with calcitonin, glucagon or the diphosphonates and appears to have additive effects (Hadjipavlou et al, 1977; Ryan and Schwartz, 1980; Figure 7.61).

Actinomycin D is another inhibitor of RNA synthesis which has also been used in the treatment of Paget's disease (Fennelly and Groarke, 1971; Fennelly, 1971; Somerville and Evans, 1975; Ryan, 1977). It is given intravenously, at a dose of 500 μg daily for 5 days or weekly. It has been less widely used than mithramycin but appears to have similar effects. Hepatotoxicity is not, however, a feature.

Gallium nitrate, another chemotherapeutic agent, also has some activity in Paget's disease (Bockman et al, 1989). It accumulates in osteoclasts and appears to inhibit osteoclast-mediated bone resorption (Mills et al, 1988a). Early studies in Paget's disease suggest that doses much smaller than those used for chemotherapy (such as 0.5 mg/kg iv daily for 7–14 days) decrease bone resorption with a later fall in alkaline phosphatase (Bockman et al, 1989). A recent report using a dose of 100 mg/m^2 daily for 5 days showed marked suppression of both alkaline phosphatase and hydroxyproline. As might be predicted, the fall in bone resorption preceded the decrease in formation (Matkovic et al, 1990). Treatment was associated with transient falls in haemoglobin and haematocrit.

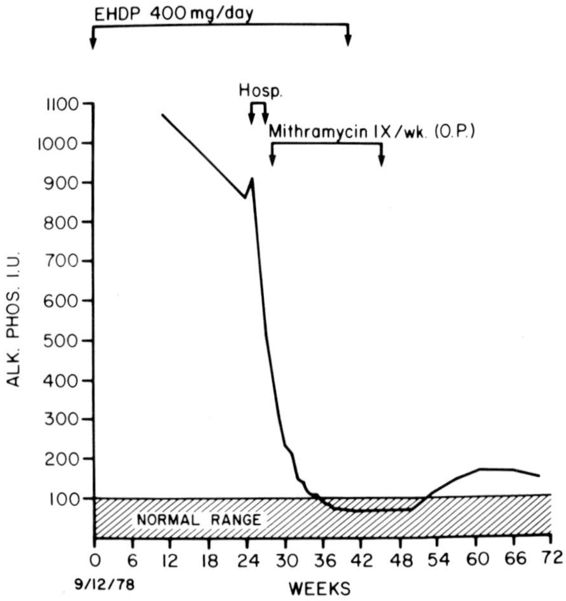

Figure 7.61

Effect of etidronate and mithramycin on disease activity in a patient with extensive disease. Note the accelerated response when mithramycin was added to treatment and the marked suppression of disease activity. (From Ryan and Schwartz, 1980.)

Glucagon

Glucagon has been used in Paget's disease and has been shown to relieve bone pain and

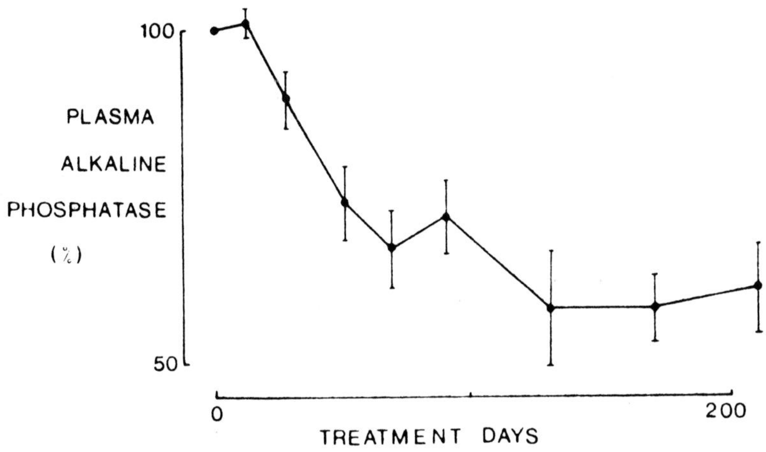

Figure 7.62

Mean biochemical response (± SEM) in nine patients with Paget's disease treated with a low phosphate diet (and aluminium hydroxide), calcium and a thiazide diuretic. Mean value of alkaline phosphatase fell to 58 per cent of pretreatment values. (From Evans, 1977.)

decrease biochemical indices of disease activity (Condon, 1971; Hadjipavlou et al, 1977). Experimentally it has been shown to stimulate the secretion of calcitonin, and this is thought to be its mechanism of action. The drug must be given intravenously and causes significant nausea and diarrhoea.

Calcium and thiazides

A method of stimulating the endogenous secretion of calcitonin was attempted by Evans (1977a), who administered a high calcium intakc, low phosphorus diet, aluminium hydroxide and a thiazide diuretic (chlorthialidone). This produced a decrease in disease activity and in bone pain (Evans et al, 1982). Similar results were obtained when the aluminium hydroxide was omitted from the regimen (Evans, 1983). The effects on alkaline phosphatase are modest and values are rarely suppressed below 70 per cent of pretreatment levels (Figure 7.62). Moreover the responses are transient, particularly in patients with the less marked suppression of disease activity. If values are suppressed to less than 70 per cent of initial values, the effects appear to be more sustained and gradual relapse occurs over 5 years.

No radiographic improvements have been reported. Side effects are confined to mild gastrointestinal upset in a minority of patients. Similar effects have been noted with the use of calcium infusions (Sekel, 1973). It may be that these effects are due to an increase in plasma calcium, stimulation of endogenous calcitonin production or suppression of parathyroid hormone.

Analgesics

Simple analgesics and non-steroidal anti-inflammatory drugs are of obvious value in bone pain. However, large doses of aspirin (5 g/day) have been shown to reduce bone turnover in some patients with Paget's disease (Nagant de Deuxchaisnes and Krane, 1964, 1977; Figure 7.63). An early fall in hydroxyproline is followed by a later fall in activity of serum alkaline phosphatase. Serum and urinary calcium decrease, consistent with an early effect on bone resorption. Kinetic studies have also shown a decrease in bone turnover, and histological studies have shown a reduction in the number of osteoblasts and osteoclasts. These effects are less consistent than those seen with calcitonins or the diphosphonates. In view of the high doses

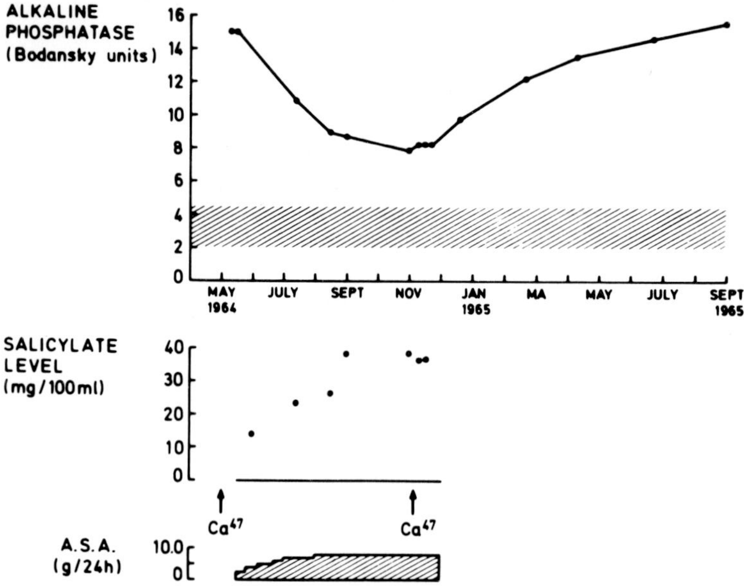

Figure 7.63

Sequential measurements of alkaline phosphatase in a patient treated with high doses of aspirin (ASA) (from Nagant de Deuxchaisnes and Krane, 1977).

required and the adverse effects of aspirin, its use as an inhibitor of bone resorption has been abandoned. Aspirin is, nevertheless, useful as a simple analgesic, and it is the impression of some that the response of bone pain to aspirin is better than to other non-steroidal anti-inflammatory drugs (Smith, 1979).

Of the drugs reviewed all manner of combinations have been tested, usually on a limited basis. They include sequential use of calcitonins with diphosphonates (Adami et al, 1984; Perry et al, 1984) or mithramycin (Hadjipavlou et al, 1977; Avramides et al, 1982). These and other combinations have not gained widespread acceptance.

Other drugs and regimens

Other drugs (listed on page 159) appear to have less specific effects on bone remodelling, but have, in the past, been thought to be of value, usually in a limited proportion of patients.

Amylin is a 37-amino-acid peptide secreted by the β-cells of the pancreas and co-secreted with insulin. It has calcium-lowering effects similar to calcitonin (Datta et al, 1989) and, like calcitonin, appears to have direct effects on osteoclasts. Very recent studies in man suggest that it decreases bone resorption in Paget's disease (S. Gilby et al, unpublished work).

Comparative aspects

The comparative effects of treatment regimens on the symptoms and complications of Paget's disease are reviewed in Chapter 8, and the present chapter has dealt largely with the characteristics of the drugs used and their effects on the biochemical indices of disease activity. As is apparent, few studies have directly compared the efficacy of different treatments and in many cases there is little information on dose-response with any one treatment.

With respect to the comparative evaluation of

treatments using biochemical techniques, the response most frequently assessed is serum activity of alkaline phosphatase. There are a number of problems, however, in making valid comparisons, both within centres and between centres.

In populations of patients the activity of alkaline phosphatase has a unimodal log-normal distribution (Walton et al, 1977a). This compounds the difficulty of assessing biochemical responses between regimens in populations of patients or within patients treated with the same regime. Expressing response as a decrement in activity of alkaline phosphatase or as a percentage fall has its limitations. For example, a decrease in alkaline phosphatase from 120 to 80 IU may represent complete suppression of disease activity, but only a 33 per cent reduction in initial value. A similar percentage fall in a patient with more extensive disease would represent an incomplete response. Similar problems arise with the use of z scores or logarithmic transformation. There are also problems in assessing response in terms of the number of patients achieving normal turnover, again because this is highly dependent on case selection and initial disease activity.

In consequence, it is very difficult to make strict comparisons between the experience of different centres using different regimens when patient populations are not matched for initial disease activity. Where individual responses are reported, or where patients have been matched for disease activity, some comparison of treatment regimens is possible and is provided in the figures shown throughout this chapter.

The increasing use of the diphosphonates will compound the problems of evaluation using biochemical indices because of the prolonged remission that may be obtained and the slow relapse. The effect of an incomplete relapse and the response to further treatment is illustrated in Figure 7.64. The fall in disease activity that might have been achieved during a second course of treatment will be dependent in part on the degree of biochemical relapse. Some, but not all, studies take this into account.

In general, there is a remarkable similarity in response between diphosphonates as judged by changes in biochemical indices of disease activity. As for calcitonin, the proportion of patients in whom disease activity is restored to normal is dependent upon the initial disease activity. With

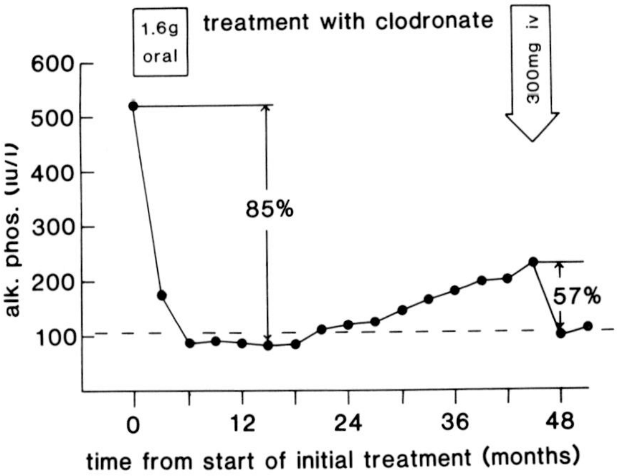

Figure 7.64

Effect of incomplete relapse on biochemical responses to diphosphonates in a patient with Paget's disease. During both courses of treatment alkaline phosphatase values fell to normal (dotted line). In contrast, the apparent response when expressed as a percentage of the value immediately before treatment was less marked after the second course. (From Yates et al, 1985.)

extensive disease a higher proportion of diphosphonate treatments attain normal values than is seen with the calcitonins (Table 7.7). The choice of diphosphonate is likely to relate more to side effects than to differences in efficacy so far as the degree of disease suppression is concerned (Table 7.8).

Despite the similarity between many treatment regimens in the degree of biochemical suppression of disease activity, there appear to be some differences, not only in the proportion of patients attaining a 'remission', but also in the duration of the response evoked (Table 7.3). In general, short treatments appear to give less prolonged remissions. An unexplained observation is that patients given low doses of etidronate remain in remission for significantly longer than patients given higher doses, even though remission is induced in a lower proportion of patients with the smaller doses (Table 7.3). The reasons for differences in the duration of response or remission between

Table 7.7 Comparative responses to diphosphonates (DP: etidronate and clodronate) and calcitonins (CT: SCT and HCT) in Paget's disease. Partial response was a fall in alkaline phosphatase values to 25 per cent or more of initial values. Complete response was a decrease in alkaline phosphatase values to within the normal range. Note that the vast majority of patients show a partial response, irrespective of the type of treatment. As disease activity increased, the complete response rate decreased, a phenomenon much more marked with the use of calcitonins. (Data from Hamilton et al, 1974; MacIntyre et al, 1980; Gray et al, 1987; O'Donoghue and Hosking, 1987 and an unpublished series.)

Pretreatment alkaline phosphatase (IU/l)	*Agent*	*No of patients*	*Partial response (% patients)*	*Complete response (% patients)*	*DP/CT response rate*
<200	DP	46	91 ± 4	87 ± 5	
	CT	18	94 ± 4	88 ± 6	1.0
200–500	DP	53	94 ± 3	57 ± 7	
	CT	36	81 ± 5	25 ± 5	2.3
>500	DP	48	94 ± 4	25 ± 6	
	CT	28	79 ± 6	7 ± 2	3.6

Table 7.8 Some comparative properties of the diphosphonates used in Paget's disease.

	Etidronate	*Clodronate*	*Pamidronate*
Suppression of disease activity	++	++	++
Potency	+	+	++
Prolonged remission	++	++	++
Osteomalacia	+	–	–
Gastrointestinal effects (by mouth)	+	+	++
Transient proteinuria (iv)	–	+	+
Fever	–	–	+
Rash	Occ	Occ	Occ
Local thrombophlebitis (iv infusion)	–	–	+
Bone pain	+	–	+
Parenteral formulation	+	+	+
Oral formulation available	+	+	–

+ = effect; ++ = marked effect; Occ = occasional effect.

diphosphonate regimens are unknown. They do not appear to be due to differences in the initial disease activity nor to the prior exposure of patients to other medical treatments.

The length of remission after treatment with diphosphonates appears to be related in part to the degree of suppression of Paget's disease induced over the first few months of treatment. Thus, in those patients who attain normal activities of alkaline phosphatase with etidronate or clodronate, remission is more prolonged, irrespective of the extent of disease activity (Gray et al, 1987; Figure 7.65). Similar observations have been made following treatment with pamidronate (Harinck et al, 1987a). This effect has some analogies with tumour chemotherapy in the sense that the greater the decrease in tumour burden, the longer the remission expected. The more durable remissions obtained in Paget's disease in patients with the more complete

Table 7.9 Comparative effects of therapeutic regimens in patients with high activities of alkaline phosphatase. The number of patients (*n*) is shown and the proportion of patients in whom a normal phosphatase was observed following treatment (%*N*). Data are provided only where the sample size is 10 or more. The source refers to the figure number.

Agent	*Regimen*	*Pre-treatment alkaline phosphatase (ratio of normal reference range)*						*Source*
		3–5		*>3*		*>5*		
		n	*%N*	*n*	*%N*	*n*	*%N*	
Salmon CT	50–100 IU daily or ×3/week for 6 months	—	—	22	9	17	6	Figure 7.13
Human CT	100 IU daily for 3–34 months	—	—	18	11	10	10	Figure 7.14
Etidronate	5–10 mg/kg per day for 6 months	—	—	38	10	31	6	Figure 7.35
	2.5–5 mg/kg per day for 6 months	—	—	15	7	11	9	Figure 7.29, 7.35
	20 mg/kg per day for 1–6 months	31	45	70	27	39	13	Figure 7.29, 7.37*
	300–500 mg i/v for 5 days	—	—	9	22	—	—	Figure 7.37
Clodronate	0.8–1.6 g daily for 1–6 months	14	57	44	43	30	37	Figure 7.44
	300 mg i/v for 5 days	10	30	20	15	10	0	Figure 7.44
Pamidronate	15 mg i/v for 5–12 days	—	—	11	36	—	—	Figure 7.47
	30 mg i/v weekly for 12 weeks	—	—	—	—	15	53	Richardson et al, 1990
Alendronate	5–10 mg i/v for 5 days	12	58	18	44	—	—	Figure 7.53
Mithramycin	15–25 mg/kg per day for 10 days	—	—	10	0	—	—	Figure 7.60
Etidronate + calcitonin	400 mg + 100 IU ×3/week for 6 months	—	—	18	28	11	18	Figure 7.57

*Includes a personal unpublished series.

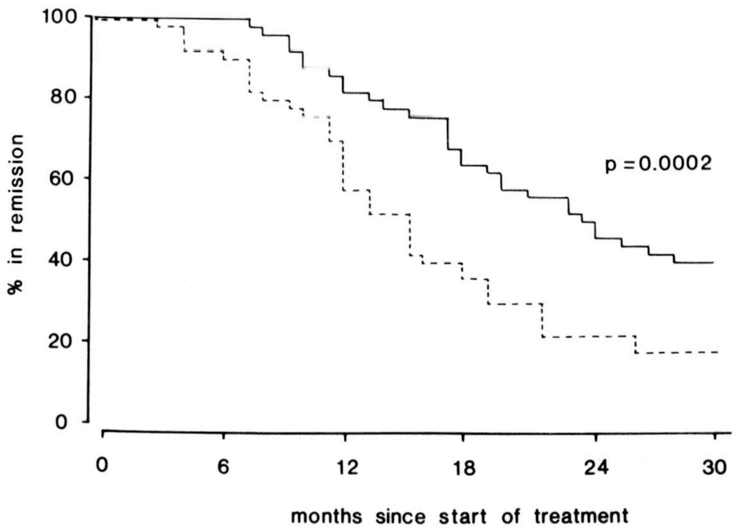

Figure 7.65

Actuarial plot showing the duration of remission from diphosphonate treatment (clodronate or etidronate). Patients were divided into those in whom activity of alkaline phosphatase had suppressed to normal and those who had reached stable remission with values above the reference range. Patients who reached the laboratory reference range (solid line) remained in remission for significantly longer than patients in whom values were not suppressed to normal. (From Gray et al, 1987.)

biochemical responses may reflect the ablation of an abnormal osteoclast population. This suggests that treatment strategies for the future might include meticulous attention to maximal suppression of disease activity.

If the degree of disease suppression is a valid criterion of efficacy, then clodronate and the aminodiphosphonates seem to be the most effective, followed by etidronate in high doses or combined with calcitonin (Table 7.9). If the duration of remission is important, the most impressive long-term remissions have been observed thus far with clodronate (Figure 7.43), but are to be expected with the other diphosphonates. The extent to which biochemical control can be translated to clinical benefit is reviewed in Chapter 8.

CHAPTER 8

Management and assessment of response

There is no cure for Paget's disease, but a variety of treatments (Chapter 7) induce a substantial decrease in disease activity. The use of the calcitonins and diphosphonates has gained most widespread acceptance, but mithramycin, fluoride and the combined use of thiazides and calcium supplements are still used.

The aims of treatment are not to suppress abnormal biochemistry or scintigraphic findings, but to treat or prevent the complications that occur because of Paget's disease. Questions arise whether the biochemical control of Paget's disease modifies the clinical consequences of the disorder. These questions are difficult to answer. In the case of bone pain, for example, placebo-controlled trials are required, and there is the additional difficulty of ascribing pain to Paget's disease itself rather than to its attendant complications such as osteoarthrosis. There are even more problems in the assessment of treatment on fracture rates, sarcoma, deformity, etc.

The following sections review to what extent our current knowledge can answer these questions. Are the symptoms and complications of Paget's disease significantly modified by treatment, and if so, which regimens are most suited to the specific aims of treatment? The surgical aspects of Paget's disease lie within the province of orthopaedics and occasionally of neurosurgery, but the optimal management of Paget's disease often requires a combined medical and surgical approach. Where appropriate this too is indicated. Some additional comments on the biochemical and scintigraphic assessment of treatment are also included.

Clinical features and complications of Paget's disease.

Common
- Bone pain – pagetic
  - – articular
- Fracture – long bones, vertebral bodies
- Neurological – deafness
- Deformity and enlargement of bones

Uncommon
- Pain – fissure fracture, avulsion fracture
- Spinal neurological syndromes
- Hypercalcaemia and calciuria of immobilization or fracture
- Cardiovascular disease
- Vascular bleeding from bone during surgery
- Extraskeletal calcification and urolithiasis

Rare
- Gout
- Epidural haematoma
- Osteosarcoma and other bone tumours
- Cranial nerve lesions (except VIII)
- Brain stem and cerebellar syndromes
- Hypercalcaemia
- Extramedullary haematopoiesis

Significance uncertain
- Pseudogout
- Angioid streaks
- Hyperparathyroidism
- Chondrocalcinosis

Laboratory assessment of treatment

Since serum activity of alkaline phosphatase and urinary excretion of hydroxyproline provide reproducible and reasonably accurate indices of the extent of disease activity, they have found widespread acceptance as tools for monitoring the response to treatment. Additional methods more appropriate to the clinical evaluation of new treatments include assessment of bone scans, tracer kinetic studies, bone histology and detailed skeletal radiography (Table 8.1). Bone biopsy may be of limited value in the routine assessment of patients, but has a place for excluding other pathology (such as osteomalacia, sarcoma, etc).

Table 8.1 Direct and indirect methods used to assess responses to long-term treatment of Paget's disease (from Kanis and Gray, 1987).

Estimate of disease activity	*Focal changes*	*Integrated effects*
Focal signs and symptoms	+	–
Biochemical markers	–	+
Bone histology	+	–
Quantitative scintigraphy	+	+
Whole body ^{99m}Tc-diphosphonate retention	–	+
Radiography	+	–
Quantitative thermography	+	–
Bone blood flow	+	–
Tracer kinetics	–	+
Limb volumes	+	–
Facial stereomorphometry	+	–
Audiology	+	–

Alkaline phosphatase

Serum activity of alkaline phosphatase is the most frequently used index of response to treatment. In Paget's disease in the absence of liver disease, the total serum activity of alkaline phosphatase may be used as an index of the number of functioning osteoblasts and hence disease activity. Since the turnover of bone-derived alkaline phosphatase is of the order of 2 days (Walton et al, 1975), changes in serum alkaline phosphatase reflect fairly precisely the changes in osteoblast release of the enzyme. In evaluating response to treatment, the failure of alkaline phosphatase to change within the first few weeks of treatment, for example with etidronate or clodronate, reflects therefore the delayed response of the osteoblast cell population (Figure 8.1). Similarly, a progressive increase in serum alkaline phosphatase is likely to reflect accurately the integrated changes in osteoblast activity.

Serum alkaline phosphatase measured at intervals in untreated patients remains relatively constant (Woodard, 1959; Nagant de Deuxchaisnes and Krane, 1964). The coefficient of variation of repeated measurements in untreated Paget's disease measured over a period of many months is less than 10 per cent, and is similar during the plateau phase of treatment (Gray et al, 1987). This suggests that any deviation in serum alkaline phosphatase greater than 25 per cent has a high probability of indicating a significant change, and

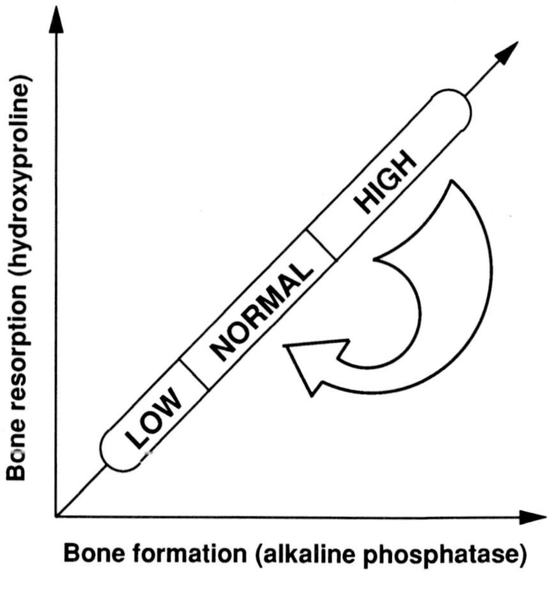

Figure 8.1

Schematic diagram to illustrate the changes in the relationship between indices of bone formation and resorption in Paget's disease with time during treatment with inhibitors of bone resorption. The early effect of treatment is a decrease in bone resorption and a later decrease in bone formation. Thus, patients go through a transient state where formation exceeds resorption. When the new steady state is reached after 3 to 6 months, formation once more matches resorption, albeit at a lower level of bone turnover.

we have found this a useful guide for the assessment of response and relapse to treatment.

Hydroxyproline

Measurements of hydroxyproline in urine provide the other major biochemical marker used to monitor the effects of treatment of Paget's disease. For reasons reviewed in Chapter 4, it is a less satisfactory index than alkaline phosphatase. Because hydroxyproline provides an index of bone resorption there is a different pattern of response and relapse to that seen with alkaline phosphatase, and this provides a useful method for assessing the early effects of treatment until responses are complete. At this time the slope of the relationship between alkaline phosphatase and urinary hydroxyproline does not differ markedly from that in untreated patients (Figure 8.2; Walton et al, 1977) which suggests that in the long-term assessment for treatment either measurement can be used for routine purposes.

Scintigraphy

As reviewed in Chapter 4, scintigraphic activity as assessed by bone scans shows a high correlation with biochemical estimates of disease activity. Moreover, the calcitonins, mithramycin and the diphosphonates all decrease scan uptake and changes correlate closely with changes in serum activity of alkaline phosphatase. This might suggest that scintigraphy is of little additional value in assessing response to treatment. Symptoms and complications of Paget's disease are, however, focal and not solely dependent on the extent of disease. Scintigraphy is useful, therefore, in identifying focal problems at presentation, during treatment and after relapse, particularly with the use of the diphosphonates where relapse may be slow and symptoms of uncertain significance may reappear with only modest increments in disease activity. For these reasons relapse may be detected on scintigraphy before biochemical evidence of relapse, a sequence of events reported in about a third of patients (Vellenga et al, 1981). In patients where biochemical measurements of disease activity lie within the laboratory

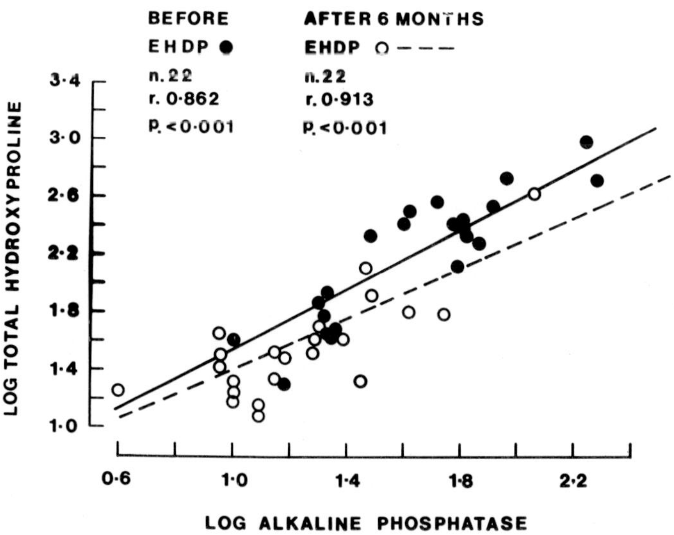

Figure 8.2

Relationship between serum alkaline phosphatase and urinary hydroxyproline excretion in 22 patients with Paget's disease before and after 6 months of treatment with etidronate (5–10 mg/kg per day). Treatment decreased mean values of both measurements, but the relationship between alkaline phosphatase and hydroxyproline before and after treatment is similar.

reference range, bone scanning may be the only objective index of response to treatment.

It is important to recognize that scintigraphic uptake may be abnormally increased despite complete suppression of disease activity. This is probably because of the residual architectural abnormalities in bone.

Clinical responses to treatment for pain

Bone pain

Pain is a common complication of Paget's disease, but its cause is heterogeneous. Pain of bony origin often responds to simple analgesics or to one of the non-steroidal anti-inflammatory drugs. We prefer to give specific treatment such as calcitonin or diphosphonate for bone pain, since a short treatment may induce prolonged relief from pain even in the presence of biochemical evidence of relapse.

Pain relief has been noted in the vast majority of patients in response to treatment with calcitonins, mithramycin and the diphosphonates. Most studies report improvements in approximately 80 per cent of patients in whom pain was attributed to their Paget's disease. In patients with an increase in skin temperature over an affected site, pain relief coincides with a fall in temperature (Woodhouse et al, 1971; Camus et al, 1973). There is a wide variation in response (30–80 per cent) and this almost certainly reflects different causes for pain (Hosking, 1981a). Pain arising from the tibia more commonly responds to treatment than that from the spine (Evans et al, 1977a) which is likely to reflect the heterogeneous cause for pain. It should be recognized that a placebo response is a prominent feature and in some series has been as high as 30 per cent (Khairi et al, 1974; Canfield et al, 1977). There have been relatively few placebo-controlled trials, but the persistence of pain relief suggests that in most instances pain relief is not a placebo effect.

Several controlled trials have shown analgesic effects of calcitonin in other disorders associated with bone pain (Chapter 7). In Paget's disease, a single controlled clinical trial has also shown a significant analgesic effect of calcitonin (Bouvet, 1977). Pain relief occurs within 2–6 weeks and may persist for long periods despite the withdrawal of treatment and a biochemical relapse (Woodhouse et al, 1971; Kanis et al, 1974; Bastian et al, 1977; Martin et al, 1977; Plehwe et al, 1977; Hosking, 1981). For this reason it has been suggested that short courses of calcitonin (such as 50 IU thrice weekly for 6 weeks), repeated as necessary, can be used irrespective of the degree of biochemical control, where treatment is desired solely for pain relief (Kanis et al, 1974).

The rapidity of the effect of calcitonin on bone pain suggests that this cannot be due to its effect on bone remodelling. Calcitonin appears to have inherent analgesic properties and this may provide an explanation in part. There is some evidence that the analgesic effects of salmon calcitonins are greater than those of mammalian calcitonins (Gennari et al, 1983). Skin temperature also falls rapidly over affected sites (Camus et al, 1973; Bouvet, 1977) after calcitonin treatment, as does bone blood flow (Wooton et al, 1978), suggesting that the vascular responses may be important for pain relief.

Similar degrees of pain relief are reported following the use of mithramycin (Hadjipavlou et al, 1977; Ryan and Schwartz, 1980) and the diphosphonates (Altman et al, 1973; Canfield et al, 1977; Khairi et al, 1977; Frijlink et al, 1979; Douglas et al, 1980a; Mautalen et al, 1985; Cantril et al, 1986).

During treatment with diphosphonates pain relief generally occurs later than with the calcitonins and may not be observed until several months after the start of treatment (Altman et al, 1973; Johnston et al, 1980; Delmas et al, 1982). In this respect it is interesting that the rate of decrease in bone blood flow induced by the diphosphonates is slower than with calcitonin, suggesting a vascular basis for bone pain. The relationship between the duration of pain relief and the duration of biochemical control has not been adequately explored with the diphosphonates, but is likely to be related.

With the exception of etidronate, controlled studies of pain relief with the use of diphosphonates have not been undertaken in Paget's disease. However, pain relief has been observed in a number of double-blind studies in other bone disorders, particularly neoplastic disease affecting the skeleton (Elomaa et al, 1983; Siris et al,

1983). Controlled studies using etidronate in Paget's disease have shown a dose-dependent response in bone pain (Altman et al, 1973; Canfield et al, 1977; Ibbertson et al, 1979). The response rate is significantly greater in patients given higher doses of etidronate (10 mg/kg per day) than those given lower doses or placebo treatment (Figure 8.3).

The degree of suppression of bone turnover and its relationship to symptoms has also not been formally explored, but there is anecdotal evidence to suggest a marked degree of heterogeneity between patients. Some patients attain useful remission of pain with modest degrees of suppression of disease activity. In others, the converse is true. We have observed a patient recently in whom many trials of treatment have been given with significant suppression of disease activity, but no effect on bone pain. Pain relief was obtained with more aggressive treatment when serum activity of alkaline phosphatase lay within the normal laboratory reference range, an effect which we (and the patient) have noted with each relapse and treatment irrespective of the agent used (Figure 8.4).

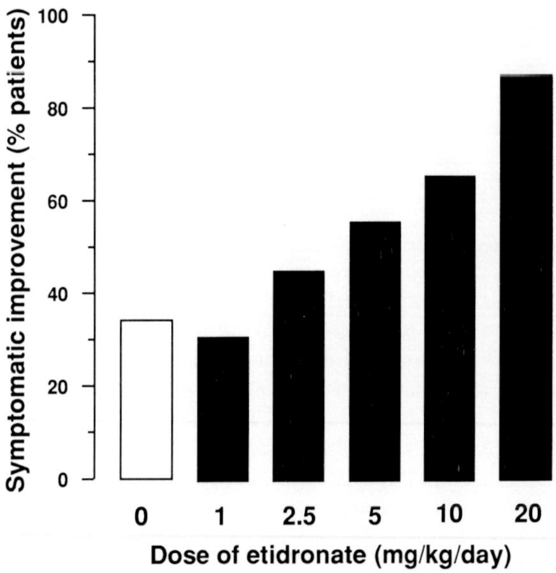

Figure 8.3

Symptomatic response in Paget's disease after 6 months of treatment at the doses shown. In this double-blind study there was a dose-dependent effect between 2.5 and 20 mg/kg per day. (Data from Altman et al, 1973.)

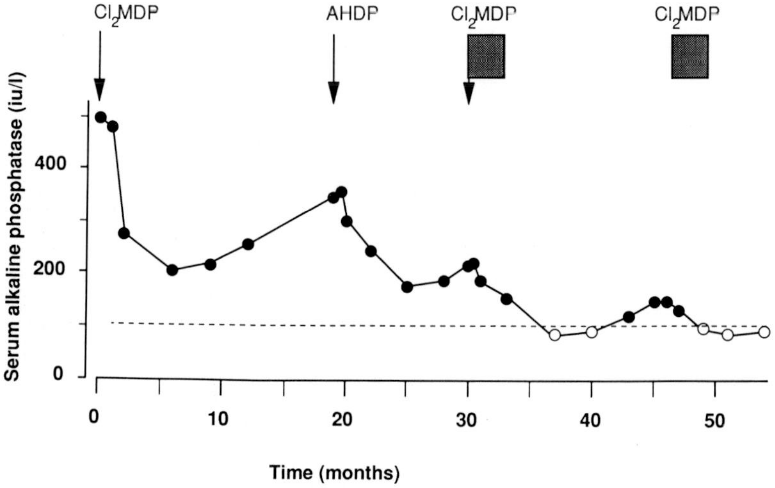

Figure 8.4

Sequential estimations of serum alkaline phosphatase in a patient with a painful pagetic tibia. The patient had fissure fractures which caused pain on weight bearing, but also had pain at rest. Disappearance of rest pain coincided only with suppression of disease activity to normal (open circles). More modest suppressions of disease activity were without effect (AHDP = aminohexane diphosphonate 50 mg iv daily for 5 days; clodronate 300 mg iv daily for 5 days or 1600 mg daily by mouth for the times shown.

Several investigators have reported increases in bone pain following treatment with etidronate or pamidronate, particularly with higher doses when used for prolonged periods (Chapter 7). The incidence of new pain appears to be greater in patients with monostotic disease (Fromm et al, 1979), and in patients who have received multiple treatments with etidronate (Altman, 1985). In addition, most patients with this complication have predominantly osteolytic disease of the long bones of the lower limbs and for this reason and because of possible concerns about fracture we avoid the use of etidronate in such patients.

In those centres where the development of bone pain after treatment is a common problem (Nagant de Deuxchaisnes et al, 1979; Boyce et al, 1984), hyperphosphataemia is frequently observed, suggesting a higher intestinal absorption or unusual sensitivity to etidronate. For this reason the occurrence of hyperphosphataemia during low-dose treatment may alert the physician to future problems, and the dose should be reduced. On the other hand, high serum phosphate values during short-term treatment with high doses (such as 20 mg/kg per day for one month) provide a useful index of compliance (Kanis, 1984). If bone pain occurs during treatment the drug should be stopped.

Headache

It is argued whether Paget's disease of the skull ever gives rise to bone pain, though this has been reported by a number of observers (Davies, 1968; Hamdy, 1981). It has been suggested that much higher doses of calcitonin than commonly recommended should be used to treat headache effectively and to induce radiographic improvement (Hamdy, 1981), but this may be related to the presence of more extensive disease elsewhere (see Chapter 3, Table 3.15).

Non-communicating hydrocephalus may present with chronic headache and is relieved by ventriculo-atrial shunting (Hausser et al, 1984). In other patients it may be relieved by any specific treatment and occasionally patients are seen in whom there appears to be a specific relationship between headache and the degree of biochemical control (Kanis and Gray, 1987; Figure 8.5).

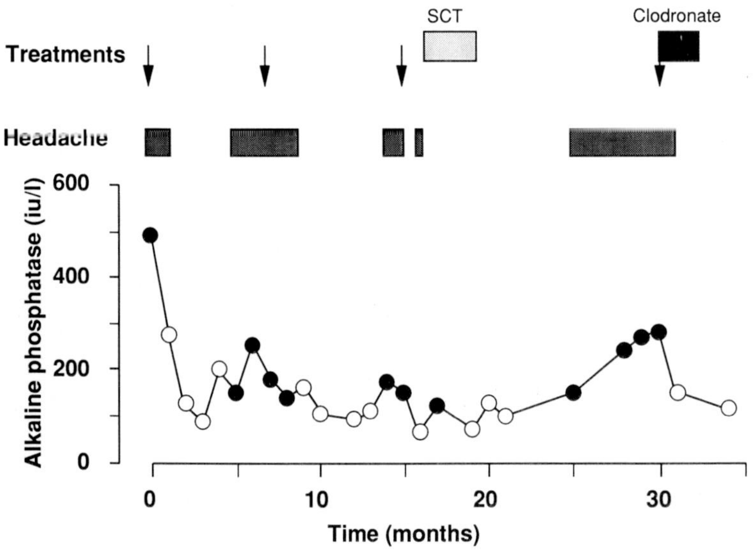

Figure 8.5

Relationship between headache and serum activity of alkaline phosphatase in a patient repeatedly treated with diphosphonates and calcitonin. Note that the remission from pain (signified by open circles) coincided with low disease activity irrespective of the treatments given. Arrows denote intravenous treatments with clodronate (300 mg for 5 days).

Migraine has been reported to respond to calcitonin when associated with Paget's disease (Hamilton and Queseda, 1973) but this may be a chance association. The vascular effects of calcitonin suggest, however, that this phenomenon would merit further investigation.

Osteoarthrosis

The mechanism and thus the treatment of bone pain in Paget's disease is heterogeneous and other causes are the presence of fissure fractures, osteoarthrosis and neurological syndromes.

In practice, the greatest difficulties arise in distinguishing between pain due to Paget's disease, pain due to coexistent osteoarthrosis and joint pain arising from deformity with a change in leg length. Joint pain at the hip, knee or back associated with deformity may be relieved by an appropriate shoe raise.

In the case of suspected osteoarthritic pain it is possible to establish the source by injection of local anaesthetic into the joint space (Stevens, 1981). Our own practice is to give a course of specific treatment, either calcitonin or diphosphonate, and to reassess pain once disease activity has been adequately controlled. We have been surprised by the number of patients with

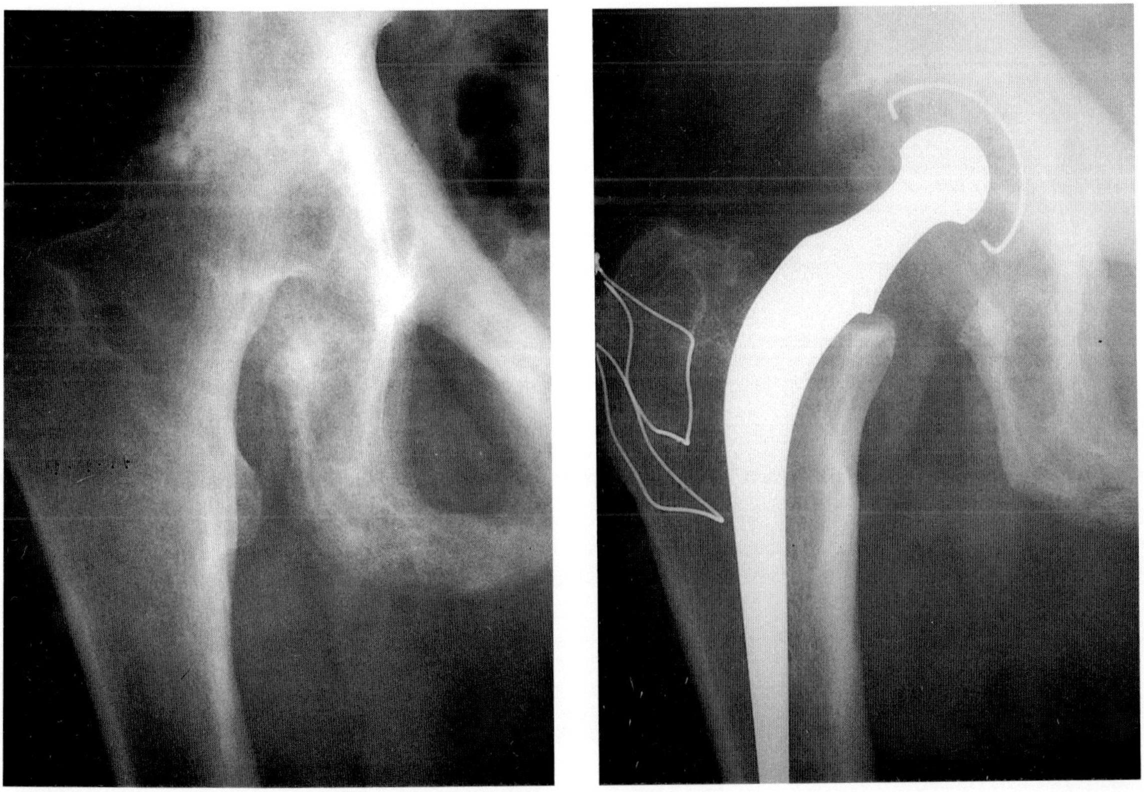

Figure 8.6

Marked coxa plana associated with hip pain and Paget's disease of the pelvis but not the femur. Pain relief occurred after hip replacement. (From Bowie and Kanis, 1977.)

pain thought to be due to osteoarthropathy in whom significant and sustained remission from pain was obtained by medical treatment.

In patients in whom osteoarthrosis at the hip is of sufficient severity not to be controlled by analgesics then replacement arthroplasty is the treatment of choice. The results of surgery are generally excellent, with marked pain relief and restoration of function. Protusio may be corrected by acetabular rings to support the acetabular cup or by the insertion of bone grafts at the acetabular floor (Stauffer and Sim, 1976; Merkow et al, 1984; Broberg and Cass, 1986; McDonald and Sim, 1987; Figure 8.6). An alternative procedure at the hip is subtrochanteric osteotomy (Roper, 1971a). Replacement surgery may also be valuable in patients with osteoarthrosis at the knee, but tibial osteotomy may be considered in young patients with arthrosis of one compartment. There have been significant recent advances in joint replacement surgery of the knee with the use of constrained (linked) or unconstrained prostheses. Surgery is technically easier than at the hip, but revision surgery is more problematic. If the life of knee prostheses proves durable, then it is likely that knee replacement will assume a much more important role in the management of pagetic osteoarthrosis at this site than is presently the case.

Pagetic bone is highly vascular so that bleeding may be profuse (Dove, 1980) and adequate provision for transfusion is a wise precaution. Blood loss from total hip replacement surgery is on average twice that observed at unaffected hips (Goutallier et al, 1984). For this reason it has been suggested that pretreatment of underlying Paget's disease would be an advantage (Bowie and Kanis, 1976). If rapid effects are required, then

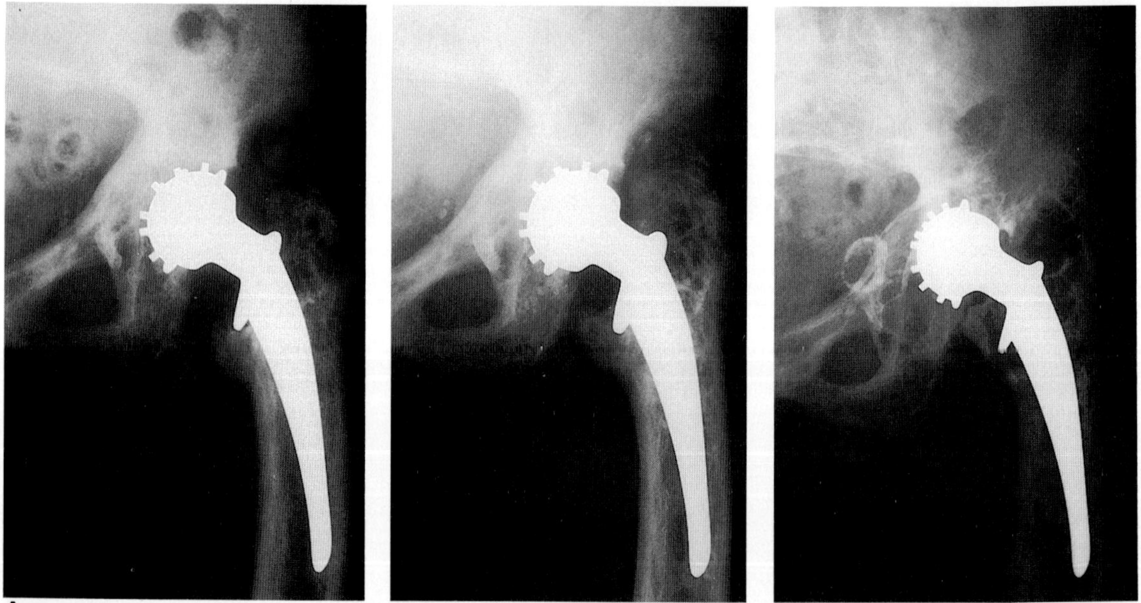

A B C

Figure 8.7

Sequential radiographs in a patient with Paget's disease of the femur and acetabular wall. The patient had surgery for pain (McKee–Farrar arthroplasty). (A) shows the immediate postoperative result. Over the ensuing 18 months the patient developed pain and the prosthesis sank into the femoral shaft (B). Two years later the prosthesis had sunk still further and there was medial migration through the acetabular wall (C).

calcitonin is the preferred agent since its effects on bone blood flow occur over weeks rather than over months, as seen with the diphosphonates (Wooton et al, 1978).

Prostheses may be difficult to fit because of deformity or sclerotic bone, or more arguably difficult to maintain in place when fixed within the soft bone that is found in 25 per cent of cases (Dove, 1980; Figure 8.7). It may be desirable, therefore, to pretreat patients medically for longer periods before surgical intervention. It is not known whether the outcome of surgery can be improved by prolonged pre-operative or post-operative treatment, but this seems possible since the need for revision is somewhat greater in pagetic arthroplasty than in the general community (McDonald and Sim, 1987). On the other hand, coxarthropathy is likely to be progressive if left, even with good medical management (Figure 8.8), and surgical intervention should not be unnecessarily delayed.

In patients with extensive osteophytosis there may be an increased risk of heterotopic ossification (Merkow et al, 1984). In such cases etidronate, if used early enough, preferably at the time of surgery, appears to decrease the extent of heterotopic calcification but does not prevent it (Bijvoet et al, 1974). Large doses are required (20 mg/kg per day) for several weeks until the patient is fully mobile. Although calcification reappears when treatment is stopped, the ultimate effects on mobilization are improved by avoiding calcification in the early postoperative period.

Other causes of pain

The management of fissure fractures, sarcoma and neurological syndromes are discussed later.

Bony quality, enlargement and deformity

Woven bone formation, enlargement and deformity of bones give rise to many of the mechanical complications of Paget's disease. It is clear that disease activity can be controlled for many years when diphosphonates are given intermittently or calcitonin given continuously. There is now good evidence to suggest that suppression of disease activity significantly improves the quality of bone.

The decrease in bone turnover induced by treatment appears to be associated with a resumption of formation of lamellar rather than woven bone formation, irrespective of the agent given (Woodhouse et al, 1971; Khairi et al, 1977; Alexandre et al, 1981a; Meunier et al, 1982; Russell et al, 1984; Yates et al, 1985; Plates 28 and 29). If lamellar bone formation were to continue with adequate long-term management and to be subject to the normal factors that regulate the modelling and remodelling of bone, it might be supposed that long-term treatment would result in the gradual improvement of bony enlargement and deformity. Any such improvement in skeletal architecture would, however, be a slow process because these agents reduce bone turnover towards normal and correspondingly increase the turnover time of the affected skeleton.

Radiographic change

Few centres have been involved in the precise radiographic assessment of Paget's disease and its response to treatment. Such centres have emphasized that radiographic changes that are designated as improvements should not occur in the natural history of the untreated disorder. A reduction in bone size, a widening of the medullary cavity, improved corticomedullary differentiation and more uniform cortical density are all changes which, if found, have been considered to be due to treatment. In addition, a halt in the resorption front or increased radiographic density of the resorption phase of Paget's disease may also be taken to indicate a treatment-dependent effect (Doyle et al, 1974a, 1980; Nagant de Deuxchaisnes et al, 1977, 1979, 1982). In assessing radiographic changes, it is important to ensure that serial radiographs are reproducibly positioned because small rotational errors will give rise to large but spurious changes (Figure 3.65).

An increase in radiodensity is well documented with the use of calcitonins as is an improvement in cortico-medullary differentiation (Nagant de Deuxchaisnes et al, 1977, 1980b; Doyle et al, 1980; Murphy et al, 1980; Whyte et al, 1985;

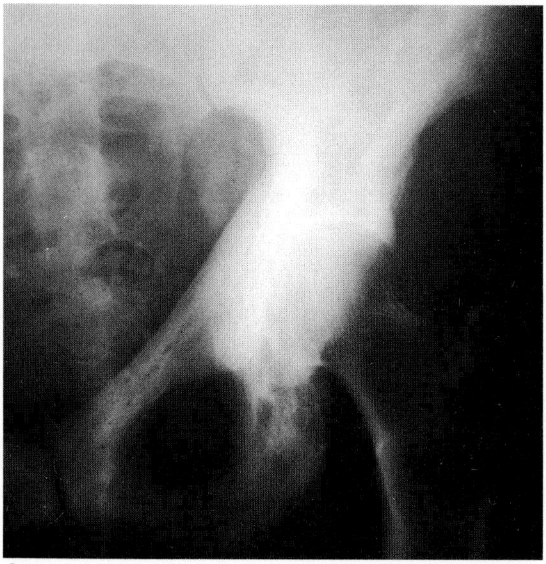
A

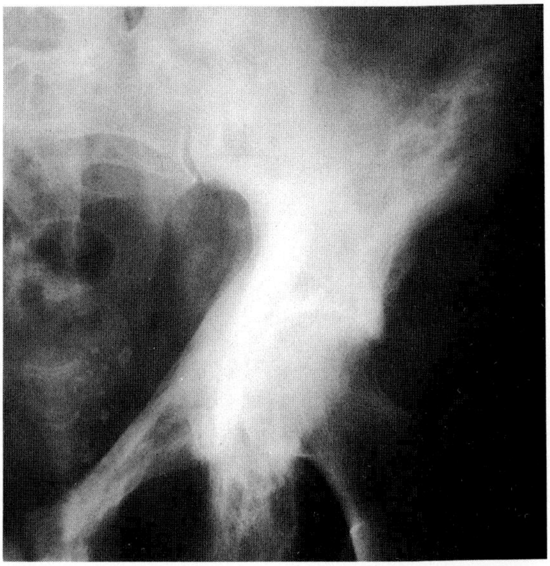
B

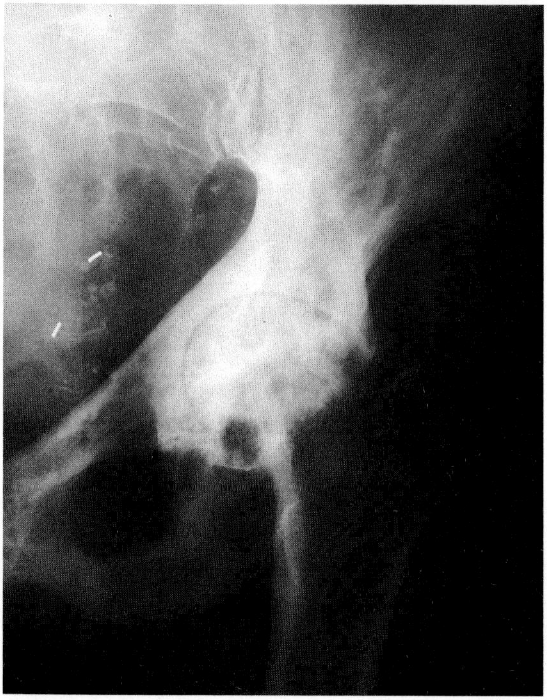
C

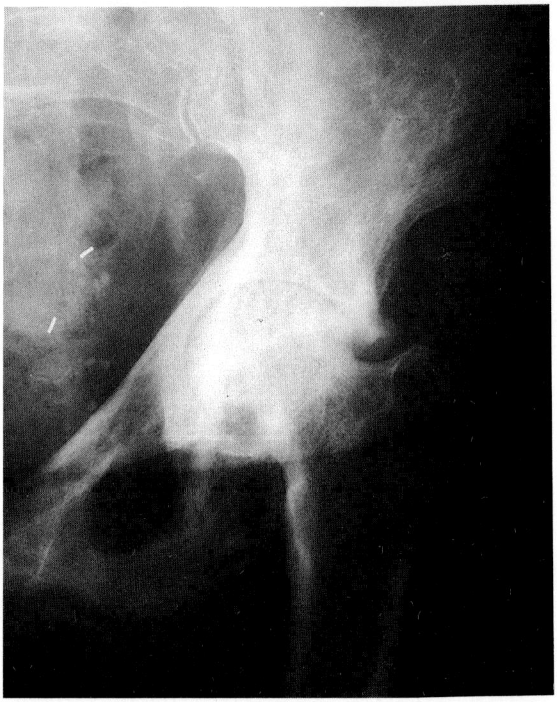
D

Figure 8.8

Sequential radiographs of the hip in a patient with Paget's disease of both sides of the hip joint. The first film (A) shows hypertrophy of the medial wall of the hip and concentric narrowing of the hip joint space. Two years later the appearances remained unchanged except that the medial wall had increased in width (B). Over the next 12 years there was progressive medial migration of the femoral head (C,D,E) seen by the decreasing width of the acetabular wall. There was also progressive coxa plana. During the 3-year span between (C) and (E) the patient's disease was well controlled with diphosphonates.

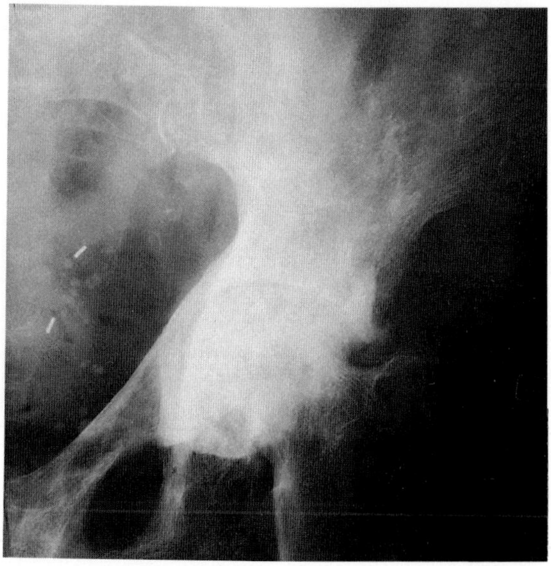

E

Figure 8.8 *(continued)*

Figures 8.9 and 8.10). This is an expected consequence of a decrease in bone turnover (Chapter 2). Prolonged treatment may alter bone shape (Doyle et al, 1980), an effect more marked and rapid in young patients (Doyle et al, 1974a). A decrease in external diameter has been observed in untreated patients (Lander and Hadjipavlou, 1986a) but this is very rare and a decrease, therefore, suggests a treatment-specific response.

As might be predicted, the radiographic changes with calcitonin are particularly evident with osteolytic Paget's disease (Figure 8.11; Woodhouse et al, 1972, 1977; DeRose et al, 1974; Doyle et al, 1974a; Nagant de Deuxchaisnes et al, 1977, 1980b; Murphy et al, 1980a,b; Whyte et al, 1981, 1985).

Short courses of calcitonin do not halt the advance of the resorption front, although the junction between abnormal and normal bone may become less distinct (Nagant de Deuxchaisnes et al, 1977). More prolonged treatment appears to prevent extension in almost all patients in whom this has been evaluated when doses of 50–100 IU daily are used (Doyle et al, 1974a; Nagant de Deuxchaisnes et al, 1977; Woodhouse et al, 1977; Nagant de Deuxchaisnes, 1989).

It has been suggested that the doses needed to halt the resorption front are greater than those needed to obtain maximal biochemical suppression (Doyle et al, 1974; Singer et al, 1980), particularly for osteoporosis circumscripta (Woodhouse et al, 1971; Whyte et al, 1981). The halt of disease extension contrasts with observations made on untreated patients in whom radiographic advance of the disease occurred in 20–30 per cent of patients followed over two years (Woodhouse et al, 1977).

Less work has been undertaken to evaluate the radiographic effects of the diphosphonates and mithramycin. In the case of mithramycin, radiographic improvements have been noted but probably occur less frequently than with calcitonin (Ryan, 1977), perhaps due to the shorter and less marked suppression of disease activity.

Radiographic improvements have been observed in osteolytic disease following treatment with etidronate (Murphy et al, 1980b; Altman, 1985). Intracortical resorption areas may become less radiotranslucent with low doses of etidronate (5–10 mg/kg; Dodd et al, 1987). More frequently they increase in size with a 10 mg dose. In one series 20 per cent of lesions improved but 50 per cent deteriorated (Dodd et al, 1987). Marked increases in radiographic translucency may be observed with doses of 20 mg/kg when given for long periods (3–6 months), particularly in patients with pre-existing osteolysis due to the impairment of mineralization of osteoid (see Plate 26).

In contrast, others have shown a consistent failure of etidronate to heal intracortical resorption clefts using recommended doses (Table 8.2; Lander and Hadjipavlou, 1986; Nagant de Deuxchaisnes et al, 1979, 1980b). In addition, no halt of resorption fronts was observed (Figure 8.12). However, one of these centres has unusual experience with the use of etidronate with, as mentioned previously, a higher apparent incidence of treatment-related bone pain and hyperphosphataemia. It seems possible, therefore, that these radiographic effects (observed in other centres with the use of high doses of etidronate) (Finerman et al, 1976) may be due to an increased susceptibility to or greater bioavailability of the drug. These investigators suggest that etidronate

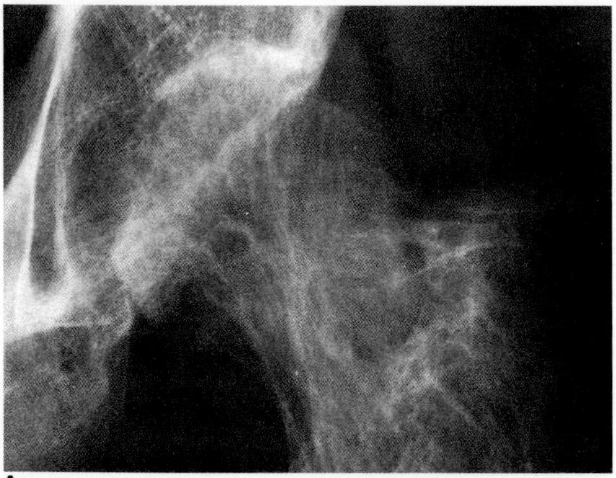
A

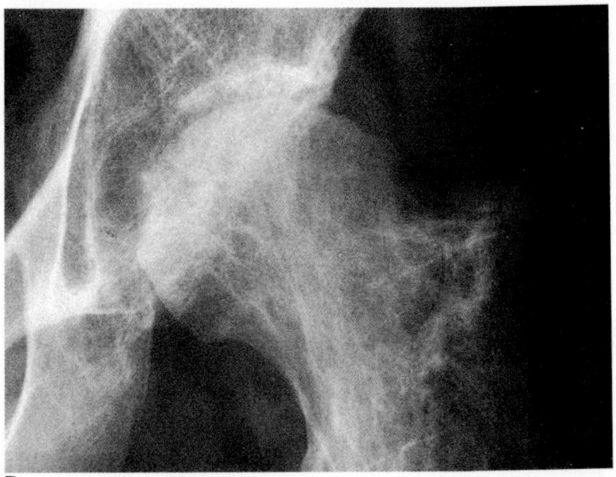
B

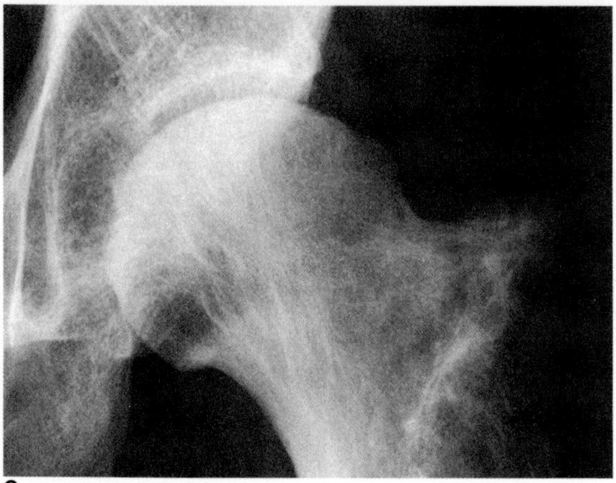
C

Figure 8.9

Anteroposterior radiograph of left hip in a 28-year-old patient before and during treatment with human calcitonin (0.5 mg daily). Note marked osteopaenia before treatment (A) so that the joint space is barely definable. After 1 month of treatment (B) there was increased radiographic density with redefinition of the joint. (C) After 6 months of continuous treatment there was a further increase in density, particularly of the medial cortex of the femoral neck. (From Whyte et al, 1985.)

has 'adverse effects on skeletal architecture', but it seems more likely that the apparent osteolysis is due to the formation of unmineralized bone rather than to a change in skeletal architecture.

Remineralization of osteoid occurs rapidly after short courses of treatment (Preston et al, 1986), but may be delayed after stopping more prolonged treatment (Finerman et al, 1976; Nagant de Deuxchaisnes et al, 1979). Where marked osteolysis has been induced, the drug should be stopped. Treatment with calcitonin appears to reverse the lesion (Figure 7.39; Table 8.2; Nagant de Deuxchaisnes et al, 1979) and is worthy of trial if osteopaenia is associated with bone pain.

The other diphosphonates also halt the resorption front and more consistently increase skeletal radiodensity. Changes have been well documented with pamidronate (Nagant de Deuxchaisnes et al, 1982b; Vellenga et al, 1985; Cantrill et al, 1986; Dodd et al, 1987; Figures 8.13 and 8.14). The resorption front is consistently halted in addition to the expected consequences of

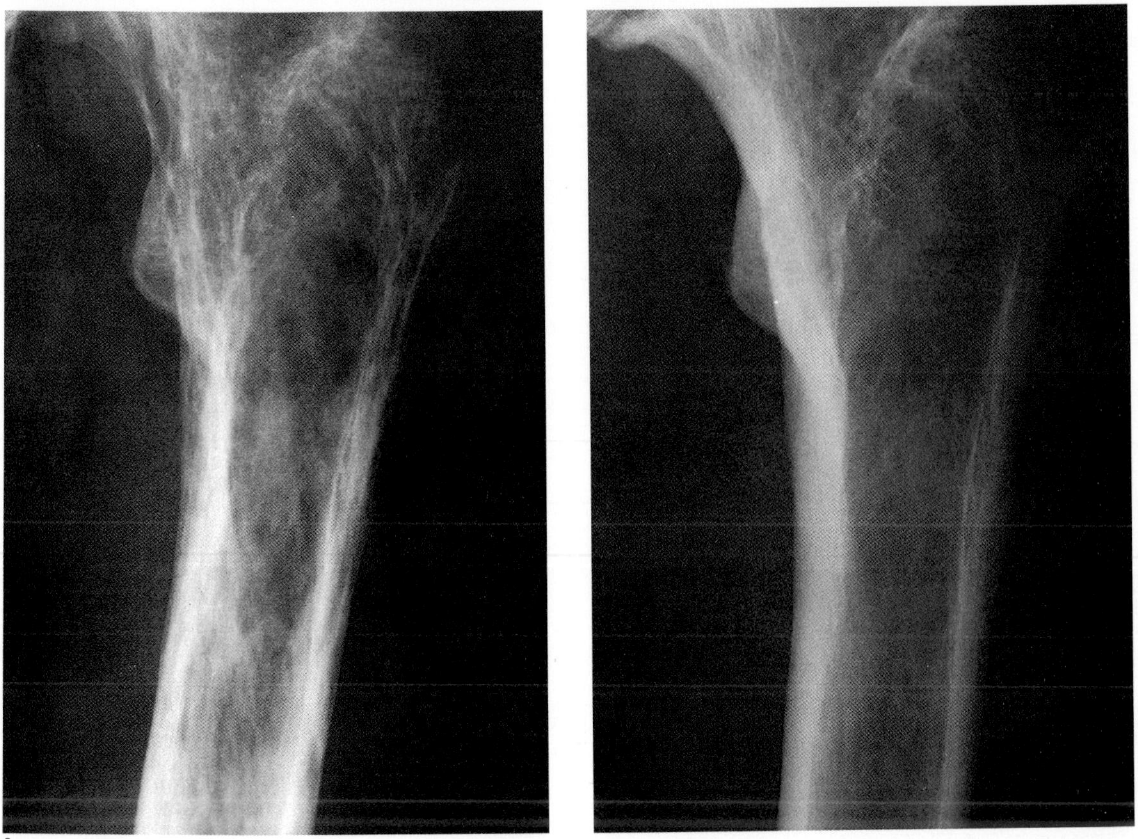

A B

Figure 8.10

Radiograph of the proximal shaft of the left femur (A) before and (B) after 10 months of continuous treatment with human calcitonin, 0.5 mg daily. Note the increased corticomedullary definition and more normal trabecular architecture. (From Whyte et al, 1985.)

Table 8.2 Radiographic changes interpreted as improvements or deterioration in (a) patients sequentially treated with calcitonin or etidronate and (b) patients given calcitonin alone or in combination with etidronate (from Nagant de Deuxchaisnes et al, 1980).

Treatment	*Improvement*		*Deterioration*	
	No of sites	*No of sites/ patient*	*No of sites*	*No of sites/ patient*
(*a*) Calcitonin	36	7.2	0	0
Etidronate	1	0.2	22	4.4
(*b*) Calcitonin	35	5.8	0	0
Calcitonin + etidronate	13	2.2	14	2.3

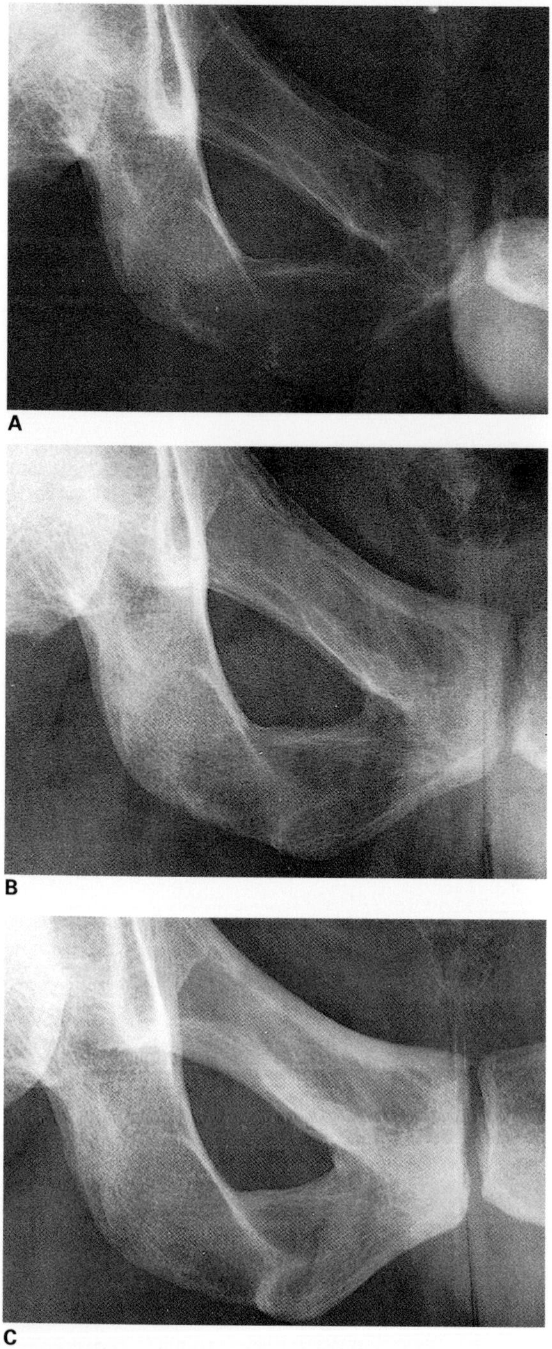

A

B

C

Figure 8.11

Anteroposterior radiograph of the right ischium and pubis before (A) and after 1 (B) and 6 (C) months of treatment with human calcitonin, 0.5 mg daily. Note the progressive disappearance of the resorption front and reconstitution of the cortex. (From Whyte et al, 1985.)

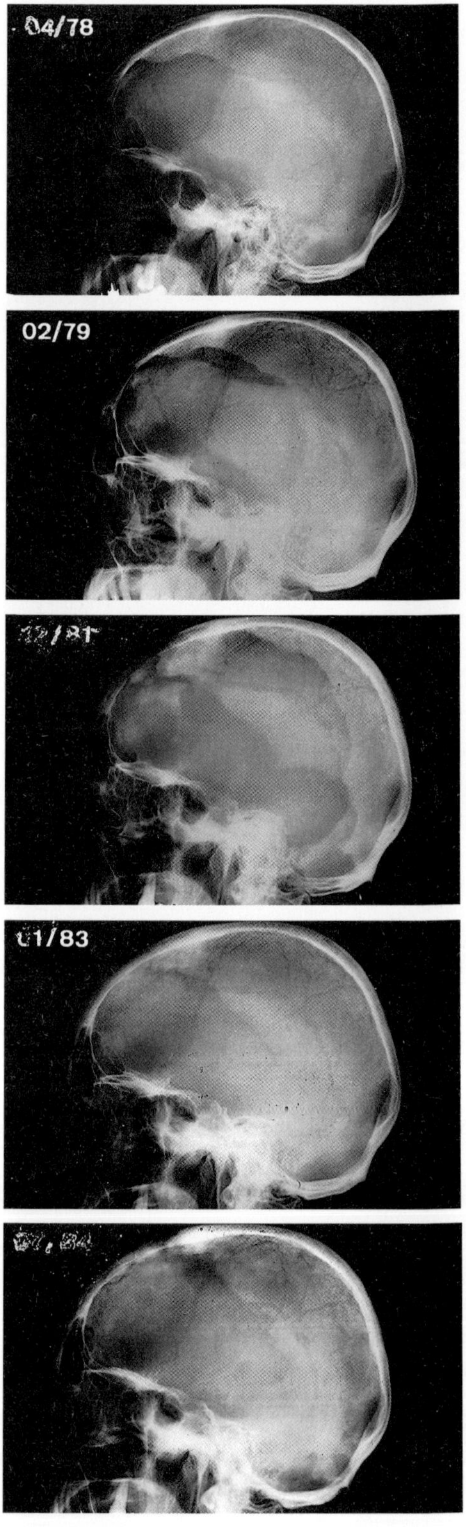

A

B

C

D

E

Figure 8.12 (facing page)

Sequential radiographs showing osteoporosis circumscripta of the skull in a patient (A) before and (B) after 10 months of treatment with etidronate (5.5 mg/kg per day). Note the increase in radiodensity but the advance of the resorption front. Following a period of treatment for 28 months (C), extension of the front occurred with resorption of the radiodense islands. Following treatment with pamidronate (400 mg daily for 1 year; D) there was a marked decrease in radiotranslucency and an apparent regression of the resorption front. During an 18-month treatment-free period patchy regression occurred giving a mottled appearance (E). (From Nagant de Deuxchaisnes, 1989.)

decreased bone remodelling. Similar changes have been noted with clodronate and aminobutane diphosphonate (Altman, 1985; Kanis and Gray, 1987; Figures 8.15, 8.16). When relapse occurs after diphosphonate treatment there may be a characteristic rim of radiotranslucency evident at the resorption front (Gray et al, 1987; Anderson et al, 1988; Figure 8.16). Infilling of intracortical resorption clefts appears to be a less consistent effect with pamidronate than with calcitonin (Nagant de Deuxchaisnes et al, 1982b; Dodd et al, 1987). With the exception of etidronate, other diphosphonates have not been compared with calcitonin.

Deformity and enlargement

The favourable histological and radiographic effects observed with treatment suggest that progressive enlargement and deformity of Paget's disease might be prevented with effective long-term treatment, but do not help us to determine whether deformity may be reversed. The potential techniques available for examining this question are limited. The improvement of neurological syndromes in Paget's disease might be taken as evidence for the reversal of structural

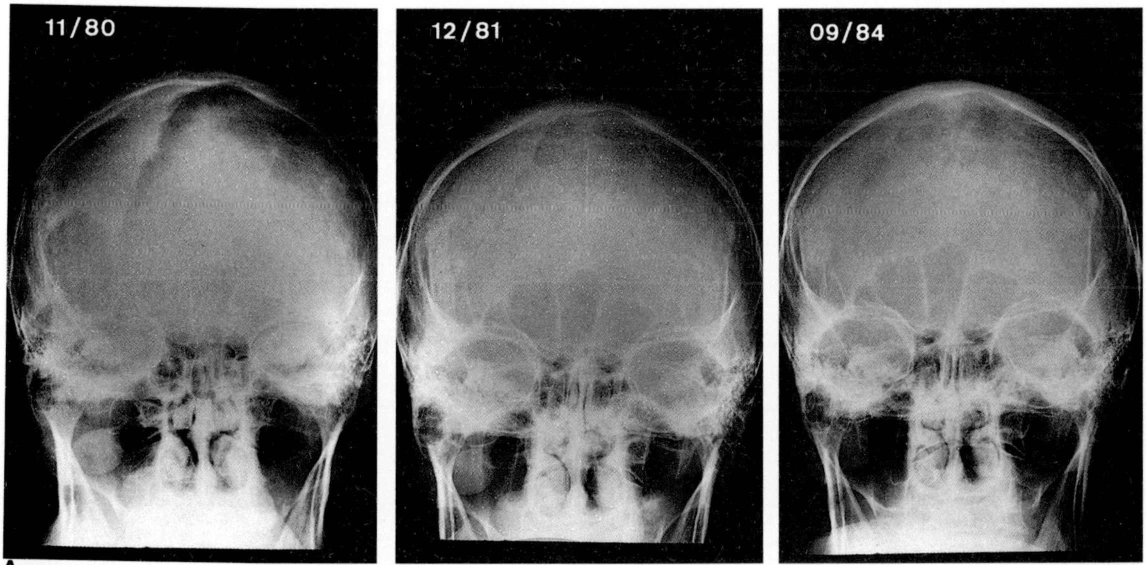

A B C

Figure 8.13

Partial regression of osteoporosis circumscripta during treatment with pamidronate. (A) before treatment, (B) after 12 months of treatment (600 mg daily) and (C) 3 years after treatment was stopped. (From Nagant de Deuxchaisnes, 1989.)

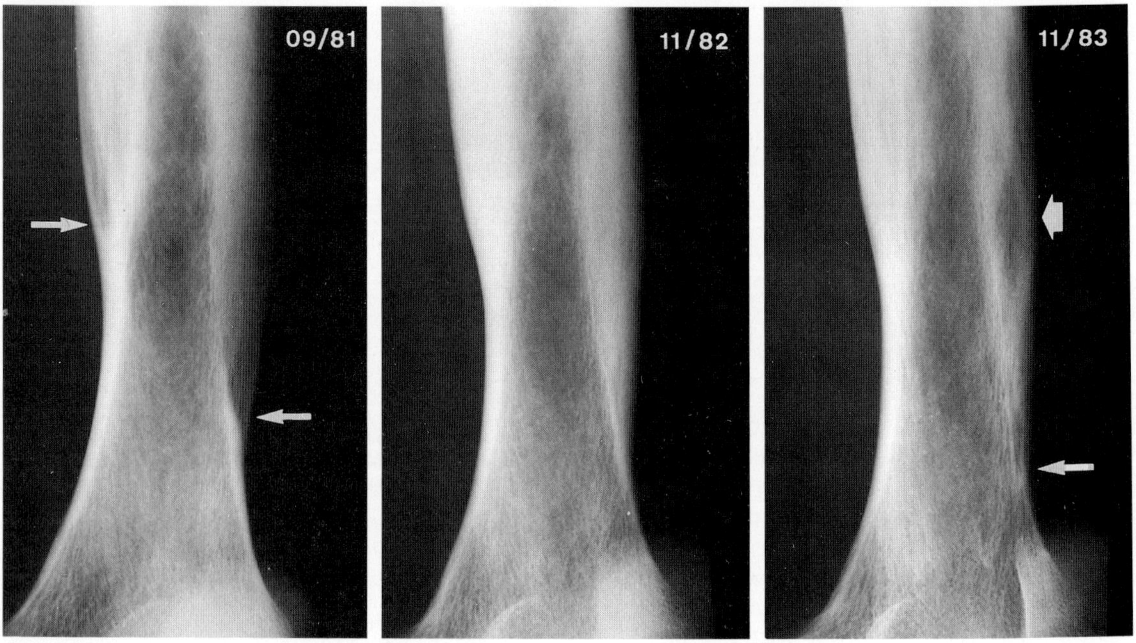

Figure 8.14

Sequential radiographs of the distal femur at the dates shown (A) before and (B) after 12 months' treatment with pamidronate, 600 mg daily. Note the infilling of the resorption front (thin arrows). After treatment was stopped (C) a new area of osteolysis appeared (thick arrow) with extension of the resorption front. (From Nagant de Deuxchaisnes, 1989.)

abnormalities, but in many instances these syndromes are related to the abnormal vascularity of pagetic bone, and clinical improvement in neurological complications cannot necessarily be taken as evidence for structural improvement (reviewed later).

As mentioned previously, bone size may be decreased following treatment with the calcitonins (Doyle et al, 1974, 1980) and this may also occur with the diphosphonates (Figure 8.17). However, the changes are often unconvincing because of the difficulties of ensuring radiographic reproducibility. An interesting technique has recently been developed which may help in the sequential assessment of bone shape or volume. This is the use of serial computerized axial tomography and the subtraction of sequential images (Bone et al, 1990; Figure 8.18).

An approach that we have used to minimize repositional errors is to undertake stereophotography of superficial bony sites affected by Paget's disease (Burke, 1971). These techniques have been applied to patients with disease of the facial bones or the skull, since the deformity is in

Figure 8.15

Sequential lateral (A,B,C) and anteroposterior (D,E,F) radiographs of the tibia before (left and centre) and following a 5-day treatment with alendronate (right). Before treatment a resorption front and intracortical resorption clefts were evident and progressed during the 8 months between X-ray examinations (16.5 mm/year). Eight months after treatment the resorption front and clefts were infilled.

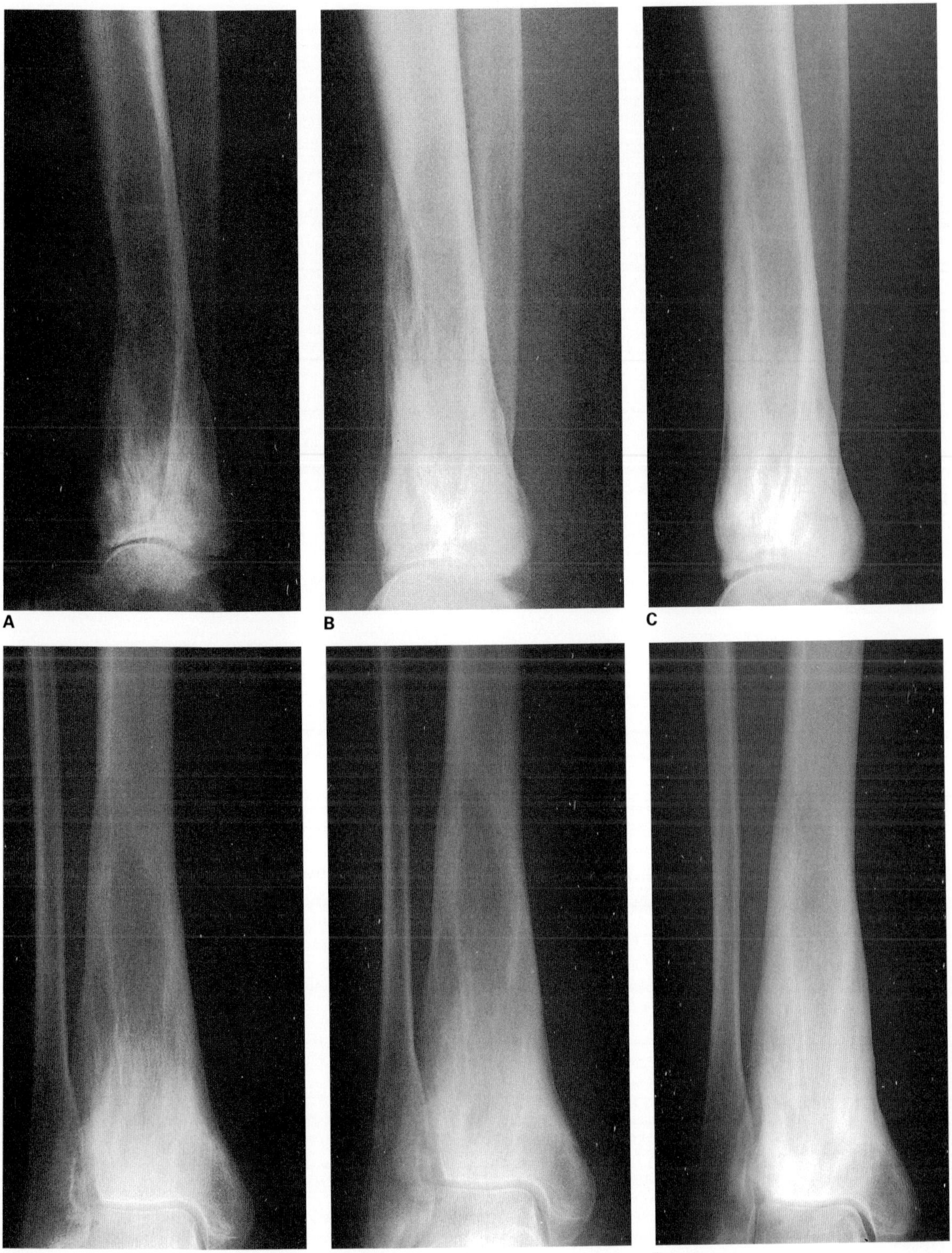
A
B
C
D
E
F

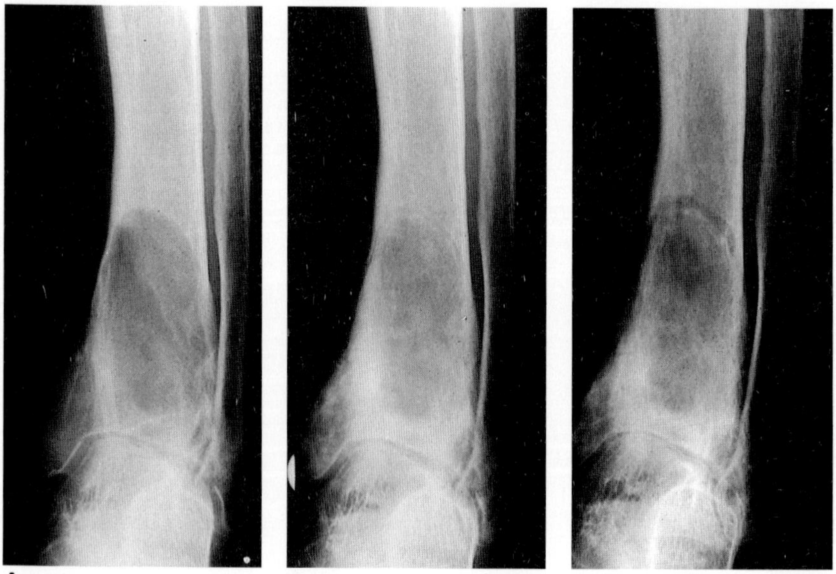

A B C

Figure 8.16

Radiographic effects of clodronate in osteolytic Paget's disease of the tibia. Before treatment (A) a marked resorption front is observed. The patient was treated with intravenous clodronate for one week, which resulted in biochemical suppression of disease activity and a halt in the resorption front and increased radiodensity (B). Biochemical relapse was associated with progression of the resorption front (C). Note the small osteolytic rim at the interface between normal and pagetic bone at the start of relapse. (From Kanis and Gray, 1987.)

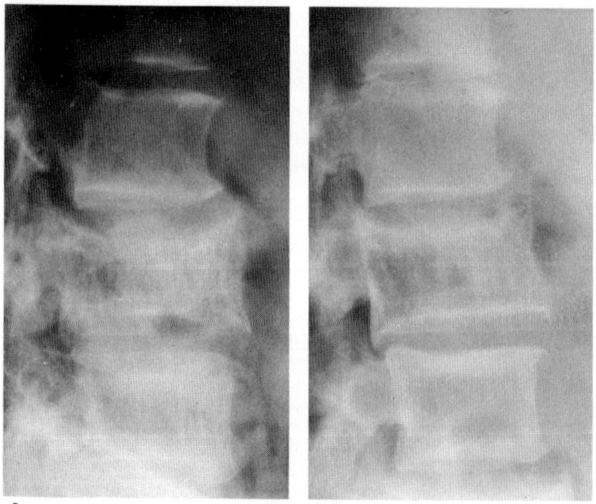

A B

Figure 8.17

Radiographs of the lumbar spine before (A) and during treatment (B) with intermittent courses of clodronate. During the 44-month interval disease activity was consistently suppressed by 60 per cent or greater. No changes in vertebral dimensions were observed at the upper vertebral site (L2). The expanded vertebra at L2 showed a decrease in width of 4 mm during treatment.

part due to the underlying changes in the shape of the bone. These studies suggest that long-term suppression of disease activity is associated with a decrease in skull or facial volume and the restoration of a more normal shape (Bickerstaff et al, 1990; Figures 8.19 and 8.20). Comparable changes are not observed at sites unaffected by Paget's disease. These observations have extremely important implications for long-term medical management, because not only may progressive deformity be arrested, but adequate modelling of bone may also occur.

Well-established deformities are clearly not correctable by medical management alone. The occurrence of fracture in a long bone presents an opportunity to correct deformity. Elective surgical correction of deformity has been undertaken to reduce abnormal mechanical loads on adjacent joints, to relieve pain from fissure fractures and for cosmetic and dental reasons (Merle d'Aubigne and Witvoet, 1966; Meyers et al, 1978). In our own experience, surgical osteotomy at the tibia has produced excellent results both cosmetically and when deformity has been associated with pain

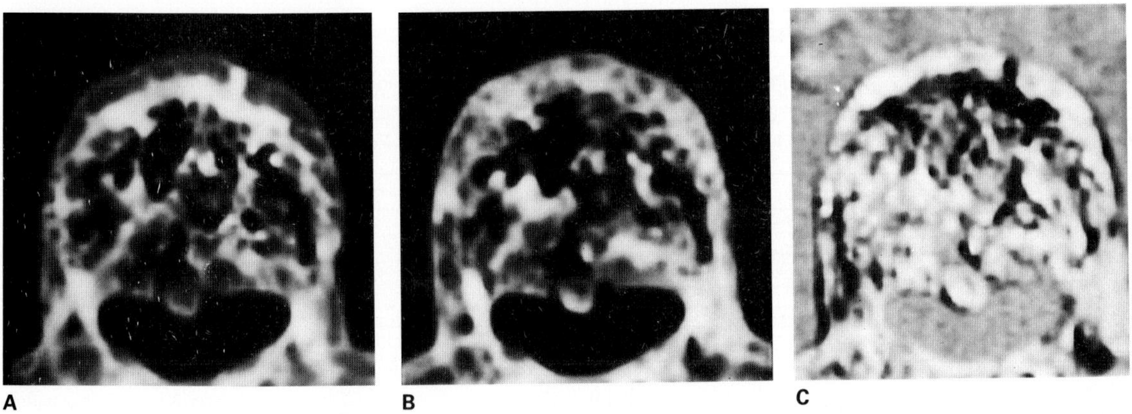

Figure 8.18

High-resolution axial tomography of the lumbar spine in Paget's disease and the effect of treatment. (A) shows the pretreatment image (1 mm thick) of the fourth lumbar vertebra at the midvertical level. The image shows lytic and sclerotic lesions characteristic of Paget's disease. Note in particular the low density of the anterior cortical rim. (B) shows the CAT image at the same site 6 months after daily injections of 0.5 mg human calcitonin. Areas of sclerosis have become less dense, and lytic regions have increased in density. The anterior cortical edge has been filled in with new bone. (C) shows the subtraction scan where the first image has been digitally subtracted from the second, so that white regions represent bone gain and dark regions indicate bone loss. (From Bone et al, 1989.)

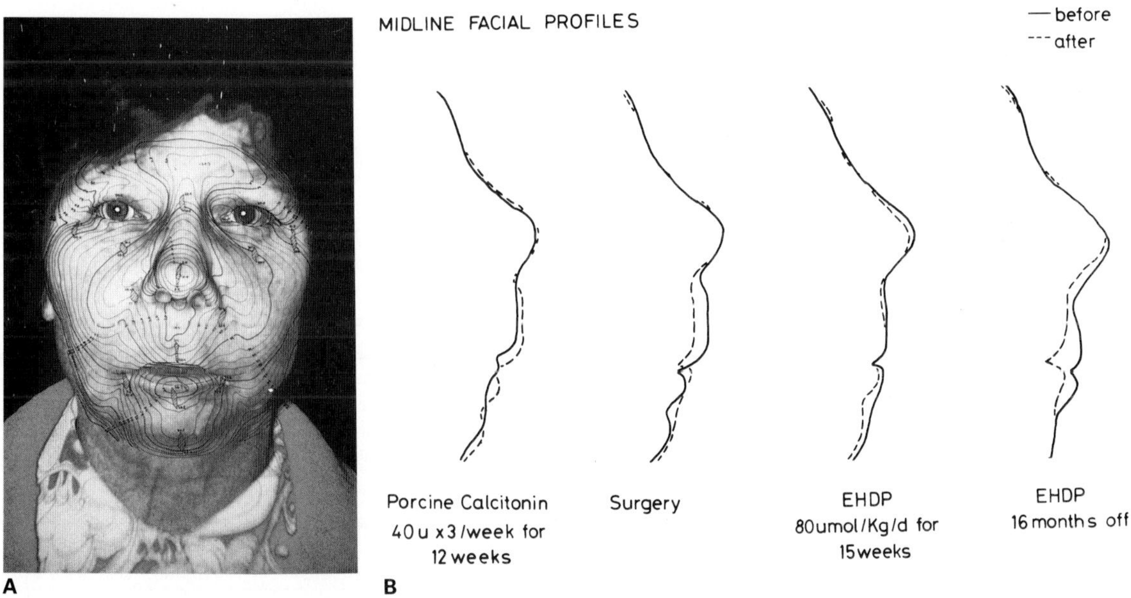

Figure 8.19

Stereological evaluation of Paget's disease. (A) The patient had Paget's disease of the maxilla. Stereologically derived contour lines of the face are superimposed. These enabled contour profiles to be computed and sequential estimations of the mid-line facial profile are shown on (B). A short course of calcitonin had little significant effect; the effects of maxillary surgery are more evident. Whereas a short course of subsequent treatment with etidronate (EHDP) had little effect, significant improvement in mid-line facial profile occurred following a sustained biochemical remission of disease activity. (From Kanis and Gray, 1987.)

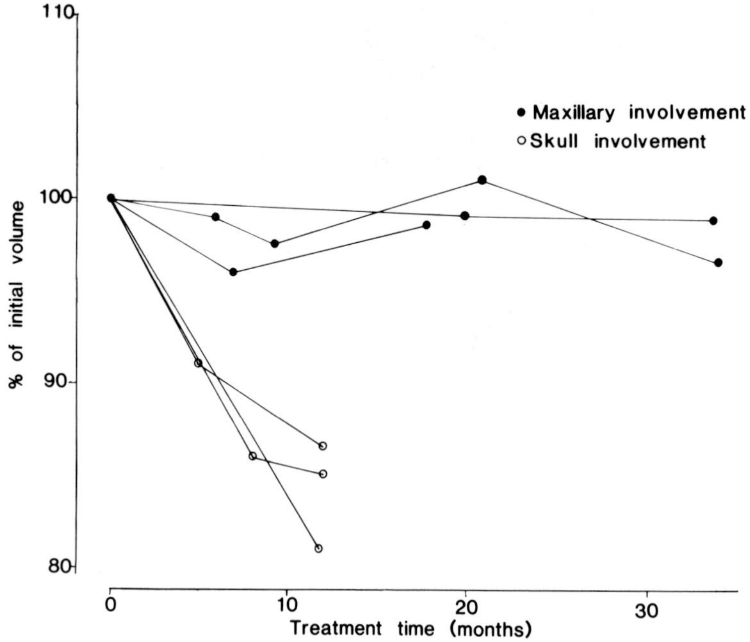

Figure 8.20

Effects of suppression of disease activity in six patients with Paget's disease treated with diphosphonates. Three patients with Paget's disease affecting the anterior skull vault (○) showed a decrease in volume whereas skull volume did not change in those patients with Paget's disease elsewhere (●). (Adapted from Bickerstaff et al, 1990.)

(Figure 8.21). As for hip surgery, medical treatment before and after elective surgery for deformity may be advantageous (Meyers et al, 1978).

Fracture

Fissure fracture

There is no formal evidence that medical treatment, with the calcitonins, the diphosphonates or any other agent, significantly alters the natural history of fissure fractures (Hosking, 1977; Redden et al, 1981). In contrast, we and others have observed healing during treatment with calcitonin in the occasional patient, despite the persistence of fissure fracture for many years before treatment (Figures 8.22 and 8.23). In most instances fissure fractures do not heal spontaneously (Figure 8.24) and it is tempting to suggest that calcitonin may have accelerated healing. It is difficult to be sure however that the association of healing with treatment is not fortuitous. This is a question that can only be addressed by controlled trials, but in the absence of information from prospective studies, it seems reasonable to give a trial of treatment with calcitonin for fissure fractures associated with pain or at sites vulnerable to complete fracture. There is some clinical and experimental evidence that calcitonin accelerates fracture healing (reviewed later), which strengthens this opinion.

Fortunately, most fissure fractures are asymptomatic, but bone pain caused by fissure fracture which persists after otherwise adequate medical treatment is a very difficult problem to manage. The sudden development of bone pain at the site of a fissure fracture may herald its extension, and prophylactic surgical intervention is the treatment of choice where feasible. Complete fractures of the femoral neck carry an increased risk of

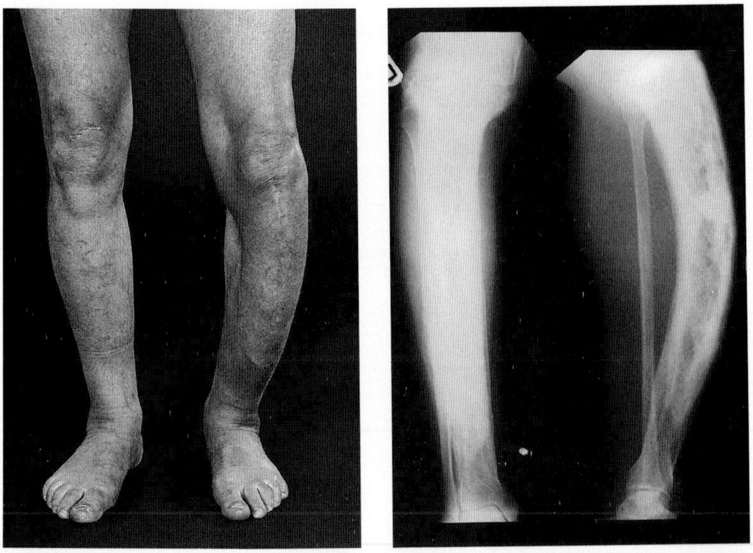

A B

Figure 8.21

(A) Clinical photograph and (B) radiograph of a patient with deformity of the left tibia due to Paget's disease. Following suppression of disease activity with diphosphonates, the patient underwent elective surgical osteotomy (C,D,E).

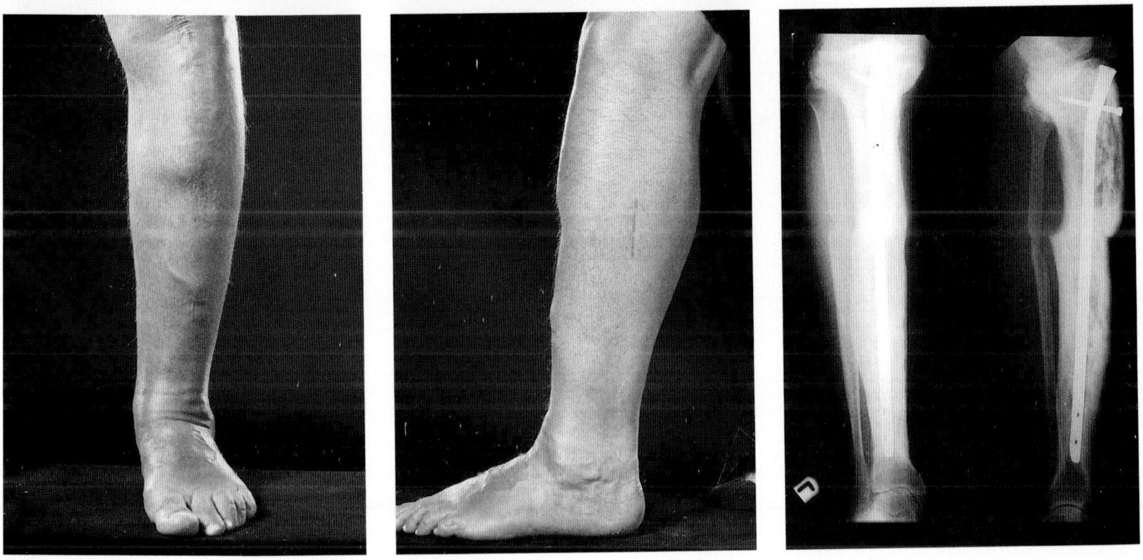

C D E

delayed union (Chapter 5) and some consider that even asymptomatic fissure fracture at this site should be managed surgically.

Persistent pain at the site of fissure fractures may be managed by external splinting, which is more readily applied to the tibia than to the femur. This commonly improves symptoms, but healing of fractures is rare, and symptoms reappear when splinting is discontinued (Figure 8.24). In a small series of patients with multiple fissure fractures and bone pain we have been impressed by the pain relief and the occasional

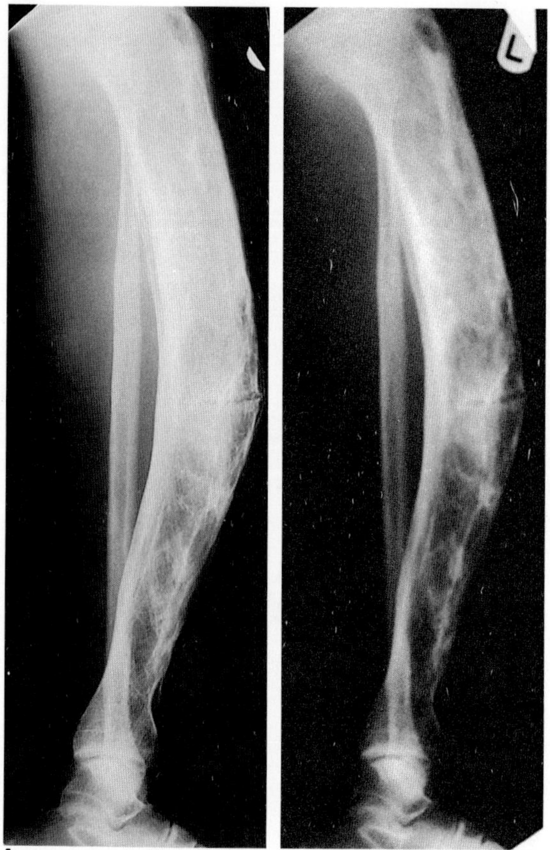

A B

Figure 8.22

Lateral radiograph of the leg showing anterior bowing deformity of the left tibia with an extensive fissure fracture of the anterior aspect (A). The fracture had been present for 12 years and was treated by external splinting with a cast brace. Two years later (B) the fracture had healed. In the intervening time the patient was treated with intramuscular porcine calcitonin (160 MRC units daily im, six times weekly for 2 months followed by thrice weekly injections for 23 months).

healing of other fissure fractures that occurred after surgical osteotomy (Figures 8.25 and 8.26). The healing of adjacent fissure fractures has also been noted after accidental fracture (Barry, 1969; Figure 8.27) and this would argue for a more aggressive surgical approach to the management of painful fissures than is generally adopted.

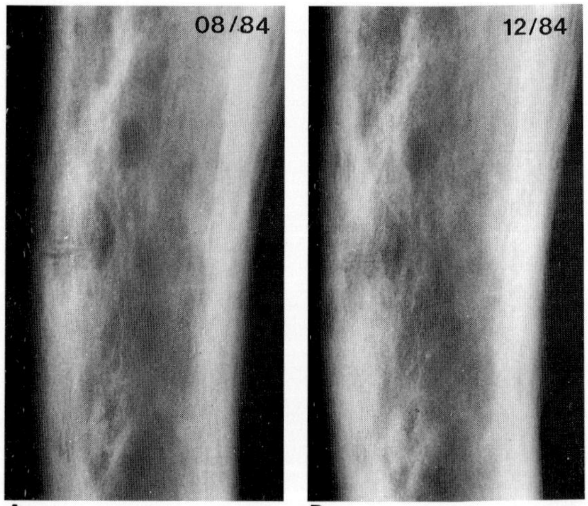

A B

Figure 8.23

A fissure fracture in a tibia (A) before and (B) after treatment with salmon calcitonin (100 IU/day) for 4 months. Note the partial healing by its walling off within cortical bone. (From Nagant de Deuxchaisnes, 1989.)

Complete fracture

Pathological fractures of long bones are the most common presentation to orthopaedic surgeons. They are usually transverse and occur more commonly in the femur than the tibia. About one-half of patients give no history of trauma and in the remainder trauma is slight. Complete fractures can be treated conventionally except that the changes in quality (brittleness or softness), and vascularity of bone may present technical problems for the orthopaedic surgeon (Bowie and Kanis, 1977; Dove, 1980; Stevens, 1981; Figure 8.28). There may also be poor differentiation between cortical and medullary bone which together with deformity presents problems for intramedullary fixation. In addition, the use of plates is often difficult when bone architecture is abnormal or where there is a marked deformity (Figures 8.29 and 8.30). Following complete fracture, a marked rarefaction of surrounding bone

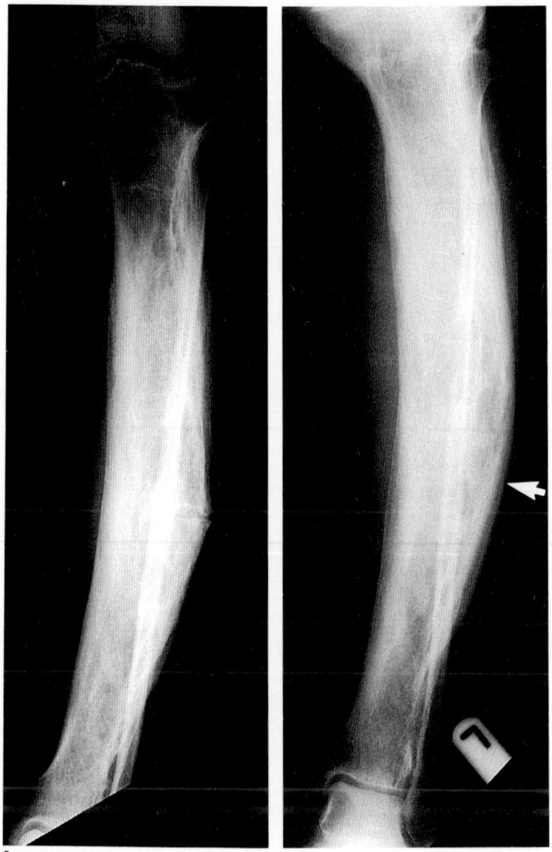

Figure 8.24

Sequential radiographs of the left leg over a 10-year period. Note the fissure fracture and angular deformity of the lateral aspect of the tibia (A). Ten years later (B) the tibia has undergone remodelling but the fissure fracture (arrowed) is still present, although its lateral border is walled off. Disease activity was controlled throughout this period with courses of clodronate or calcitonin and the symptoms managed by external splinting.

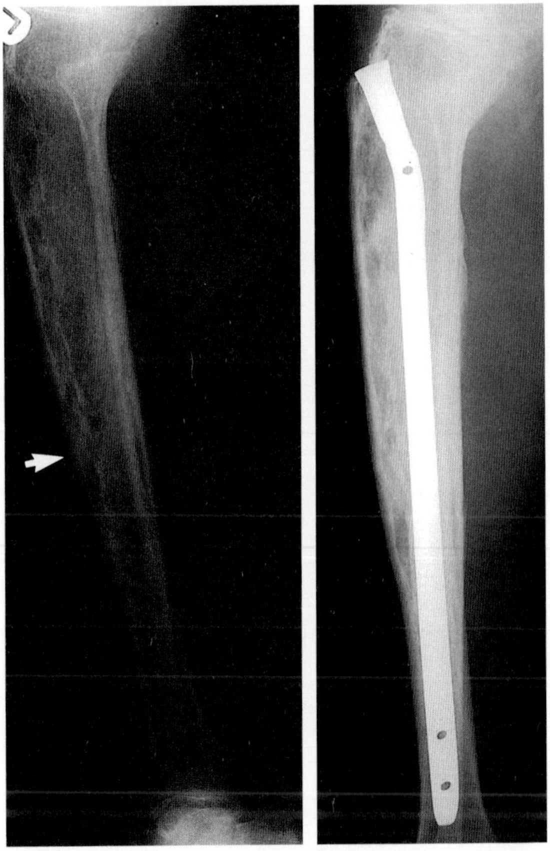

Figure 8.25

Lateral view of left tibia (A) before and (B) 6 months after nailing. The patient complained of pain on weight bearing at the site of the fissure fracture (arrowed) despite control of disease activity with medical treatment. Surgery was associated with immediate pain relief but without apparent healing of the fracture.

occurs that may be confused with malignant changes (Chapter 5). Nevertheless, pathological fracture may occur at the site of pre-existing sarcoma.

Many fractures heal well with conservative treatment (Hosking, 1977; Barry, 1980) but there is a high incidence of non-union (Chapter 5). This is most marked for fractures of the neck of the femur, where there appears to be a very high incidence (Grundy, 1970; Dove, 1980). Fortunately this is a relatively rare site for fracture in Paget's disease, and it may be best managed, where possible, by total hip replacement. In the combined figures of Grundy (1970) and Barry (1969)

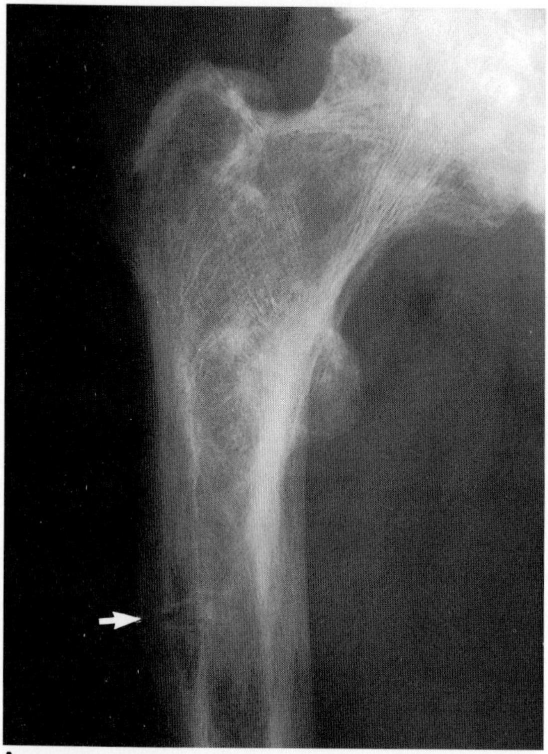

A

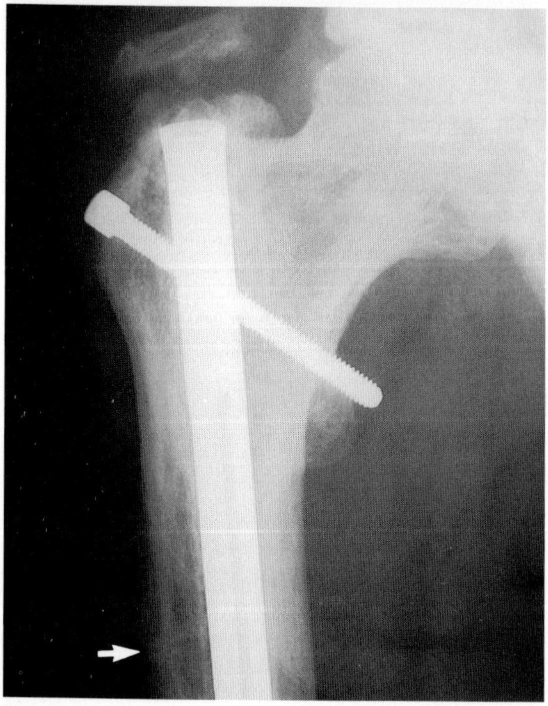

B

Figure 8.26

Serial radiographs of the right hip to show the presence of a fissure fracture (arrowed) and the effects of nailing with a locking pin. (A) Before surgery the fissure fracture had caused chronic pain on bearing weight and was uninfluenced by medical treatment. Surgery gave immediate pain relief. (B) Note the partial healing of the fracture 6 months after surgery.

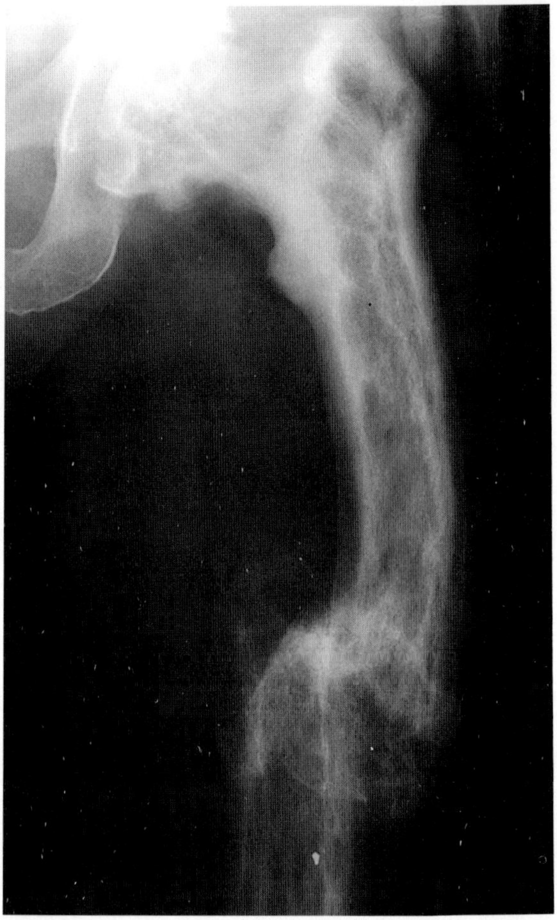

Figure 8.27

Radiograph of the femur. The patient had persistent pain on weight bearing attributed to a fissure fracture. Following osteotomy at the site of the fissure and conservative management, the fracture united with complete pain relief thereafter.

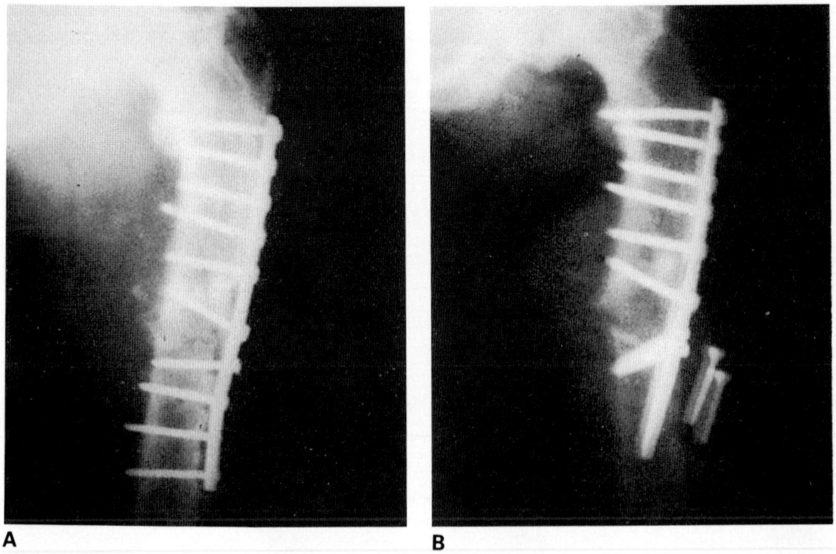

Figure 8.28

Transverse fracture of a pagetic femur fixed by means of a long plate which was bent to accommodate the deformity. Several of the screws previously transfixing pagetic bone (A) became dislodged (B) because of fixation through very soft bone. (From Bowie and Kanis, 1977.)

30 per cent of 112 femoral fractures excluding cervical fractures had failed to unite at 6 months, indicating that the incidence of delayed union is appreciable at other sites.

Problems often arise in choosing between conservative treatment and open reduction and fixation. The choice will depend upon a number of factors which must be weighed up in each case. Conservative management may involve prolonged immobilization in patients who are often elderly, and the 3-month mortality rate is high (Dove, 1980). Surgical management is therefore preferable, where feasible, in the elderly. In addition, immobilization is associated with substantial morbidity, including bone loss. In normal subjects more bone may be lost in one month due to immobilization than in a whole year under normal circumstances due to osteoporosis. In Paget's disease, immobilization bone loss is accelerated, and this increases the risk of hypercalciuria, hypercalcaemia and nephrolithiasis. On the other hand there are, as previously mentioned, considerable technical problems to be overcome with surgical intervention. In patients who are managed conservatively there is a good case to be made for treatment with either calcitonin or a diphosphonate other than etidronate to prevent bone loss, hypercalciuria and hypercalcaemia.

The occurrence of fracture provides an opportunity to correct deformity when managed conservatively. The same is true for surgical management but again this is not without technical difficulties due to variations in medullary width, variable quality of bone, increased vascularity and the deformity itself (Figures 8.29 and 8.30).

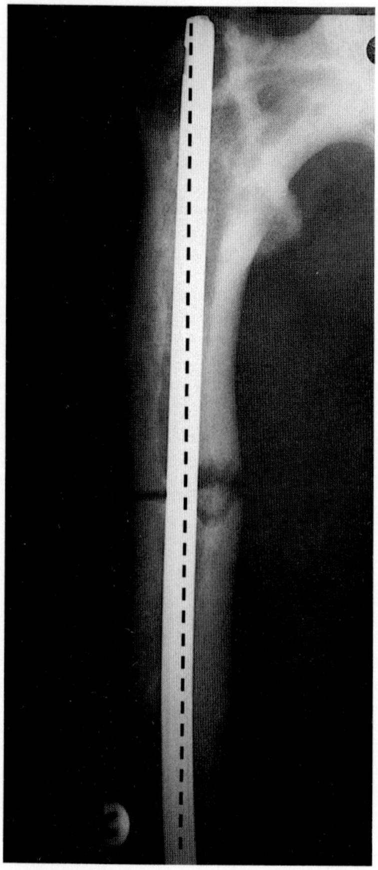

Figure 8.29

Multiple fissure fractures on the lateral aspect of a pagetic femur. A complete transverse fracture occurred at the site of a previous fissure and was internally fixed with an intramedullary nail. The fixation has corrected the deformity in part, but the superimposed black line shows the extent that the nail was bent to conform to the femoral deformity. (From Bowie and Kanis, 1977.)

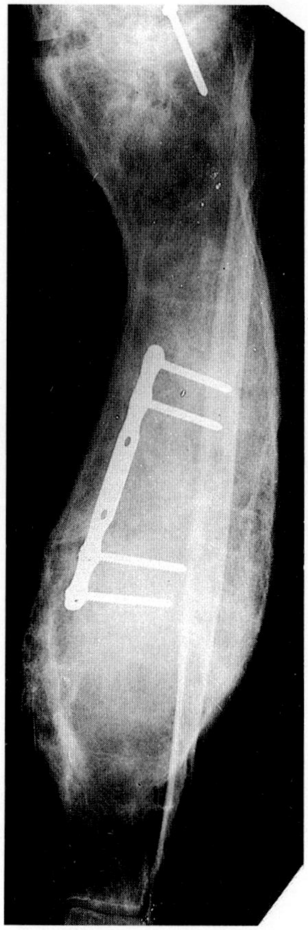

Figure 8.30

A fracture of a grossly deformed and osteolytic tibia treated with a plate screwed on either side of the fracture site. Despite the soft bone the plate maintained its fixation and the fracture healed normally.

Questions arise whether medical treatment affects the healing of complete fractures and whether long-term treatment might prevent their occurrence. These questions have not been absolutely resolved. Apparently normal rates of fracture healing have been observed in patients given either calcitonin or clodronate immediately before their fracture or throughout their conservative management (Evans and Slee, 1977; Douglas et al, 1980). In contrast, large doses of etidronate (20 mg/kg per day) impair fracture healing (Khairi et al, 1977; Finerman et al, 1986). Indeed, fracture of the pelvis has occurred during bone biopsy in etidronate-treated patients. Fracture healing does

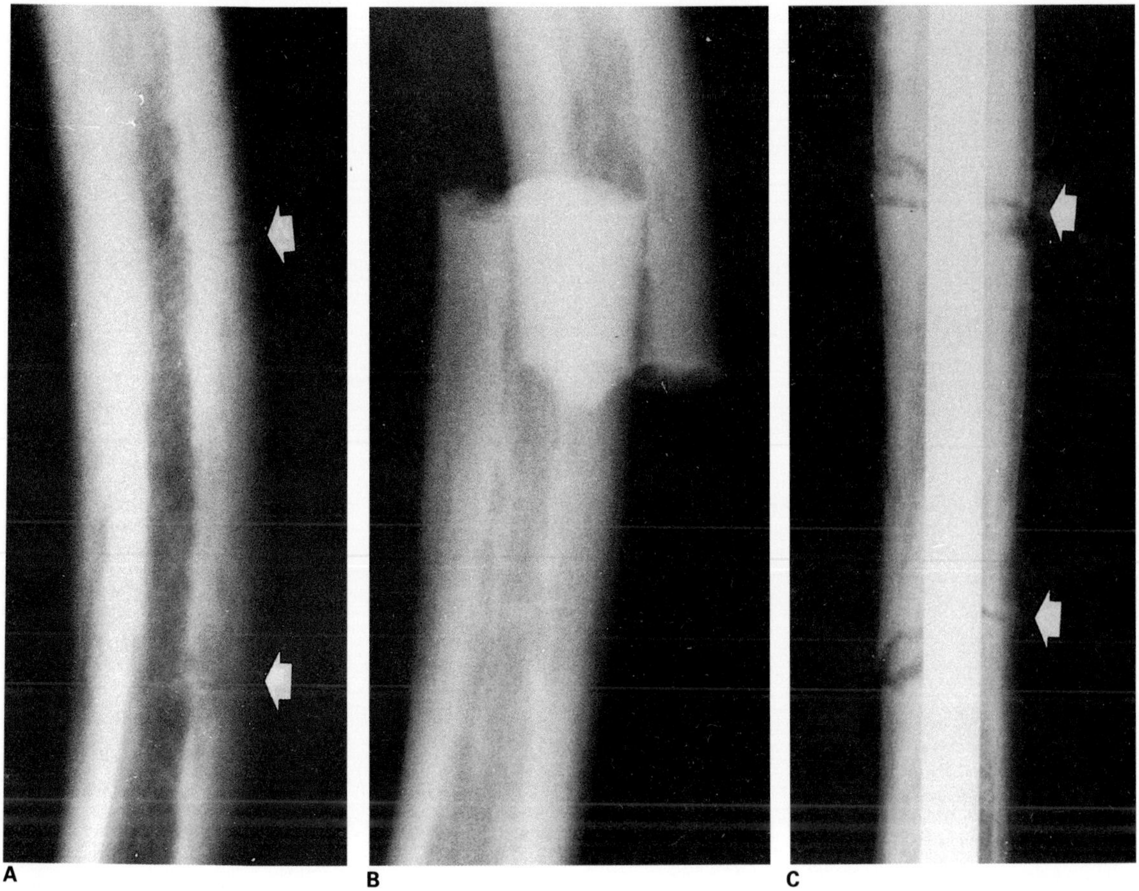

Figure 8.31

Fissure fractures of the convex aspect of the femoral diaphysis. The occurrence of a complete fracture was due to extension of the proximal fissure (upper arrow). Intramedullary nailing and iatrogenic extension of the distal fissure (lower arrow) provided an opportunity to correct the deformity. (From Maldague and Malghem, 1989.)

not appear to be a problem at lower doses, but in view of the wide variation in absorption and thus in bioavailability, it seems prudent to withdraw treatment in patients with fracture unless continued treatment is required, for example for heterotopic ossification.

There are very few studies examining whether long-term medical treatment of Paget's disease favourably alters the risk of subsequent fracture. In addition, none of the studies is controlled. The risk of fracture appears to be increased in the presence of marked osteolytic disease, particularly of the lower limb (O'Reilly and Race, 1933; Dickson et al, 1945) and the reversal of such

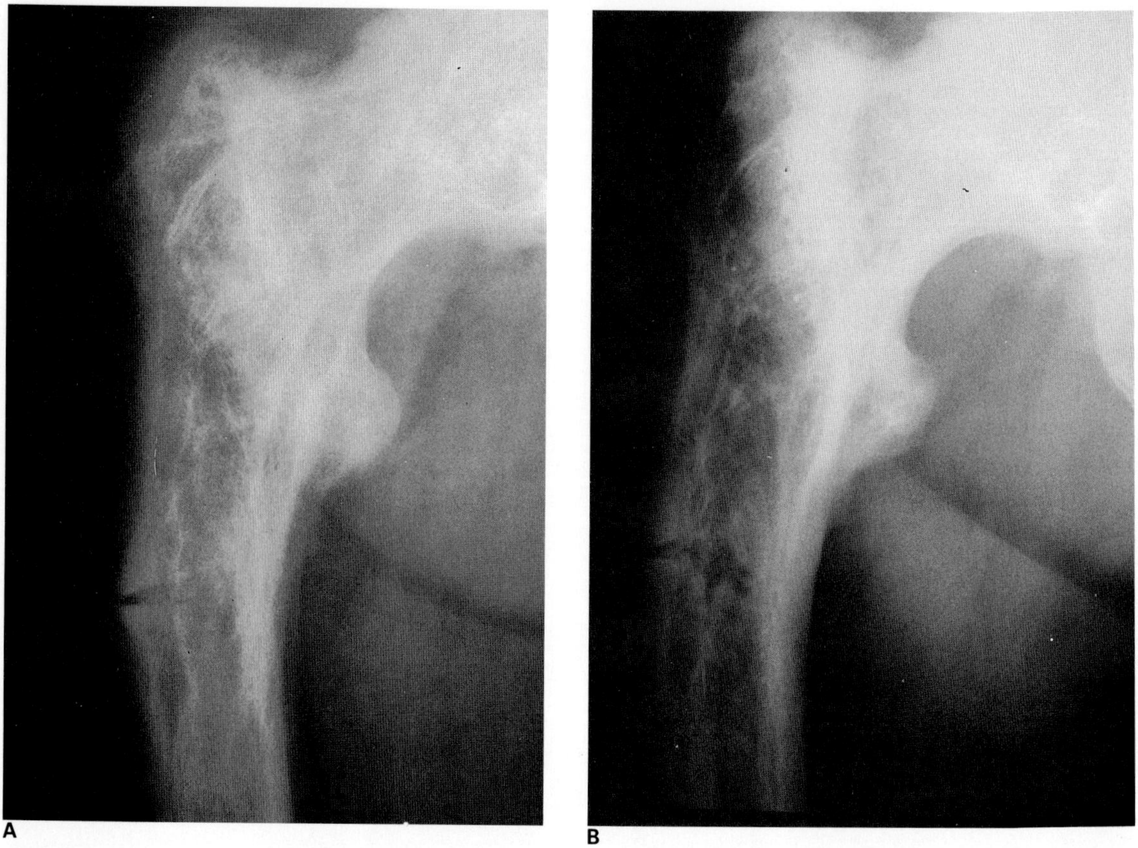

Figure 8.32

Sequential radiographs of the proximal femur in a patient with a fissure fracture at the lateral aspect of the femoral shaft (A). Following treatment with high doses of etidronate (20 mg/kg per day) the patient developed pain and marked radiolucency at the site (B). This reversed when treatment was stopped.

abnormalities with medical treatment suggests the risk of fracture should decrease. In addition, there is some evidence that calcitonin stimulates embryonic bone growth (Burch, 1984) and accelerates fracture healing in experimental animals (Delling et al, 1970). There is also some evidence that calcitonin accelerates fracture repair as judged by callus formation in patients without Paget's disease.

Several authors have shown that treatment with etidronate may increase the incidence of fractures in patients with Paget's disease using doses of 20 mg/kg per day for 6 months or longer (Kantrowitz et al, 1975; Finerman et al, 1976; Canfield et al, 1977; Nagant de Deuxchaisnes et al, 1979). For these reasons, high doses for these extended periods are not recommended. The effects of recommended doses on fracture are uncertain due to inadequate data on the natural history of fracture in Paget's disease. We avoid the use of etidronate in patients who are at high risk from fracture, particularly patients with extensive osteolytic disease or fissure fractures in the long bones of the lower limbs (Figure 8.32).

Estimates of the occurrence of fracture in untreated patients vary between 9 and 28 per cent. One survey which evaluated the incidence of fracture in patients given etidronate suggested that the fracture rate was not significantly different from that observed in the normal aging population (Johnston et al, 1983). The authors' interpretation was that etidronate given in recommended doses (5 mg/kg per day) decreased the risk of fracture. The absence of an adequate control population makes this conclusion tentative. More recently, a survey using each patient as their own control examined the apparent fracture risk before and after treatment. The authors (Nagant de Deuxchaisnes et al, 1985) obtained much lower figures for fracture rate than those of Johnston et al (1983). Unfortunately, this survey was undertaken at the centre with an atypical experience of the use of etidronate, and their conclusion that etidronate in low doses may increase the risk from fracture does not help resolve these questions.

Neurological syndromes

Deafness and cranial nerve lesions

Since the pathogenesis of deafness is multifactorial, it is not surprising that the effects of medical treatment on deafness in Paget's disease have been variable. Improved hearing has been reported after calcitonin and diphosphonate treatment, but this is not a consistent observation, and most authors report no change in hearing with medical treatment (Shai et al, 1971; Grimaldi et al, 1975; Moffat, 1975; Khairi and Johnston, 1977; Lando et al, 1988). Several groups have found that patients receiving continuous treatment showed less deterioration during long-term treatment as assessed by audiometry than those not receiving treatment (Solomon et al, 1977; Samman et al, 1986). It thus seems probable that long-term treatment will at least decrease the rate of progression of deafness.

Many patients are helped by hearing aids, and in a few patients with conductive deafness stapedectomy has led to improved hearing (Waltner, 1965; Henkin et al, 1972). Cranial nerve palsies may also improve with medical treatment (Frank et al, 1982).

Cranial and spinal syndromes

Acute brain-stem compression caused by herniation of the cerebellar tonsils requires urgent neurological decompression. More chronic central neurological syndromes such as dementia may also benefit from decompression procedures (Ray, 1942; Wycis, 1944; Culebras et al, 1974; Taggart et al, 1978). Obstructive hydrocephalus is more appropriately managed by ventriculo-atrial or peritoneal shunting (Friedman et al, 1971). Normal pressure hydrocephalus may also respond to shunt procedures (Botez et al, 1977; Goldhammer et al, 1979; Hausser et al, 1984; Martin et al, 1985).

The sudden onset of paraparesis requires urgent neurological assessment and decompression if appropriate. Sudden onset of cord syndromes may not always be associated with myelographic abnormalities, suggesting an acute vascular insufficiency.

Until recently, most patients with progressive spinal syndromes underwent surgery, and this appears to have been of benefit in about 85 per cent of patients (Sadar et al, 1972; David-Chausse et al, 1974). The operation is not without difficulties due to the vascularity of bone and the fact that multiple sites may be involved (Schmidek, 1977). Symptoms may recur and be the result of progressive disease, vascular steal syndrome, postoperative scarring or occasionally involvement of bone grafts by adjacent pagetic disease (Jaffe, 1933; Hartman and Dohn, 1966; Klenerman, 1966; Stevens, 1981). Mortality is significant and occurs in about 10 per cent of patients (Douglas et al, 1981b).

There is now considerable evidence to suggest that effective medical management can improve spinal neurological syndromes observed in Paget's disease where symptoms and signs are slowly progressive (Shai et al, 1971; DeRose et al, 1974; Melick et al, 1976; Alexandre et al, 1979; Chen et al, 1979; Meunier et al, 1979; Walpin and Singer, 1979; Herzberg and Bayliss, 1980; Douglas et al, 1981a,b; Delmas et al, 1982). Irrespective of the agent used, substantial clinical improvement occurs in the majority of patients provided that disease activity is adequately controlled. The response in spinal root and cord syndromes is comparable to that observed following laminectomy, without the hazards of a surgical intervention and without the mortality (Sadar et al, 1972;

Hadjipavlou et al, 1977; Walpin and Singer, 1979; Douglas et al, 1981b). After medical treatment the clinical improvement correlates remarkably with the degree of disease activity as judged by biochemical estimates of turnover (Douglas et al, 1980a, 1981a,b; Figures 8.33 and 8.34), and provides perhaps the most convincing evidence for the relationship between the clinical and biochemical indices of disease activity.

The rate of neurological improvement seen with drug treatment is surprisingly rapid, occurring within days or weeks of starting treatment, and is not invariably associated therefore with changes in spinal canal diameter (Douglas et al, 1981b; Charhon et al, 1982; Figure 8.33). It is unlikely that improvements are a result of the natural history of the disorder because spontaneous recovery from cord compression due to Paget's disease has not been reported. The rapidity of response to medical treatment suggests that the response cannot have been due to remodelling of bone, but rather to a decrease in soft-tissue swelling (where improvements in myelography have been demonstrated) (Figures 8.34–8.38), or to a redistribution of blood flow (Douglas et al, 1981b). This latter mechanism is consistent with the known anatomical relationship between blood supply to the vertebrae and the cord (Crock and Yoshizana, 1977). Case reports draw attention to the rapid reversal of paraparesis in patients given calcitonin who had no demonstrable cord compression on myelography (Douglas et al, 1980a; Herzberg and Bayliss, 1980; Porrini et al, 1987; Figure 8.35).

Whereas the acute onset of paraparesis or quadriparesis in the presence of myelographic evidence of occlusion is an indication for immediate surgical decompression, medical treatment is probably of first choice in slowly evolving syndromes. In our patients in whom improvements have occurred on medical treatment, surgical intervention has not been required with adequate control of disease activity in an experience of more than 20 patients. Such patients require life-long supervision to ensure that disease suppression is maintained either with intermittent courses of diphosphonate or large and continuous doses of calcitonin (50–100 IU daily).

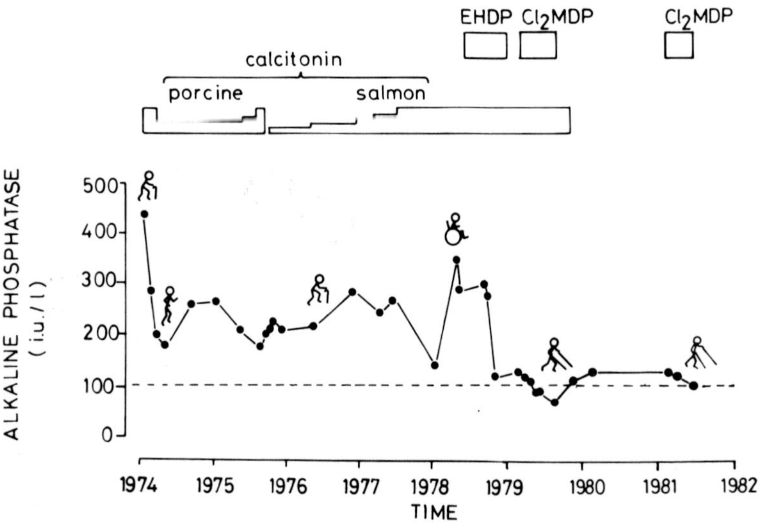

Figure 8.33

Long-term effects of treatment of paraparesis caused by Paget's disease. Improvement in mobility occurred during long-term treatment with calcitonin within 2 months, but was eventually associated with a biochemical relapse that heralded clinical deterioration. The addition of the diphosphonate, clodronate (Cl_2MDP), and etidronate (EHDP) suppressed alkaline phosphatase values to normal and improved neurologic signs and symptoms. (From Douglas et al, 1981b.)

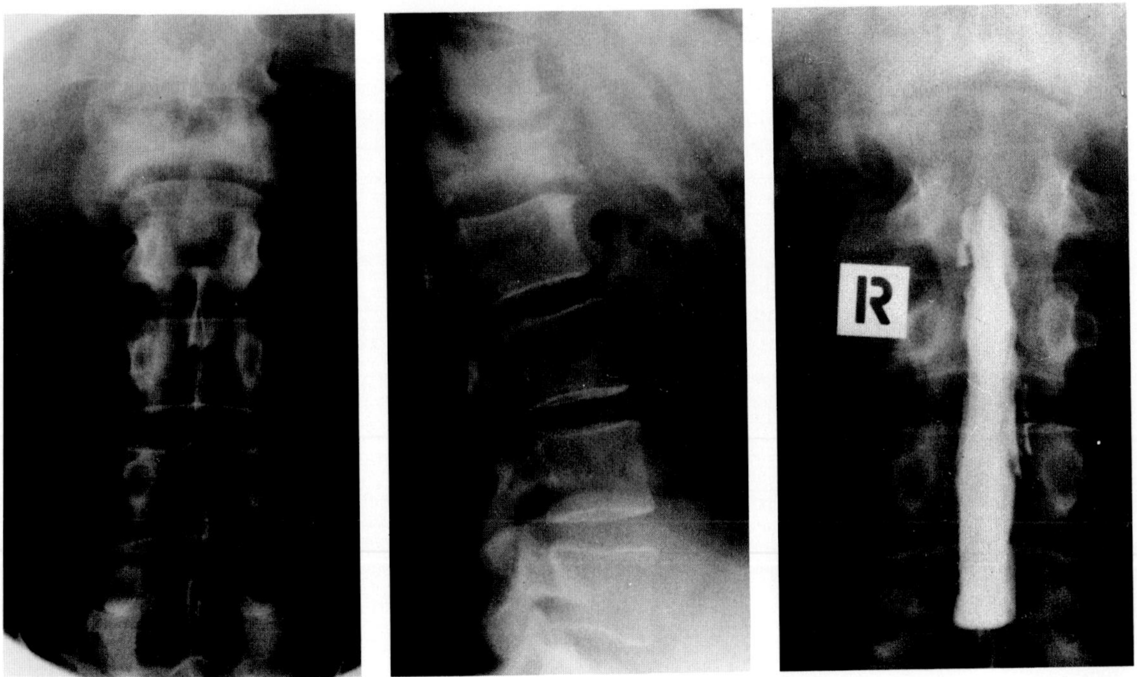

A B C

Figure 8.34

(A/B) Radiographs of a patient with slowly progressive paraparesis (same patient as in Figure 8.35). There is marked expansion and collapse of the first lumbar vertebra, and the myelogram (C) showed complete obstruction below L1, the site of a previous laminectomy. (From Douglas et al, 1981a.)

Sarcoma

Patients with sarcoma may present with bone pain, swelling or pathological fracture. The prognosis of these patients is extremely poor (Price and Goldie, 1969). There is no evidence that medical treatment alters the natural history of established sarcoma (Russell and Smith, 1973; Walton and Strong, 1973; DeVries et al, 1974; Kanis et al, 1974). Indeed, the role of chemotherapeutic or surgical intervention is not established, except for symptomatic treatment (Price and Goldie, 1969). Radiation therapy or amputation may be used to reduce bone pain.

Table 8.3 Survival of patients (expressed as a percentage) with osteosarcoma (combined data of Haibach et al, 1985; Price and Goldie, 1969; McKenna et al, 1966).

After year	*Pagetic sarcoma (n = 189)*	*Non-pagetic sarcoma (n = 605)*
1	42	67
2	16	40
3	8	37
5	6	25

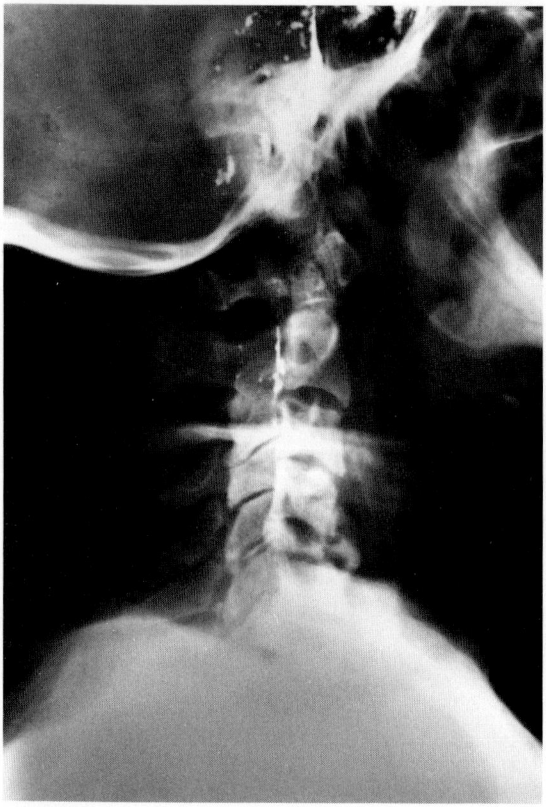

Figure 8.35

Patient with Paget's disease of C4, C5 and C6 with collapse at C5. Note the marked sclerosis at C4 and C5, but no obvious enlargement. The patient presented with tetraplegia mistakenly attributed to prostatic carcinoma. Myelography showed no obstruction and radiographs elsewhere indicated the diagnosis of Paget's disease confirmed by biopsy. The patient was treated with salmon calcitonin, 100 IU daily. Improvement was noted in muscle power in 3 days and full power was restored within 7 months. (From Douglas et al, 1981b.)

Most patients die within 12 months and the 5-year survival is 5–8 per cent (Table 8.3; Price and Goldie, 1969; Wick et al, 1981). Patients commonly develop pulmonary and skeletal metastases and there may be extensive local extension of disease. Recently, the prognosis of sarcoma in childhood has improved with the combination of aggressive chemotherapy and surgery in specialist centres (Goorin et al, 1985; Souhami and Craft, 1988). The referral of our fitter and younger patients for such treatment has not yet produced worthwhile dividends, but the numbers are few.

Immobilization and hypercalcaemia

Immobilization bone loss and hypercalciuria, and hypercalcaemia have been effectively treated with clodronate and calcitonin (see Figure 4.4; Woodhouse, 1972; Auld et al, 1979). In the presence of coexisting hyperparathyroidism the fall in serum calcium is incomplete (Hamdy et al, 1987), and this may alert the physician to the additional underlying disorder. Medical treatment with calcitonin or the newer diphosphonates should be considered in patients with fractures who are managed conservatively, not necessarily to prevent hypercalcaemia, but to prevent bone loss which in Paget's disease may be very marked during immobilization.

Cardiovascular complications

Paget's disease significantly increases the cardiac output when the disorder is extensive, but cardiac failure is more likely to occur in patients with intrinsic heart disease which should be treated conventionally. In the presence of extensive disease, cardiac index decreases following treatment with calcitonin or etidronate (Woodhouse et al, 1975; Khairi and Johnston, 1977; Henley et al, 1979; Figure 8.39), presumably an effect related mainly to the decrease in bone blood flow. A fall in cardiac output is not invariably observed (Crosbie et al, 1975), perhaps due to the heterogeneous causes of cardiovascular disease in an elderly population. As might be expected, cardiac output rises when treatment with calcitonin is stopped, but remains suppressed for longer after stopping diphosphonates.

It is of interest that calcitonin is a potent diuretic. Indeed, it is more potent than frusemide

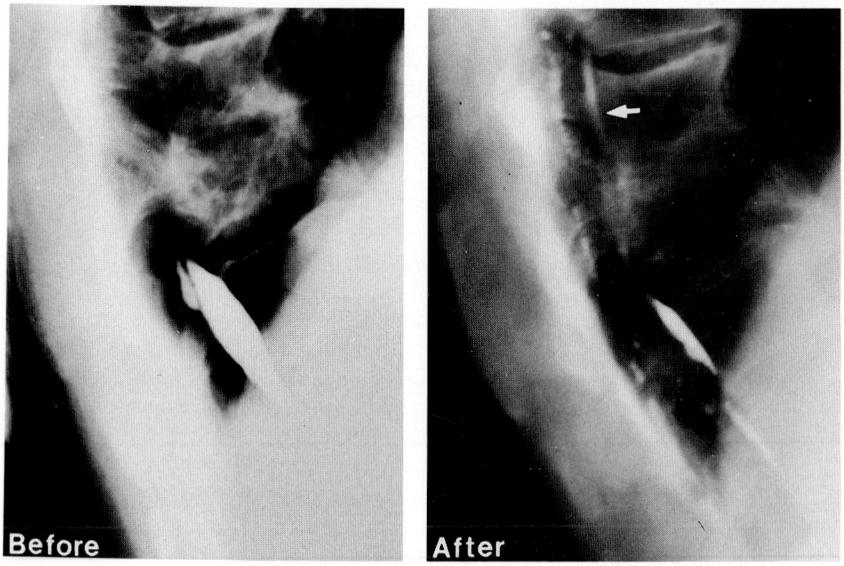

Figure 8.36

Myelographic examination before and 6 months after a 7-month course of clodronate (see Figure 8.39). Complete block of flow of contrast was noted before treatment. Thirteen months later there was contrast (arrowed) beyond the previous level of obstruction. (From Douglas et al, 1980b.)

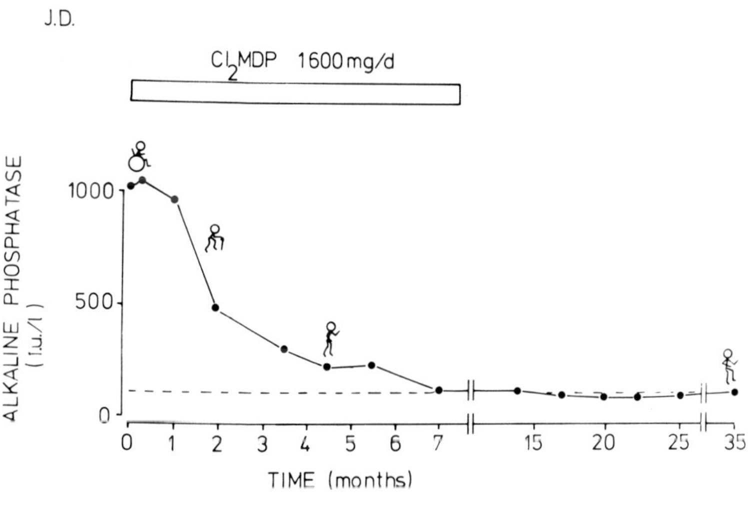

Figure 8.37

Sequential changes in alkaline phosphatase in a patient with slowly progressive paraparesis (Figure 8.38). Improvement in motor power occurred within 1 month and was completely restored by 5 months. The patient has remained in remission now for 10 years. (From Douglas et al, 1981b.)

(furosemide) on a molar basis, and this may contribute to the rapidity of effect (Figure 8.40). The occasional patient with Paget's disease is reported whose failure was resistant to digoxin but who improved markedly with calcitonin (Shai et al, 1971; DeRose et al, 1974). In such cases long-term treatment is required.

Current indications for medical and surgical treatment

Despite the difficulties of assessing the effects of medical treatment on the complications of Paget's disease, a number of considerations

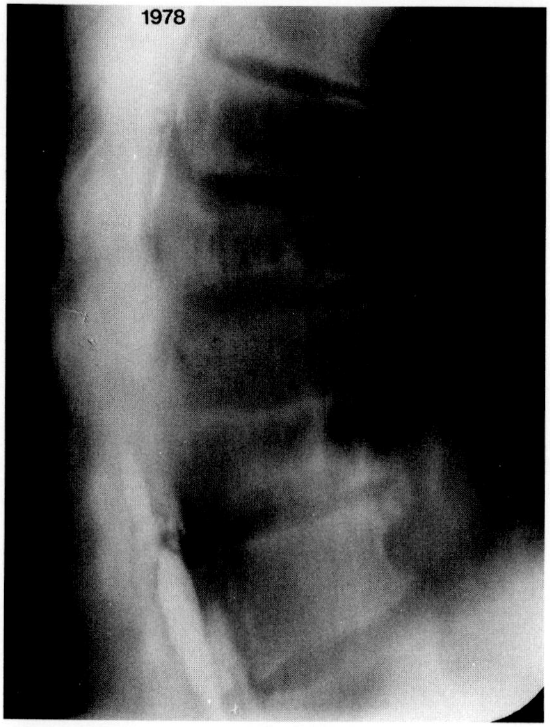

Figure 8.38

Myelogram in a patient with progressive weakness of the lower limbs. On admission, X-ray examination and myelography showed Paget's disease of T9, T10 and T11, with complete blockage at the level of T10. The patient was treated with salmon calcitonin, 100 IU daily. The patient was able to walk in 9 days, at which time this myelogram showed free flow.

suggest that suppression of disease activity significantly alters the natural history of Paget's disease. In addition to the histological and radiographic improvements observed, the most convincing and dramatic clinical example is the sustained remission from neurological syndromes. There appears to be a good correlation between the degree of biochemical control and the attainment of remission, and this in turn helps to validate the biochemical monitoring of disease activity.

Nevertheless, a need clearly exists for well-designed, long-term prospective studies to determine whether or not the suppression of disease activity, now attainable with medical management, improves the incidence of complications, particularly of fracture.

Suggested indications for the treatment of Paget's disease are summarized in Table 8.4. The decision whether or not to offer long-term treatment depends not only upon the evidence for efficacy of a specific treatment regimen on specific complications, but also upon considerations such as side effects, convenience and cost. The use of the different drugs is not mutually exclusive and their respective value needs to be assessed on an individual basis. The most widely available options are the calcitonins and etidronate. Calcitonin is preferred in rapidly advancing osteolysis of long bones, but etidronate provides a better option for long-term control of disease activity. Both have problems with their use. With

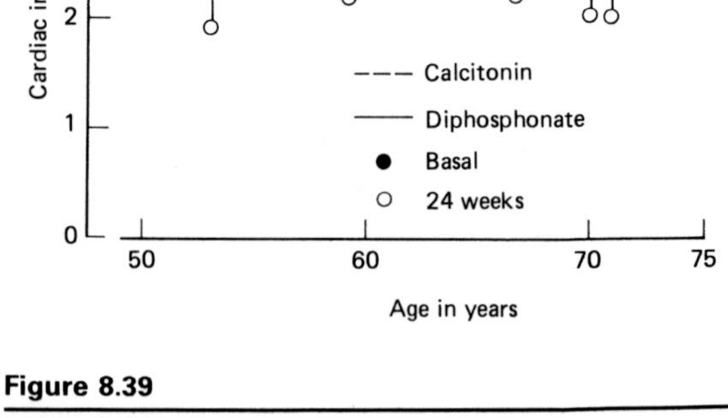

Figure 8.39

Effect of treatment with calcitonin (dotted lines) or etidronate on cardiac index. The lines join values before (●) and after (○) treatment for 24 weeks. (From Henley et al, 1979.)

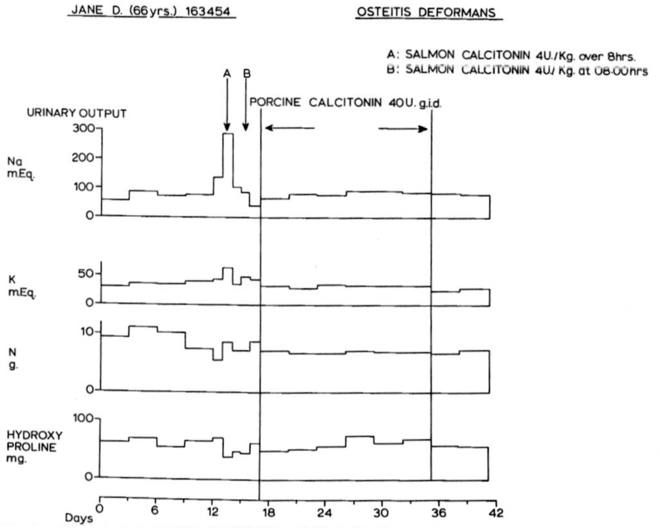

Figure 8.40

Urinary electrolyte excretion in a patient treated with calcitonin. The patient had cardiac failure and the first injection of calcitonin was associated with a marked sodium diuresis. (Kanis and Strong, unpublished work.)

Table 8.4 Suggested indications for specific medical treatment of Paget's disease (from Kanis and Gray, 1987).

Indication	*Evidence of efficacy*
(*a*) Long-term suppression of disease activity	
Progressive neurological syndromes:	
Vascular steal	Yes, rapid improvement
Cord compression	Yes, slow improvement
Root compression	Yes, probably slow Improvement
Nerve compression	Stabilized
Deafness and tinnitus	Rarely improves but stabilized
Progressive deformity of skull or weight-bearing bones, especially in young	Likely
Healing of fissure fractures	Unproven, but unlikely
Prophylaxis:	
Juvenile hyperphosphatasia	Unproven, but likely
Familial expansile osteolysis	Unproven, but likely
Severe disease in young patients	Probable
Extensive osteolysis in weight-bearing long bones	Yes, especially with calcitonin
In preparation for orthopaedic surgery (more stable or normal skeletal environment)	Unproven but likely
High output cardiac failure	Yes
Reduce risk of fracture	Unproven but likely
(*b*) Short-term treatment	
Bone pain	Yes
Immobilization hypercalcaemia, hypercalciuria and bone loss	Yes, not with etidronate
Before orthopaedic surgery (to decrease bone vascularity)	Anecdotal, but bone blood flow known to diminish
Improve fracture healing	No evidence
Sarcoma	No evidence

the increasing availability of second- and third-generation diphosphonates, it is likely that the use of both the calcitonins and etidronate will decrease in the future.

Until a few years ago the only non-controversial indication for medical treatment of Paget's disease was bone pain. As new and effective inhibitors of bone resorption have become available and long-term experience with their use is gained, the indications for treatment have widened and may widen still further in the future. This will pose additional questions, particularly who not to treat. It is clear that patients with no clinical expression of their disorder have little to gain from medical treatment, unless it can be shown that such patients are at high risk of developing complications in the future. Such questions will need to be answered by well-designed epidemiological studies as well as the evaluation of new treatments as they become available.

Despite the advances in the medical management of Paget's disease, many patients present with complications which require surgery (Table 8.5). The hope that medical treatment avoids the need for surgery is fulfilled only in part, and there are well recognized indications where surgery is the treatment of choice. Nevertheless, medical treatments have avoided the need for surgery, particularly in the case of hip pain and some of the spinal neurological syndromes. Of equal significance, the advent of effective medical treatments has meant that surgical intervention can be more readily undertaken in a larger proportion of patients than previously feasible. It is likely, but not proven, that the results of surgery will be more durable with concurrent medical treatments. These observations suggest that a combined medical and surgical approach provides the optimal management for what is now increasingly recognized as an eminently treatable disorder.

Table 8.5 Indications for surgical treatment.

Diagnosis	– biopsy
Fissure fracture	– risk of complete fracture
	– pain
Complete fracture	
Osteoarthrosis	– hips
	– knee
Deformity	
Neurological syndromes	
Sarcoma (rarely)	

CHAPTER 9

Aetiology

The aetiology of Paget's disease is not known. Unfortunately there are no animal models of Paget's disease and speculation has been based on information derived from a variety of disciplines including epidemiology, histopathology, radiology, biochemical assessment and clinical observation. It is for this reason that the subject of aetiology is left to last!

The major theories advanced for its aetiology are summarized in Table 9.1 and many are of historical interest only. Paget himself described the disease as osteitis deformans, reasoning that it had an inflammatory cause. Apart from its response to large doses of aspirin and to corticosteroids, there is no evidence for a chronic inflammatory process. The evidence for and against many of the hypotheses has been reviewed earlier, as shown in Table 9.1. The purpose of this chapter is to argue the relative merits of the more plausible rather than to re-review in detail the observations on which the improbable were based.

Table 9.1 Factors proposed to be of importance in the aetiology of Paget's disease. The table also refers to the relevant chapter where the evidence for the theory is discussed.

	Discussion in Chapter
Inflammatory	8
Autoimmune	5
Abnormal vasculature	2
Collagen defect	5
Viral infection	2
Mechanical stress	9
Vitamin D deficiency	4
Benign neoplasm	5
Endocrinology	4
Environmental – unknown	1, 3

The osteoclast

The aetiology of Paget's disease can be considered from many points of view. We have little insight into the way bone-cell metabolism is disturbed, even though morphology indicates that it is grossly abnormal. Histological and biochemical investigation is thus in its infancy, but there are data to indicate at least the cell types which are disturbed (see page 254).

Most evidence would suggest that abnormal osteoclast behaviour is responsible for the disorder. The osteoclasts look abnormal and histomorphometric observations suggest that the functional capacity of these cells is markedly impaired. It can be argued that the osteoblast is also abnormal and, in addition to morphological abnormalities, the osteoblasts at pagetic sites clearly assemble collagen and possibly other bone proteins in an abnormal manner. On the

Some histopathological features of Paget's disease.

Abnormal osteoclast morphology and function
Osteoblast dysfunction – malorientation of lamellar collagen
– woven bone formation
Disturbed bone remodelling – activation frequency
– focal imbalance
– ? coupling
Stromal fibrosis
Increased vascularity of bone and surrounding tissues
Focal and sharp demarcation from normal bone
Association with – sarcoma
– giant cell tumour
– ? abnormal collagen of skin and eye
Site susceptibility

other hand, pagetic osteoblasts appear to synthesize normal amounts of collagen and many of their abnormal features disappear where osteoclast numbers are decreased with treatment, irrespective of the agent used. Moreover, similar pleomorphism and abnormalities in collagen assembly are found in all disorders associated with increased activation of bone remodelling; so too is an increase in the vascularity and fibrosis of marrow. These considerations suggest that it is the osteoclast, its precursor or signals to these which are disrupted, and that the changes in osteoclast function are secondary consequences of an increase in the activation frequency of bone (Figure 9.1).

This conclusion is supported by the reversal of many abnormalities of osteoblast function by specific inhibitors of osteoclast-mediated bone resorption. The calcitonins and diphosphonates may well exert effects, direct or indirect, on osteoblasts in vivo, but this has yet to be convincingly shown. Much more evidence points to a dominant activity of these agents on osteoclast performance and recruitment. The limited domain of the osteoclast and its 'immortality' (discussed below) might also suggest the osteoclast as the cell which is primarily disturbed, but we know little of the precursor cells and less about signals which might induce focal changes in bone-cell metabolism.

If osteoclast precursors derive from circulating precursor cells, as current fashion suggests, the

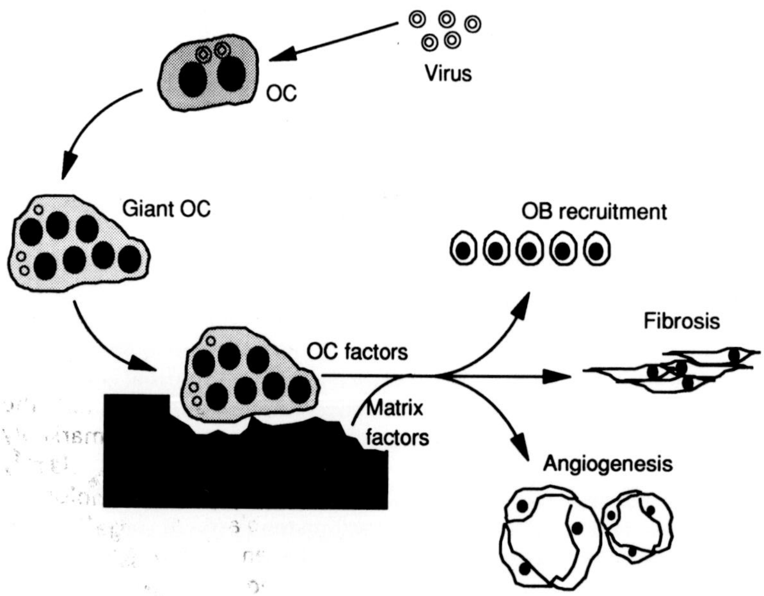

Figure 9.1

Diagram illustrating the infection of osteoclasts with a viral agent. The schema depicts the increased fibrosis, vascularity and osteoblast numbers as secondary consequences of osteoclast mediated bone turnover.

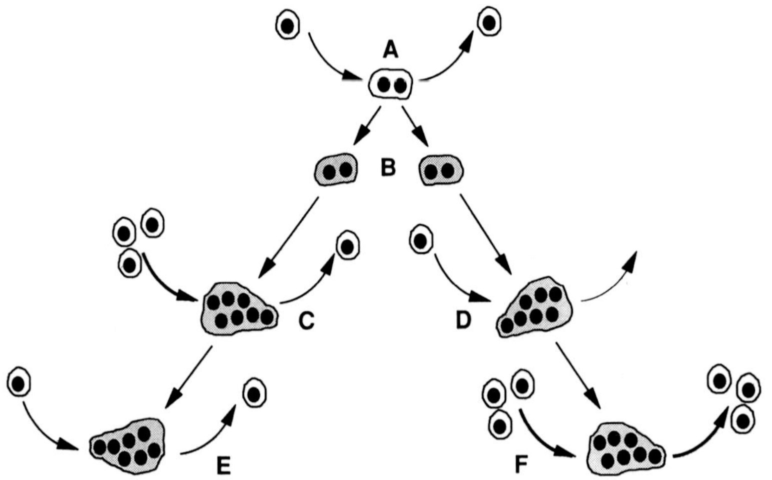

Figure 9.2

Postulated steps in the induction and maintenance of Paget's disease. The schema depicts the transformation of a normal osteoclast by an unknown factor (B) but the continued recruitment of normal osteoclast precursors. Induction induces functional incompetence and a transient change in nuclear turnover, either by accelerating their accession (C) or decreasing their removal (D). In the established disorder nuclear turnover may remain normal (E) or increased (F), but at the expense of an increase in osteoclast nuclearity.

focal nature of the disorder would argue against an abnormality of the osteoclast precursor, or argue for a local factor which altered the predisposition of precursors to behave abnormally. The latter seems to be the more plausible, given our current knowledge, but if so, it is not necessary to postulate that abnormal local factors maintain the disorder, only that they were responsible for the initiation of the disorder. The concept of the 'immortal osteoclast' with its limited functional domain is attractive in this regard. An abnormal pagetic osteoclast, like all osteoclasts, would incorporate new but normal precursor cells and shed other nuclei indefinitely without altering its phenotypic characteristics. This notion is attractive since it accommodates the focal nature of Paget's disease, the sharp spatial demarcation between normal and affected sites, the slow spread of the disorder through marrow or bony elements, the infrequency with which the disorder crosses joints, the failure to observe new pagetic foci, and the pattern of recurrence of the disease after treatment.

It is not necessary to invoke that accession of new or shedding of old nuclear material is abnormal, only that at one time this was so – otherwise no increase in cell nuclearity would be observed. It is possible, however, that once this disorder is established, nuclear turnover could be normal (Figure 9.2).

The gross abnormalities exhibited by pagetic osteoclasts and the presence of inclusions of viral origin have suggested that the disorder is a slow viral infection. A viral infection with the incorporation of viral RNA into nuclear material is an attractive hypothesis to account for an initiating event to cause the transformation of osteoclasts. Whereas there seems little doubt that the inclusions are viral in origin, there is no direct evidence that their presence causes abnormal osteoclast metabolism. There is, however, some indirect evidence to support this view.

Viral aetiology

Paget's disease is generally multi-focal, but there is little evidence to suggest that new foci occur in patients after presentation. This is consistent with a single episode of dissemination to multiple sites. The number of pagetic foci per patient in an affected population approximates a log-normal distribution (Chapter 3). The frequency distribution of the number of sites is similar in both sexes and all ages. This is consistent with a similar sensitivity to a causal agent for all ages and both sexes.

Patients with a family history of Paget's disease have nearly twice as many pagetic foci as those patients with no family history. The distribution of the lesions of these two groups of patients within the skeleton is, however, very similar (Chapter 3). This is consistent with a difference in sensitivity of patients with a family history to exposure to a viral agent. These considerations do not pertain to familial expansile osteolysis where the distribution of skeletal lesions is markedly different from the more straightforward pagetic patient.

There are a number of problems to be resolved in forwarding a viral aetiology. The first relates to the nature of the virus and reasons for positive immunofluorescence for measles, RSV and canine distemper (Chapter 2). The rate of mutation of RNA viruses is high and it is possible that an infecting virus many years ago may have had different antigenic sites. Alternatively, mutant strains or multiple viruses might cause osteoclast dysfunction.

A second problem relates to the difficulties in passaging, which again may be related to a high mutation rate of viral RNA.

Third, there is little serological evidence for infection. Serological studies have shown no differences in antibody profiles between pagetic and control populations. Antibodies tested include measles, mumps, parainfluenza 1, 2 and 3, RSV, herpes, influenza, adenovirus and canine distemper (Mills et al, 1980; Rebel et al, 1980a; Morgan-Capner et al, 1981; Baslé et al, 1983; Pringle et al, 1985). This is in marked contrast with subacute sclerosing panencephalitis (SSPE), where antibody titres for measles are very high. The lack of a systemic or measurable immune response does not, however, exclude a viral pathogenesis nor a viral initiation.

The immune modulator inosiplex has some activity in SSPE over a period of several months (Huttenlocher and Mattson, 1979). It has been given to patients with Paget's disease, but no evidence was found for the suppression of disease activity (Figure 9.3). Indeed, the drug had no effect on the proportion of osteoclasts or their nuclei expressing the viral protein (Kanis et al, 1985a).

None of these observations argue against a viral aetiology, but only increase the complexity of the case. There are a number of further observations, however, which are more difficult to reconcile.

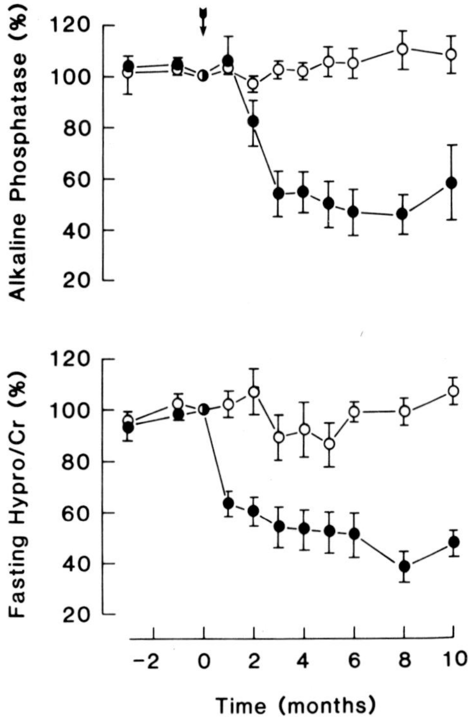

Figure 9.3

Comparison of the effects of the antiviral agent inosiplex (○) and clodronate (●) on disease activity (mean ± SEM) in 4 patients with Paget's disease (from Kanis et al, 1985a).

A major uncertainty is whether the viral proteins might cause osteoclast dysfunction in Paget's disease or merely reflect the consequence of abnormal osteoclast metabolism due to other causes. The presence of viral-like inclusions has not been seen in osteoclasts from normal subjects. Nuclear inclusions have been observed, however, in giant cell tumours (associated with giant osteoclasts) even in patients without Paget's

Table 9.2 Relationship between osteoclast size, bone resorption and functional competence in disorders associated with viral-like nuclear inclusions.

Disorder	*Osteoclast size and nuclearity*	*Bone resorption at affected sites*	*Resorbing capacity of osteoclasts*	*Distribution of disease*
Paget's disease	Giant	Markedly enhanced	Impaired	Focal
Pycnodysostosis	Large	Decresed	Impaired	Generalized
Osteopetrosis	Small	Decreased	Possibly impaired	Generalized
Giant cell tumour	Giant	Markedly enhanced	Unknown	Focal
Expansile osteolysis	Giant	Markedly increased	Unknown	Focal

disease (Welsh and Meyer, 1970; Mirra et al, 1981; Abelanet et al, 1982). More recently, paramyxoviridal inclusions have been observed in osteopetrosis (Mills et al, 1988), pycnodysostosis (Benéton et al, 1987; Figure 9.4) and familial expansile osteolysis (Dickson et al, 1990; Figure 9.5). It appears therefore that viral-like inclusions may be associated with a number of bone disorders, and there appears to be no consistency between their presence and the size or degree of bone resorption. There may be a closer relationship, however, between the presence of inclusions and the functional activity of individual osteoclasts (Table 9.2).

Whereas viral-like inclusion particles are not observed in normal osteoclasts, their presence in several bone disorders indicates that they are not specific for a particular disease nor related consistently to focal bone disease or the morphology of osteoclasts. Although the presence of viral RNA might alter osteoclast metabolism, these collective observations would suggest that the expression of viral protein could be an incidental finding or the result of abnormal osteoclast dysfunction rather than its cause.

It is of interest that the canine distemper virus belongs to the paramyxoviridae in that a recent survey showed an apparent association between Paget's disease and dog ownership (O'Driscoll and Anderson, 1985; Figure 9.6). A further unpublished survey by the same authors and one in New Zealand has confirmed this observation and very recently positive in situ hybridization has been shown with probes of the canine distemper nucleocapsid (Gordon et al, 1990). Other surveys also undertaken in the UK have failed to find this association (Barker and Detheridge, 1985; Stamp et al, 1986). Serological tests for canine distemper virus have not shown increased titres (Hamill et al, 1986). A recent survey in Spain found an association of the disorder with pets and also with eating lamb or goat not subject to sanitary control (Piga et al, 1988). Unlike pet exposure, the risk associated with eating lamb or goat persisted

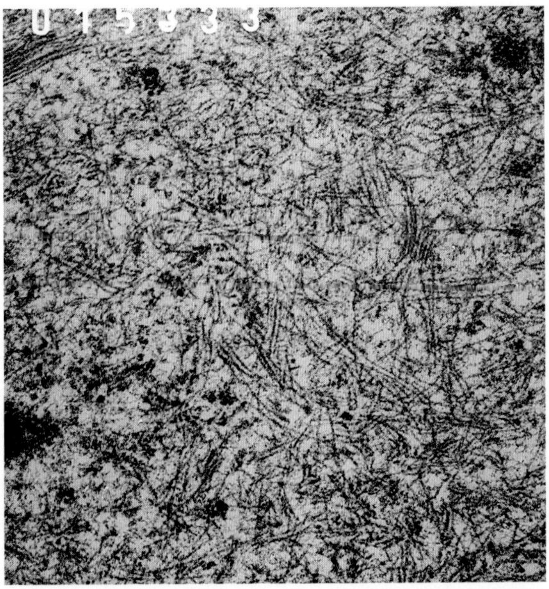

Figure 9.4

Electron micrograph showing intranuclear viral-like filamentous lesions in a patient with pycnodysostosis.

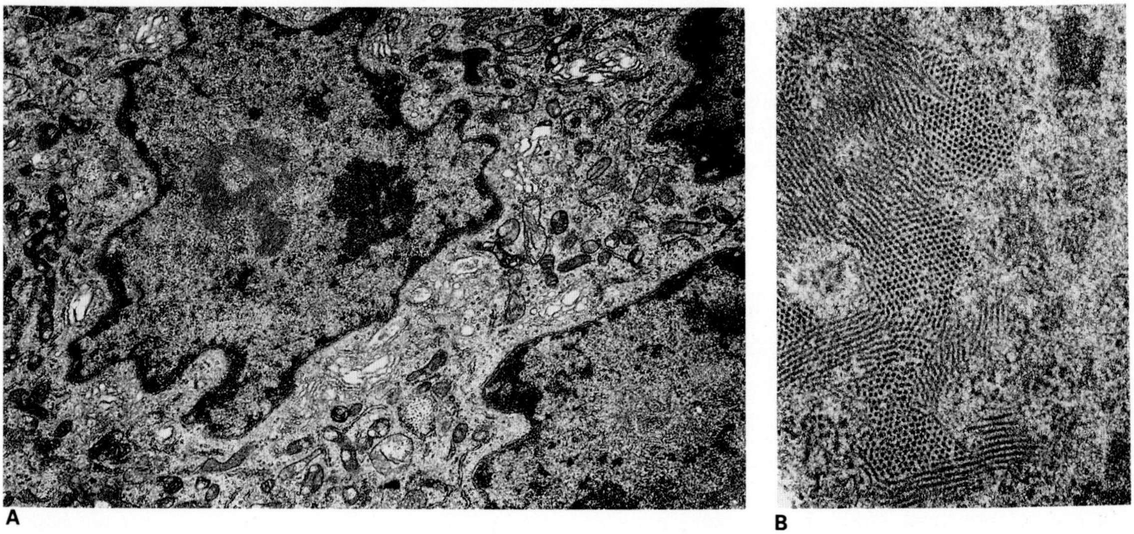

Figure 9.5

Viral-like microcylindrical inclusions found in the nucleus of an osteoclast from a patient with expansile osteolysis (A, × 530). The higher-power electron micrograph (B) (× 20 000) shows their paracrystalline arrangement in cross-section.

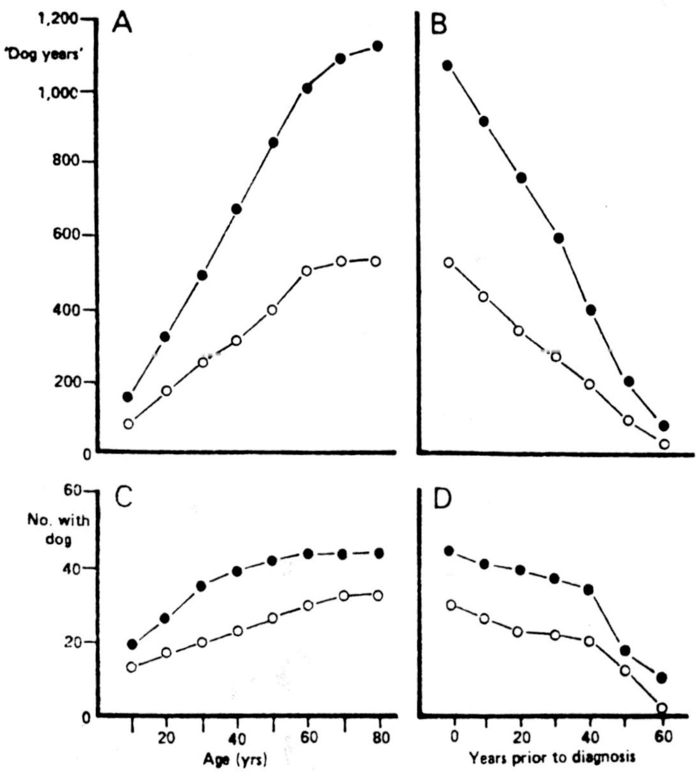

Figure 9.6

Relationship between past pets and Paget's disease. Note the apparent association between dog ownership and the duration of dog ownership in patients with Paget's disease (●) compared with hospital controls (○). (From O'Driscoll and Anderson, 1985.)

after controlling for the confounding variables considered. The causal relationship of any association, even if real, is of course speculative.

Other environmental factors

The probability of a given skeletal site being infected might be expected to depend upon the numbers of normal osteoclasts within that bone at the time of exposure. It has been argued that bones with abundant trabecular tissue or more red marrow, such as the spine and pelvis, are more prone to the disorder (Guyer and Clough, 1978; Harinck et al, 1986). As a generalization this seems to be true (Table 9.2). Thus the frequency of lesions in the long bones is less than might be expected from skeletal volume, more in keeping with their low trabecular bone content. This may also explain the marked difference in disease prevalence at different spinal sites, but would not explain the high frequency of sacral involvement, nor the increased susceptibility for the skull in women (Chapter 3).

On this basis it would be necessary to invoke a difference in sex- and site-specific sensitivity. A number of observations have been made to support site-specific factors, particularly mechanical stress (Lievre, 1974). Pagetic sites are more frequent in the load-bearing axial skeleton and lower limbs (Guyer and Sheperd, 1980). But when sites are examined according to skeletal volume the femur is not over-represented, and both the tibia and fibula seem to be relatively protected (Table 9.3; Figure 9.7). It would be of interest to relate susceptibility of sites to the osteoclast population normally resident at those sites. In this way, it might be possible to examine to what extent random or non-random events determined the susceptibility to Paget's disease. Sparing of pagetic involvement in a paralysed limb due to polio in a patient with extensive disease (Barry, 1969) and the occasional anecdote of an unusual distribution at sites of repeated stress (for example billiard-player's fingers, Solomon, 1979) support the view that biomechanical factors might alter susceptibility.

Several further problems need to be reconciled with a viral aetiology (Table 9.4). The first is the

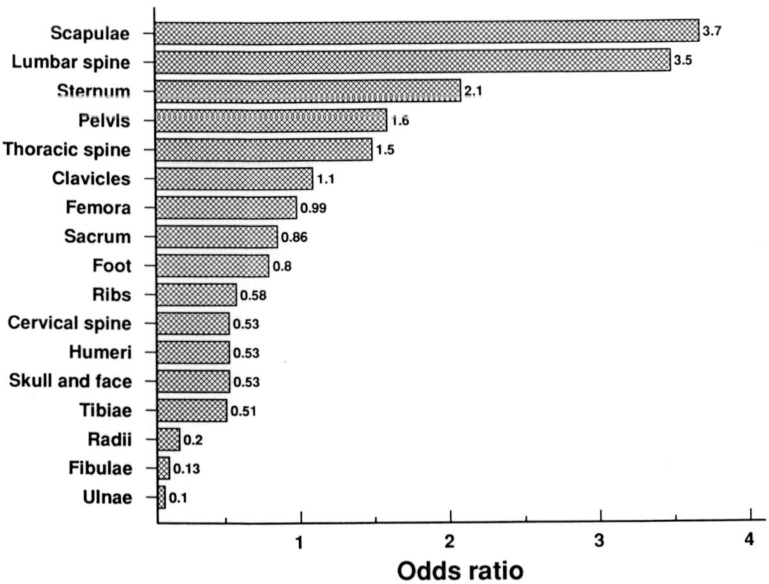

Figure 9.7

Frequency of pagetic lesions in 197 patients at the sites shown divided by the skeletal volume (Coutris et al, 1975) at that site. Thus the scapulae are affected 3.7 times more frequently than is accounted for by skeletal volume, and the ulna is 10 times less susceptible than expected.

Table 9.3 Distribution of pagetic lesions in 197 patients and their relationship with skeletal volume. Skeletal volume is assessed by the method of Coutris et al, 1975.

Site	*No of lesions*	*% of all lesions (A)*	*% skeletal volume (B)*	*A/B*
Scapulae	48	3.7	1	3.70
Lumbar spine	226	17.5	5	3.50
Sternum	27	2.1	1	2.10
Pelvis	208	16.1	10	1.61
Dorsal spine	232	18.0	12	1.50
Feet	39	3.0	2	1.50
Clavicles	14	1.1	1	1.10
Femora	128	9.9	10	0.99
Sacrum	55	4.3	5	0.86
Ribs	45	3.5	6	0.58
Skull and face	83	6.4	12	0.53
Humeri	41	3.2	6	0.53
Tibiae	53	4.1	8	0.51
Cervical spine	45	3.5	7	0.50
Hands and forearms	22	1.7	10	0.17
Fibulae	6	0.5	4	0.13

Table 9.4 Population characteristics of Paget's disease which must be accommodated in aetiological theories.

Late onset
Geographic variation in prevalence
Familial tendency
Genetic substrate, eg HLA DQW1 A9 B15
Dog ownership/viral exposure

striking variation in geographical distribution of the disorder compared with the ubiquity of the paramyxoviridae. The second relates to the latency between exposure and clinical expression. A long latency is generally consistent with a slow virus and if the virus were originally measles or RSV the latency must be several decades. The occasional finding of Paget's disease in teenagers suggests that a fixed latency is not invariable.

At present, the case for a viral aetiology is not entirely convincing. If true, a hypothesis must accommodate a variable latency and marked differences in susceptibility of sites and sex. It must also explain why similar inclusions alter osteoclast behaviour differently in different disorders. Differences in prevalence around the world might be explained in part by differences in exposure, the differences between races within the same country again suggest differences in susceptibility. In addition, the question arises as to what extent familial clustering is related to genetic or environmental factors.

Genetic factors

The family studies in Paget's disease suggest an autosomal dominant pattern of inheritance. A striking pattern of inheritance is seen only in a very small minority of patients. However, evidence for familial association is found in a substantial minority of patients, and due to the difficulties in screening for Paget's disease may well be underestimated. The family studies of Sofaer et al (1983) were unable to identify environmental differences between affected and unaffected siblings of their patients.

Early studies typing human leukocyte antigens, ABO blood groups or secretor status in pagetic populations showed no significant associations with Paget's disease (Blotman et al, 1975; Roux et al, 1975; Simon et al, 1975; Cullen et al, 1976; Mercier and Seignal, 1976; Galbraith et al, 1977). Other studies in affected families have suggested a family linkage (Fotino et al, 1977; Tilyard et al, 1982). More recent studies in populations have suggested weak associations with the DR antigens (Singer et al, 1985; Foldes et al, 1987). Our own studies have not confirmed this, but rather suggested an association with A9 and B15 (Figure 9.8). The frequency of these antigens is not markedly different around the world and cannot account therefore for the marked geographic variation. The lack of consistency in the pattern of HLA antigens might indicate different genetic patterns of susceptibility to external and internal agencies.

The interaction between genetic and environmental factors is not understood. Patients with a family history of Paget's disease have more pagetic lesions than those giving no family history, but the distribution of these lesions is comparable (Chapter 3). This observation might suggest a single disease process with a common aetiology where genetic factors alter the susceptibility to the disorder and perhaps its severity,

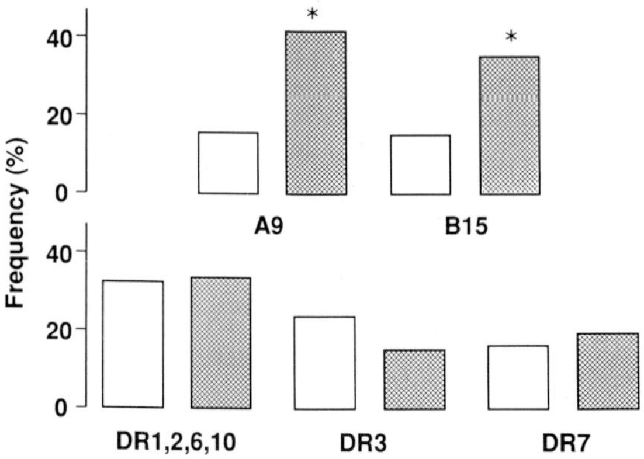

Figure 9.8

Pattern of HLA-antigens in 59 patients with Paget's disease (hatched), compared with a reference population (unhatched). There was a significant increase in the frequency of HLA A9 and B15 compared with the normal Sheffield population ($p < 0.005$).

rather than the natural history of the disorder once established. In contrast, the distribution of lesions in expansile osteolysis is markedly different, as too is the natural history of the disorder.

The interrelationships between environmental and genetic factors may be amenable to investigation. Very recently it has been shown that mice which are transgenic for the HTLV-1 transactivating factor (tax) have a form of bone disease which shares several characteristics of Paget's disease (Ruddle et al, 1990). In these mice all the elements of the remodelling sequence are augmented, woven bone formation and marrow fibrosis are marked, and giant osteoclasts are present. The gene product normally regulates viral protein synthesis, but in infected cells and in the transgenic mice it upregulates a variety of proteins through its interaction with NF-κB, a DNA binding protein. The proteins which are upregulated include a number of bone active agents including β_2-microglobulin, lymphotoxin, interleukin-2 (IL-2), tumour necrosis factor (TNFα), β-interferon and the α chain of the IL-2 receptor. The model might help provide some insight into the complex interrelationships between viral infection, genetic susceptibility and abnormal cytokine and skeletal metabolism.

The cause of Paget's disease is still elusive.

REFERENCES

Abe T, Kawamuki K, Kudo M et al, Biological activity of a new bisphosphonate, YM 084, in animals, *J Bone Miner Res* (1989) **4**(Suppl 1):538

Abelanet R, Forest M, Vacher-Lavenu MC et al, Inclusions paramyxovirus-like intranucléaires dans les tumeures à cellules géantes des ostéoclastes, *Rhumatologie* (1982) **12**:156–9.

Acar J, Delbarre F, Waynberger N, Les complications cardiovasculaires de la maladie osseuse de Paget, *Arch Mal Coeur* (1968) **61**:849–68.

Adami S, Bhalla AK, Dorizzi R et al, The acute phase response after bisphosphonate administration, *Calcif Tissue Int* (1987) **41**:326–31.

Adami S, Frijlink WB, Bijvoet OLM et al, Regulation of calcium absorption by 1,25,di-hydroxy-vitamin D. Studies of the effects of a bisphosphonate treatment, *Calcif Tissue Int* (1982) **34**:317–20.

Adami S, Guarrera G, Salvagna G et al, Sequential treatment of Paget's disease with human calcitonin and dichloromethylene diphosphonate (Cl_2MDP), *Metab Bone Dis Relat Res* (1984) **5**:265–7.

Adami S, Salvagno G, Dorizz R et al, The acute phase response after administration of bisphosphonates in humans, *Calcif Tissue Int* (1985) **38**(Suppl):21.

Adami S, Salvagna G, Guarrera G et al, Treatment of Paget's disease of bone with intravenous 4-amino-1-hydroxybutylidene-1,1-bisphosphonate, *Calcif Tissue Int* (1986) **39**:262–9.

Agha FP, Norman A, Hirschi S et al, Paget's disease. Coexistence with metastatic carcinoma, *NY State J Med* (1976) **76**:734–5.

Aitken JM and Lindsay R, Mithramycin in Paget's disease, *Lancet* (1973) **i**:1177–8.

Albright F and Henneman PH, The suppression of Paget's disease with ACTH and cortisone, *Trans Assoc Am Physicians* (1955) **68**:238–46.

Albright JA and Skinner HCW, Bone remodelling dynamics. In: Albright JA, Brand RA, eds. *The scientific basis of orthopaedics*. (Appleton–Century–Crofts: New York 1979) 185–229.

Alexandre C, Chapuy MC and Meunier PJ, Le test d'hypocalcemie aux calcitonines synthétiques de saumon et humaine. Réponses paradoxales hypercalcemiques chez les pagétiques traités par l'EHDP, *Rev Rhum Mal Osteoartic* (1979a) **46**:335–42.

Alexandre CM, Chapuy MC, Vignon E et al, Treatment of Paget's disease of bone with ethane-1 hydroxy-1,1-diphosphonate (EHDP) at a low dosage (5 mg/kg/day), *Clin Orthop* (1983) **174**:193–205.

Alexandre CM, Matthews JL, Meunier PJ et al, Ultrastructural aspects of osteoclasts and osteoblasts in Paget's disease of bone treated with dichloromethylene diphosphonate (Cl_2MDP), In: Cohn DV, Talmage RV, Matthews JL, eds. *Hormonal control of calcium metabolism*. (Excerpta Medica: Amsterdam 1981b) 335.

Alexandre C, Meunier PJ, Edouard C et al, Effects of ethane-1 hydroxy-1,1 diphosphonate on quantitative bone histology in Paget's disease of bone, *Metab Bone Dis Relat Res* (1981a) **3**:309–15.

Alexandre C, Trillet M, Meunier P et al, Traitement des paraplégies pagétiques traitées par les diphosphonates, *Rev Neurol* (1979b) **135**:625–32.

Altman RD, Long-term follow up of therapy with intermittent etidronate disodium in Paget's disease of bone, *Am J Med* (1985) **79**:583–90.

Altman RD, Brown M and Gargano F, Low back pain in Paget's disease of bone, *Clin Orthop* (1987) **217**:152–61.

Altman RD and Collins B, Musculoskeletal manifestations of Paget's disease of bone, *Arthritis Rheum* (1980) **23**:1121–7.

Altman RD and Collins-Yudiskas B, Synthetic human calcitonin in refractory Paget's disease of bone, *Arch Intern Med* (1987) **147**:1305–8.

Altman RD, Johnston CC, Khairi MRA et al, Influence of disodium etidronate on clinical and laboratory manifestations of Paget's disease of bone (osteitis deformans), *N Engl J Med* (1973) **289**:1379–84.

Amara SG, Jonas V, Rosenfeld MG et al, Alternative RNA processing in calcitonin gene expression generates mRNAs encoding different polypeptide products, *Nature* (1982) **298**:240–4.

Amor B, Nguyen N, Treves R et al, Treatment of Paget's disease of bone with (4-chlorophenyl) thiomethylene bisphosphonic acid, a new bisphosphonate, *Calcif Tissue Int* (1989) **44**(Suppl):102.

Anderson DC and Cantrill JC, Treatment of Paget's disease of bone, *Br Med J* (1988) **296**:291.

Anderson DC, O'Driscoll JB, Buckler HM et al, Relapse of osteoporosis circumscripta as a lytic ring after treatment of Paget's disease with 3-amino-hydroxypropylidene-1,1-bisphosphonate (APD), *Br J Radiol* (1988) **61**:996–1001.

Arlet J and Mazieres B, La circulation dans l'os pagétique. Revue générale et données personnelles, *Rev Rhum Mal Osteoartic* (1975) **42**:643–6.

Arlot ME and Meunier PJ, Effects of two diphosphonates (EHDP and Cl_2MDP) on serum uric acid in Pagetic patients, *Calcif Tissue Int* (1981) **33**:195–8.

Arnalich F, Plaza I, Sobrino JA et al, Cardiac size and function in Paget's disease of bone, *Int J Cardiol* (1984) **5**:491–505.

Ashton BA, Hohling HJ and Triffitt JT, Plasma proteins present in human cortical bone: enrichment of the alpha-2-HS-glycoprotein, *Calcif Tissue Res* (1976) **22**:27–33.

Ashton BA and Smith R, Plasma alpha-2-HS-glycoprotein concentration in Paget's disease of bone: its possible significance, *Clin Sci* (1980) **58**:435–8.

Astre G, Maladie osseuse pagétoïde d'un crane gallo-romain, *Rev Pathol Genérale et Comparée* (1957) **57**:955–61.

Atkins RM, Yates AJP, Gray RES et al, Aminohexane diphosphonate in the treatment of Paget's disease of bone, *J Bone Miner Res* (1987) **2**:273–9.

Audran M, Renier JC, Clochon P et al, Treatment of Paget's disease with SR41319B a new diphosphonate, *Calcif Tissue Int* (1985) **38**(Suppl):124a.

Auld WHR, Simpson RH and Smyth M, Hypercalcaemia in Paget's disease of bone, *Lancet* (1979) **i**:562–3.

Avioli LV, The benefits of long-term calcitonin treatment in Paget's disease of bone, In: Pecile A, ed. *Calcitonin.* (Elsevier: Amsterdam 1985) 325–8.

Avramides A, Salmon and porcine calcitonin treatment of Paget's disease of bone, *Clin Orthop* (1977) **127**:78–85.

Avramides A, Flores A, DeRose J et al, Treatment of Paget's disease of bone with once a week injections of salmon calcitonin, *Br Med J* (1975) **3**:632.

Avramides A, Flores A, DeRose J et al, Paget's disease of bone. Observations after cessation of long-term synthetic salmon calcitonin treatment, *J Clin Endocrinol Metab* (1976) **42**:459–63.

Avramides A, Flores A and Wallach S, Treatment of Paget's disease of bone (osteitis deformans) using synthetic salmon calcitonin alone and in combination with mithramycin, *Acta Endocrinol* (1982) **248**(Suppl):26–7.

Azria M, *The calcitonins. Physiology and pharmacology.* (Karger: Basel 1989).

Bannister P, Roberts M and Sheridan P, Recurrent hypercalcaemia in a young man with monostotic Paget's disease, *Postgrad Med J* (1986) **62**:481–3.

Baker DJP, The epidemiology of Paget's disease, *Metab Bone Dis Relat Res* (1981) **3**:231–4.

Barker DJP, The epidemiology of Paget's disease of bone, *Br Med Bull* (1984) **40**:396–400.

Barker DJP, Chamberlain AT, Guyer AB et al, Paget's disease of bone: the Lancashire focus, *Br Med J* (1980) **280**:1105–7.

Barker DJP, Clough PLW, Guyer PB et al, Paget's disease of bone in 14 British towns, *Br Med J* (1977) **i**:1181–3.

Barker DJP and Detheridge FM, Dogs and Paget's disease, *Lancet* (1985) **ii**:1245.

Barker DJ and Gardner MJ, Distribution of Paget's disease in England Wales and Scotland and a possible relationship with vitamin D deficiency in childhood, *Br J Prev Social Med* (1974) **28**:226–32.

Baron R and Saffar JL, A quantitative study of the effect of prolonged calcitonin treatment on alveolar bone remodelling in the golden hamster, *Calcif Tissue Res* (1977) **22**: 265–74.

Baron R and Vignery A, Behaviour of osteoclasts during a rapid change in their number induced by high doses of parathyroid hormone or calcitonin in intact rats, *Metab Bone Dis Relat Res* (1981) **2**:339–43.

Baron R, Vignery A and Horowitz M, Lymphocytes, macrophages and the regulation of bone remodelling, In: Peck WA, ed. *Bone and mineral research*. (Elsevier: Amsterdam 1983) 175–84.

Barry HC, Sarcoma in Paget's disease of bone in Australia, *J Bone Joint Surg* (1961) **43A**:1122–34.

Barry HC, *Paget's disease of bone*. (Churchill–Livingstone: Edinburgh and London 1969).

Barry HC, Orthopaedic aspects of Paget's disease of bone, *Arthritis Rheum* (1980) **23**:1128–30.

Baslé M, Fournier JG, Rozenblatt S et al, Measles virus RNA detected in Paget's disease of bone tissue by in situ hybridization, *J Gen Virol* (1986) **67**:907–13.

Baslé MF, Rebel A, Fournier JG et al, On the trail of paramyxoviruses in Paget's disease of bone, *Clin Orthop* (1987) **217**:9–15.

Baslé MG, Rebel A, Filmon R et al, Maladie osseuse de Paget. Anticorps sériques antirougeole, *Nouv Presse Med* (1983) **12**:769–70.

Baslé MG, Rebel A, Renier C et al, Bone tissue in Paget's disease treated by ethane-1-hydroxy-1,1-diphosphonate EHDP. Structure ultrastructure and immunocytology, *Clin Orthop* (1984) **184**:281–8.

Bastian JW, Aldred JP, Lesh JB et al, Clinical experience in Paget's disease with porcine and salmon calcitonin, In: Hioco DJ ed. *La maladie de Paget*. (Lab Armour Montagu: Paris 1977) 270–99.

Bell NH, Avery S and Johnston CC, Effects of calcitonin in Paget's disease and polyostotic fibrous dysplasia, *J Clin Endocrinol* (1970) **31**:283–90.

Benéton MNC, Harris S and Kanis JA, Paramyxovirus-like inclusions in two cases of pycnodysostosis, *Bone* (1987) **8**:211–17.

Bickerstaff D, Douglas DL, Burke PH et al, Improvement in facial deformity of Paget's disease treated with diphosphonates, *J Bone Joint Surg* (1990) **72B**:132–6.

Bijvoet OLM, Frijlink WB, Jie K et al, APD in Paget's disease of bone. Role of the mononuclear phagocyte system?, *Arthritis Rheum* (1980a) **23**:1193–204.

Bijvoet OLM, Hosking DJ, Frijlink WB et al, Treatment of Paget's disease with combined calcitonin and diphosphonate (EHDP), *Metab Bone Dis Relat Res* (1978a) **1**:251–61.

Bijvoet OLM, Hosking DJ, Lemkes HHPJ et al, Development in the treatment of Paget's disease. In: Copp DH, Talmage RV, eds. *Endocrinology of calcium metabolism*. (Excerpta Medica: Amsterdam and Oxford 1978b) 48–54.

Bijvoet OLM, Hosking DJ, van Aken J et al, The treatment of Paget's disease. Combination of calcitonin and diphosphonates, In: Kanis JA, ed. *Bone disease and calcitonin*. (Armour Pharmaceutical: Eastbourne 1977) 25–37.

Bijvoet OLM and Jansen A, Thyrocalcitonin in Paget's disease, *Lancet* (1967) **ii**:472.

Bijvoet OLM, Nollen AJG, Sloof TJJH et al, Effects of a diphosphonate on para-articular ossification after total hip replacement, *Acta Orthop Scand* (1974) **45**:926–34.

Bijvoet OLM, Reitsma PH and Frijlink WB, Bisphosphonates and Paget's disease, *Lancet* (1980b) **i**:1416–17.

Bijvoet OLM, Reitsma PH, Frijlink WB et al, APD, bisphosphonates, the bone resorbing and the mononuclear phagocyte system. In: Donath A, Courvoisier B, eds. *Diphosphonates and bone*. (Editions Medicine et Hygiene: Geneva 1982) 328–36.

Bijvoet OLM, van der Sluys Veer J, DeVries H et al, Natriuretic effect of calcitonin in man, *N Engl J Med* (1971) **284**:681–8.

Bijvoet OLM, van der Sluys Veer JD and Jansen AP, Effects of calcitonin on patients with Paget's disease, thyrotoxicosis or hypercalcaemia, *Lancet* (1968) **i**:876–81.

Bilezikian JP, Canfield RE, Jacobs TP et al, Response of 1,25-dihydroxyvitamin D to hypocalcemia in human subjects, *N Engl J Med* (1978) **299**:437–41.

Blanco O, Stivel M, Mautalen C et al, Familial idiopathic hyperphosphatasia. A study of two young siblings treated with porcine calcitonin, *J Bone Joint Surg* (1977) **59B**:421–7.

Bloch-Michel H, Benoist M, Cophigon J et al, Tumeurs benignes à cellules géantes associées à une maladie de Paget, *Rev Rhum Mal Osteoartic* (1975) **42**:681–7.

Blomqvist C, Malignant hypercalcemia – a hospital survey, *Acta Med Scand* (1986) **220**:455–63.

Bloom RA, Libson E, Blank P et al, Prevalence of Paget's disease of bone in hospital patients in Jerusalem: an epidemiologic study, *Israel J Med Sci* (1985) **21**:954–6.

Blotman F, Blard JM, Labauge R et al, Exploration ultrasonique de la circulation encephalique chez le pagetique, *Rev Rhum Mal Osteoartic* (1975) **42**:647–50.

Blotman F, Suquet P, Labauge R et al, L'hémodétournement carotidien externe par le crane pagétique. In: Hioco DJ, ed. *La maladie de Paget. Symposium international.* (Lab Armour Montagu: Paris 1974) 79–87.

Bockman R, Warrell R, Bosco B et al, Treatment of Paget's disease of bone with low-dose subcutaneous gallium nitrate, *J Bone Miner Res* (1989) **4**(Suppl 1):167.

Bohrer SP, Osteitis deformans in Nigerians, *African J Med Sci* (1970) **1**:109–13.

Bone HG, Cody D, Ellis B et al, Assessment of healing in Paget's disease of bone using high resolution quantitative computed tomography, *Proc 71st Annual Meeting of the Endocrine Society* (1989), abstract 451.

Boonekamp PM, van der Wee Pals LJA, van Wij-van Lennep MLL et al, Two modes of action of bisphosphonates on osteoclastic resorption of mineralised matrix, *Bone Miner* (1986) **1**:27–39.

Bordier P, Hioco D, Tun-Chot S, Calcitonin: acute effects upon serum calcium urinary hydroxyproline excretion and osteoclasts in man. In: Taylor S, Foster G, eds. *Calcitonin 1969*. (Heinemann: London 1970) 339–47.

Borgstrom GH, Elomaa I, Blomqvist C et al, Cytogenetic investigations of patients on clodronate therapy for Paget's disease of bone, *Bone* (1987) **8**(Suppl 1):85–6.

Boris A, Hurley JF, Trmal T et al, Inhibition of diphosphonate blocked bone mineralisation. Evidence that calcitonin promotes mineralisation, *Acta Endocrinol* (1979) **91**:351–61.

Botez MI, Bertrand G, Leveille J et al, Parkinsonism – dementia complex, hydrocephalus and Paget's disease, *J Can Sci Neurol* (1977) **4**:139–42.

Boudreau RJ, Lisbona R, Hadjipavlou A, Observations on serial radionuclide blood-flow studies in Paget's disease, *J Nucl Med* (1983) **24**:880–5.

Bounameaux HM, Schifferli J, Montani J-P et al, Renal failure associated with intravenous diphosphonates, *Lancet* (1983) **i**:471.

Boussina I, Gerster JC, Epiney J et al, A study of the incidence of articular chondrocalcinosis in Paget's disease of bone, *Ann Rheum Dis* (1975) **34**:198.

Bouvet JP, Traitment de la maladie de Paget par la thyrocalcitonine du saumon, *Nouv Presse Med* (1977) **6**:1447–50.

Bowerman JW, Altman J, Hughes JL et al, Pseudomalignant lesions in Paget's disease of bone, *AJR* (1975) **124**:57–61.

Bowie HIC and Kanis JA, Calcitonin in the assessment and preparation of patients with Paget's disease for surgery. In: Kanis JA, ed. *Bone disease and calcitonin.* (Armour Pharmaceutical: Eastbourne 1977) 61–9.

Boyce BF, Fogelman I, Ralston S et al, Focal osteomalacia due to low dose diphosphonate therapy in Paget's disease, *Lancet* (1984) **i**:821–4.

Braga P, Ferri S, Santagostino A et al, Lack of opiate receptor involvement in centrally induced calcitonin analgesia, *Life Sci* (1978) **22**:971–8.

Brailsford JF, Paget's disease of bone, *Br J Radiol* (1954) **27**:435–42.

Broberg MA and Cass JR, Total knee arthroplasty in Paget's disease of the knee, *J Arthroplasty* (1986) **1**:139–42.

Brook RI, Giant cell tumour in patients with Paget's disease, *J Oral Surg* (1970) **30**:230–41.

Brown HP, LaRocca H and Wickstrom JK, Paget's disease of the atlas and axis, *J Bone Joint Surg* (1971) **53A**:1441–4.

Brown JP, Delmas PD, Malaval L et al, Serum bone-gla protein: a specific marker for bone formation in postmenopausal osteoporosis, *Lancet* (1984) **i**:1091–3.

Buckler HM, Cantrill JA and Anderson DC, The use of intravenous 3-amino-1-hydroxy-propylidene-1,1-bisphosphonate (APD) in forty patients with Paget's disease of bone, *Bone* (1986) **7**:307.

Buclin T, Randin JP, Jacquet AF et al, The effect of rectal and nasal administration of salmon calcitonin in normal subjects, *Calcif Tissue Int* (1987) **41**:252–8.

Bull JWD, Nixon WLB, Pratt RTC et al, Paget's disease of the skull and secondary basilar impression, *Brain* (1959) **82**:10–22.

Burch WM, Calcitonin stimulates growth and maturation of embryonic chick pelvic cartilage in vitro, *Endocrinology* (1984) **114**:1196–1201.

Burckhardt P, Ducommun J and Hessler, C, Treatment of Paget's disease with human calcitonin. In: MacIntyre I, ed. *Human calcitonin and Paget's disease*. (Hans Huber: Berne 1977) 155–66.

Burckhardt PM, Singer FR and Potts JT, Parathyroid function in patients with Paget's disease treated with salmon calcitonin. *Clin Endocrinol* (1973) **2**:15–22.

Burgener FA and Perry PE, Pitfalls in the radiographic diagnosis of Paget's disease of the pelvis, *Skeletal Radiol* (1978) **2**:231–8.

Burke PH, Stereophotogrammetric measurement of normal facial asymmetry in children, *Hum Biol* (1971) **43**:536–48.

Butlin HT, Pathological Society of London, Osteitis deformans, *Lancet* (1885) **i**:519.

Buxbaum JN and Kammerman S, Immunoglobulin abnormalities in Paget's disease of bone, *Clin Exp Immunol* (1984) **55**:200–204.

Camus JP, Tricoire J, Mariel L et al, La maladie de Paget. Poussées evolutives traitées par la calcitonine. Etude thermographique, *Nouv Presse Med* (1973) **2**:2517–19.

Canalis E, McCarthy T and Cantrella M, The regulation of bone formation by local growth factors, *Bone Miner Res Ann* (1989) **6**:27–56.

Canfield R, Rosner W, Skinner J et al, Diphosphonate therapy of Paget's disease of bone, *J Clin Endocrinol Metab* (1977) **44**:96–106.

Canfield RE, Siris ES, Jacobs TP et al, EHDP treatment of Paget's disease of bone, *Br J Clin Pract* (1981) **13**(Suppl):58–63.

Caniggia A, Nuti R, Galli M et al, Effect of a long-term treatment with the amino-suberic analog of eel calcitonin on osteocalcin in Paget's disease, *Panminerva Med* (1987) **29**:1–5.

Cantalamessa L, Catania A, Reschini E et al, Inhibitory effect of calcitonin in man, *Metabolism* (1978) **27**:987–92.

Cantrill JA, Buckler HM and Anderson DC, Low dose intravenous 3-amino-1-hydroxypropylidene-1,1-bisphosphonate (APD) for the treatment of Paget's disease of bone, *Ann Rheum Dis* (1986) **45**:1012–18.

Carano A, Teitelbaum SL, Kousek JD et al, Bisphosphonates directly inhibit the bone resorption activity of isolated avian osteoclasts in vitro, *J Clin Invest* (1990) **85**:456–61.

Care AD, The direct measurement of thyrocalcitonin secretion in vivo. In: Talmage RV, Belanger LF, eds. *Parathyroid hormone and thyrocalcitonin (calcitonin)*. (Excerpta Medica: Amsterdam 1968) 417–27.

Chambers TJ, Diphosphonates inhibit bone resorption by macrophages in vitro, *J Pathol* (1980) **132**:255–62.

Chambers TJ and Magnus CJ, Calcitonin alters behaviour of isolated osteoclasts, *J Pathol* (1982) **82**:27–39.

Chandler PT and Chandler SA, Bone density as a parameter of Paget's disease, *Postgrad Med* (1982) **71**:57–9.

Chao WH and Forte LR, Rat kidney cells in primary culture: hormone mediated desensitization of the adenosine-3′,5′-monophosphate response to parathyroid hormone and calcitonin, *Endocrinology* (1982) **111**:252–9.

Chao WH and Forte LR, Rat kidney cells in primary culture: interaction of salmon calcitonin with receptor sites, *Endocrinology* (1983) **112**:745–52.

Chapuy M-C, Charhon SA and Meunier PJ, Sustained biochemical effects of short treatment of Paget's disease of bone with dichloromethylene diphosphonate, *Metab Bone Dis Relat Res* (1983) **4**:325–8.

Chapuy M-C and Meunier PJ, Comparison of the acute effect of eel and salmon calcitonins in Pagetic patients, *Horm Metab Res* (1982) **14**:559–60.

Chapuy M-C, Meunier PJ and Alexandre C, Comparison of the acute effects of human and salmon calcitonins in Pagetic patients: relation with plasma calcitonin levels, *Metab Bone Dis Relat Res* (1980) **2**:93–7.

Chapuy M-C, Meunier P, Terrier M et al, Effets biologiques à court terme de la calcitonine synthétique de saumon dans la maladie de Paget. Influence de la posologie, *Pathol Biol* (1975) **23**:349–59.

Chapuy M-C, Zucchelli P and Meunier PJ, Parathyroid function in Paget's disease of bone, *Miner Electrolyte Metab* (1981) **6**:112–18.

Charhon S, Chapuy MC, Valentin-Opran A et al, Intravenous etidronate for spinal cord dysfunction due to Paget's disease, *Lancet* (1982) **i**:391–2.

Cheah KSE, Collagen genes and inherited connective tissue disease, *Biochem J* (1985) **229**:287–303.

Chen JR, Rhee R, Wallach S et al, Neurologic disturbances in Paget's disease of bone: response to calcitonin, *Neurology* (1979) **29**:448–57.

Cheung HS, Singer FR, Mills B et al, In vitro synthesis of normal bone (type 1) collagen by bones of Paget's disease patients, *Proc Soc Exp Biol Med* (1980) **163**:547–52.

Chierichetti SM, Gennari C, Piolini M et al, Comparative biological activities of different calcitonins in man. In: Pecile A, ed. *Calcitonin*. (Elsevier Science Publishers: Holland 1985) 173–81.

Clarke PRR and Williams HI, Ossification in extradural fat in Paget's disease of the spine, *Br J Surg* (1975) **62**:571–2.

Collins AJ, Ring F, Bacon PA et al, Thermography and radiology: Complimentary methods for the study of inflammatory diseases, *Clin Radiol* (1976) **27**:237–43.

Collins D, *Pathology of bone*. (Butterworths: London 1966).

Collins DH, Paget's disease of bone: incidence and subclinical forms, *Lancet* (1956) **ii**:51–7.

Condon JR, Glucagon in the treatment of Paget's disease of bone, *Br Med J* (1971) **4**:719–21.

Condon JR, Reith SBM, Nassim JR et al, Treatment of Paget's disease of bone with mithramycin, *Br Med J* (1972) **1**:421–3.

Cone SM, The pathology of osteitis deformans Paget's disease, *J Bone Joint Surg* (1922) **4**:751–88.

Conget JI, Vendrell J, Halperin I et al, Widespread tremor after injection of sodium calcitonin, *Br Med J* (1989) **298**:189.

Cooke BED, Paget's disease of the jaws: fifteen cases, *Ann R Coll Surg Engl* (1956) **19**:223–40.

Cooper CW, Schwesinger WH, Mahgoub AM et al, Thyrocalcitonin: stimulation of secretion by pentagastrin, *Science* (1971) **172**:1238–40.

Cooper CW, Obie JF, Toverud SV et al, Elevated serum calcitonin and serum calcium during suckling in the baby rat, *Endocrinology* (1977) **101**:1657–64.

Copp DH, Crocford DW and Kuch Y, Calcitonin from ultimo-branchial glands of dogfish and chickens, *Science* (1967) **158**:924–6.

Coulton LA, Preston CJ, Couch M et al, An evaluation of serum osteocalcin in Paget's disease of bone, *Arthritis Rheum* (1988) **31**:1142–7.

Coutris G, Gayla J, Rondier J et al, Analyse des pertubations des voies principales du metabolisme calcique dans la maladie de Paget. Effets de l'administration de calcitonine, *Rev Rhum Mal Osteoartic* (1975) **42**:757–9.

Crisp AJ, Pizotifen to prevent side-effects of calcitonin, *Lancet* (1981) **i**:775.

Crock HV and Yoshizawa H, *The blood supply of the vertebral column and spine in man*. (Springer: Berlin 1977).

Crosbie WA, Mohamedally SM and Woodhouse NJY, Effect of salmon calcitonin on cardiac output oxygen transport and bone turnover in patients with Paget's disease, *Clin Sci Mol Med* (1975) **48**:537–40.

Culebras A, Feldman RG and Fager CA, Hydrocephalus and dementia in Paget's disease of the skull, *J Neurol Sci* (1974) **23**:307–21.

Cullen P, Russell RGG, Walton RJ et al, Frequencies of HLA-A and HLA-B histocompatibility antigens in Paget's disease of bone, *Tissue Antigens* (1976) **7**:55–6.

Czerny V, Eine lokale Malacie des Unterschenkels, *Wien Med Wochenschr* (1873) **1**:1–3.

D'Agostino HR, Barnett CA, Zielinski XJ et al, Intranasal salmon calcitonin treatment of Paget's disease of bone: results in nine patients, *Clin Orthop* (1988) **230**:223–8.

Dahniya MH, Paget's disease of bone in Africans, *Br J Radiol* (1987) **60**:113–16.

Dalinka MK, Aronchick JM and Haddad JG, Paget's disease, *Orthop Clin North Am* (1983) **14**:3–19.

Dastur FD and Kaji DM, Paget's disease of bone, *J Postgrad Med* (1971) **17**:43–6.

Datta HK, Zaida M, Winalawansa SJ et al, In vivo and in vitro effects of amylin and amylin-amide on calcium metabolism in the rat and rabbit, *Biochem Biophys Res Commun* (1989) **162**:876–81.

David-Chausse J, Vallat JM and Dehais J, Deux cas de compression de la queue de cheval d'origine pagétique. Role du rétrécissement du canal lombaire osseux. In: Hioco DJ, ed. *La maladie de Paget. Symposium International.* (Lab Armour Montagu: Paris 1974) 59–69.

Davies DJ, Paget's disease of the temporal bone. A clinical and histopathological survey, *Acta Otolaryng* (1968) **242**(Suppl):7–43.

Deftos LJ, Roos BA, Bronzert D et al, Immunochemical heterogeneity of calcitonin in plasma, *J Clin Endocrinol Metab* (1975) **40**:409–12.

Deftos LJ, Weisman MH, Williams GW et al, Influence of age and sex on plasma calcitonin in human beings, *N Engl J Med* (1980) **302**:1351–3.

Delling G, Shafer A and Ziegler R, The effect of calcitonin on fracture healing and ectopic bone formation in the rat. In: Taylor S, ed. *Calcitonin 1969.* (Heinemann: London 1970) 175–81.

Delling GR, Schulz A and Ziegler R, Changes of bone remodelling surfaces and bone structure in Paget's disease following long-term treatment with calcitonin, *Calcif Tissue Int* (1977) **22**:359–61.

Delmas P, Chapuy M-C, Edouard C et al, Beneficial effects of aminohexane diphosphonate in patients with Paget's disease of bone resistant to sodium etidronate, *Am J Med* (1987) **83**:276–82.

Delmas PD, Chapuy M-C, Vignon E et al, Long-term effects of dichloromethylene diphosphonate in Paget's disease of bone, *J Clin Endocrinol Metab* (1982) **54**:837–44.

Delmas PD, Demiaux B, Malaval L et al, Serum bone gla-protein is not a sensitive marker of bone turnover in Paget's disease of bone, *Calcif Tissue Int* (1986) **38**: 60–1.

Denninger HS, Paleopathological evidence of Paget's disease, *Ann Med Hist* (1933) **5**:73–81.

DeQueker J, Paget's disease in a painting by Quintein Metsys (Massys) (1465–1530) in the National Gallery London, *Br Med J* (1989) **299**:1579–81.

DeRose J, Singer F, Avramides A et al, Response of Paget's disease to porcine and salmon calcitonins – effects of long-term treatment, Am J Med (1974) **56**:858–66.

Detheridge FM, Guyer PB and Barker DJP, European distribution of Paget's disease of bone, *Br Med J* (1982) **285**:1005–8.

Detheridge FM, Barker DJP and Guyer PB, Paget's disease of bone in Ireland, *Br Med J* (1983) **287**:1345–6.

DeVernejoul MC, Pointillart A, Bordeau A et al, Effect of calcitonin administration on young pig trabecular bone remodelling, *Bone* (1990) **11**:29–33.

Devogelaer JP, Esselinckx W and Nagant de Deuxchaisnes C, The effect of the bisphosphonate tiludronic acid (SR 41319 B) in Paget's disease of bone, *Calcif Tissue Int* (1989) **44**(Suppl):104.

DeVries E, van der Weij JP, Veen CJP et al, In vitro effect of (3-amino-1-hydroxypropylidene)-1,1-bisphosphonic acid (APD) on the function of mononuclear phagocytes in lymphocytic proliferation, *Immunology* (1982) **47**:157–63.

DeVries HR and Bijvoet OLM, Results of prolonged treatment of Paget's disease of bone with disodium ethane-1-hydroxy-1,1-diphosphonate (EHDP), *Neth J Med* (1974) **17**:281–97.

Dewis P, Prasad BK, Anderson DC et al, Clinical experience with the use of two diphosphonates in the treatment of Paget's disease, *Ann Rheum Dis* (1985) **44**:34–8.

Dickson DD, Camp JD and Ghormley RK, Osteitis deformans: Paget's disease of the bone, *Radiology* (1945) **44**:449–70.

Dickson GR, Osterberg PH, Wallace RGH et al, Familial expansile osteolysis (FEO): an ultrastructural investigation, *Bone* (1991) in press.

Dinarello CA, Interleukin 1, *Rev Infect Dis* (1984) **6**:51–95.

Direkze M and Milnes JN, Spinal cord compression in Paget's disease, *Br J Surg* (1970) **57**:239–40.

Dodd GW, Ibbertson HK, Fraser TRC et al, Radiological assessment of Paget's disease of bone after treatment with the bisphosphonates EHDP and APD, *Br J Radiol* (1987) **60**:849–60.

Douglas DL, *Effects of dichloromethylene diphosphonate on Paget's disease of bone*, MD thesis, University of Sheffield (1983).

Douglas DL, Duckworth T, Kanis JA et al, Biochemical and clinical responses to dichloromethylene diphosphonate (Cl_2MDP) in Paget's disease of bone, *Arthritis Rheum* (1980a) **23**:1185–92.

Douglas DL, Duckworth T, Kanis JA et al, Spinal cord dysfunction in Paget's disease of bone: has medical treatment a vascular basis? *J Bone Joint Surg* (1981a) **63B**:495–503.

Douglas DL, Kanis JA, Duckworth T et al, Paget's disease: improvement of spinal cord dysfunction with diphosphonates and calcitonin, *Metab Bone Dis Relat Res* (1981b) **3**:327–36.

Douglas DL, Russell RGG, Preston CJ et al, Effect of dichloromethylene diphosphonate in Paget's disease of bone and in hyperparathyroidism or malignant disease, *Lancet* (1980b) **i**:1043–7.

Dove J, Complete fractures of the femur in Paget's disease of bone, *J Bone Joint Surg* (1980) **62B**:12–17.

Doyle FH, Banks LM and Pennock JM, Radiologic observations on bone resorption in Paget's disease, *Arthritis Rheum* (1980) **23**:1205–14.

Doyle FH, Pennock J, Greenberg PB et al, Radiological evidence of a dose-related response to long-term treatment of Paget's disease with human calcitonin, *Br J Radiol* (1974a) **47**:1–8.

Doyle FH, Woodhouse NJY, Glen ACA et al, Healing of the bones in juvenile Paget's disease treated by human calcitonin, *Br J Radiol* (1974b) **47**:9–15.

Drapkin AJ, Epidural hematoma complicating Paget's disease of the skull: a case report, *Neurosurgery* (1984) **14**:211–14.

Edeiken J, Roentgen diagnosis of diseases of bone. In: Harris JH, ed. *Golden's diagnostic radiology*. (Williams and Wilkins: Baltimore and London 1982).

Editorial, Paget's disease of bone, *Br Med J* (1977) **1**:1427–8.

Editorial, Osteolytic Paget's disease, *Lancet* (1986) **i**:1255.

Eisinger J, Comparison de l'effet hypocalcémiant immediat de la calcitonine de saumon par voie veineuse et par voie nasale, *Rev Rhum Mal Osteoartic* (1985a) **52**:195.

Eisinger J, Action de la calcitonine en spray nasal chez les pagétiques, *Lyon Mediterranée Médicale* (1985b) **21**:9631–4.

Eisinger J and Laponche AM, Traitement discontinu de la maladie de Paget par la calcitonine. Etude histologique, *Rev Rhum Mal Osteoartic* (1976) **43**:511–16.

Elomaa I, Blomqvist C, Grohn P et al, Long-term controlled trial with diphosphonate in patients with osteolytic bone metastases, *Lancet* (1983) **i**:146–9.

Ende JJ and van Rooijen HJM, Some effects of EHDP and Cl_2MDP on the metabolism of mouse calvaria in tissue culture, *Proc Kon Ned Akad Wet* (1979) **C82**:43–53.

Eretto P, Krohel GB, Shihab ZM et al, Optic neuropathy in Paget's disease, *Am J Ophthalmol* (1984) **97**:505–10.

Eriksen EF, Normal and pathological remodelling of human trabecular bone. Three dimensional reconstruction of the remodelling sequence in normals and in metabolic bone disease, *Endocr Rev* (1986) **4**:379–408.

Espinasse D, Mathieu L, Alexandre C et al, The kinetics of ^{99m}Tc labelled EHDP in Paget's disease before and after dichloromethylene-diphosphonate treatment, *Metab Bone Dis Relat Res* (1981) **2**:321–4.

Evans GA and Slee GC, Calcitonin for multiple fractures in Paget's disease, *Br Med J* (1977) **1**:357.

Evans IMA, Human calcitonin in the treatment of Paget's disease: long-term trials. In: McIntyre I, ed. *Human calcitonin and Paget's disease*. (Hans Huber: Berne 1977a) 111–23.

Evans IMA, Banks L, Doyle FH et al, Paget's disease of bone: the effect of stopping long term human calcitonin and recommendations for future treatment, *Metab Bone Dis Relat Res* (1980) **2**:87–91.

Evans RA, A cheap oral therapy for Paget's disease of bone, *Aust NZ J Med* (1977b) **7**:259–61.

Evans RA, Treatment of Paget's disease of bone, *Med J Aust* (1983) **1**:159–63.

Evans RA, Dunstan CR, Wong WYP et al, Long-term experience with a calcium-thiazide treatment for Paget's disease of bone, *Miner Electrolyte Metab* (1982) **8**:325–33.

Evens RG and Bartter FC, The hereditary aspects of Paget's disease (osteitis deformans), *JAMA* (1968) **205**:900–2.

Eyre DR, Koob TJ and van Ness KP, Quantitation of hydroxypyridinium crosslinks in collagen by high performance liquid chromatography, *Anal Biochem* (1984) **137**:380–8.

Fahrenkrug J, Hornum I and Rehfeld JF, Effect of calcitonin on serum gastrin concentration and component pattern in man, *J Clin Endocrinol Metab* (1975) **41**:149–52.

Falch JA, Paget's disease in Norway, *Lancet* (1979) **ii**:1022.

Fast DK, Felix R, Dowse C et al, The effects of diphosphonates on growth and glycolysis of connective tissue cells in culture, *Biochem J* (1978) **172**:97–107.

Fedou P, Codine P and Simon L, Ostéolyse pseudotumorale sous diphosphonates, *Rev Rhum Mal Osteoartic* (1986) **53**:293–4.

Felix R, Bette J and Fleisch H, Effect of disphosphonate on the synthesis of prostaglandins in cultured calvaria cells, *Calcif Tissue Int* (1981) **33**:549–52.

Felix R and Fleisch H, Increase in fatty acid oxidation in calvaria cells cultured with diphosphonates, *Biochem J* (1981) **196**:237–45.

Felix R and Fleisch H, The effects of bisphosphonates on glycolysis in cultured cells and their homogenate, *Experientia* (1983) **39**:1293–5.

Felix R, Guenther HL and Fleisch H, The subcellular distribution of ^{14}C-dichloromethylenebisphosphonate and ^{14}C 1-hydroxyethylidene-1,1-bisphosphonate in cultured calvaria cells, *Calcif Tissue Int* (1984) **36**:108–13.

Fennelly JJ, Clinical and biochemical studies of Paget's disease of bone with emphasis on the effect of RNA inhibitors actinomycin A and mithramycin, *Ir J Med Sci* (1971) **140**:431–48.

Fennelly JJ and Groarke JF, Effect of actinomycin D on Paget's disease of bone, *Br Med J* (1971) **1**:423–6.

Fennelly JJ and Hogan A, Pseudouridine excretion – a reflection of high RNA turnover in Paget's disease, *Ir J Med Sci* (1972) **141**:103–7.

Finerman GAM, Gonick HC, Smith RK et al, Diphosphonate treatment of Paget's disease, *Clin Orthop* (1976) **120**:115–24.

Finerman GAM and Stover SL, Heterotopic ossification following hip replacement on spinal cord injury. Two clinical studies with EHDP, *Metab Bone Dis Relat Res* (1981) **3**:337–42.

Fiore CE, Castorina F, Malatino LS et al, Antalgic activity of calcitonin: effectiveness of the epidural and subarachnoid routes in man, *Int J Clin Pharmacol Res* (1983) **3**:257–60.

Fischer JA, Tobler PH, Henke H et al, Salmon and human calcitonin-like peptides coexist in the human thyroid and brain, *J Clin Endocrinol Metab* (1983) **57**:1314–16.

Fisher AK, Additional paleopathological evidence of Paget's disease, *Ann Med Hist* (1935) **7**:197–8.

Fleisch H, Diphosphonates: history and mechanisms of action, *Metab Bone Dis Relat Res* (1981) **3**:279–87.

Fleisch H, Experimental basis for the use of bisphosphonates in Paget's disease of bone, *Clin Orthop* (1987) **217**:72–8.

Fleisch H, Bisphosphonates: mechanisms of action and clinical applications. In: Peck WA, ed. *Bone and mineral research, annual 1.* (Excerpta Medica: Amsterdam 1989) 319–57.

Flora L, Hassing GS, Cloyd GG et al, The long-term skeletal effects of EHDP in dogs, *Metab Bone Dis Relat Res* (1981) **3**:289–300.

Flora L, Hassing GS, Parfitt AM et al, Comparative skeletal effects of two diphosphonates in dogs, *Metab Bone Dis Relat Res* (1980) **2**:389–407.

Fogelman I and Carr D, A comparison of bone scanning and radiology in the assessment of patients with symptomatic Paget's disease, *Eur J Nucl Med* (1980) **5**:417–21.

Fogelman I, Carr D and Boyle IT, The role of bone scanning in Paget's disease, *Metab Bone Dis Relat Res* (1981a) **3**:243–54.

Fogelman I, Pearson DW, Bessent RG et al, A comparison of skeletal uptake of 3 diphosphonates by whole body retention, *J Nucl Med* (1981b) **22**:880–3.

Fogelman I, Smith L, Mazess R et al, Absorption of oral diphosphonate in normal subjects, *Clin Endocrinol* (1986) **24**:57–62.

Foldes J, Shamir S, Scherman L et al, Histocompatibility antigens and Paget's disease of bone, *Calcif Tissue Int* (1987) **41**(Suppl 2):59.

Fon GT, Wong WS, Gold RH et al, Skeletal metastases of melanoma: radiographic, scintigraphic and clinical review, *AJR* (1981) **137**:103–8.

Fornasier VL, Stapleton K and Williams CC, Histologic changes in Paget's disease treated with calcitonin, *Hum Pathol* (1978) **9**:455–61.

Foster GV, Doyle FH, Bordier P et al, Effects of thyrocalcitonin on bone, *Lancet* (1966) **ii**:1428–31.

Fotino M, Haymovits A and Falk CT, Evidence for linkage between HLA and Paget's disease, *Transplant Proc* (1977) **9**:1867–8.

Fournie A, Valverde C, Tap G et al, Test d'hypocalcémie aiguë à la calcitonine de porc et de saumon, *Rev Rhum* (1977) **44**:91–8.

Fraioli F, Fabbri A, Genessi L et al, Subarachnoid injection of salmon calcitonin induces analgesia in man, *Eur J Pharmacol* (1982) **78**:381–2

Francis MD, Russell RGG and Fleisch H, Diphosphonates inhibit formation of calcium phosphate crystals in vitro and pathological calcification in vivo, *Science* (1969) **165**:1264–6.

Francis MJO and Smith R, Evidence of a generalised connective tissue defect in Paget's disease of bone, *Lancet* (1974) **i**:841–2.

Franck WA, Bress NM, Singer FR et al, Rheumatic manifestation of Paget's disease of bone, *Am J Med* (1974) **56**:592–603.

Frank MS, Brandt LJ, Kaufman DM et al, Oropharyngeal dysphagia in Paget's disease of bone (osteitis deformans): response to calcitonin, *Am J Gastroenterol* (1982) **77**:450–6.

Fraser KB and Martin SJ, *Measles virus and its biology*, (Academic Press: London 1978).

Fraser TRC, Ibbertson HK, Holdaway IM et al, Effective oral treatment of severe Paget's disease of bone with APD (3-amino-1-hydroxypropylidene-1,1- bisphosphonate): a comparison with combined calcitonin and EHDP (1-hydroxyethylidene-1,1-bisphosphonate), *Aust NZ J Med* (1984) **14**:811–18.

Friedman J and Raisz LG, Thyrocalcitonin. Inhibitor of bone resorption in tissue culture, *Science* (1965) **150**:1465–7.

Friedman P, Sklaver P and Klawans HL, Neurologic manifestations of Paget's disease of the skull, *Dis Nerv Sys* (1971) **32**:809–17.

Frijlink WB, te Velde J, Bijvoet OLM et al, Treatment of Paget's disease with 3-amino-1-hydroxypropylidene-1,1-bisphosphonate (APD), *Lancet* (1979) **i**:799–803.

Fromm GA, Roca JF, Mautalen CA et al, Osteitis deformante de Paget. Manifestaciones clinicas y humorales en 148 pacientes, *Medicina (B Aires)* (1980) **40**:635–42.

Fromm GA, Schajowicz F, Casco C et al, The treatment of Paget's bone disease with sodium etidronate, *Am J Med* (1979) **277**:29–37.

Frost AM, *Bone remodelling and its relationship to metabolic bone disease*. (Thomas: Springfield, Illinois 1973).

Frost HM, Some effects of basic multicellular unit-based remodelling on photon absorptiometry of trabecular bone, *Bone Miner* (1989) **7**:47–65.

Fuss M, Bergans A and Corvilain J, Hypercalcaemia due to immobilisation in Paget's disease of bone, *Lancet* (1978) **ii**:941.

Galante L, Joplin GF, MacIntyre I et al, The calcium lowering effect of synthetic human porcine and salmon calcitonin in patients with Paget's disease, *Clin Sci* (1973) **44**:605–10.

Galbraith HJB, Evans E and Lacey J, Paget's disease of bone. A clinical and genetic study, *Postgrad Med J* (1977) **53**:33–9.

Gardner WJ and Dohn DF, Trigeminal neuralgia – hemifacial spasm – Paget's disease. Significance of this association, *Brain* (1966) **89**:555–62.

Gardner MJ and Barker DJP, Mortality from malignant tumours of bone and Paget's disease in the United States and in England and Wales, *Int J Epidemiol* (1978) **7**:121–30.

Gardner MJ, Guyer PB and Barker DJ, Radiological prevalence of Paget's disease of bone in British migrants to Australia, *Br Med J* (1978) **i**:1655–7.

Gattereau A, Vinay P, Bielmann P et al, Effect of acute administration of salmon and human calcitonin on blood urate and renal excretion of uric acid in patients with Paget's disease of bone, *J. Clin Endocrinol Metab* (1979) **49**:635–7.

Gennari C, Agnusdei D, Gonelli S et al, La calcitonina di salmone spray nasale nel dolore osseo. In: Christiansen C, ed. *Advances in osteoporosis. Diagnosis and treatment today.* (Masson Italia Editori: Milan 1989) 85–9.

Gennari C, Chierichetti SM, Gonnelli S et al, Analgesic activity and side effects of different calcitonins in man. In: Pecile A, ed. *Calcitonin.* (Elsevier: Holland 1985) 183–8.

Gennari C, Chierichetti SM, Vibelli C et al, Acute effects of salmon human and porcine calcitonins on plasma calcium and cyclic AMP levels in man, *Current Therapeutic Research* (1981) **30**:1024–32.

Gennari C, Passeri M, Chierichetti SM et al, Side-effects of synthetic salmon and human calcitonin, *Lancet* (1983) **i**:594–5.

Genuth SM and Klein L, Hypoparathyroidism and Paget's disease: the effect of parathyroid hormone administration, *J Clin Endocrinol Metab* (1972) **35**:693–9.

Gershberg H, Girgis M, Goldberg L et al, The acute response to calcitonin in Paget's disease: its relationship to the serum alkaline phosphatase level and the effect of phosphate treatment, *J Clin Endocrinol Metab* (1973) **36**:691–6.

Gibbs CJ, Aaron JE and Peacock M, Osteomalacia in Paget's disease treated with short term high dose sodium etidronate, *Br Med J* (1986) **292**:1227–9.

Goldhammer Y, Braham J and Kosary IZ, Hydrocephalic dementia in Paget's disease of the skull: treatment by ventriculoatrial shunt, *Neurology* (1979) **29**:513–16.

Golding D, Beethoven's deafness, *JAMA* (1971) **215**:119.

Goldman AB, Braunstein P, Wilkinson D et al, Radionuclide uptake studies of bone – quantitative method of evaluating response of patients with Paget's disease to diphosphonate therapy, *Radiology* (1975) **117**:365–9.

Goldman AB, Bullough P, Kammerman S et al, Osteitis deformans of the hip joint, *AJR* (1977) **128**:601–6.

Goldsmith RS, Treatment of Paget's disease with phosphate, *Semin Drug Treat* (1972) **2**:69–75.

Gonzalez D, Vega E, Ghiringhelli G et al, Comparison of the acute effect of the intranasal and intramuscular administration of salmon calcitonin in Paget's disease, *Calcif Tissue Int* (1987) **41**:313–15.

Goorin AM, Abelson HT and Frei E, Osteosarcoma: fifteen years later, *N Engl J Med* (1985) **313**:1637–43.

Gordon MT, Sharpe PT and Anderson DC, Evidence from in situ hybridisation that canine distemper but not measles virus may be involved in Paget's disease of bone, *Bone* (1991) in press.

Goutallier D, Sterkers Y and Cadeau F. Expérience de la prothèse totale au cours de la coxopathie pagétique, *Rhumatologie* (1984) **36**:81–82.

Graham J and Harris WH, Paget's disease involving the hip joint, *J Bone Joint Surg* (1971) **53B**:650–9.

Gray RES, Yates AJP, Preston CJ et al, Duration of effect of oral diphosphonate therapy in Paget's disease of bone, *Q J Med* (1987) **64**:755–67.

Greditzer HG, McLeod RA, Unni KK et al, Bone sarcomas in Paget's disease, *Radiology* (1983) **146**:327–33.

Greenberg PB, Doyle FH, Fisher MT et al, Treatment of Paget's disease of bone with synthetic human calcitonin: biochemical and roentgenologic changes, *Am J Med* (1974) **56**:867–70.

Greene GS and Maurer AH, Solitary vertebral body uptake on bone scintigraphy: the black ivory vertebrae sign, *Semin Nucl Med* (1985) **15**:317–21.

Greenfield GB, *Radiology of the bone disease*, 3rd edn (JB Lippincott Company: Philadelphia and Toronto 1980) Chapter 3.

Grimaldi PMGB, Mohamedally SM and Woodhouse NJY, Deafness in Paget's disease. Effect of salmon calcitonin treatment, *Br Med J* (1975) **2**:726.

Groh JA, Mono-ostotic Paget's disease as a clinical entity: roentgenologic observations in nine cases, *Am J Radiol* (1943) **50**:235–48.

Grundy M, Fractures of the femur in Paget's disease of bone, *J Bone Joint Surg* (1970) **52B**:252–63.

Grunstein HS, Clifton-Bligh P and Posen S, Paget's disease of bone. Experiences with 100 patients treated with salmon calcitonin, *Med J Aust* (1981) **2**:278–80.

Gudmundsson TV, Galante L, Horton R et al, Human plasma calcitonin. In: Taylor S, Foster G, eds. *Calcitonin 1969.* (Heinemann: London 1969) 102–9.

Guilland-Cumming DF, Beard DJ, Douglas DL et al, Abnormal vitamin D metabolism in Paget's disease of bone, *Clin Endocrinol* (1985) **22**:559–66.

Guncaga J, Lauffenburger T, Lentner C et al, Diphosphonate treatment of Paget's disease of bone, *Horm Metab Res* (1974) **6**:62–9.

Gundberg CM, Lian JB, Gallop PM et al, Urinary gamma-carboxyglutamic acid and serum osteocalcin as bone markers: studies in osteoporosis and Paget's disease, *J Clin Endocrinol Metab* (1983) **57**:1221–5.

Gutman AB and Kasabach H, Paget's disease (osteitis deformans): analysis of 116 cases, *Am J Med Sci* (1936) **191**:361–80.

Guyer PB, The clinical relevance of radiologically revealed Paget's disease of bone (osteitis deformans), *Br J Surg* (1979) **66**:438–43.

Guyer PB, Paget's disease of bone: The anatomical distribution, *Metab Bone Dis Relat Res* (1981) **3**:239–42.

Guyer PB and Chamberlain AT, Paget's disease of bone in two American cities, *Br Med J* (1980) **280**:985.

Guyer PB and Chamberlain AT, Paget's disease of bone in South Africa, *Clin Radiol* (1988) **39**:51–2.

Guyer PB, Chamberlain AT, Ackery DM et al, The anatomic distribution of osteitis deformans, *Clin Orthop* (1981) **156**:141–4.

Guyer PB and Clough PWL, Paget's disease of bone: some observations on the relation of the skeletal distribution to pathogenesis, *Clin Radiol* (1978) **29**:421–6.

Guyer PB and Sheperd DFC, Paget's disease of the lumbar spine, *Br J Radiol* (1980) **53**:286–8.

Haddad JG, Birge S and Avioli L, Effects of prolonged thyrocalcitonin administration on Paget's disease of bone, *N Engl J Med* (1970b) **283**:549–55.

Haddad JG and Caldwell JG, Calcitonin resistance: clinical and immunologic studies in subjects with Paget's disease of bone treated with porcine and salmon calcitonin, *J Clin Invest* (1972) **51**:3133–41.

Haddad JG Jr, Couranz S and Avioli LV, Nondialyzable urinary hydroxyproline as an index of bone collagen formation, *J Clin Endocrinol Metab* (1970a) **30**:282–7.

Hadjipavlou A, Shaffer N, Lander P et al, Pagetic spinal stenosis with extradural pagetoid ossification. A case report, *Spine* (1988) **13**:128–30.

Hadjipavlou AG, Tsoukas GM, Siller TN et al, Combination drug therapy in Paget's disease of bone, *J Bone Joint Surg* (1977) **59A**:1045–51.

Hagg E, Eklund M and Torring O, Disodium etidronate in hypercalcaemia due to immobilisation, *Br Med J* (1984) **288**:607–8.

Haibach H, Farrell C and Dittrich FJ, Neoplasma arising in Paget's disease of bone: a study of 82 cases, *Am J Clin Pathol* (1985) **83**:594–600.

Haining SA, Guilland-Cumming CF, Taylor CM et al, Investigations into the metabolism of 24,25-dihydroxyvitamin D_3 in patients with Paget's disease of bone, *J Endocrinol* (1987) **112**(Suppl):174.

Hamdy NAT, Gray RES, McCloskey E et al, Clodronate in the medical management of hyperparathyroidism, *Bone* (1987) **8**(Suppl 1):69–78.

Hamdy RC, *Paget's disease of bone: assessment and management*. (Praeger: New York 1981).

Hamill RJ, Baughn RE, Mallette LE et al, Serological evidence against role for canine distemper virus in pathogenesis of Paget's disease of bone, *Lancet* (1986) **2**:1399.

Hamilton CR, Effects of synthetic salmon calcitonin in patients with Paget's disease of bone, *Am J Med* (1974) **56**:315–22.

Hamilton CR and Quesada O, Paget's disease of the skull and migraine headache, *J Hopkins Med J* (1973) **132**:179–85.

Harinck HIJ, Bijvoet OLM, Blanksma HJ et al, Efficacious management with aminobisphosphonate (APD) in Paget's disease of bone, *Clin Orthop* (1987a) **217**:79–98.

Harinck HIJ, Bijvoet OLM, Vellenga CJRL et al, Relation between signs and symptoms in Paget's disease of bone, *Q J Med* (1986) **58**:133–51.

Harinck HIJ, Papapoulos SE, Blanksma HJ et al, Paget's disease of bone: early and late responses to three different modes of treatment with amino-hydroxypropylidene bisphosphonate (APD), *Br Med J* (1987b) **295**:1301–5.

Harris WH and Heaney RD, Skeletal renewal and metabolic bone disease, *N Engl J Med* (1969a) **280**:193–202.

Harris WH and Heaney RD, Skeletal renewal and metabolic bone disease, *N Engl J Med* (1969b) **280**:253–9.

Harris WH and Heaney RD, Skeletal renewal and metabolic bone disease, *N Engl J Med* (1969c) **280**:303–11.

Hartman JT and Dohn DF, Paget's disease of the spine with cord or nerve-root compression, *J Bone Joint Surg* (1966) **48A**:1079–84.

Harvey L, Gray T, Benéton MNC et al, Ultrastructural features of the osteoclasts from Paget's disease of bone in relation to a viral aetiology, *J Clin Pathol* (1982) **35**:771–9.

Hausser C, Ouaknine GE and Sylvestre J, Hydrocephalus and headache in Paget's disease of the skull: complete relief by ventriculo-atrial shunt, *Can J Neurol Sci* (1984) **11**:69–72.

Heath DA, The role of mithramycin in the management of Paget's disease, *Metab Bone Dis Relat Res* (1981) **3**:343–5.

Hedlund T, Hulth A and Johnell O, Early effects of parathormone and calcitonin on the number of osteoclasts and on serum-calcium in rats, *Acta Orthop Scand* (1983) **54**:802–4.

Heistad DD, Abboud FM, Schmid PG et al, Regulation of blood flow in Paget's disease of bone, *J Clin Invest* (1975) **55**:69–74.

Henkin RI, Lifschitz MD and Larson AL, Hearing loss in patients with osteoporosis and Paget's disease of bone, *Am J Med Sci* (1972) **263**:383–92.

Henley JW, Croxson RS and Ibbertson HK, The cardiovascular system in Paget's disease of bone and the response to therapy with calcitonin and diphosphonate, *Aust NZ J Med* (1979) **9**:390–7.

Herzberg L and Bayliss E, Spinal cord syndrome due to non-compressive Paget's disease of bone. A spinal artery steal phenomenon reversible with calcitonin, *Lancet* (1980) **ii**:13–15.

Hesch RD, Huefner M, Hasenyager M et al, Inhibition of gastric secretion by calcitonin, *Acta Endocrinol Scand* (1971) **155**(Suppl):216.

Heynen G, Brassine A, Daubresse JC et al, Lack of clinical and physiological relationship between gastrin and calcitonin in man, *Eur J Clin Invest* (1981) **11**:331–5.

Heynen G, Delwaide P, Bijvoet OLM et al, Clinical and biological effects of low doses of (3-amino-1-hydroxypropylidene)-1,1-bisphosphonate (APD) in Paget's disease of bone, *Eur J Clin Invest* (1982) **11**:29–35.

Heynen G, Franchimont P, Kanis JA et al, Human calcitonin. Some physiopathological aspects. In: Pecile A, ed. *Calcitonin 1980: Chemistry Physiology Pharmacology and Clinical aspects.* (Excerpta Medica: Amsterdam 1981) 208–16.

Heynen G, Hendrick JC and Franchimont P, Heterogeneity of calcitonin in human serum. In: Norman AW, Schaefer K, Grigoleit HG et al, eds. *Vitamin D and problems related to uremic bone disease.* (Berlin 1975) 475–81.

Heynen G, Kanis JA, Oliver D et al, Evidence that endogenous calcitonin protects against renal bone disease, *Lancet* (1976) **ii**:1322–6.

Hillyard CJ, Cooke TJ, Coombes RC et al, Normal plasma calcitonin: circadian variation and response to stimuli, *Clin Endocrinol* (1977) **6**:291–8.

Hirsch PF, Voelkel EF and Munson PL, Thyrocalcitonin: hypocalcemic hypophosphatemic principle of the thyroid gland, *Science* (1964) **146**:412–14.

Holtrop ME, Raisz LG and Simmons HA, The effects of parathyroid hormone, colchicine and calcitonin on the ultrastructure and the activity of osteoclasts in organ culture, *J Cell Biol* (1974) **60**:346–55.

Hornum I, Fahrenkrug J, Rehfeld JF, Gastrointestinal effect of calcitonin: inhibition of gastrin secretion. In: Pors Nielsen J and Hjorting-Hansen E, eds. *Calcified Tissues.* (Fadl's Forlag: Copenhagen 1975) 299–303.

Hosking DJ, Structural complications of Paget's disease of bone. In: Kanis JA, ed. *Bone disease and calcitonin.* (Armour Pharmaceutical: Eastbourne 1977) 49–59.

Hosking DJ, Calcitonin and diphosphonate in the treatment of Paget's disease of bone, *Metab Bone Dis Relat Res* (1981a) **3**:317–26.

Hosking DJ, Paget's disease of bone, *Br Med J* (1981b) **281**:686–8.

Hosking DJ, *Paget's disease of bone.* (Update Publications: London 1982).

Hosking DJ, Practical implications of calcitonin antigenicity. In: Gennari C and Segre G, eds. *The effects of calcitonins in man.* (Masson Italia Editori: Milan 1983) 67–74.

Hosking DJ, Bijvoet OLM, van Aken J et al, Paget's bone disease treated with diphosphonate and calcitonin, *Lancet* (1976) **i**:615–17.

Hosking DJ, Denton LB, Cadge B et al, Functional significance of antibody formation after long-term salmon calcitonin therapy, *Clin Endocrinol* (1979) **10**:243–52.

Hosking DJ, Vennart W and Huddlestone LB, Bone turnover in Paget's disease. Biochemical and kinetic measurements during salmon calcitonin therapy, *Calcif Tissue Int* (1981) **31**:471–6.

Howarth S, Cardiac output in osteitis deformans, *Clin Sci* (1953) **12**:271–5.

Howatson AF and Fornasier VL, Microfilaments associated with Paget's disease of bone: comparison with nucleocapsids of measles virus and respiratory syncytial virus, *Intervirology* (1982) **18**:150–9.

Huaux JP, Esselinckx W, Noel H et al, Paget's sarcoma with two illustrative cases, *Clin Rheumatol* (1984) **3**:459–66.

Hurley DL, Tiegs RD, Wahner HW et al, Axial and appendicular bone mineral density in patients with long-term deficiency or excess of calcitonin, *N Engl J Med* (1987) **317**:537–41.

Hutchinson J, The Bradshaw lecture on museums, *Br Med J* (1888) **2**:1263

Hutchinson J, On osteitis deformans, *Illustr Med News* (1889) **2**:169–80.

Huttenlocher PR and Mattson RH, Isoprinosine in subacute sclerosing panencephalitis, *Neurology* (1979) **29**:763–71.

Hutter RVP, Foote FW, Frazell EL et al, Giant cell tumours complicating Paget's disease of bone, *Cancer* (1963) **16**:1044–56.

Huwyler R, Born W, Ohnhaus E et al, Plasma kinetics and urinary excretion of exogenous human and salmon calcitonin in man, *Am J Physiol* (1979) **236**:E15–E19.

Ibbertson HK, Fraser TRC, Scott DJ et al, Paget's disease of bone: Assessment and management, *Drugs* (1979a) **18**:33–47.

Ibbertson HK, Henley JW, Fraser TR et al, Paget's disease of bone – clinical evaluation and treatment with diphosphonate, *Aust NZ J Med* (1979b) 9:31–5.

Irvine RE, Familial Paget's disease with early onset, *J Bone Joint Surg* (1953) **35B**:106–12.

Itoyama Y, Fukumura A, Ito Y et al, Acute-epidural hematoma complicating Paget's disease of the skull, *Surg Neurol* (1986) **25**:137–41.

Iwasaki Y and Koprowski M, Cell to cell transmission of virus in the central nervous system. I. Subacute sclerosing panencephalitis, *Lab Invest* (1974) **31**:187–96.

Jacobs JW, Goodman RH, Chin WW et al, Calcitonin messenger RNA encodes multiple polypeptides in a single precursor, *Science* (1981) **213**:457–9.

Jacobs TP, Michelsen J, Polay JS et al, Giant cell tumor in Paget's disease of bone. Familial and geographic clustering, *Cancer* (1979) **44**:742–7.

Jaeger P, Jones W, Clemens TL et al, Evidence that calcitonin stimulates 1,25-dihydroxyvitamin D production and intestinal absorption of calcium in vivo, *J Clin Invest* (1986) **78**:456–61.

Jaffe ML, Paget's disease of bone, *Arch Pathol* (1933) **15**:83–131.

Jaffe HL, The Classic: Paget's disease of bone, *Clin Orthop* (1977) **127**:4–23.

Jaworski ZFG, Parameters and indices of bone resorption. In: Meunier PJ, ed. *Bone histomorphometry. Proc 2nd Int Workshop*. (Armour Montague: Paris 1976) 193–235.

Jaworski ZFG, Physiology and pathology of bone remodelling. Cellular basis of bone structure in health and in osteoporosis, *Orthop Clin North Am* (1981) **12**:485–512.

Jaworski ZFG and Hooper C, Study of cell kinetics within evolving secondary Haversian Systems, *J Anat* (1980) **131**:91–102.

Jaworski ZFG, Meunier PJ and Frost HM, Observations on two types of resorption cavities in human lamellar cortical bone, *Clin Orthop* (1972) **83**:279–85.

Johnson LC, Morphologic analysis in pathology: the kinetics of disease and general biology of bone. In: Frost HM ed. *Bone Biodynamics*. (Little Brown and Co: Boston 1964) 543–654.

Johnson LC, The kinetics of skeletal remodelling. In: *Structural organisation of the skeleton. Birth defects original article series*. (National Foundation: New York 1966.)

Johnston CC, Altman RD, Canfield RE et al, Review of fracture experience during treatment of Paget's disease of bone with etidronate disodium (EHDP), *Clin Orthop* (1983) **172**:186–94.

Johnston CC, Khairi MRA and Meunier PJ, Use of etidronate (EHDP) in Paget's disease of bone, *Arthritis Rheum* (1980) **23**:1172–6.

Jones JV and Reed MF, Paget's disease: a family with 6 cases, *Br Med J* (1967) **iv**:90–1.

Jones PBB, McCloskey EV and Kanis JA, Transient taste-loss during treatment with etidronate, *Lancet* (1987) **ii**:637.

Jorgens J, The radiographic characteristics of carcinoma of the prostate, *Surg Clin North Am* (1965) **45**:1427–40.

Jowsey J, Quantitative microradiography, *Am J Med* (1966) **40**:485–91.

Kadir S, Kalisher L and Schiller AL, Extramedullary hematopoiesis in Paget's disease of bone, *AJR* (1977) **129**:493–5.

Kallio DM, Garant PR and Minkin C, Ultrastructural effects of calcitonin on osteoclasts in tissue culture, *J Ultrastruct Res* (1972) **39**:205–16.

Kanehisa J, Time course of escape from calcitonin-induced inhibition of motility and resorption of disaggregated osteoclasts, *Bone* (1989) **10**:125–9.

Kanis JA, Bone and collagen diseases. In: Dieppe PA, Bacon PA, Baniji AN et al, eds. *Slide atlas of rheumatology*. (Gower Medical Publishing Ltd: London 1984a) Chapter 22.

Kanis JA, Monitoring the treatment of Paget's disease with etidronate, *Calcif Tissue Int* (1984b) **36**:629–31.

Kanis JA, Adams ND, Cecchetin M et al, Ethanol induced secretion of calcitonin in chronic renal disease, *Clin Endocrinol* (1979) **10**:155–61.

Kanis JA, Cundy T, Heynen G et al, The pathophysiology of hypercalcaemia, *Metab Bone Dis Relat Res* (1980) **2**:151–9.

Kanis JA, Evanson JM and Russell RGG, Paget's disease of bone: diagnosis and management, *Metab Bone Dis Relat Res* (1981) **3**:219–30.

Kanis JA, Fitzpatrick K and Strong JA, Treatment of Paget's disease of bone with porcine calcitonin: clinical and metabolic responses, *Q J Med* (1975) **44**:399–413.

Kanis JA and Gray RES, Long-term follow-up observations on treatment in Paget's disease of bone, *Clin Orthop* (1987) **217**:99–125.

Kanis JA, Gray RES, Murray SA et al, Short term high doses of etidronate in Paget's disease of bone, *Br Med J* (1986) **292**:1667

Kanis JA, Heynen G, Cundy T et al, An estimate of the endogenous secretion rate of calcitonin in man, *Clin Sci* (1982) **63**:145–52.

Kanis JA, Heynen G, Paterson A et al, Endogenous secretion of calcitonin in physiological and pathological conditions. In: Pecile A ed. *Calcitonin*. (Elsevier: Amsterdam 1985b) 81–8.

Kanis JA, Heynen G and Walton RJ, Plasma calcitonin in Paget's disease of bone, *Clin Sci Mol Med* (1977) **52**:329–32.

Kanis JA, Horn DB, Scott RDM et al, Treatment of Paget's disease of bone with synthetic salmon calcitonin, *Br Med J* (1974) **3**:727–31.

Kanis JA, Preston CJ, Beard M et al, Comparative effects of an antiviral drug, inosiplex and diphosphonates in Paget's disease of bone, *Bone* (1985a) **6**:69–72.

Kanis JA, Preston CJ, Yates AJP et al, Effects of intravenous diphosphonates on renal function, *Lancet* (1983) **i**:1328.

Kanis JA, Urwin GH, Gray RES et al, Effects of intravenous etidronate disodium on skeletal and calcium metabolism, *Am J Med* (1987) **82**(Suppl 2A):55–70.

Kantrowitz FG, Byrne MH, Schiller AI et al, Clinical and biochemical effects of diphosphonates in Paget's disease of bone, *Arthritis Rheum* (1975) **18**:407.

Kaplan RA. Geho WB, Poindexter C et al, Metabolic effects of diphosphonates in primary hyperparathyroidism, *J Clin Pharmacol* (1977) **17**:410–19.

Kattapuram SV and Phillips WC, Paget's disease of bone mimicking metastases, *J Can Assoc Radiol* (1982) **33**:239–45.

Kawashima H, Torikai S and Kurokawa K, Calcitonin selectively stimulates 25-hydroxyvitamin D_3-1-alpha-hydroxylase in proximal straight tubule of rat kidney, *Nature* (1981) **291**:327–9.

Kennedy BJ, Metabolic and toxic effects of mithramycin during tumour therapy, *Am J Med* (1970) **49**:494–503.

Kerley ER and Bass WM, Paleopathology: meeting ground for many disciplines, *Science* (1967) **157**:638–44.

Khairi MRA, Altman RD, DeRosa GP et al, Sodium etidronate in the treatment of Paget's disease of bone. A study of long-term results, *Ann Intern Med* (1977) **87**:656–63.

Khairi MRA and Johnston CC, Treatment of Paget's disease of bone (osteitis deformans) with sodium etidronate (EHDP), *Clin Orthop* (1977) **127**:94–105.

Khairi MRA, Johnston CC, Altman RD et al, Treatment of Paget's disease of bone (osteitis deformans). Results of a one year study with sodium etidronate. *JAMA* (1974a) **230**:562–7.

Khairi MRA, Robb JA, Wellman HN et al, Radiographs and scans in diagnosing symptomatic lesions of Paget's disease of bone (osteitis deformans), *Geriatrics* (1974b) **29**:49–54.

Khairi MRA, Wellman HN, Robb JA et al, Paget's disease of bone (osteitis deformans): symptomatic lesions and bone scan, *Ann Intern Med* (1973) **79**:348–51.

Khokker MA and Dandona P, Diphosphonates inhibit human osteoblast secretion and proliferation, *Metabolism* (1989) **38**:184–7.

Klenerman L, Cauda equina and spinal cord compression in Paget's disease, *J Bone Joint Surg* (1966) **48B**:365–70.

Knaggs RL, On osteitis deformans (Paget's disease) and its relation to osteitis fibrosa and osteomalacia, *Br J Surg* (1925) **13**:206–379.

Krane S, Paget's disease of bone, *Calcif Tissue Int* (1986) **38**:309–17.

Krane S, Paget's disease of bone. In: Braunwald E et al, eds. *Harrison's principles of internal medicine*. (McGraw-Hill 1987.)

Krane SM, Paget's disease of bone, *Clin Orthop* (1977) **127**:24–36.

Krane SM, Skeletal metabolism in Paget's disease of bone, *Arthritis Rheum* (1980) **23**:1087–94.

Krane SM, Etidronate disodium in the treatment of Paget's disease of bone, *Ann Intern Med* (1982) **96**:619–25.

Krane SM, Harris ED, Singer FR et al, Acute effects of calcitonin on bone formation in man, *Metabolism* (1973) **22**:51–8.

Krane SM, Kantrowitz FG, Byrne M et al, Urinary excretion of hydroxylysine and its glycosides as an index of collagen degradation, *J Clin Invest* (1977) **59**:819–27.

Krane SM, Munoz AJ and Harris ED, Urinary polypeptides related to collagen synthesis, *J Clin Invest* (1970) **49**:716–29.

Krane SM and Simon LS, Metabolic consequences of bone turnover in Paget's disease of bone, *Clin Orthop* (1987) **217**:26–36.

Kraszeski JL, Avramides A, Wallach S et al, Three adult cases resembling hereditary bone dysplasia, *Metab Bone Dis Relat Res* (1981) **3**:9–16.

Kumar K, Paget's disease of bone, *J Indian Med Assoc* (1986) **84**:316–18.

Kurose H, Seino Y, Shima M et al, Intranasal absorption of salmon calcitonin, *Calcif Tissue Int* (1987) **41**:249–51.

Labat ML, Florentin I, Davigny M et al, Dichloromethylene diphosphonate (Cl_2MDP) reduces natural killer (NK) cell activity in mice, *Metab Bone Dis Relat Res* (1984) **5**:281–98.

Lander PH and Hadjipavlou AG, A dynamic classification of Paget's disease, *J Bone Joint Surg* (1986a) **68B**:431–8.

Lander PH and Hadjipavlou AG, Paget's disease with contraction of long bones, *Radiology* (1986b) **159**: 471–2.

Lando M, Hoover, LA and Finerman G, Stabilization of hearing loss in Paget's disease with calcitonin and etidronate, *Arch Otolaryngol Head Neck Surg* (1988) **114**:891–4.

Lang R, Milkman M, Jensen PS et al, Chronic treatment of Paget's disease of bone with synthetic human calcitonin, *Yale J Biol Med* (1981) **54**:355–65.

Lauffenberger T, Olah AJ, Dambacher MA et al, Bone remodelling and calcium metabolism: A correlated histomorphometric, calcium kinetic and biochemical study in patients with osteoporosis and Paget's disease, *Metabolism* (1977) **26**:589–605.

Lavender JP, Evans MA, Arnot R et al, A comparison of radiography and radioisotope scanning in the detection of Paget's disease and in the assessment of response to human calcitonin, *Br J Radiol* (1977) **50**:243–50.

Lawrence GD, Loeffler RG and Martin LC, Immobilisation hypercalcemia, *J Bone Joint Surg* (1973) **55A**:87–92.

Lawrence JS, Paget's disease in population samples, *Ann Rheum Dis* (1970) **29**:562.

Lawson-Matthew PJ, Guilland-Cumming DF, Yates AJP et al, Contrasting effects of intravenous and oral etidronate on vitamin D metabolism in man, *Clin Sci* (1988) **74**:101–6.

Lebbin D, Ryan W and Schwarz TB, Outpatient treatment of Paget's disease of bone with mithramycin, *Ann Intern Med* (1974) **81**:635–7.

Lee WR, Bone formation in Paget's disease: a quantitative microscopic study using tetracycline markers, *J Bone Joint Surg* (1967) **49B**:146–53.

Lesh JB, Aldred JP, Bastian JW et al, Clinical experience with porcine and salmon calcitonins. In: Taylor S, ed. *Endocrinology 1973* (Heinemann: London 1974) 409–24.

Levine RB, Rao VM, Karasick D et al, Paget's disease: unusual radiographic manifestations, *CRC Crit Rev Diagn Imaging* (1986) **25**:209–32.

Levison V, The treatment of Paget's disease of bone by radiotherapy, *Ann Physical Med* (1970) **10**:230–5.

Levy F, Muff R, Dotti-Sigrist S et al, Formation of neutralizing antibodies during intranasal synthetic salmon calcitonin treatment of Paget's disease, *J Clin Endocrinol Metab* (1988) **67**:541–5.

Lievre JA, Données cliniques et étio-pathogèniques sur la maladie osseuse de Paget, *Acta Orthop Belg* (1974) **40**:454–64.

Lindsay JR and Lehman RH, Histopathology of the temporal bone in advanced Paget's disease, *Laryngoscope* (1969) **79**:213–27.

Lloyd GAS, Phelps PD and DuBoulay GH, High-resolution computerized tomography of the petrous bone, *Br J Radiol* (1980) **53**:631–41.

Lluberas-Acosta G, Hansell J and Schumacher R, Paget's disease of bone in patients with gout, *Arch Intern Med* (1986) **146**:2389–92.

Lockwood DR, Vogel JM, Schneider US et al, Effect of the diphosphonate EHDP on bone mineral metabolism during prolonged bed rest, *J Clin Endocrinol Metab* (1975) **41**:533–41.

Looij BJ, Roelfsema F, Heide D et al, The effect of calcitonin on growth hormone secretion in man, *Clin Endocrinol* (1988) **29**:517–27.

Louyot P, Pourel J, Delagoutte JP et al, Quelques aspects inhabituels des fractures d'os pagétique, *Rev Rhum Mal Osteoartic* (1975) **42**:653–60.

Lucas RB, the jaws and teeth in Paget's disease of bone, *J Clin Pathol* (1955) **8**:195–200.

Lunn JR, Osteitis deformans, *Illustr Med News* (1889) **2**:182–6.

McCloskey EV, Yates AJP, Benéton MNC et al, Comparative effects of intravenous diphosphonates on calcium and skeletal metabolism in man, *Bone* (1987) **8**(Suppl 1):35–42.

McCloskey EV, Yates AJP, Gray RES et al, Diphosphonates and phosphate homeostasis, *Clin Sci* (1988) **74**:607–12.

McDonald DJ and Sim FH, Total hip arthroplasty in Paget's disease. A follow-up note, *J Bone Joint Surg* (1987) **69A**:766–72.

McGavack TH, Seegers W and Reifenstein FC, The influence of anabolic steroid (DeLadumone) therapy on the clinical and metabolic aspects of Paget's disease, *J Am Geriatr Soc* (1961) **9**:533–8.

MacIntyre I, *Human calcitonin and Paget's disease.* (Hans Huber: Bern 1977).

MacIntyre I, Alevizaki M, Bevis PJR et al, Calcitonin and the peptides from the calcitonin gene, *Clin Orthop* (1987) **217**:45–55.

MacIntyre I, Evans IMA, Hobitz HHG et al, Chemistry physiology and therapeutic applications of calcitonin, *Arthritis Rheum* (1980) **23**:1139–47.

McKenna RJ, Schwinn CP, Soong KY et al, Osteogenic sarcoma arising in Paget's disease, *Cancer* (1964) **17**:42–66.

MacKenzie A, Court-Brown WM, Doll R et al, Mortality from primary tumours of bone in England and Wales, *Br Med J* (1961) **i**:1782–90.

Mackenzie S, An arrested case of osteitis deformans in which fracture of the affected bones took place, *Illustr Med News* (1889) **2**:186–7.

McKusick VA, *Heritable disorders of connective tissue.* (CV Mosby Co: St Louis 1972) 718.

Maier R, Neher R, Rittel W et al, Comparison of the hypocalcaemic response between human and porcine calcitonins. In: Taylor S, Foster G, eds. *Calcitonin 1969* (Heinemann: London 1970) 381–5.

Mailander JC, The black beard sign of monostotic Paget's disease of the mandible, *Clin Nucl Med* (1986) **11**:325–7.

Maldague B and Malghem J, Dynamic radiological patterns of Paget's disease of bone, *Clin Orthop* (1987) **217**:126–51.

Maldague B and Malghem J, Imagerie médicale de la maladie de Paget, *Rev Pract (Paris)* (1989) **39**:1113–24.

Malkani K, Baslé M and Rebel A, Goniometric observation of nuclear inclusions in osteoclasts in Paget's bone disease, *J Submicrosc Cytol* (1976) **8**:229–36.

Marotti G and Muglia MA, A scanning electron microscope study of human bony lamellae – proposal for a new model of collagen lamellar organization, *Arch Ital Anat Embriol* (1988) **93**:163–75.

Marotti GP, Map of bone formation rate values recorded throughout the skeleton of the dog. In: Jaworski ZFG, ed. *Proc 1st workshop on bone histomorphometry.* (University of Ottawa Press: Ottawa 1976) 202–7.

Martin BJ, Roberts MA and Turner JW, Normal pressure hydrocephalus and Paget's disease of bone, *Gerontology* (1985) **31**:397–402.

Martin TJ, Treatment of Paget's disease with calcitonins, *Aust NZ J Med* (1979) **9**:36–43.

Martin TJ, Jerums G, Melick R et al, Clinical, histological and biochemical observations on the effect of porcine calcitonin in Paget's disease of bone, *Aust NZ J Med* (1977) **7**:36–43.

Martin TJ and Woodhouse NJY, Calcitonin in the treatment of Paget's disease. In: Kanis JA, ed. *Bone disease and calcitonin.* (Armour Pharmaceutical: Eastbourne 1977) 11–24.

Marx SJ, Woodard CJ and Aurbach GD, Calcitonin receptors of kidney and bone, *Science* (1972) **178**:999–1001.

Mathe JF, Delobel R, Resche F et al, Syndromes médullaires au cours de la maladie de Paget. Role du facteur vasculaire, *Nouv Presse Med* (1976) **39**:2619–21.

Matkovic V, Apseloff G, Shepard DR et al, Use of gallium to treat Paget's disease of bone: a pilot study, *Lancet* (1990) **335**:72–4.

Maurice PF, Lynch TN, Bastomsky CH et al, Metabolic evidence for suppression of Paget's disease of bone by aspirin, *Trans Assoc Am Physicians* (1962) **75**:208–12.

Mautalen C, Gonzalez D, Blumenfeld E et al, Spontaneous fractures of uninvolved bones in patients with Paget's disease during unduly prolonged treatment with disodium etidronate (EHDP), *Clin Orthop* (1986) **207**:150–5.

Mautalen CA, Treatment of Paget's bone disease with the bisphosphonate APD, *Henry Ford Hosp Med J* (1983) **31**:244–8.

Mautalen CA, Casco CA, Gonzalez D et al, Side-effects of disodium aminohydroxypropylidene diphosphonate (APD) during treatment of bone diseases, *Br Med J* (1984) **288**:828–9.

Mautalen CA, Gonzalez D and Ghiringhelli G, Efficacy of the bisphosphonate APD in the control of Paget's bone disease, *Bone* (1985) **6**:429–32.

Mazieres B, Jung-Rozenfarb M and Arlet J, Rapport de la maladie de Paget avec l'hyperostose vertébrale ankylosante et l'hyperostose frontale interne, *Semin Hop Paris* (1978) **54**:521–5.

Mazzuoli GF, Passeri M, Gennari C et al, Effects of salmon calcitonin in postmenopausal osteoporosis: a controlled double-blind clinical study, *Calcif Tissue Int* (1986) **38**:3–8.

Melick R, Ebeling P and Hjorth RJ, Improvement in paraplegia in vertebral Paget's disease treated with calcitonin, *Br Med J* (1976) **1**:627–8.

Melick RA and Martin TJ, Paget's disease in identical twins, *Aust NZ J Med* (1975) **5**:564–5.

Mercier P and Seignalet J, First HLA and disease symposium, Paris, 23–25 June 1976.

Merkow RL, Pellicci PM, Holy DP et al, Total hip replacement for Paget's disease of the hip, *J Bone Joint Surg* (1984) **66A**:752–8.

Merle d'Aubigne R and Witvoet J, Correction chirugicales des déformations pagétiques des membres inférieurs, *Rev Rhum Mal Osteoartic* (1966) **33**:163–70.

Merrick MV and Merrick JM, Observations on the natural history of Paget's disease, *Clin Radiol* (1985) **36**:169–74.

Meunier P, Chapuy M-C, Courpron P et al, Effects cliniques, biologiques et histologiques de l'éthane-1-hydroxy-1,1-diphosphonate (EHDP) dans la maladie de Paget, *Rev Rhum Mal Osteoartic* (1975) **42**:699–705.

Meunier PJ, Chapuy M-C, Alexandre C et al, Effects of

disodium dichloromethylene diphosphonate on Paget's disease of bone, *Lancet* (1979) **ii**:489–92.

Meunier PJ, Chapuy M-C, Alexandre C et al, Effects of ethane-1-hydroxy-1,1-diphosphonate (EHDP) and dichloromethylene diphosphonate (Cl_2MDP) in Paget's disease of bone. In: Donath A, Courvoisier B, eds. *Diphosphonates and bone*. (Editions Medicine et Hygiene: Genève 1982) 300–301.

Meunier PJ, Coindre J, Edouard CM et al, Bone histomorphometry in Paget's disease. Quantitative and dynamic analysis of Paget's disease and nonpagetic bone tissue, *Arthritis Rheum* (1980) **23**:1095–1103.

Meunier PJ, Salson C, Mathieu L et al, Skeletal distribution of Paget's disease, *Clin Orthop* (1987) **217**:37–44.

Meyers MH, Downey MD and Singer FR, Osteotomy for tibia vara in Paget's disease under cover of calcitonin, *J Bone Joint Surg* (1978) **60A**:810–14.

Michael WR, King WR and Wakim JM, Metabolism of disodium ethane-1-hydroxy-1,1-diphosphonate (disodium etidronate) in the rat, rabbit, dog and monkey, *Toxicol Appl Pharmacol* (1972) **21**:503–15.

Milgram JW, Radiographical and pathological assessment of the activity of Paget's disease of bone, *Clin Orthop* (1977) **127**:43–54.

Miller SC and Jee WSS, The bone lining cell: a distinct prototype? *Calcif Tissue Int* (1987) **41**:1–5.

Mills BG, Masuoka LS, Graham CC Jr et al, Gallium-67 citrate localization in osteoclast nuclei of Paget's disease of bone, *J Nucl Med* (1988a) **29**:1083–7.

Mills BG and Singer FR, Nuclear inclusions in Paget's disease of bone, *Science* (1976) **194**:201–2.

Mills BG, Singer FR, Weiner LP et al, Cells cultured from bone affected by Paget's disease, *Arthritis Rheum* (1980) **23**:1115–20.

Mills BG, Singer FR, Weiner LP et al, Immunohistological demonstration of respiratory syncytial virus antigens in Paget's disease of bone, *Proc Natl Acad Sci USA* (1981) **78**:1209–13.

Mills BG, Singer FR, Weiner LP et al, Evidence for both respiratory syncytial virus and measles virus antigens in the osteoclasts of patients with Paget's disease of bone, *Clin Orthop* (1984) **183**:303–11.

Mills BG, Yabe J and Singer FR, Osteoclasts in human orteopetrosis contain viral-nucleocaspid-like material. *J Bone Miner Res* (1988b) **3**:101–6.

Minaire P, Depassio J, Berard E et al, Effects of clodronate on immobilization bone loss, *Bone* (1987) **8**(Suppl 1):63–8.

Mirra JM, Pathogenesis of Paget's disease based on viral aetiology, *Clin Orthop* (1987) **217**:162–70.

Mirra JM, Bauer FCH and Grant TT, Giant cell tumour with viral-like intranuclear inclusions associated with Paget's disease, *Clin Orthop* (1981) **158**:243–51.

Moffat WH, Effects of calcitonin therapy in deafness associated with Paget's disease of bone, *Br Med J* (1975) **2**:203.

Molleson T, Bones of contention, *Bone* (1988) **5**:19–21.

Monson DK, Finn HA, Dawson PJ et al, Pseudosarcoma in Paget's disease of bone. A case report, *J Bone Joint Surg* (1989) **71A**:453–5.

Morgan-Capner P, Robinson P, Clewley G et al, Measles antibody in Paget's disease, *Lancet* (1981) **i**:733.

Muhlbauer RC, Stutzer A, Schenk R et al, 1-Hydroxy-3-(methylpentylamino) propylidene bisphosphonate, a potent new inhibitor of bone resorption, *J Bone Miner Res* (1989) **4**(Suppl 1):168.

Mundy GR, Differential diagnosis of osteopenia, *Hosp Pract* (1978) November, 65–72.

Murphy WA, Whyte MP and Haddad JG, Healing of lytic Paget's disease of bone with diphosphonate therapy, *Radiology* (1980a) **134**:635–7.

Murphy WA, Whyte MP and Haddad JG, Paget's bone disease: radiologic documentation of healing with human calcitonin therapy, *Radiology* (1980b) **136**:1–4.

Nagant de Deuxchaisnes C, Calcitonin in the treatment of Paget's disease, *Triangle* (1983) **22**:103–28.

Nagant de Deuxchaisnes C, Medical management of Paget's disease of bone. In: De Groot, ed. *Endocrinology*, 2nd edn, Vol 2. (WB Saunders: Philadelphia 1989) 1211–44.

Nagant de Deuxchaisnes C, Devogelaer JP, Huaux JP et al, New modes of administration of salmon calcitonin in Paget's disease. Nasal spray and suppository, *Clin Orthop* (1987) **217**:56–71.

Nagant de Deuxchaisnes C, Dufour JP, Devogelaer JP et al, Etidronate and the risk of fracture, *Lancet* (1985) **ii**:610–11.

Nagant de Deuxchaisnes C and Krane SM, Paget's disease of bone: clinical and metabolic observations, *Medicine* (1964) **43**:233–66.

Nagant de Deuxchaisnes C and Krane SM, Le traitement de la maladie de Paget par l'acide acétylsalicylique et le fluorure de sodium. In: Hioco DJ, ed. *La Maladie de Paget* (Lab Armour Montagu: Paris 1977) 196–213.

Nagant de Deuxchaisnes C, Maldague B, Malghem J et al, The action of the main therapeutic regimes on Paget's disease of bone with a note on the effect of vitamin D deficiency, *Arthritis Rheum* (1980a) **23**:1215–34.

Nagant de Deuxchaisnes C, Rombouts-Lindemans C, Huaux JP et al, Diphosphonates and inhibition of bone mineralisation, *Lancet* (1982a) **ii**:607–8.

Nagant de Deuxchaisnes C, Rombouts-Lindemans C, Huaux JP et al, Effets comparés des traitements à la calcitonine, au diphosphonate EHDP et à l'association calcitonine–diphosphonate sur les lésions radiologiques de la maladie de Paget, *Acta Rhumatol* (1980b) **4**:425–57.

Nagant de Deuxchaisnes C, Rombouts-Lindemans C, Huaux JP et al, Relative vitamin D deficiency in Paget's disease, *Lancet* (1981) **i**:833–4.

Nagant de Deuxchaisnes C, Rombouts-Lindemans C, Huaux JP et al, Treatment of Paget's disease with the diphosphonate APD. A biological and radiological study. In: Donath A, Courvoisier B, eds. *Diphosphonates and bone*. (Editions Medicine et Hygiene: Geneva 1982b) 303–27.

Nagant de Deuxchaisnes C, Rombouts-Lindemans C, Huaux JP et al, Roentgenologic evaluation of the efficacy of calcitonin in Paget's disease of bone. In: MacIntyre I, Szelke M, eds. *Molecular endocrinology*. (Elsevier: Amsterdam 1977) 213–33.

Nagant de Deuxchaisnes C, Rombouts-Lindemans C, Huaux JP et al, Roentgenologic evaluation of the action of the diphosphonate EHDP and of combined therapy (EHDP and calcitonin) in Paget's disease of bone. In: MacIntyre I, Szelke M, eds. *Molecular endocrinology*. (Elsevier, Amsterdam 1979) 405–33.

Nagant de Deuxchaisnes and Rombouts-Lindemans C, Exploration biologique de la maladie de Paget, *Journal Belge de Medecine Physique et de Rehabilitation (Acta Med Belg Med Phys)* (1974) **29**:243–93.

Nager GT, Paget's disease of the temporal bone, *Ann Otol Rhinol Laryngol* (1975) **84**(Suppl 22):1–32.

Naiken VS, Did Beethoven have Paget's disease of bone? *Ann Intern Med* (1971) **74**:995–9.

Nathan AW, Ludlam HA, Wilson DW et al, Hypercalcaemia due to immobilisation of a patient with Paget's disease of bone, *Postgrad Med J* (1973) **58**:714–15.

Neuman H, Beethovens gehorleiden, *Wien Med Wochenschr* (1927) **77**:1015–19.

Newman FW, Paget's disease: a statistical study of eighty-two cases, *J Bone Joint Surg* (1946) **28A**:798–804.

Newmark III H, Paget's disease of a vertebral body seen on computerised tomography, *Comput Radiol* (1982) **6**:7–9.

Nicholas JA and Killoran P, Fracture of the femur in patients with Paget's disease, *J Bone Joint Surg* (1965) **47A**:450–61.

Nicholas JJ, Srodes CH, Herbert D et al, Metastatic cancer in Paget's disease of bone. A case report, *Orthopaedics* (1987) **10**:725–9.

Nicholson GC, Moseley JM, Sexton PM et al, Abundant calcitonin receptors in isolated rat osteoclasts, *J Clin Invest* (1986) **78**:355–60.

Nuti R, Multicentre trial on carbocalcitonin (Turbocalcitonin) in Paget's bone disease, *Clin Trials J* (1986) **23**(Suppl 1):53–72.

O'Doherty DP, Bickerstaff DR, McCloskey EV et al, A comparison of the acute effects of subcutaneous and intranasal calcitonin, *Clin Sci* (1990a) **78**:215–19.

O'Doherty DP, Bickerstaff DR, McCloskey EV et al, The treatment of Paget's disease of bone with aminohydroxybutylidene bisphosphonate, *J Bone Miner Res* (1990b) **5**:483–91.

O'Donoghue DJ and Hosking DJ, Biochemical response to combination of disodium etidronate with calcitonin in Paget's disease, *Bone* (1987) **8**:219–25.

O'Driscoll JB and Anderson DC, Past pets and Paget's disease, *Lancet* (1985) **ii**:919–21.

Ohya K, Yamada S, Felix R et al, Effect of bisphosphonates on prostaglandin synthesis by rat bone cells and mouse calvaria in culture, *Clin Sci* (1985) **69**:403–11.

O'Reilly TJ and Race J, Osteitis deformans, *Q J Med* (1933) **1**:471–92.

Oreopoulos DG, Dudsan H, Harrison J et al, Metabolic balance studies in patients with Paget's disease receiving salmon calcitonin over long periods, *Can Med Assoc J* (1977) **116**:851–5.

O'Riordan JLH and Aurbach GD, Mode of action of thyrocalcitonin, *Endocrinol* (1968) **82**:377–83.

Osterberg PH, Wallace RGH, Adams DA et al, Familial expansile osteolysis – a new dysplasia, *J Bone Joint Surg* (1988) **70B**:255–60.

Overgaard K, Riis B, Christiansen C et al, Effect of salcatonin given intranasally on early postmenopausal bone loss, *Br Med J* (1989) **299**:477–9.

Oyanang S, te Meulen V, Katz M et al, Comparison of subacute sclerosing panencephalitis and measles virus: an electron microscope study, *J Virol* (1971) **7**:176.

Paget J, On a form of chronic inflammation of bones (osteitis deformans), *Medico-Chirurgical Transactions of London* (1877) **60**:37–63.

Paget J, Additional cases of osteitis deformans, *Medico-Chirurgical Transactions of London* (1882) **65**:225–36.

Paget J, Remarks on osteitis deformans, *Illus Med News* (1889) **2**:181–2.

Pales L, Maladie de Paget préhistorique, *Anthropologie* (1929) **39**:263–70.

Palmieri GMA, Beahm DE, Joel W et al, Calcitonin and vitamin D in Paget's disease. In: Frame B, et al, eds. *Clinical aspects of bone disease*. (Excerpta Medica: Amsterdam 1973) 547–50.

Pankovich AM, Simmons DJ and Kulkani VV, Zonal osteons in cortical bone, *Clin Orthop* (1974) **100**:356–63.

Papapoulos SE, Frolich M, Mudde AH et al, Serum osteocalcin in Paget's disease of bone: basal concentrations and response to biphosphonate treatment, *J Clin Endocrinol Metab* (1987) **65**:89–94.

Papapoulos SE, Frolisch M, Hoekman K et al, Dimethyl-APD treatment modifies osteoblastic function in patients with Paget's disease, *Calcif Tissue Int* (1989) **44**(Suppl): 108.

Papapoulos SE, Harinck HIJ, Bijvoet OLM et al, Effects of decreasing serum calcium on circulating parathyroid hormone and vitamin D metabolites in normocalcaemic and hypercalcaemic patients treated with APD, *Bone Miner* (1986) **1**:69–78.

Parfitt AM, The action of parathyroid hormone on bone. Relation to bone remodelling and turnover, calcium homeostatis and metabolic bone disease, *Metabolism* (1976) **25**:909–55.

Parfitt AM, The quantum concept of bone remodelling and turnover. Implications for the pathogenesis of osteoporosis, *Calcif Tissue Int* (1979) **28**:1–5.

Parfitt AM, Morphologic basis of bone mineral measurements. Transient and steady state effects of treatment in osteoporosis, *Miner Electrolyte Metab* (1980) **4**:273–87.

Parfitt AM, The physiologic and clinical significance of bone histomorphometric data. In: Recker R, ed. *Bone histomorphometry techniques*. (CRC Press: Boca Raton, Florida 1983) 143–223.

Parfitt AM, Simon LS, Villaneuva AR et al, Procollagen type I carboxy-terminal extension peptide in serum as a marker of collagen biosynthesis in bone. Correlation with iliac bone formation rates and comparison with total alkaline phosphatase, *J Bone Miner Res* (1987) **2**:427–36.

Parvainen MT, Galloway JH, Towers JH et al, Alkaline phosphatase isoenzymes in serum determined by high performance anion-exchange liquid chromatography with detection by enzyme reaction, *Clin Chem* (1988) **34**:2406–9.

Paterson CR, Paget's disease of bone. In: *Metabolic disorders of bone*. (Blackwell Scientific Publications: Oxford 1974) 240–52.

Paton D, *The relation of angioid streaks to systemic disease*. (Thomas: Springfield, Illinois 1972).

Pecile A, Ferri S, Sbraga PC et al, Effects of intracerebroventricular calcitonin in the conscious rabbit, *Experientia* (1975) **31**:332–33.

Perry HM, Droke DM and Avioli LV, Alternate calcitonin and etidronate disodium therapy for Paget's bone disease, *Arch Intern Med* (1984) **144**:929–33.

Petralito A, Lunetta M, Liuzzo A et al, Effects of salmon calcitonin on blood glucose and insulin levels under basal conditions and after intravenous glucose load, *J Endocrinol Invest* (1979) **2**:209–11.

Piga AM, Lopez-Abente G, Ibanez AE et al, Risk factors for Paget's disease: a new hypothesis, *Int J Epidemiol* (1988) **17**:198–201.

Pinnell SR, Fox R and Krane SM, Human collagens:

differences in glycosylated hydroxylysines in skin and bone, *Biochim Biophys Acta* (1971) **229**:119–22.

Plehwe WE, Hudson J, Clifton-Bligh P et al, Porcine calcitonin in the treatment of Paget's disease of bone, *Med J Aust* (1977) **1**:577–81.

Pluijm van der G, Lowik C, Binderup L et al, Effects of disodium 1-hydroxy-3-1(1-pyrodinyl)-propylidene-1,1-bisphosphonate on bone resorption in vitro and in vivo, *J Bone Miner Res* (1989) **4**(Suppl 1):358.

Polednak AP, Rates of Paget's disease of bone among hospital discharges by age and sex, *J Am Geriatr Soc* (1987) **35**:550–3.

Pompe van Meerdervoort HF and Richter GG, Paget's disease of bone in South African Blacks, *S Afr Med J* (1976) **50**:1897–9.

Pontiroli AE, Alberetto M and Pozza G, Intranasal calcitonin and plasma calcium concentrations in normal subjects, *Br Med J* (1985) **290**:1390–1.

Porretta C, Daklin D and Jones J, Sarcoma in Paget's disease of bone, *J Bone Joint Surg* (1957) **39A**:1314–29.

Porrini AA, Cocco JAM and Morteo OG, Spinal artery steal syndrome in Paget's disease of bone, *Clin Exp Rheumatol* (1987) **5**:377–8.

Porter RW, Wicks M and Ottewell D, Measurement of the spinal canal by diagnostic ultrasound, *J Bone Joint Surg* (1976) **60B**:481–4.

Posen S, Clifton-Bligh P and Wilkinson M, Paget's disease of bone and hyperparathyroidism: coincidence or causal relationship? *Calcif Tissue Res* (1978) **26**: 107–9.

Posen S and Grunstein HS, Turnover rate of skeletal alkaline phosphatase in humans, *Clin Chem* (1982) **28**:153–4.

Preston CJ, Yates AJP, Benéton MNC et al, Effective short term treatment of Paget's disease with oral etidronate, *Br Med J* (1986) **292**:79–80.

Price CHG, The incidence of osteogenic sarcoma in south-west England and its relationship to Paget's disease of bone, *J Bone Joint Surg* (1962) **44B**:366–76.

Price CHG and Goldie W, Paget's sarcoma of bone – a study of 80 cases, *J Bone Joint Surg* (1969) **51B**:205–24.

Price JL, The radiology of excavated Saxon and medieval human remains from Winchester, *Clin Radiol* (1975) **26**:363–70.

Price PA, Nishimoto S, Parthemore JG et al, A new biochemical marker for bone metabolism, *Calcif Tissue Int* (1979) **28**:159.

Price PA, Parthemore JG and Deftos LJ, New biochemical marker for bone metabolism, *J Clin Invest* (1980) **66**:878–83.

Pringle CR, Wilkie ML and Elliott RM, A survey of respiratory syncytial virus and para-influenza virus type 3 neutralising and immuno-precipitating antibodies in relation to Paget's disease, *J Med Virol* (1985) **17**:377–86.

Prockop DJ and Kivirikko KI, Heritable diseases of collagen, *N Engl J Med* (1984) **311**:376–86.

Prockop DJ, Kivirikko KI, Tuderman L et al, The biosynthesis of collagen and its disorders, *N Engl J Med* (1979a) **301**:13–23.

Prockop DJ, Kivirokko KI, Tuderman L et al, The biosynthesis of collagen and its disorders, *N Engl J Med* (1979b) **301**:77–85.

Proops D, Bailey D and Hawke M, Paget's disease and the temporal bone – a clinical and histopathological review of six temporal bones, *J Otolaryngol* (1985) **14**:20–9.

Pun KK and Chan LWL, Analgesic effect of intranasal calcitonin in the treatment of osteoporotic vertebral fractures, *Clin Ther* (1989) **11**:205–9.

Purves MJ, Some effects of administering sodium fluoride to patients with Paget's disease, *Lancet* (1962) **ii**:1188–9.

Pygott F, Paget's disease of bone: the radiological incidence, *Lancet* (1957) **i**:1170–1.

Raine CS, Feldman LA, Sheppard RD et al, Subacute sclerosing panencephalitis virus in cultures of organised nervous tissue, *Lab Invest* (1973) **28**:627–40.

Ralston SH, Boyce BF, Cowan RA et al, The effect of 1α-hydroxyvitamin D_3 on the mineralization defect in disodium etidronate-treated Paget's disease. A double blind randomized clinical study, *J Bone Miner Res* (1987) **2**:5–12.

Rao VM and Karasick D, Hypercementosis – an important clue to Paget's disease of the maxilla, *Skeletal Radiol* (1982) **9**:126–8.

Rasmussen H and Bordier P, *The cellular basis of metabolic bone disease*, (Williams and Wilkins: Baltimore, 1974).

Rauis A, Etude statistique sur la maladie de Paget. Ses complications et leur traitement, *Acta Orthop Belg* (1974) **40**:499–530.

Ravault PP, Lejeune E, Bouvier M et al, L'Osteoporose circonscrite des os longs au cours de la maladie de Paget, *J Radiol Electrol* (1970) **51**:499–502.

Ray BS, Platybasia with involvement of central nervous system, *Ann Surg* (1942) **116**:231–50.

Reasbeck JC, Goulding A, Campbell DR et al, Radiological prevalence of Paget's disease in Dunedin, New Zealand, *Br Med J* (1983) **286**:1937.

Rebel A, Baslé M and Malkani K, Towards a viral aetiology for Paget's bone disease, *Br J Clin Pract* (1981) **13**(Suppl):9–12.

Rebel A, Baslé M, Pouplard A et al, Viral antigens in osteoclasts from Paget's disease of bone, *Lancet* (1980a) **ii**:344–6.

Rebel A, Baslé MF, Minard MF et al, Actions de la calcitonine sur les ostéoclastes de la maladie de Paget au cours d'un traitement de longue durée, *Pathol Biol* (1977) **95**:611–16.

Rebel A, Baslé M, Pouplard A et al, Bone tissue in Paget's disease of bone. Ultrastructure and immunocytology, *Arthritis Rheum* (1980b) **23**:1104–14.

Rebel A, Bregeon C, Baslé M et al, Les inclusions des ostéoclastes dans la maladie osseuse de Paget, *Rev Rhum Mal Osteoartic* (1975) **42**:637–41.

Rebel A, Malkani K and Baslé M, Anomalies nucléaires des ostéoclastes de la maladie osseuse de Paget, *Nouv Presse Med* (1974) **3**:1299–1301.

Rebel A, Malkani K, Baslé M et al, Osteoclast ultrastructure in Paget's disease, *Clin Orthop* (1987) **217**:4–8.

Recker RR, Hassing GS, Lau JB et al, The hyperphosphatemic effect of disodium ethane-1-hydroxy-1,1-diphosphonate (EHDP); renal handling of phosphorus and the renal response to parathyroid hormone, *J Lab Clin Med* (1973) **81**:258–66.

Recker RR and Saville PD, Intestinal absorption of disodium ethane-1-hydroxyl-1,1-diphosphonate (disodium etidronate) using a deconvolution technique, *Toxicol Appl Pharmacol* (1973) **24**:580–9.

Redden JF, Dixon J, Vennart W et al, Management of fissure fractures in Paget's disease, *Int Orthop* (1981) **5**:103–6.

Reginster J-Y, Albert A and Franchimont P, Salmon-calcitonin nasal spray in Paget's disease of bone: preliminary results in five patients, *Calcif Tissue Int* (1985a) **37**:577–80.

Reginster J-Y, Denis D and Albert A, One year controlled randomised trial of prevention of early postmenopausal bone loss by intranasal calcitonin, *Lancet* (1987) **ii**:1481–3.

Reginster J-Y and Franchimont P, Side effects of synthetic salmon calcitonin given by intranasal spray compared with intramuscular injection, *Clin Exp Rheum* (1985b) **3**:155–7.

Reginster J-Y, Gritten C, Diverse P et al, Traitement de la maladie de Paget par l'étidronate disodique (EHDP) a faible dose (5 mg/kg par jour), *Rev Rhum Mal Osteoartic* (1985c) **52**:145–50.

Reginster J-Y, Jeugmans-Huynen AM, Albert A et al, Biological and clinical assessment of a new bisphosphonate (chloro-4 phenyl) thiomethylene bisphosphonate, in the treatment of Paget's disease of bone, *Bone* (1988a) **9**:349–54.

Reginster J-Y, Jeugmans-Huynen AM, Albert A et al, One year's treatment of Paget's disease of bone by synthetic salmon calcitonin as a nasal spray, *J Bone Miner Res* (1988b) **3**:249–52.

Resnick CS, Garver P and Resnick D, Bony expansion in skeletal metastases from carcinoma of the prostate as seen by bone scintigraphy, *South Med J* (1984) **77**:1331–5.

Resnick CS, Walter RD, Haghighi P et al, Case report 218, *Skeletal Radiol* (1982) **9**:145–7.

Resnick D, Paget's disease of bone: current status and a look back to 1943 and earlier, *AJR* (1988) **150**:249–56.

Resnick D and Niwayama G, Paget's disease. In: Resnick D, Niwayama G, eds. *Diagnosis of bone and joint disorders.* (Saunders: Philadelphia 1981) 1721–54.

Reynolds JJ and Dingle JT, A sensitive in vitro method for studying the induction and inhibition of bone resorption, *Calcif Tissue Res* (1970) **4**:339–49.

Rhodes BA, Greyson ND, Hamilton CR et al, Absence of anatomic arteriovenous shunts in Paget's disease of bone, *N Engl J Med* (1972) **287**:686–9.

Richardson PC, Cantrill JA and Anderson DC, Experience of treating 218 patients with Paget's disease of bone using intravenous 3-aminohydroxypropylidene 1-

1 bisphosphonate (pamidronate, APD), *J Bone Miner Res* (1989) **4**(Suppl 1):S198.

Riggs BL and Jowsey J, Treatment of Paget's disease with fluoride, *Semin Drug Treat* (1972) **2**:65–8.

Ring EFJ, Davies J and Barker JR, Thermographic assessment of calcitonin therapy in Paget's disease. In: Kanis JA, ed. *Bone disease and calcitonin*. (Armour Pharmaceutical: Eastbourne 1977) 39–48.

Rojanasathit S, Rosenberg E and Haddad JG, Paget's bone disease. Response to human calcitonin in patients resistant to salmon calcitonin, *Lancet* (1974) **ii**:1412–15.

Rondier J, Huchet B and Cayla J, Ostéolyse pseudo-sarcomateuse chez un pagétique traité par étidronate disodique (EHDP), *Rev Rhum Mal Osteoartic* (1984) **51**:49–54.

Roper BA, Paget's disease at the hip with osteoarthritis: results of intertrochanteric osteotomy, *J Bone Joint Surg* (1971a) **53B**:660–2.

Roper BA, Paget's disease involving the hip joint. A classification, *Clin Orthop* (1971b) **80**:33–8.

Rosenfeld MG, Mermod JJ, Amara SG et al, Production of a novel neuropeptide encoded by the calcitonin gene via tissue-specific RNA processing, *Nature* (1983) **304**:129–35.

Rosenkrantz JA, Wolf J and Kaicher JJ, Paget's disease (osteitis deformans): review of 111 cases, *Arch Intern Med* (1952) **90**:610–33.

Ross FGM, Middlemiss JH and Fitton JM, Paget's sarcoma in bone – a radiological study. In: Price CHG, Ross FGM, eds. *Bone – certain aspects of neoplasia*. (Butterworths: London 1973.)

Roth A and Kolaric K, Analgetic activity of calcitonin in patients with painful osteolytic metastases of breast cancer, *Oncology* (1986) **43**:283–7.

Roux H, Mercier P, Maestracci D et al, HLA et maladie de Paget, *Rev Rhum Mal Osteoartic* (1975) **42**:661–2.

Ruddle NH, Paul N, Horowitz M et al, HTLV-1 activation of lymphotoxin (TNFβ) production and high-turnover bone disease, *Calif Tissue Int* (1990) **46**(Suppl 2):A58.

Russell AS, Chalmers IM, Percy JS et al, Long term effectiveness of low dose mithramycin for Paget's disease of bone, *Arthritis Rheum* (1979) **22**:215–18.

Russell RGG, Paget's disease. In: Nordin BEC, ed. *Metabolic bone and stone disease*. (Churchill–Livingstone: Edinburgh 1984) 190–233.

Russell RGG, Beard DJ, Cameron EC et al, Biochemical markers of bone turnover in Paget's disease, *Metab Bone Dis Relat Res* (1981) **3**:255–62.

Russell RGG and Fleisch H, Inorganic pyrophosphate and pyrophosphatases in calcification and calcium homeostasis, *Clin Orthop* (1970) **69**:101–17.

Russell RGG and Smith R, Diphosphonates. Experimental and clinical aspects, *J Bone Joint Surg* (1973) **55B**:66–8.

Russell RGG, Smith R, Preston C et al, Diphosphonates in Paget's disease, *Lancet* (1974) **i**:894–8.

Ryan WG, Mithramycin in Paget's disease of bone, *Lancet* (1973) **i**:1319.

Ryan WG, Breaking the back of Paget's disease, *Arch Intern Med* (1990) **149**:2639.

Ryan WG, Treatment of Paget's disease of bone with mithramycin, *Clin Orthop* (1977) **127**:106–10.

Ryan WG and Schwartz TB, Mithramycin treatment of Paget's disease of bone, *Arthritis Rheum* (1980) **23**:1155–61.

Sadar ES, Walton RJ and Gossman HM, Neurological dysfunction in Paget's disease of the vertebral column, *J Neurosurg* (1972) **37**:661–5.

Sakadura T, Tsukamoto T, Shimizu T et al, Biological activities of (Asu 1.7)-eel calcitonin. In: Cohn DV, Talmage RV, Matthews J, eds. *Hormonal control of calcium metabolism* (Excerpta Medica: Amsterdam 1981) 398.

Salson C, Distribution squelettique de la maladie de Paget évaluée par la scintigraphie osseuse quantitative dans 170 cas, thesis, Université Claude-Bernard, Lyons (1981).

Samman MEL, Linthiaum FH, House HP et al, Calcitonin as treatment for hearing loss in Paget's disease, *Am J Otol* (1986) **7**:241–3.

Schajowicz F, Araujo ES and Berenstein M, Sarcoma complicating Paget's disease of bone. A clinicopathological study of 62 cases, *J Bone Joint Surg* (1983) **65B**:299–307.

Schenk R, Eggli P, Fleisch H et al, Quantitative morphometric evaluation of the inhibitory activity of new amino bisphosphonates on bone resorption in the rat, *Calcif Tissue Int* (1986) **38**:342–9.

Schmidek HH, Neurologic and neurosurgical sequelae of Paget's disease of bone, *Clin Orthop* (1977) **127**:70–7.

Schmitt J, Barrncand D and Duc M, Manifestations neurologiques intraéraniennes de la maladie de Paget, *Rev Otoneurolophthalmol* (1968) **40**:196–203.

Schmorl G, Über osteitis deformans Paget, *Virchows Arch* (1932) **283**:694–751.

Schubert F, Siddle KJ and Harper JS, Diaphyseal Paget's disease: an unusual finding in the tibia, *Clin Radiol* (1984) **35**:71–4.

Seaman WB, The roentgen appearance of early Paget's disease, *AJR* (1987) **16**:587–94.

Segrest JP and Cunningham LW, Variations in human urinary O-hydroxylysyl glycoside levels and their relationship to collagen metabolism, *J Clin Invest* (1970) **49**:1497–1509.

Sekel R, Calcium infusion in painful Paget's disease of bone, *Lancet* (1973) **i**:372–3.

Seret P, Baslé MF, Rebel A et al, Sarcomatous degeneration in Paget's bone disease, *Cancer Res Clin Oncol* (1987) **113**:392–9.

Shai F, Baker RK and Wallach S, The clinical and metabolic effects of porcine calcitonin on Paget's disease of the bone, *J Clin Invest* (1971) **50**:1927–40.

Shier CK, Ellis BI, Tennyson G et al, Nineteen-year radiographic follow-up of untreated Paget's disease of bone, *Henry Ford Hosp Med J* (1986) **34**:127–9.

Shinoda H, Adamek G, Felix R et al, Structure–activity relationship of various bisphosphonates, *Calcif Tissue Int* (1983) **35**:87–99.

Shirazi PH, Ryan WG and Fordham EW, Bone scanning in evaluation of Paget's disease of bone, *CRC Crit Rev Clin Radiol Nucl Med* (1974) **5**:523–58.

Simon L, Blotman F, Seignalet J et al, Etiologie de la maladie de Paget, *Rev Rheum Mal Osteoartic* (1975) **42**:535–44.

Singer FR, Human calcitonin treatment of Paget's disease of bone, *Clin Orthop* (1977a) **127**:86–93.

Singer FR, *Paget's disease of bone*. (Plenum Medical Publishers; New York 1977b).

Singer FR, Aldred P, Neer RM et al, An evaluation of antibodies and clinical resistance to salmon calcitonin, *J Clin Invest* (1972) **51**:2331–8.

Singer FR, Fredericks RS and Minkin C, Salmon calcitonin therapy for Paget's disease of bone, *Arthritis Rheum* (1980) **23**:1148–53.

Singer FR and Habener JF, Multiple immunoreactive forms of calcitonin in human plasma, *Biochem Biophys Res Commun* (1974) **61**:710–16.

Singer FR, Melvin KEW and Mills BG, Acute effects of calcitonin on osteoclasts in man, *Clin Endocrinol* (1976) **5**(Suppl):333–40.

Singer FR and Mills BG, Paget's disease of bone: etiologic and therapeutic aspects. In: Peck WA, ed. *Bone and mineral research, annual 2*. (Elsevier Science: Amsterdam 1983a) 394–421.

Singer FR and Mills BG, Evidence for a viral etiology of Paget's disease of bone, *Clin Orthop* (1983b) **178**:245–51.

Singer FR, Mills BG, Park MS et al, Increased HLA-DQWI antigen pattern in Paget's disease of bone, *Clin Res* (1985) **33**:574A.

Singer FR, Neer RM, Goltzman D et al, Treatment with Paget's disease of bone and hypercalcaemia with salmon calcitonin. In: Taylor S, ed. *Endocrinology. Proc 4th Int Symp*. (W Heinemann: London 1974) 397–408.

Singer FR, Rude PK and Mills BG, Studies in the treatment and etiology of Paget's disease of bone. In: MacIntyre I, ed. *International symposium on human calcitonin and Paget's disease. Ciba Foundation Symposium*. (Hans Huber: Berne 1977) 93–110.

Singer FR, Woodhouse NJY, Parkinson DK et al, Some acute effects of administered porcine calcitonin in man, *Clin Sci* (1969) **37**:181–90.

Siris ES, Canfield RE, Jacobs TE et al, Long-term therapy of Paget's disease of bone with EHDP, *Arthritis Rheum* (1980) **23**:1177–83.

Siris ES, Canfield RE, Jacobs TP et al, Clinical and biochemical effects of EHDP in Paget's disease of bone: patterns of response to initial treatment and long-term therapy, *Metab Bone Dis Relat Res* (1981) **3**:301–8.

Siris ES, Clemens TP, McMahon D et al, Parathyroid function in Paget's disease of bone, *J Bone Miner Res* (1989) **4**:75–9.

Siris ES, Hyman GA and Canfield RE, Effects of dichloromethylene diphosphonate in women with breast carcinoma metastatic to the skeleton, *Am J Med* (1983) **74**:401–6.

Siris ES, Jacobs TPJ and Canfield RE, Paget's disease of bone, *Bull NY Acad Med* (1980) **56**:285–304.

Sissons HA, Epidemiology of Paget's disease, *Clin Orthop* (1966) **45**:73–9.

Sjoberg HE, Torring O, Granberg B et al, Postmenopausal osteoporosis: response of immunoextracted calcitonin to a calcium clamp, *Bone* (1989) **10**:15–18.

Sleeboom HP, Bijvoet OLM, van Oosterom AT et al, Comparison of intravenous (3-amino-1-hydroxypropylidene)-1,1-bisphosphonate and volume repletion in tumour induced hypercalcaemia, *Lancet* (1983) **ii**:239–43.

Smith BJ and Eveson JW, Paget's disease of bone with particular reference to dentistry, *J Oral Pathol* (1981) **10**:233–47.

Smith J, Botet JF and Yeh SDJ, Bone sarcomas in Paget's disease: a study of 85 patients, *Radiology* (1984a) **152**:583–90.

Smith ML, Fogelman I, Ralston S et al, Correlation of skeletal uptake of ^{99m}Tc-diphosphonate and alkaline phosphatase before and after oral diphosphonate therapy in Paget's disease, *Metab Bone Dis Relat Res* (1984b) **5**:167–70.

Smith R, Paget's disease of bone. In: Apley AG, ed. *Biochemical disorders of the skeleton*. (Butterworths: London 1979) 133–60.

Smith R, Disorders of the skeleton. In: Weatherall DJ, Ledingham JGG, Warrell DA, eds. *Oxford textbook of medicine*. (Oxford University Press: Oxford 1986) 17.1–17.36.

Smith R, Russell RGG and Bishop M, Diphosphonates and Paget's disease of bone, *Lancet* (1971) **i**:945–7.

Smith R, Russell RGG and Bishop M, Paget's disease of bone: experience with a diphosphonate (disodium etidronate) in treatment, *Q J Med* (1973) **42**:235–56.

Sofaer JA, Dental extractions in Paget's disease of bone, *Int J Oral Surg* (1984) **13**:79–84.

Sofaer JA, Holloway SM and Emery AEH, A family study of Paget's disease of bone, *J Epidemiol Community Health* (1983) **37**:226–31.

Solomon LR, Billiard-player's fingers: an unusual case of Paget's disease of bone, *Br Med J* (1979) **1**:931.

Solomon LR, Evanson JM, Canty DP et al, Effect of calcitonin treatment on deafness due to Paget's disease of bone, *Br Med J* (1977) **2**:485–7.

Somerville PJ and Evans RA, Actinomycin D in the treatment of Paget's disease of bone, *Med J Aust* (1975) **2**:13–16.

Souhami R and Craft A, Letter to the editor, *Lancet* (1988) **i**:931–2.

Sparrow NA and Duvall AJ, Hearing loss and Paget's disease, *J Laryngol Otol* (1967) **81**:601–11.

Spinks TJ, Joplin GF, Evans IMA et al, Long term measurements of skeletal and lean body mass in Paget's disease of bone treated with synthetic human calcitonin, *Calcif Tissue Int* (1982) **34**:459–64.

Stamp TCB, Mackney PH and Kelsey CR, Innocent pets and Paget's disease? *Lancet* (1986) **ii**:917.

Stauffer RN and Sim FH, Total hip arthroplasty in Paget's disease of the hip, *J Bone Joint Surg* (1976) **58A**:476–8.

Steber J and Wierich P, Properties of hydroxyethane diphosphonates affecting its environmental fate: degradability, sludge absorption, mobility in soils and bioconcentration, *Chemosphere* (1986) **15**:929–45.

Stegmann R, Offizielles Protokol der k. k. Gesellschaft der Aerzte in Wein, *Wien Klin Wochenschr* (1905) **18**:619–21.

Steinbach HL, Some roentgen features of Paget's disease, *AJR* (1961) **86**:950–64.

Stevens J, Orthopaedic aspects of Paget's disease, *Metab Bone Dis Relat Res* (1981) **3**:271–8.

Stevenson J, Paget's Disease, *Hospital Update* (1984) **10**:431–43.

Stevenson JC, Abeyasekera G, Hillyard CJ et al, Calcitonin and the calcium-regulating hormones in postmenopausal women: effect of oestrogens, *Lancet* (1981) **i**:693–5.

Stevenson JC and Evans IMA, Pharmacology and therapeutic use of calcitonin, *Drugs* (1981) **21**:257–72.

Stevenson JC, Evans IMA, Colston KW et al, Serum prolactin after subcutaneous human calcitonin, *Lancet* (1977) **ii**:711–12.

Stevenson JC, Hillyard CJ, MacIntyre I et al, A physiological role of calcitonin: protection of the maternal skeleton, *Lancet* (1979) **ii**:769–70.

Stout SD and Teitelbaum SL, Histological analysis of undecalcified thin sections of archeological bone, *Am J Phys Anthrop* (1977) **44**:263–70.

Stover SL, Hahn HR and Miller JM, Disodium etidronate in the prevention of heterotopic ossification following spinal cord injury, *Paraplegia* (1976a) **14**:146–56.

Stover SL, Neumann KMW and Miller JM, Disodium etidronate in the prevention of postoperative recurrence of heterotopic ossification in spinal cord injury patients, *J Bone Joint Surg* (1976b) **58A**:683–8.

Strickberger S, Schulman S and Hutchins G, Association of Paget's disease of bone with calcific aortic valve disease, *Am J Med* (1987) **82**:953–6.

Stuart C, Aspects radiologique dynamiques de la maladie de Paget. In: Hioco DJ, ed. *La Maladie de Paget.* (Lab Armour Montagu: Paris 1977) 27–42.

Sturtridge WC, Harrison JE and Wilson DR, Long-term treatment of Paget's disease of bone with salmon calcitonin, *Can Med J* (1977) **117**:1031–46.

Stutzer Z, Muhlbauer RC, Janner M et al, Inhibitory effect of bone resorption of a new bisphosphonate 1-hydroxy-3-(methylpentylamino) propylidene-bisphosphonate (BM 21-0955), *Calcif Tissue Int* (1989) **44**(Suppl):107.

Suchett-Kaye AI, Paget's disease of bone, *Gerontol Clin* (1970) **122**:241–55.

Taggart H, Gordon DS and Roberts SD, Basilar impression in a case of Paget's disease treated with calcitonin and surgery, *Ir J Med Sci* (1978) **147**:435–6.

Talmage RV, Cooper CW and Toverud SU, The physiological significance of calcitonin. In: Peck WA, ed. *Bone and mineral research, annual 1.* (Excerpta Medica: Amsterdam 1983) 74–143.

Taubman MB, Kammerman S and Goldberg B, Radioimmunoassay of procollagen in serum of patients with Paget's disease of bone, *Proc Soc Exp Biol Med* (1976) **152**:284–7.

Taylor AK, Linkhart SG, Mohan S et al, Presence of a unique fragment of osteocalcin in serum and urine of Paget's disease patients: Possible marker for the disease, *Am J Bone Mineral Research* (1989) **4**(Suppl 17):s198.

Taylor AR and Chakravorty BC, Clinical syndromes associated with basilar impression, *Arch Neurol* (1964) **10**:475–84.

Theodors A, Askari AD and Wieland RG, Colchicine in the treatment of Paget's disease of bone: A new therapeutic approach, *Clin Ther* (1981) **3**:365–73.

Thiebaud D, Jaeger P and Burckhardt P, Paget's disease of bone treated in five days with AHPrBP (APD) per os, *J Bone Miner Res* (1987) **2**:45–52.

Thiebaud D, Jaeger P, Gobelet C et al, A single infusion of the bisphosphonate AHPrBP (APD) as treatment of Paget's disease of bone, *Am J Med* (1988) **85**:207–12.

Thompson RC Jr, Gaull GE, Horwitz SJ et al, Hereditary hyperphosphatasia. Studies of three siblings, *Am J Med* (1969) **47**:209–19.

Tilyard MW, Gardner RJM, Milligan L et al, A probable linkage between familial Paget's disease and the HLA loci, *Aust NZ J Med* (1982) **12**:498–500.

Tjon-A-Tham RTO, Bloem JL, Falke THM et al, Magnetic resonance imaging in Paget's disease of the skull, *Am J Nuc Roentgenol* (1985) **6**:879–81.

Toh SH, Claunch BC and Brown PH, Effects of calcitonin treatment on the natural course of bone demineralization in Paget's disease, *J Clin Endocrinol Metab* (1983) **56**:405–9.

Traver CA, The association of fractures in Paget's disease (osteitis deformans), *NY State J Med* (1936) **36**:242–6.

Troehler U, Bonjour JP and Fleisch H, Renal secretion of diphosphonates in rats, *Kidney Int* (1975) **8**:6–13.

Upchurch KS, Simon LS, Schiller AL et al, Giant cell reparative granuloma of Paget's disease of bone: a unique clinical entity, *Ann Intern Med* (1983) **98**:35–40.

Urwin GH, Yates AJP, Gray RES et al, Treatment of the hypercalcaemia of malignancy with intravenous clodronate, *Bone* (1987) **8**(Suppl 1):43–51.

Valentin-Opran A, Risedronate: Preliminary results of a pharmacological study in pagetic patients, *J Bone Miner Res* (1990) **5**:S119.

Van Breukelen FJM, Bijvoet OLM and van Oosterom AT, Inhibition of osteolytic bone lesions by APD, *Lancet* (1979) **i**:803–6.

Van Meedervoort E and Richter G, Paget's disease of

bone in South African blacks, *S Afr Med J* (1976) **50**:1897–9.

Vega E, Gonzalez D, Ghiringhelli G et al, Intravenous aminopropylidene, bisphosphonate (APD) in the treatment of Paget's bone disease, *J Bone Miner Res* (1987) **2**:267–71.

Vellenga CJLR, Mulder JD and Bijvoet OLM, Radiological demonstration in healing in Paget's disease of bone treated with APD, *Br J Radiol* (1985c) **58**:831–7.

Vellenga CJLR, Pauwels EKJ and Bijvoet OLM, Comparison between visual assessment and quantitative measurement of radioactivity on the bone scintigram in Paget's disease of bone, *Eur J Nucl Med* (1984a) **9**: 533–7.

Vellenga CJLR, Pauwels EKJ and Bijvoet OLM, Some characteristics of local scintigraphic and radiologic patterns of Paget's disease of bone (osteitis deformans), *Diagn Imaging Clin Med* (1985a) **54**:273–81.

Vellenga CLJR, Pauwels EKJ, Bijvoet OLM et al, Scintigraphic aspects of the recurrence of treated Paget's disease of bone, *J Nucl Med* (1981) **22**:510–17.

Vellenga CLJR, Pauwels EKJ, Bijvoet OLM et al, Bone scintigraphy in Paget's disease treated with combined calcitonin and diphosphonate (EHDP), *Metab Bone Dis Relat Res* (1982) **4**:103–11.

Vellenga CJLR, Pauwels EKJ, Bijvoet OLM et al, Untreated Paget's disease of bone studied by scintigraphy, *Radiology* (1984b) **153**:799–805.

Vellenga CJLR, Pauwels EKJ, Bijvoet OLM et al, Quantitative bone scintigraphy in Paget's disease treated with APD, *Br J Radiol* (1985b) **58**:1165–72.

Villiaumey J and Larget-Piet B, Le dégénerescence sarcomateuse de l'os pagétique. In: Hioco DJ, ed. *La Maladie de Paget*. (Lab Armour Montagu: Paris 1977) 103–18.

Wall RM, Pearce A and Murray JR, Clinical aspects of Paget's disease, *Br J Clin Pract* (1981) **13**(Suppl):1–2.

Wallach S, Comparative effects of salmon, human and eel calcitonins on skeletal turnover in human disease. In: Gennari C, Segre G, eds. *The effects of calcitonins in man*. (Masson Italia Editori: Milan 1983) 141–51.

Walpin LA and Singer FR, Paget's disease – reversal of severe paraparesis using calcitonin, *Spine* (1979) **4**:213–19.

Waltner JG, Stapedectomy in Paget's disease, *Arch Otolaryngol* (1965) **82**:355–8.

Walton JG and Strong JA, Calcitonin and osteogenesic sarcoma, *Lancet* (1973) **i**:887–8.

Walton KR, Green JR, Reeve J et al, Reduction in skeletal blood flow in Paget's disease with disodium etidronate therapy, *Bone* (1985) **6**:29–31.

Walton RJ, Studies on phosphate metabolism in man with special reference to the effects of a diphosphonate in Paget's disease of bone, D Phil thesis, Magdalen College, Oxford (1978).

Walton RJ, Preston CJ, Bartlett M et al, Biochemical measurements in Paget's disease of bone. Distribution and correlations, *Eur J Clin Invest* (1977a) **7**:37–9.

Walton RJ, Preston C, Russell RGG et al, An estimate of the turnover rate of bone derived plasma alkaline phosphatase in Paget's disease of bone, *Clin Chim Acta* (1975) **63**:227–9.

Walton RJ, Russell RGG and Smith R, Changes in renal and extrarenal handling of phosphate induced by disodium etidronate (EHDP) in man, *Clin Sci Mol Med* (1975) **49**:45–56.

Walton RJ, Woods CG, Russell RGG et al, Histological measurements in Paget's disease of bone, *Calcif Tissue Res* (1977b) **22**(Suppl):295–7.

Warshowsky H, Goltzman D, Rouleau MF et al, Direct in vivo demonstration by radioautography of specific binding for calcitonin in skeletal and renal tissues of the rat, *J Cell Biol* (1980) **85**:682–94.

Waxman AD, McKee D, Siemsen JK et al, Gallium scanning in Paget's disease of bone. Effect of calcitonin, *Am J Radiol* (1980) **134**:303–6.

Wellman HN, Schauwecker D, Robb JA et al, Skeletal scintimaging and radiography in the diagnosis and management of Paget's disease, *Clin Orthop* (1977) **127**:55–62.

Wells C and Woodhouse NJY, Paget's disease in an Anglo-Saxon, *Med Hist* (1975) **19**:396–400.

Welsh RA and Meyer AT, Nuclear fragmentations and associated fibrils in giant cell tumour of bone, *Lab Invest* (1970) **22**:63–72.

Welzel D, Analgesic potential of salmon calcitonin in postoperative pain. In: Gennari C, Segre G, eds. *The effects of calcitonins in man*. (Masson Italia Editori: Milan 1983) 223–32.

Wener JA, Gorton SJ and Raisz LG, Escape from inhibition of resorption in cultures of fetal bone treated with calcitonin and PTH, *Endocrinology* (1972) **90**: 752–9.

Whiteley J, Francis MJO, Walton RJ et al, Serum proline imino-peptidase activity in normal subjects and in patients with Paget's disease of bone, *Clin Chim Acta* (1976) **71**:157–63.

Whyte MP, Alkaline phosphatase: physiological role explored in hypophosphatasia, *Bone Miner Res Ann* (1989) **6**:175–218.

Whyte MP, Daniels EH and Murphy WA, Osteolytic Paget's bone disease in a young man, *Am J Med* (1985) **78**:326–32.

Whyte MP, Murphy WA, Haddad JG et al, In: Pecile A, ed. *Calcitonin 1980. Chemistry, physiology, pharmacology and clinical aspects.* (Excerpta Medica: Amsterdam 1981) 217–21.

Wick MR, McLeod RA, Siegal GP et al, Sarcomas of bone complicating osteitis deformans (Paget's disease). Fifty years experience, *Am J Surg Pathol* (1981) **5**:47–59.

Wilder-Smith CH, Raue F, Holz-Gottswinter G et al, Procollagen III peptide serum levels in Paget's disease of the bone, *Klin Wochenschr* (1987) **65**:174–8.

Wilks S, Case of osteoporosis or spongy hypertrophy of the bones (calvaria clavicle os femoris and rib exhibited at the Society), *Trans Path Soc London* (1869) **20**:273–7.

Wilks S, Osteitis deformans (letter), *Lancet* (1909) **ii**:1627.

Williams CP, Meachim G and Taylor WH, Effect of calcitonin treatment on osteoclast counts in Paget's disease of bone, *J Clin Pathol* (1978) **31**:1212–17.

Wilner D and Sherman RS, Roentgen diagnosis of Paget's disease (osteitis deformans), *Med Radiogr Photogr* (1966) **42**:35–78.

Winfield J and Stamp TCB, Bone and joint symptoms in Paget's disease, *Ann Rheum Dis* (1984) **43**:769–73.

Woodard HQ, Long-term studies of the blood chemistry in Paget's disease of bone, *Cancer* (1959) **12**:1226–37.

Woodhouse NJY, Paget's disease of bone, *Clin Endocrinol Metab* (1972) **1**:125–41.

Woodhouse NJY, Paget's disease: a review and indications for treatment with calcitonin. In: Kanis JA, ed. *Bone disease and calcitonin.* (Armour Pharmaceutical: Eastbourne 1976) 3–9.

Woodhouse NJY, Historical and epidemiological aspects of Paget's disease. In: MacIntyre I, ed. *Human calcitonin and Paget's disease.* (Hans Huber: Bern 1977) 50–65.

Woodhouse NJY and Barnes ND, The response of athyroidal patients to calcium infusion. Evidence for an action of calcitonin. In: Taylor S, ed. *Calcitonin. Proc Symp on Thyrocalcitonin and the C-cells.* (Heinemann: London 1968) 361–3.

Woodhouse NJY, Bordier P, Fisher M et al, Human calcitonin in the treatment of Paget's disease, *Lancet* (1971) **i**:1139–43.

Woodhouse NJY, Chalmers A, Wells I et al, Paget's disease. Radiological changes occurring in untreated patients and those on therapy with salmon calcitonin during two years observations, *Br J Radiol* (1977a) **50**:699–705.

Woodhouse NJY, Crosbie WA and Mohamedally SM, Cardiac output in Paget's disease: response to long-term salmon calcitonin therapy, *Br Med J* (1975) **4**:686.

Woodhouse NJY, Fisher MT, Sigurdsson G et al, Paget's disease in a 5 year old: acute response to human calcitonin, *Br Med J* (1972a) **iv**:267–9.

Woodhouse NJY, Joplin GR, MacIntyre I et al, Radiological regression in Paget's disease treated with human calcitonin, *Lancet* (1972b) **ii**:992–4.

Woodhouse NJY, Mohamedally SM, Saed Nejad F et al, Development and significance of antibodies to salmon calcitonin in patients with Paget's disease on long term treatment, *Br Med J* (1977b) **2**:928–9.

Woodhouse NJY, Reiner H, Kalu DN et al, Some effects of acute and chronic calcitonin administration in man. In: Taylor S, ed. *Calcitonin 1969* (Heinemann: London 1970) 504–13.

Wooton R, Reeve J, Spellacy E et al, Skeletal blood flow in Paget's disease of bone and its response to calcitonin therapy, *Clin Sci Mol Med* (1978) **54**:69–74.

Wooton R, Reeve J and Veall N, Measurement of skeletal blood flow in normal man and in patients with Paget's disease of bone. In: Pors Nielsen S, Hjorting-Hansen E, eds. *Calcified tissues 1975. Proc XIth Europ symp on calcified tissues.* (FADL's Forlag: Copenhagen 1975) 380–5.

Wooton R, Tellez M, Green JR et al, Skeletal blood flow in Paget's disease of bone, *Metab Bone Dis Relat Res* (1981) **3**:263–70.

Wrany H, Hyperostosis maxillarum. In: *Prager Viertel-jahrschrift*, quoted by Paget 1877 (1867).

Wycis H, Platybasia secondary to advanced osteitis deformans with severe neurologic manifestations. Successful surgical result: report of a case, *Arch Neurol Psychiat* (1945) **1**:68–73.

Yakatan GL, Poynor WJ, Talbert RL et al, Clodronate kinetics and bioavailability, *Clin Pharmacol Ther* (1982) **31**:402–10.

Yarbro JW, Kennedy BJ and Barnum CP, Mithramycin inhibition of ribonucleic acid synthesis, *Cancer Res* (1966) **26**:36–9.

Yates AJP, Jones TH, Mundy KI et al, Immobilisation hypercalcaemia in adults and treatment with clodronate, *Br Med J* (1984) **289**:1111–12.

Yates AJP, Percival RC, Gray RES et al, Intravenous clodronate in the treatment and retreatment of Paget's disease of bone, *Lancet* (1985) **i**:474–7.

Yeh S, Rosen G and Benua RS, Gallium scans in Paget's sarcoma, *Clin Nucl Med* (1982) **7**:546–52.

Zadek RE and Milgram JW, Progression of Paget's disease in the tibia, *J Bone Joint Surg* (1977) **58A**:876–8.

Ziegler R, Bellwinkel S, Schmidtchen D et al, Effect of hypercalcaemia, hypocalcaemia and calcitonin on glucose stimulated insulin release, *Horm Metab Res* (1972) **4**:60.

Ziegler R, Holz G, Raue F et al, Nasal application of human calcitonin in Paget's disease of bone. In: MacIntyre I, Szelke M, eds. *Molecular endocrinology*. (Elsevier: Amsterdam 1979) 293–300.

Ziegler R, Holz G, Rotzler B et al, Paget's disease of bone in West Germany, *Clin Orthop* (1985) **194**:199–204.

Zlatkin MB, Lander PH, Hadjipavlou AG et al, Paget's disease of the spine: CT with clinical correlation, *Radiology* (1986) **160**:155–9.

I N D E X

Page numbers in *italic* refer to the illustrations